To Morton

I owe you much, this
is a small thing for your
kindness at the crucial
moment.
With fondness.

Ali.

East Grinstead
May 2006

Ward's
Anaesthetic
Equipment

Commissioning Editor: Natasha Andjelkovic
Project Development Managers: Cecilia Murphy
Project Manager: Glenys Norquay
Illustration Manager: Mick Ruddy
Design Manager: Jayne Jones
Illustrator: Tim Loughhead
Marketing Manager (UK): Brant Emery
Marketing Manager (USA): Emily Christie

Ward's Anaesthetic Equipment

FIFTH EDITION

Edited by

Andrew J Davey LRCP & SI FRCA
Consultant Anaesthetist
Rex Binning Department of Anaesthesia
Royal Sussex County Hospital
Brighton and Sussex University Hospitals NHS Trust
Brighton, UK

Ali Diba BM FRCA
Consultant Anaesthetist
Anaesthetic Department
Queen Victoria Hospital NHS Trust
East Grinstead, West Sussex, UK

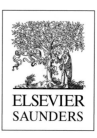

ELSEVIER
SAUNDERS

ELSEVIER
SAUNDERS

An imprint of Elsevier Limited

© 2005, Elsevier Limited. All rights reserved.
© Paul D Davis for Chapters 1 and 2.

First published 2005

First edition 1975
Second edition 1985
Third edition 1992
Fourth edition 1998

The right of Andrew J Davey and Ali Diba to be identified as editors of this work has been asserted by him/her/them in accordance with the Copyright, Designs and Patents Act 1988.

ISBN 1 4160 2558 8

British Library Cataloguing in Publication Data
A catalogue record for this book is available from the British Library

Library of Congress Cataloging in Publication Data
A catalog record for this book is available from the Library of Congress

Notice
Medical knowledge is constantly changing. Standard safety precautions must be followed, but as new research and clinical experience broaden our knowledge, changes in treatment and drug therapy may become necessary or appropriate. Readers are advised to check the most current product information provided by the manufacturer of each drug to be administered to verify the recommended dose, the method and duration of administration, and contraindications. It is the responsibility of the practitioner, relying on experience and knowledge of the patient, to determine dosages and the best treatment for each individual patient. Neither the Publisher nor the editors nor contributors assume any liability for any injury and/or damage to persons or property arising from this publication.
The Publisher

Printed in China

Last digit is the print number: 9 8 7 6 5 4 3 2 1

Working together to grow
libraries in developing countries

www.elsevier.com | www.bookaid.org | www.sabre.org

ELSEVIER   BOOK AID International   Sabre Foundation

Contents

CONTENTS

List of Contributors

Chris J Barham MBBS FRCA
Consultant Anaesthetist
Department of Anaesthesia
The Queen Victoria Hospital NHS
Trust
East Grinstead, UK

Paul Beatty BSc MSc PhD CEng FIPEM
Senior Lecturer in Biomedical
Engineering
Imaging Science and Biomedical
Engineering
The University of Manchester
Manchester, UK

Hubert Bland MBChB
Clinical Director
BOC Medical
The Priestley Centre
Surrey Research Park
Guildford, UK

John A Carter MBBS FRCA
Consultant in Anaesthesia and
Intensive Care Medicine
Department of Anaesthesia
Frenchay Hospital
Bristol, UK

Matthew R Checketts MBChB FRCA
Consultant Anaesthetist
University Department of Anaesthesia
Ninewells Hospital
Dundee, UK

Richard PD Cooke FRCP FRCPath Dip HIC
Consultant Medical Microbiologist
Department of Clinical Microbiology
University Hospital Aintree
Liverpool, UK

Andrew J Davey LRCP & SI FRCA
Consultant Anaesthetist
Rex Binning Department of
Anaesthesia
Royal Sussex County Hospital
Brighton and Sussex University
Hospitals NHS Trust
Brighton, UK

Paul D Davis BSc DipAdvStSc CSci MIPEM CPhys MInstP
Principal Physicist
Department of Clinical Physics and
Bioengineering
Southern General Hospital
Glasgow, UK

Ali Diba BM FRCA
Consultant Anaesthetist
Anaesthetic Department
Queen Victoria Hospital NHS Trust
East Grinstead, West Sussex, UK

Stephen Fenlon BM BS FRCA
Consultant Anaesthetist
Department of Anaesthesia
Queen Victoria Hospital
East Grinstead, UK

Nicholas P Gall MSc MD MRCP
Consultant Electrophysiologist
Department of Cardiology
King's College Hospital
London, UK

Mark T Kearney MD
Senior Lecturer in Cardiology
British Heart Foundation Intermediate
Fellow
King's College London
London, UK

Trevor A King FRCA
Consultant Anaesthetist
Department of Anaesthestics
East Sussex Hospitals NHS Trust
Eastbourne, UK

Robert Sekun Kong MBBS FRCA EDIC
Consultant Cardiac Anaesthetist
Department of Anaesthesia
Royal Sussex County Hospital
Brighton, UK

Patrick T Magee MSc FRCA MIEE AMI MechE
Consultant in Anaesthesia
Department of Anaesthesia
Royal United Hospital;
Visiting Senior Lecturer
Department of Mechanical
Engineering
University of Bath
Bath, UK

Andrew Morley FRCA
Consultant Anaesthetist
Anaesthetic Department
Guy's and St Thomas' NHS
Foundation Trust
London, UK

John TB Moyle MB BS CEng MInstMC DPallMed FRCA
Consultant in Palliative Medicine
Chartered Engineer
Milton Keynes Hospital
Milton Keynes, UK

Nilesh Nanavati MBBS FFARCSI
SpR Anaesthetics
South East Thames rotation
London, UK

Chetan Patel MBBS FRCA
Consultant Anaesthetist
Department of Anaesthesia
The Queen Victoria Hospital NHS
Foundation Trust
East Grinstead, UK

Martin Street FJFICM
Consultant Intensivist
Department of Intensive Care
Royal Sussex County Hospital
Brighton, UK

Nicole Svatek
Manager
Virgin Human Factors
Virgin Atlantic Airways Ltd
Crawley, UK

Daniel W Wheeler MA MRCP FRCA BM BCh ILTM
Clinical Lecturer in Anaesthesia
University Department of Anaesthesia
University of Cambridge
Cambridge, UK

J A W Wildsmith MD FRCA FRCP Ed
Foundation Professor of Anaesthesia
University Department of Anaesthesia
Ninewells Hospital & Medical School
Dundee, UK

Antony R Wilkes PhD MSc BSc
Senior Research Fellow
Department of Anaesthetics and
Intensive Care Medicine
Wales College of Medicine
Cardiff University
Cardiff, UK

Preface to the Fifth Edition

The fifth edition of this book breaks new ground in many ways. The knowledge base of the subject matter has expanded to such a degree that it is no longer possible for a few contributors to cover all the chosen topics in depth and with up-to-date information. Advances in printing have allowed the use of colour photos and illustrations to enhance the text in a way that would have been prohibitively expensive in previous editions. There has also been a change in the editors. Sadly, this is the first edition without Dr Crispian Ward, who died in 2002. Dr John Moyle has moved on to work outside anaesthesia and Dr Ali Diba has joined this project. We hope Cris would have approved of this choice.

This book has two main purposes. The first is to provide a simple, yet comprehensive, explanation of the function of items of anaesthetic equipment to ensure their safe use in clinical practice by anaesthetists. The second is to provide a source of reference for trainee anaesthetists that covers the relevant syllabus required for the Primary and Final Fellowship Examinations in anaesthesia in the UK and Ireland.

The book will also be of interest to anaesthetic assistants, electronic and biomedical engineers in hospitals, manufacturers' representatives and those involved in anaesthesia in other countries where similar equipment is used.

The book has been extensively revised to include new developments and to eliminate obsolete items. Some chapters in the last edition have been combined for simplicity and continuity. There are new chapters on intensive care ventilators, information technology and the anaesthetic workstation, monitoring depth of anaesthesia, monitoring of cardiovascular and coagulation systems and the work of the Medicines and Healthcare products Regulatory Agency.

There has been an occasional deliberate repetition of material where the content of some chapters has overlapped. This caters for a reader who may wish to peruse individual chapters rather than read the book from cover to cover.

Andrew J Davey and Ali Diba

Acknowledgements

We are indebted to the many manufacturing companies who have provided us with essential data, illustrations, photographic material and loan equipment. Some of the illustrations have, with permission, been altered to ensure that they conform to a uniform style. We are also grateful to the many personnel of those manufacturing companies, ranging from senior technical staff to representatives and service engineers, who tirelessly answered our repeated queries and requests. Also, a particular thanks must go to the Medical Photography Department of the Queen Victoria Hospital, East Grinstead for their forbearance in graciously accommodating endless requests for photography.

Dedication

This book is dedicated to the memory of Crispian Ward, late Consultant Anaesthetist, Huddersfield Royal Infirmary, who sadly died in 2002. In the early 1970's, he was one of the first anaesthetists to realise that an understanding and working knowledge of anaesthetic equipment was essential in order to provide the highest standards of safety in anaesthesia. He therefore set out to write a suitable book on the subject (the first of its kind in the UK) and applied his many talents to this work. He was a genius with the written word. He had the ability to explain and reveal in short readable sentences. Added to this were his remarkable powers of concentration, enthusiasm and meticulous attention to detail. Those copy editors employed by the pubishers were made virtually redundant as he supplied almost flawless manuscripts. He was the scourge of type-setters by insisting that text and illustrations should appear side by side even if this entailed a major revision of a chapter's layout. The first two editions were written exclusively by him whilst working as a consultant in a busy district general hospital. This was a formidable achievement.

As the subject matter expanded and Cris reached retirement, he enlisted the help of two younger anaesthetic colleagues, John Moyle (also an electrical engineer) and myself, for the next two editions. Although he retained editorial command, he did this with such great diplomacy and tact that we were not slighted by alterations that he requested. He was not in favour of books written by multiple contributors as he felt this would affect the style of the written word! Sadly, the subject matter has expanded to such an extent that in order to provide the depth of knowledge required this is no longer possible. However, the present editors have attempted to follow his style and hope he would be pleased with the result. He is greatly missed.

Andrew J Davey

Abbreviations

AAGBI	Association of Anaesthetists of Great Britain and Ireland
AC	Alternating current
ACOP	Approved Code of Practice
ADC	Analogue to digital converter
AEP	Auditory evoked potential
AGSS	Anaesthetic gas scavenging system
AICD	Automatic implantable cardioverter-defibrillator
ANSI	American National Standards Institute
APL	Adjustable pressure-limiting (valve)
ARX	Autoregressive model with exogenous input
ASB	Assisted spontaneous breathing
ATLS®	Advanced trauma and life support
atm	Atmosphere (unit of pressure)
AVSU	Area valved service unit
BBV	Blood borne virus
BCGA	British Compressed Gas Association
BET	Bolus elimination and transfer
BiPAP	Bi-level positive airway pressure
BIS	Bispectral index
BP	Blood pressure
BP	British Pharmacopoeia
BPEG	British Pacing and Electrophysiology Group
BPM	Breaths per minute
BS	British Standard
BSI	British Standards Institute
BSP	British Standard Pipe (screw thread)
BSR	Burst suppression ratio
BTPS	Body temperature and pressure, saturated
C	Coulomb
cmH_2O	Centimetres of water (unit of pressure)
°C	Degrees Celsius
CBF	Cerebral blood flow
CCD	Charge coupling device
CE	Conformite Européene
CEN	Comité Européene de Normalization
CFCs	Chlorofluorocarbons
CFAM	Cerebral function analysing monitor
CGO	Common gas outlet
CLAN	Closed loop anaesthesia
CLS	Cryogenic Liquid Systems
CMRR	Common mode rejection ratio
CMV	Controlled minute ventilation
CNST	Clinical Negligence Scheme for Trusts
CO	Cardiac output
COELCB	Current-operated earth-leakage circuit breaker
COSHH	Control of Substances Hazardous to Health
COPA	Cuffed Oropharyngeal Airway
CPAP	Continuous positive airway pressure
CPU	Central processing unit
CRT	Cathode ray tube
CSA	Compressed spectral array
CSSD	Central Sterile Supply Department
CVP	Central venous pressure
DAC	Digital to analogue converter
DC	Direct current
DFT	Defibrillation threshold
DLT	Double lumen tube
DoH	Department of Health (Replaces DHSS Department of Health and Social Security)
DISS	Diameter Indexed Safety System (USA)
DSA	Density spectral array
EBME	Electronic and Biomedical Engineering (Department)
ECG	Electrocardiogram
EEG	Electroencephalogram
EMG	Electromyogram
EMI	Electromagnetic interference
EMO	Epstein Macintosh Oxford
EN	Norme Européenne
EPROM	Eraseable programmable read only memory
ETT	Endotracheal tube
EU	European Union
eV	Electron volt
FDA	Food and Drug Administration (USA)
FEV	Forced expiratory volume
FEV_1	Forced expiratory volume in 1 second
FFT	Fast Fourier Transformation
FG	French gauge
FGF	Fresh gas flow
FRC	Functional residual capacity
FT	Flow time
FTc	Corrected flow time
g	Gauge pressure (as opposed to absolute pressure)
GEB	Gum-elastic bougie
GHTF	Global Harmonization Task Force
HC	Health Canada
HEI	Health Equipment Information (issued by the DoH)

HFPPV	High frequency positive pressure ventilation		**NO**	Nitric oxide
HCMs	Hundreds of cubic metres		**NPSA**	National Patient Safety Agency
HMEF	Heat and moisture exchange filter		**NRV**	Non-breathing valve
HME	Heat and moisture exchanger		**nvCJD**	New Variant Creutzfeldt–Jakob disease
ICD	Implantable cardioverter defibrillators		**O**	Ohm
ICU/ITU	Intensive care unit/Intensive therapy unit		**OD**	Outside diameter
ID	Internal diameter		**OIB**	Oxford inflating bellows
IEC	International Electrotechnical Commission		**OMV**	Oxford Miniature vaporizer
IMV	Intermittent mandatory ventilation		**Pa**	Pascal (unit of pressure)
I/O	Input or output		**PAC**	Pulmonary artery flotation catheter
IPPV	Intermittent positive pressure ventilation		**PAWP**	Pulmonary artery wedge pressure
IR	Infrared		**PCA**	Patient-controlled analgesia
ISO	International Organization for Standardization		**PCEA**	Patient-controlled epidural analgesia
K	Degrees Kelvin (always stated without degree symbol)		**PCV**	Pressure controlled ventilation
			PDPH	Post-dural puncture headache
kgf	Kilogram force		**PDT**	Percutaneous dilatational tracheostomy
kPa	Kilopascal (European standard measurement for pressure)		**PEEP**	Positive end-expiratory pressure
			PEF	Peak expiratory flow
LASER	Light Amplification by Stimulated Emission of Radiation		**PIP**	Peak inspiratory pressure
			PNS	Peripheral nerve stimulator
LCD	Liquid crystal display		**PP**	Pause pressure
LED	Light-emitting diode		**ppm**	Parts per million
LMA	Laryngeal mask airway		**PSA**	Pressure Swing Absorber
LOFT	Line Orientated Flight Training		**PSI**	Patient state index
MAP	Mean airway pressure		**psi**	Pounds per square inch (US standard measurement for pressure)
MDAPE	Median absolute performance error			
MDPE	Median performance error		**PSV**	Pressure support ventilation
MF	Median frequency		**PTFE**	Polytetrafluorethylene (Teflon)
MGPS	Medical gas pipeline services		**PV**	Peak velocity
MHRA	Medicines and Healthcare products Regulatory Agency		**PVC**	Polyvinyl chloride
			RA	Risk assessment
MHz	Megahertz		**RAM**	Random access memory
MLAEP	Mid-latency auditory evoked potential		**RCCB**	Residual current circuit breaker
mmHg	Millimetres of mercury (unit of pressure)		**RF**	Radiofrequency
MMV	Mandatory minute volume		**RMS**	Root mean squared
MORE	Manufacturers' On-line Reporting Environment		**ROM**	Read only memory
			RSA	Respiratory sinus arrhythmia
MPR	Minimum pressure retention		**SABS**	Safety Alert Broadcast System
MRI	Magnetic Resonance Imaging		**Scuba**	Self-contained underwater breathing apparatus
N	Newton			
NAO	National Audit Office		**SEF**	Spectral edge frequency
NASPE	North American Society of Pacing and Electrophysiology		**SI (units)**	Système International d'Unites (International System of Units)
NEEP	Negative end-expiratory pressure			
NELH	National Electronic Library of Health		**SIB**	Self-inflating bag
NIBP	Non-invasive blood pressure (monitoring)		**SIMV**	Synchronized intermittent mandatory ventilation
NICE	National Institute for Clinical Excellence			
NiCd	Nickel-cadmium		**SMA**	Synthetic Medical Air
NiMH	Nickel-metal hydride		**SSEP**	Somatosensory evoked potential
NIOSH	National Institute for Occupational Safety and Health (USA)		**SV**	Stroke volume
			SVP	Saturated vapour pressure
NIST	Non-interchangeable screw threaded (connection)		**swg**	Standard wire gauge
			TAP	Transoesophageal atrial pacing
NIPPV	Non-invasive positive pressure ventilation		**TCD**	Transcranial Doppler ultrasonography

TCE	Temperature compensating element	**TTJV**	Transtracheal Jet Ventilation
TCI	Target controlled infusion	**TWA**	Time-weighted average
TFT	Thin film transistor	**USP**	United States Pharmacopeia
TGA	Therapeutic Goods Administration	**UV**	Ultraviolet
TIVA	Total intravenous anaesthesia	**VF**	Ventricular fibrillation
TOF	Train of four	**VIC**	Vaporizer in circle
Torr	(Torricelli) mmHg pressure (also used for subatmospheric pressures)	**VIE**	Vacuum insulated evaporator
TSE	Transmissible Spongiform Encephalopathies	**Vmax**	Maximal velocity
TSSU	Theatre Sterile Supply Unit	**VOC**	Vaporizer out of circle

1

Physical principles

Paul D Davis

The art of anaesthesia is essentially practical. For this reason anaesthetists must have an understanding of the physical aspects of the apparatus they use, not only to use it efficiently but also to understand its limitations and to use it safely. Many avoidable accidents and near misses have occurred as the result of the misuse of equipment or misinterpretation of measurements because the anaesthetist did not understand the basic principles concerned.

One of the problems besetting the medical profession today is the clinician's inability to discuss his or her requirements with the engineer in terms that they both understand. This problem occurs not only with the development of new equipment but also with the discussion of faults and difficulties with existing equipment.

This chapter is therefore devoted to the basic physics of gases, liquids, vapours and solids, and to the principles of modern control systems, which are increasingly a part of the latest anaesthetic machines. Where reference is made to units of measurement, the International System of Units, known as the SI System (Système International d'Unités), is generally used (see Appendix).

STATES OF MATTER

An understanding of the physical principles applicable to the practice of anaesthesia can begin with a consideration of the differences between three states of matter: solid, liquid and gas. The difference between these states is best explained by considering the effects of the interactions between the atoms and molecules of which they are made. Atoms or molecules are subject to forces of attraction known as Van der Waals forces, which act to hold individual atoms or molecules near to each other.

In a solid, these intermolecular forces cause the molecules to maintain a fairly fixed position relative to each other. Although the kinetic energy of the molecules causes them to move about a mean position, these mean positions are fixed and may form a regular geometric structure or lattice. When a solid is heated, the kinetic energy of the molecules increases, so the range of movement about this mean position increases and the volume of the solid increases as expansion occurs.

As more heat is added to the solid, the range of movement of the molecules eventually becomes sufficiently great to disrupt the fixed structure and the molecules are able to move past each other. The solid has changed state to become a liquid. Nevertheless, the kinetic energy is insufficient to overcome the intermolecular forces completely and the molecules remain close to each other. Because the molecules remain near each other in a solid or a liquid, matter in either of these states is not easily compressed.

As more heat is added to the liquid, the kinetic energy of the molecules increases until the intermolecular forces are no longer sufficient to hold the molecules near each other. The state changes to the gaseous state, in which the molecules move freely throughout the volume in which they are contained. Because of the large distances between molecules in the gaseous state, matter in this state is comparatively easily compressed.

HEAT AND TEMPERATURE

Relationship between heat and temperature

The internal energy of an object is composed of the kinetic and potential energies of the molecules of which it consists. Transfer of heat energy to or from an object alters this internal energy. The temperature of an object determines the direction in which a transfer of heat energy occurs, the energy being transferred from the object with the higher temperature to the object with the lower temperature. Objects at the same temperature are in thermal equilibrium and no transfer of energy occurs.

Temperature scales

Temperature scales are based on fixed temperatures that can be reproduced by appropriate physical conditions. Two of these fixed temperatures are needed to define a temperature scale.

The SI unit of temperature is the Kelvin (K). The lower fixed point used to define the Kelvin scale is the temperature at which no further heat energy can be extracted from any object. This point is often referred to as the *absolute zero* of temperature and the Kelvin temperature as *absolute temperature*. The upper fixed point is the triple point of water, which is the temperature at which ice, water and water vapour exist in equilibrium (Fig. 1.1). The temperature range between these fixed points is

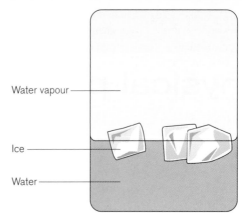

Figure 1.1 A sealed vessel containing water vapour, water and ice in equilibrium at the triple point of water.

divided into 273.16 equal parts; thus the Kelvin is defined as 1/273.16 of the temperature of the triple point of water.

This rather strange definition of the Kelvin arises from its relationship to another temperature scale, the degree Celsius (°C) scale, the latter based on the freezing and boiling points of water, which are given the values 0°C and 100°C, respectively. The Celsius temperature is now defined by the relationship:

$$\text{temperature (K)} = \text{temperature (°C)} + 273.15$$

Thus the temperature of the triple point of water is 0.01°C and a difference of one Kelvin is identical to a difference of one degree Celsius.

Heat

The SI unit of energy is the joule (J), although an alternative unit, the calorie (cal) is sometimes used specifically for heat energy. As the calorie is a rather small quantity of heat energy, the energy available from foods is often quoted in terms of kilocalories and the symbol Cal is used to represent kilocalories.

The relationship between these various units is:

1 calorie (cal) = 4.187 joule (J)
1 Calorie (Cal) = 1 kilocalorie (kcal) = 1,000 calories

Heat capacity and specific heat capacity

Objects differ in the temperature change produced by the gain or loss of a given quantity of heat energy. For example, a large object made of the same material as a small object exhibits a lesser change in temperature than the small object. Objects of the same mass but made of different materials generally also differ in the temperature change produced by the same change in heat energy. The change in heat energy and temperature are related by the *heat capacity* of the object:

change in heat energy = change in temperature × heat capacity

In order to be able to compare different objects and different materials, the term *specific heat capacity* is used. The specific heat capacity, also referred to as the *specific heat*, is the quantity of heat energy required to change the temperature of 1 kg of a substance by 1 K. The units are therefore J kg^{-1} K^{-1}.

For example, it takes 4200 J of energy to raise the temperature of 1 kg of water by 1°C. Therefore the specific heat capacity of water is 4200 J kg^{-1} K^{-1}. In comparison, it takes 910 J to raise the temperature of 1 kg of aluminium by 1°C. Therefore the specific heat capacity of aluminium is 910 J kg^{-1} K^{-1}.

Latent heat

A comparatively large alteration in the kinetic energy of molecules occurs when a substance changes state; moreover, this change of state occurs at a fixed temperature that depends on the pressure. In the case of the transition from solid to liquid, this is the *melting point* and in the case of liquid to gas, the *boiling point*. The addition of heat energy is needed for the change of state to occur, even though this change takes place at a fixed temperature. The energy is needed to increase the kinetic energy of the molecules sufficiently to overcome the forces of attraction between them and is known as *the latent heat*. These processes occur in reverse when heat energy is removed from a substance. The transition from gas to liquid is termed *the dew point* and the transition from liquid to solid, *the freezing point*.

The heat required to melt a solid is known as the *latent heat of fusion*. For ice this is 333 kJ kg^{-1} at 0°C and normal atmospheric pressure. The heat required to vaporize a liquid is called *the latent heat of vaporization*. For water, this is 2257 kJ kg^{-1} at 100°C and normal atmospheric pressure. It is noteworthy that considerably more heat is required to vaporize a liquid than to raise its temperature from room temperature to its boiling point.

Transfer of heat

Heat may be transferred from one object to another or from one part of an object to another by the processes of *conduction*, *convection* and *radiation*.

Conduction

In conduction, heat energy diffuses along an object from molecule to molecule. For example, metals such as copper are good conductors of heat, whereas glass and expanded polystyrene are poor conductors. Very poor conductors of heat are termed *thermal insulators*.

Convection

If part of a fluid is heated, it expands and becomes less dense than the fluid surrounding it. Being free to move, it rises, and as it travels upwards, its place is taken by the cooler, denser fluid from around it, which in turn is heated and rises. There is, therefore, a constant rising stream of fluid above the source of heat. These currents are known as convection currents (Fig. 1.2) and the heat energy is carried by them.

Radiation

The transfer of radiated heat energy does not require the source of heat to be in contact with any other object. The rate at which heat energy is radiated is described by Stefan's law:

$$P = \sigma \varepsilon A T^4$$

where σ is Stefan's constant, ε is the emissivity, A is the area of the radiating surface and T is the absolute temperature. The emissivity, which ranges from 0 to 1, quantifies the difference in emission from surfaces at the same temperature. A matt black surface, for example, has a greater emissivity than a reflective white surface, so the rate at which it radiates energy is greater under the same conditions.

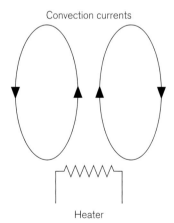

Figure 1.2 Convection currents above a heater; the arrows show the movement of fluid.

Stefan's law shows that the net transfer of heat between two objects at different temperatures is proportional to the difference between the fourth power of their temperatures, i.e. $P \propto T_1^4 - T_2^4$. Even though the ambient temperature is comparatively high, heat can still be lost to a cooler object through the radiation of heat energy.

Because of its dependence on temperature, radiated heat energy can be used as the basis of temperature measurement techniques.

PROPERTIES OF IDEAL GASES

As is the case with all substances, the smallest particle of a gas that can exist separately is a molecule, or in the case of some gases such as xenon, an atom. Gas molecules are in constant motion, moving in all directions and rebounding from each other and from the walls of the space in which they are confined. It is the change in momentum resulting from the collisions of gas molecules with the walls that appears as the pressure of the gas.

The physical properties of gases under certain conditions of temperature and pressure approximate those of a collection of non-interacting particles of negligible size that undergo collisions with each other and the walls of the container in which they are situated. These properties are known as the properties of an ideal gas. The state of such a gas in a closed container can be described by four variables: the volume of the container, the number of molecules of gas present, the temperature and the pressure. These variables are related by several gas laws, which describe the behaviour of an ideal gas.

THE GAS LAWS

Boyle's law

Boyle's law states that, at constant temperature, the volume of a fixed mass of gas is inversely proportional to its pressure:

$$V \propto \frac{1}{P} \text{ or } PV = k_B \text{ where } k_B \text{ is a constant}$$

Charles' law

Charles' law states that, at constant pressure, the volume of a fixed mass of gas is proportional to its absolute temperature:

$$V \propto T \text{ or } \frac{V}{T} = k_C \text{ where } k_C \text{ is a constant}$$

Gay-Lussac's law

Gay-Lussac's law states that, at a constant volume, the pressure of a fixed mass of gas is proportional to its absolute temperature:

$$P \propto T \text{ or } \frac{P}{T} = k_G \text{ where } k_G \text{ is a constant}$$

Combined gas law

These three gas laws can be combined to give the following relationship for a fixed mass of gas:

$$\frac{P_1 V_1}{T_1} = \frac{P_2 V_2}{T_2}$$

where P_1, V_1 and T_1 are the pressure, volume and temperature in one set of conditions and P_2, V_2 and T_2 are the corresponding quantities in a second set of conditions. The temperature, T, must be expressed on the absolute scale as a Kelvin temperature. The above formula may be used to calculate the results of a change of pressure, temperature or volume of a fixed mass of gas.

Standard temperature and pressure

Because the volume of a given mass of gas depends on temperature and pressure, comparison of gas volumes is easier if any given gas volume is converted to the volume it would have at a standard temperature and pressure. The standard temperature and pressure (STP) normally used are 0°C and 760 mm Hg (273.15 K and 101.325 kPa).

Avogadro's hypothesis

Avogadro's hypothesis states that, under conditions of constant pressure and temperature, equal volumes of gases contain equal numbers of molecules.

Mole

The SI unit for an amount of any substance is the mole. The mole is the amount of substance which contains as many elementary entities as there are atoms in 0.012 kg of carbon-12. For example, the elementary entities may be atoms, molecules, ions or electrons. The number of elementary entities in one mole is known as Avogadro's number, the value of which is 6.022×10^{23}.

Avogadro's law

Avogadro's law states that, under conditions of constant pressure and temperature, there is a direct relationship between the volume and number of moles for an ideal gas:

$V \propto n$ or $V = k_A n$ where k_A is a constant

Molar volume

The molar volume is the volume occupied by one mole of an ideal gas at STP; its value is 22.414 litres.

Ideal gas law

The gas laws described above can be combined to produce an equation of state for an ideal gas as follows:

$PV = nRT$

where R is the molar gas constant. Its value can be calculated by:

$$R = \frac{PV}{nT} = \frac{\text{standard pressure} \times \text{volume}}{\text{moles} \times \text{standard temperature}} =$$

$$\frac{\text{standard pressure} \times \text{molar volume}}{\text{standard temperature}} =$$

$$\frac{101{,}325 \text{ Pa} \times 0.022414 \text{ m}^3}{273.15 \text{ K}} = 8.314 \text{ Pa m}^3/\text{mole K}$$

Dalton's law and Amagat's law

A vessel may be occupied by more than one gas, in which case the total pressure within it is the sum of the pressures exerted independently by each of the gases. Each gas is said to exert a partial pressure. The pressure exerted by a vapour or a gas in a closed space, at a given temperature, is independent of the pressure of other vapours or gases provided they have undergone no chemical reaction with each other. When several vapours or gases having no chemical reaction with each other are present in the same space, the pressure exerted by the mixture is the sum of the pressures that would be exerted by each of its constituents if it was separately confined in the same space.

Dalton's law states that the pressure of a gas mixture is equal to the sum of the partial pressures of the gases of which it is composed.

Amagat's law states that the volume of a gas mixture is equal to the sum of the volumes of all its constituents which are at the same temperature and pressure as the mixture.

Dry gas correction

The addition of water vapour to a mixture of gases reduces the partial pressures of those gases if the total pressure of the mixture remains the same. It may be necessary to correct for this effect when determining partial pressures in humidified mixtures, for example those present in alveoli. Suppose that end tidal carbon dioxide concentration is measured in a dry gas mixture; the concentration in the alveoli will be lower because of the presence of water vapour in the mixture. The corrected value can be calculated as follows:

$$\begin{array}{l}\text{partial pressure of} \\ CO_2 \text{ in alveoli}\end{array} = \begin{array}{l}\text{partial pressure of} \\ CO_2 \text{ in dry gas}\end{array} \times$$

$$\frac{\text{atmospheric pressure} - \text{partial pressure of water vapour}}{\text{atmospheric pressure}}$$

Graham's law

The kinetic energy of a gas is dependent on its temperature and the kinetic energy is also proportional to the molecular weight and the velocity of its molecules. So for two different gases at the same temperature, which therefore have the same kinetic energy:

$$\text{kinetic energy} = 1/2 \ m_1 v_1^2 = 1/2 \ m_2 v_2^2$$

thus

$$\frac{v_1}{v_2} = \frac{\sqrt{m_2}}{\sqrt{m_1}}$$

This leads to Graham's law, which states that the rate of diffusion of a gas is inversely proportional to the square root of its molecular weight.

PROPERTIES OF REAL GASES

The properties of real gases differ from those of ideal gases because of the finite size of the molecules and the existence of intermolecular forces between them, but divergence from the behaviour of ideal gases becomes important only under conditions in which the molecules are close together. These conditions occur chiefly at lower temperatures and higher pressures. The values of temperature and pressure at which divergence from the behaviour of ideal gases becomes apparent differ from one gas to another.

Vapour pressure

A substance in the gaseous state and in contact with the same substance in the liquid or solid state is known as a vapour. The molecules in the solid, liquid or gaseous state do not all have the same kinetic energy. The more energetic or less energetic of the molecules may move between states until an equilibrium is established, with as

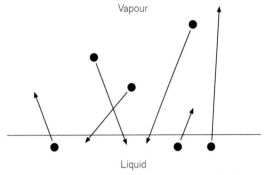

Figure 1.3 Movement of molecules between liquid and vapour states in equilibrium.

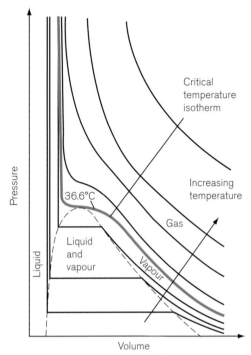

Figure 1.4 Isotherms for nitrous oxide.

many molecules changing state in one direction as those changing in the reverse direction (Fig. 1.3).

The pressure at which the gaseous state is in equilibrium with either the liquid or solid state, or with both, is known as the *saturated vapour pressure* (SVP) and is a function of temperature. The boiling point of a liquid is the temperature at which the saturated vapour pressure is equal to the atmospheric pressure, so the boiling point of a liquid depends on the ambient pressure. Since atmospheric pressure depends on altitude, the boiling point is depressed as altitude increases.

Critical temperature

A substance in the gaseous state at a pressure less than the saturated vapour pressure cannot be in equilibrium with the same substance in the liquid state; the liquid evaporates until the saturated vapour pressure is reached or until no more liquid remains. Conversely, if the pressure of a vapour is increased, liquefaction begins when the saturated vapour pressure is reached. The substance then exists as a vapour, a liquid, or a mixture of both. However, above a certain temperature, known as the *critical temperature*, liquefaction does not occur; thus it is not possible for the liquid state to exist above this critical temperature.

The relationship between pressure, volume and temperature is usually displayed as a set of isotherms, i.e. a set of curves representing the properties of the gas at constant temperature. Figure 1.4 shows isotherms for nitrous oxide. Each isotherm shows the relationship between pressure and volume at a given temperature. Nitrous oxide may exist as a liquid or a vapour below the critical temperature of 36.6°C; above this critical tempe-

rature it may exist only as a gas. It follows that if a gas is stored below its critical temperature as a mixture of liquid and vapour, determination of the contents of its container cannot be made from the pressure within. If a gas is stored above its critical temperature, the quantity of gas will be proportional to the pressure inside its container. An example is oxygen, which has a critical temperature of −118°C, and is therefore in its gaseous state at room temperature. The *critical pressure* is the pressure that is required to liquefy a gas at its critical temperature.

The Poynting effect

A mixture of 50% nitrous oxide and 50% oxygen is marketed under the name Entonox. A full cylinder of Entonox typically contains these gases at a pressure of 137 bar. According to Dalton's law, the partial pressure of the nitrous oxide in the cylinder should be 68.5 bar (i.e. 1/2 of 137 bar). Since the saturated vapour pressure of nitrous oxide at 20°C is less than this, being approximately 52 bar, one might expect liquid nitrous oxide to form when a cylinder is filled to this pressure, and an Entonox cylinder at room temperature to contain liquid nitrous oxide, but this is not the case. An effect known as the Poynting effect, or overpressure effect, alters the pressure at which liquid nitrous oxide forms in the mixture.

If a cylinder is partially filled with liquid nitrous oxide, inverted, and then further filled from a high-pressure source of oxygen, an unexpected phenomenon occurs. This may be viewed through the glass observation window of a high-pressure rig. The bubbles of oxygen diminish in size as the gas is partially dissolved in the liquid nitrous oxide through which it passes. Simultaneously, the volume of the liquid nitrous oxide diminishes as it evaporates and mixes with the oxygen. Eventually the cylinder, filled to a pressure of 13.7 MPa (137 bar), contains mixed oxygen and nitrous oxide, both in the gaseous state. Cooling of the cylinder and its contents does eventually result in the condensation of nitrous oxide at a temperature known as the pseudocritical temperature. The value of this temperature depends on the pressure of gas in the cylinder, but can be as high as −5.5°C, so precautions concerning use of cylinders of the mixture in cold conditions are necessary

Adiabatic processes

Work has to be done to compress a gas and the energy expended is converted into heat. If the process is adiabatic, i.e. there is no exchange of heat with the surroundings, the temperature of the gas rises. In some circumstances, such as the compression –ignition (diesel) engine, the compression is sufficiently rapid to cause a considerable rise in temperature, resulting in ignition of the fuel vapour. In the same way, if part of an anaesthetic apparatus were to contain oil, grease or some other flammable material and were to be subjected to a sudden rise of pressure in the presence of oxygen, as when a cylinder were turned on suddenly, an explosion could occur. For this reason all apparatus using high-pressure oxygen must be free of oil, grease or other flammable material. Pressure gauges are fitted with a constriction in the inlet to reduce the shock wave that occurs when a cylinder is turned on.

The Joule–Kelvin principle (Joule–Thompson effect)

Conversely, when a gas expands, it does work and the temperature drops. Under normal circumstances in anaesthetic practice, the expansion of a gas leaving the cylinder is not sufficiently rapid to cause a great fall in temperature. The fall in temperature is, for example, much less than that due to the latent heat of vaporization, which is the main cause of cooling of cylinders of nitrous oxide when in use.

BEHAVIOUR OF MOLECULES OF SOLIDS AND LIQUIDS

The molecules of a solid or a liquid attract each other. They may also be attracted by the molecules of another substance. The mutual attraction between molecules of a substance is termed *cohesion*, and their attraction to those of another substance is called *adhesion*.

Surface tension and capillary action

The intermolecular forces that cause liquid molecules to remain near each other (cohesion) result in a measurable tension in the surface of a liquid. The phenomenon is known as *surface tension*.

The intermolecular forces of adhesion acting between molecules of water and the glass wall of a water or saline manometer are greater than the forces of cohesion between water molecules. As a result, the attraction of the water molecules to the molecules in the wall that are above the surface of the liquid has two effects: the surface of the water forms a concave surface at its edge called a *meniscus* and the height of the water in the manometer increases. This is known as *capillary action* (Fig. 1.5). The force of adhesion acting at the walls of the tube is balanced by the force due to gravity acting on the mass of water contained in the volume that has risen above the level of water outside the manometer; the narrower the tube, the further the water rises up it.

Capillary action is the principle that causes liquid anaesthetic agent to rise up the wick in a vaporizer. The wick dips into the liquid agent, the liquid rises up the

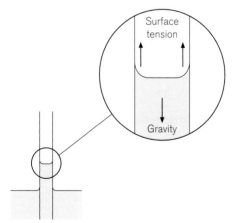

Figure 1.5 Capillary action in a tube of water due to surface tension resulting from intermolecular forces.

wick and a larger surface area is obtained from which vaporization may occur.

THE BEHAVIOUR OF FLUIDS

Fluid flow

The factors affecting fluid flow through a tube are described by the equation:

$$\text{flow} = \frac{\text{pressure difference}}{\text{resistance}}$$

It is important to distinguish between volume flow and mass flow, since the same volume flow results in a higher mass flow if the pressure of a gas is increased.

The SI unit of pressure is the Pascal (Pa) and the units of volume flow are $\text{metre}^3/\text{second}$, so in this case, the units of resistance are Pa s m^{-3}. When units other than SI units are used, resistance is typically measured as cm H_2O s l^{-1} for values encountered in anaesthetic practice. Various physical properties affect the flow of fluid through tubes; some of these are properties of the tube itself and others are properties of the fluid, such as density and viscosity.

Viscosity

Viscosity arises from friction between layers of fluid which are moving relative to each other. Although molecules in a particular layer of fluid are moving randomly in different directions, they have an average momentum in the direction of motion of the fluid layer of which they are part and this momentum is greater for a faster moving layer than for a slower moving one. Random motion causes molecules to transfer from one layer to another and this results in the transfer of momentum between layers (Fig. 1.6). The molecules that move from the faster to the slower moving layer tend to increase the speed of the slower layer and vice versa. This results in friction between the layers and the phenomenon of viscosity. The SI units of viscosity are Pa s (Pascal seconds).

Types of flow

The flow of gases or liquids can be one of two types: *laminar* or *turbulent*. In laminar flow, the fluid flows steadily in one direction; in turbulent flow, it swirls in eddies. Turbulent flow occurs at higher fluid velocities than laminar flow. The probability of turbulent rather than laminar flow occurring in a tube can be determined by calculating an index known as Reynolds number:

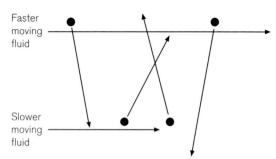

Faster moving fluid

Slower moving fluid

Figure 1.6 Molecules transfer momentum between layers of fluid moving at different rates.

$$\text{Reynolds number, } R = \frac{v\rho d}{\eta} \text{ (equation 1)}$$

where v is the linear velocity of the fluid, ρ is the density, d is the diameter of the tube and η is the viscosity. Empirical measurements with cylindrical tubes show that transition between laminar and turbulent flow occurs when Reynolds number is about 2000. If Reynolds number exceeds 2000, turbulent flow is likely to be present; if Reynolds number is below 2000, the flow is likely to be laminar. It can be seen from this formula that for a fixed set of conditions there is a critical velocity at which Reynolds number has the value 2000. When the velocity of the fluid exceeds this critical value, the character of the flow is likely to change from laminar to turbulent (Fig. 1.7). This critical velocity applies only for a given fluid in a given tube. Turbulent flow is often present where there is an orifice, a sharp bend or some other irregularity which may cause a local increase in velocity and hence an increase in Reynolds number to a value greater than 2000.

Since the volume flow (F) in a cylindrical tube can be represented by the formula:

$$F = \frac{v\pi d^2}{4} \text{ (equation 2)}$$

which may be arranged as

$$vd = \frac{4F}{\pi d} \text{ (equation 3)}$$

by substituting vd in Equation 1, Reynolds number for this type of flow can be represented as

$$R = \frac{4F\rho}{\pi d\eta}$$

This shows that, for the same volume flow (F), Reynolds number becomes smaller and laminar flow more likely as the diameter of a tube increases.

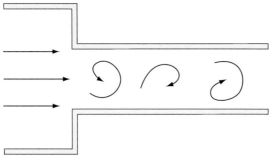

Figure 1.7 Laminar flow becoming turbulent at a sharp change in tube diameter.

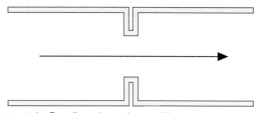

Figure 1.9 Gas flow through an orifice.

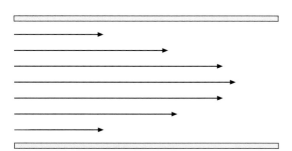

Figure 1.8 Laminar fluid flow.

Laminar flow

The behaviour of laminar flow (Fig. 1.8) in a tube is described by the equation due to Poiseuille:

$$\text{flow} = \text{pressure drop} \times \frac{\pi r^4}{8\eta l}$$

where η is the viscosity, l the length of the tube and r the radius of the tube. From this equation it can be seen that for a given pressure gradient along a tube, flow is dependent on the fourth power of the radius. Similarly, therefore, comparatively small changes in the diameter of a tube will affect the pressure drop noticeably; for example, a reduction of only 16% in the diameter of a tube doubles the pressure drop across it. Figure 1.8 shows the velocity profile of laminar flow in a tube; the velocity is greatest in the centre and decreases towards the edges.

Turbulent flow

Although the resistance can be calculated easily for laminar flow, this is not the case for turbulent flow. The analysis of turbulence is highly complex and the most important point to note is that the resistance is no longer independent of flow, so it is not possible to quote the resistance to flow of a particular item without specifying the flow itself under turbulent conditions.

Flow through an orifice

In contrast to a tube, the length of which is by definition much greater than its diameter, an orifice is an aperture, the length of which is less than its diameter

Flow through an orifice (Fig. 1.9) is described by the equation:

$$\text{Flow rate} \propto d^2 \sqrt{\frac{\Delta P}{\rho}}$$

where d is the diameter of the orifice, ΔP is the pressure difference across it and ρ is the density of the fluid. It is found, however, that if flow through an orifice reaches the speed of sound in the fluid, the rate of mass flow ceases to depend on the downstream pressure, i.e. it depends on the upstream pressure only.

Bernoulli's law, the Bernoulli effect and the venturi

There are three contributions to the energy of a moving fluid: the potential energy due to its pressure, the kinetic energy due to its movement and the potential energy due to the force of gravity on it. If its total energy does not change, Bernoulli's law applies:

$$P + \tfrac{1}{2}\rho v^2 + \rho g h = \text{constant}$$

where P is the pressure, ρ the density, v the fluid velocity, g the acceleration due to gravity and h the vertical height of an element of fluid.

If the fluid is not moving, $v = 0$, so the equation becomes

$$P + \rho g h = \text{constant}$$

indicating that the pressure at the base of a column of fluid is proportional to its height and its density. This relationship is the basis of fluid manometers.

For the case of fluid moving through a horizontal tube, the equation becomes

$$P + \tfrac{1}{2} \rho v^2 = \text{constant}$$

If the fluid flows through a tube which has a constriction within it, the velocity increases as the fluid passes the constriction. Bernoulli's law indicates that the pressure P falls as the velocity increases. A constriction with an entry and exit in which the diameter changes gradually, and which maintains laminar flow, is known as a venturi; the reduction in pressure as the fluid passes through the venturi is known as the Bernoulli effect. When the gas emerges from the constriction into the wider portion of the tube, the linear velocity of flow decreases and the pressure increases again (Fig. 1.10a). The pressure may rise to a level almost as high as that before the constriction, the extent of this rise being dependent on the design of the tube and the constriction.

If a side branch is added to the tube at the venturi, the reduction in pressure causes fluid from the branch to be entrained by the main stream (Fig. 1.10b).

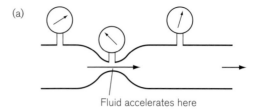

(a)

Fluid accelerates here

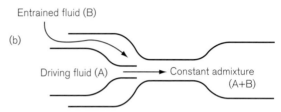

(b)

Entrained fluid (B)

Driving fluid (A)

Constant admixture (A+B)

Figure 1.10 **(a)** The Bernoulli effect and **(b)** a venturi.

FURTHER READING

Kuhn KF (1996) *Basic Physics: A Self-Teaching Guide*, 2nd edn. USA: John Wiley.

Davis PD, Kenny GNC (2003) *Basic Physics and Measurement in Anaesthesia*, 5th edn. Edinburgh: Butterworth Heinemann.

2

Basic physics of electricity

Paul D Davis

ELECTRIC CHARGE

Electricity arises from the physical properties of the elementary particles which constitute atoms and molecules. Some of these particles possess a property known as *electric charge*, of which there are two forms: a positive form and a negative form. An attractive force occurs between particles of opposite charge and a repulsive force between particles of similar charge.

Atoms comprise a positively charged nucleus surrounded by negatively charged electrons. The aggregate charge on the complete atom is normally zero because the total charge of the electrons is the same magnitude as that of the nucleus, but of opposite sign. Atoms may become charged, however, if electrons are added or removed. Such electrically charged atoms are known as *ions*. Some compounds, such as sodium chloride, dissociate into charged ions when they dissolve in water. The ions may then move through the solution as carriers of charge.

Electrons may also transport charge by moving from one atom to another through a material, but materials differ in the degree to which electrons can readily move through them. In *insulators*, electrons do not move, but remain fixed in position; in *conductors*, they move more readily; in *semiconductors*, their freedom of movement is more dependent on temperature than in conductors.

The SI unit of charge is the *coulomb* (C), which is equal to 6.2×10^{18} times the charge possessed by a single electron.

Static electricity and electric potential

Electrons can be added to an insulator or removed from it, for example, by friction with a different material, and when this takes place, the net charge due to the excess or deficit of electrons tends to remain on the insulator. This accumulation of charge is known as *static electricity* because the position of the charge is normally fixed.

Although the usual SI unit of energy, the joule (J), can be used to quantify the change that takes place when charge is moved, a different quantity, the electric potential, is normally used. The electric potential, V, is related to the potential energy (E) and the charge (Q), by the relationship:

$$V = \frac{dE}{dQ}$$

The SI unit of electric potential is the *volt* (V). An alternative term, voltage, may be used to describe the size of an electric potential.

In some circumstances the electric potential produced by static electricity may amount to thousands of volts. The rate of change of potential with distance is the potential gradient. Although air is normally an insulator, a potential gradient of sufficient magnitude can ionize air molecules, thereby causing the air to conduct, resulting in the occurrence of a spark. The energy contained in the spark may be sufficiently great to ignite a flammable mixture.

ELECTRIC CURRENT

Electric current is the flow of electrically charged particles such as electrons or ions. It occurs when an electric potential exists across a conductor or a conducting fluid. The SI unit of electric current is the *ampere* (A), which is equal to a flow of one coulomb of charge per second through any cross-section of the conductor. Current density is current flowing across unit area; its units are therefore A m^{-2} (Fig. 2.1).

Current, which flows in one direction through a conductor at a fixed rate, is known as *direct current* (DC). Current, which changes direction periodically, is known as *alternating current* (AC). An electric current may have both a direct and an alternating component. The waveform of alternating current may be of any shape, but the sine wave is the most fundamental form because all other waveforms can be constructed from a combination of sine waves of appropriate frequencies, amplitudes and phases. The range of sine wave frequencies of which any waveform consists is known as the frequency range of the waveform.

An electric circuit consists of a source of potential and one or more electrically conducting paths connected to the source that allow current to flow.

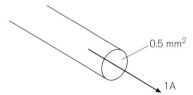

Figure 2.1 Comparison of current and current density; a current of 1 A flows through a conductor with a cross sectional area of 0.5 mm^2, so the current density is 2 A mm^{-2}.

0.5 mm^2

1 A

Resistance and Ohm's law

Materials are characterized by their electrical resistance (R), which measures the potential difference (V) required to produce a certain direct current flow (I). The relationship is given by Ohm's law:

$$I = \frac{V}{R}$$

The SI unit of resistance is the *ohm* (Ω).

Heating effect of electric currents

The power converted into heat, or some other form of energy when electric current flows through a resistance, is given by

$$P = V \times I$$

The SI unit of power is the *watt* (W). The heating effect of electric current is the principle used by the fuse, the electric component used to disconnect a supply of electricity if an excessive current flows. Under normal conditions, the current flows through the fuse without producing any noticeable effect, but when the current flow is excessive, the power converted into heat is sufficient to melt the conductor and interrupt the flow of current.

Root mean square (RMS) values

The instantaneous value of an alternating current varies throughout its cycle. It is more convenient to use a single number to specify the value of an alternating current and it is common to employ the value of direct current that would produce the same heating effect as the alternating current.

Since the heating effect depends on the power, P, this is represented by

$$P = VI \text{ (see above)}$$

and as $V = IR$, (Ohm's law)

therefore $P = I^2R$.

To obtain the equivalent direct current, the square of the alternating current is averaged over one complete cycle (Fig. 2.2), giving the mean square value. The equivalent direct current is then the square root of this and is known as the *root mean square* (RMS) value. A similar procedure is used to derive the RMS voltage of an alternating potential. The RMS voltage of the UK mains supply, for example, is 240 V, although the peak voltage occurring during the cycle is 340 V.

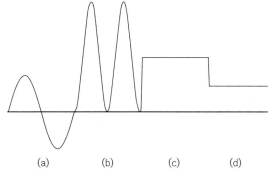

Figure 2.2 Derivation of root mean square values; **(a)** original waveform, **(b)** point by point square of amplitude, **(c)** average over one cycle of squared values, **(d)** square root of average (RMS value).

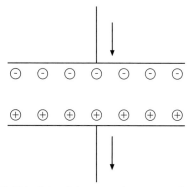

Figure 2.3 Principle of the capacitor; arrows indicate the flow of electrons that produce the change of charge on the capacitor.

Capacitance

If an electric charge is added to one of two adjacent conducting surfaces, an equal and opposite charge arises on the other conducting surface. This ability of an object to hold electric charge is the property known as *capacitance* (C). It is measured by the relationship between the charge on the conductors (Q), and the potential between them (V), as follows:

$$\text{capacitance, } C = \frac{Q}{V}$$

The SI unit of capacitance is the *farad* (F). The two conductors form a capacitor (Fig. 2.3) and the capacitance between them increases as the distance between them decreases.

An alternating potential applied across a capacitor results in the charges on the two parts of the capacitor alternating. The movement of charges to and from the conductors comprising the capacitor constitutes an alternating current. Although no charge crosses the gap between the two surfaces forming the capacitor, there is an apparent flow of current through the capacitor which is known as the *displacement current*.

Energy stored in a capacitor

The energy stored in a capacitor is a function of the potential and the charge. As the potential across a capacitor rises, it takes more energy to add the same amount of extra charge, so the total energy is not simply the product of the charge and potential. It can be shown that the stored energy, E, is represented by the equation:

$$E = 1/2\ QV \text{ (coulombs of charge x volts)}$$

and since $Q = CV$ (capacitance x volts)

$$E = 1/2 CV^2$$

A capacitor is used to store the electric energy required to produce the current pulse employed in cardiac defibrillators. Since the electrical resistance of the skin is high, the stored potential must be in the kilovolt range. As the energy required may be hundreds of joules, the capacitor typically has a value in the microfarad range. Because of the high voltage, care is needed during the operation of the equipment.

VARIABLE ELECTRIC CURRENT

The flow of a variable current in an electrical circuit produces interesting phenomena (*inductance, reactance* and *impedance*), not seen when a constant current flows. These are caused by the type of electromagnetic field created adjacent to the electrical circuit by the variable current (see below, Electric and magnetic fields). Such effects include:

Inductance

Conductors in an electric circuit passing a variable current possess a property known as inductance, which controls the rate of change of current when a voltage is applied across the conductor according to the relationship

$$\text{inductance, } L = \frac{\text{potential, } V}{\text{rate of change of current } \dfrac{dI}{dt}}$$

Inductance increases if a conductor is wound into a coil, with more turns in the coil, producing greater inductance. A component of this type is known as an inductor. Because an inductor controls the rate of change of current in a circuit, it can be used to regulate the form of the current pulse produced by a defibrillator (see Chapter 27).

Two adjacent conductors or coils possess *mutual inductance*, a property which results in a changing current in one inducing a current in the other. This property is used in transformers (see below), the components of which cause an alternating voltage at the input to be changed to a different alternating voltage at the output. Note that there is no change in frequency here.

Transformers

A transformer is made by winding two coils of wire around a ferromagnetic material (core). A changing current passing through the primary coil creates a changing magnetic field in the core. This magnetic field induces a current flow in the secondary coil. The voltage output in the secondary coil is determined by both the voltage input to the primary coil and the ratio of the number of windings (*turns*) of the two coils. If the number of turns of the two coils are identical, then the voltage output will be the same as the input. However, if the secondary coil has more windings, the voltage output will be greater (step up transformer Fig. 2.4a) and vice versa (step down transformer Fig. 2.4b).

In a well-designed transformer, the power output will be similar to the input. Therefore, if the secondary voltage is greater than the input, then the secondary current flow must be less, according to the formula:

Power in Watts (W) = Volts (V) × (I) current flow.

Reactance

The opposition to alternating current flow resulting from capacitance and inductance is called reactance. The relationship between the sine wave current flowing to and from a capacitor and the voltage across the capacitor is known as *capacitive reactance* (X_C), and is a measure of the resistance to current flow resulting from capacitance. It is measured in Ohms and is defined as

$$\text{reactance, } X_C = \frac{V}{I} = \frac{1}{2\pi f C}$$

where f is the frequency of the current and voltage, and C is the capacitance. The phase of the current is 90° in advance of the voltage. It can be seen that, for a given voltage, the current increases as the frequency or capacitance increases (Fig. 2.5).

For an inductor, *inductive reactance* (X_L), again measured in Ohms, is described by the formula:

(a)

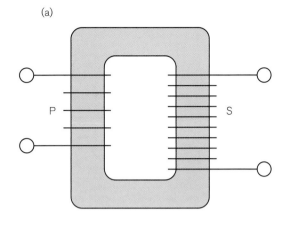

(b)

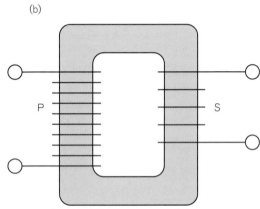

Figure 2.4 (a) Step up transformer: (P) is the primary winding and (S) is the secondary winding. **(b)** a step down transformer.

(a)

(b)

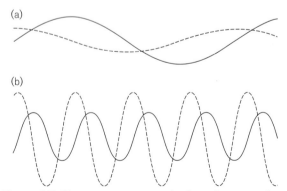

Figure 2.5 Sine wave current and voltage in a capacitor and their dependence on frequency; the dashed lines illustrate current and the solid lines voltage. (a) Low frequency. (b) High frequency.

reactance, $X_L = 2\pi f L$

where L is the inductance. An increase in frequency or increased inductance will result in an increase in reactance.

Impedance

Many components of electric circuits possess resistance, capacitance and inductance, although typically one of these properties will be more apparent than the others. The term impedance is used as a measure of the sum of all of these properties that resist the flow of an alternating current. The unit of impedance is the ohm (Ω):

$$\text{impedance, } Z = \frac{\text{voltage}}{\text{current}}$$

Because impedance includes reactance in addition to resistance, its value is a function of frequency; similarly, the phase difference between voltage and current is also a function of frequency.

ELECTRODES, CELLS AND BATTERIES

When a metallic conductor is placed in a liquid or solution containing ions, a double layer of charges forms at the interface between the conductor and the electrolyte (Fig. 2.6). A negatively charged layer at the surface of the conductor develops adjacent to a positively charged layer in the electrolyte. These charged layers are the origin of an electric potential difference between the conductor and the electrolyte which is characteristic of the particular conductor and ions present. The interface between the conductor and electrolyte is said to be *polarized*. The combination of a conductor immersed in an electrolyte is known as a *half cell* or *electrode* and the characteristic potential difference between the conductor and solution, when no current is flowing, is known as the half cell or electrode potential. An electrode can be used as a means of making an electrical contact to a solution.

If two half cells with different characteristic potentials are placed in series, the resulting potential difference can be used to drive an electric current through an external circuit, the arrangement being known as a *cell*. Several cells can be placed in series to form a *battery*.

Electric currents in the body are generally ionic currents, i.e. they comprise the movement of ions such as Na^+ and Cl^- in solution. Biological potentials measurable on the surface of the body, such as the electrocardiogram

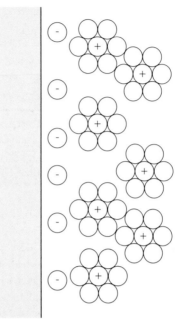

Figure 2.6 Double layer; the positive ions in solution are shown surrounded by water molecules.

(ECG), electroencephalogram (EEG), electromyogram (EMG) and others, result from the flow of these ionic currents. By contrast, in monitoring equipment, the flow of electric current comprises the movement of electrons through solid materials such as metallic conductors and nonmetallic semiconductors. An electrode is used to convert the ionic currents in the body into electronic currents which can be amplified, processed and displayed. The half cell potential of the electrode is usually many times greater than the potential to be measured, which may be a source of artefact in the measurement.

Electrodes possess a property known as *polarization resistance*, which is the change in voltage across the electrode produced by a specific change in current flowing through it. The change in voltage results from a change in thickness of the double layer. If the polarization resistance is high, the change in thickness of the double layer as current flows is greater than if the polarization resistance is low. Electrodes that are particularly suitable for monitoring the small potentials (Fig. 2.7), which comprise biopotentials, have a low polarization resistance. This avoids the signal being obsured by changes in the polarization voltage. These changes occur when the thickness of the double layer alters due to current flow or to displacement of charges in the layer when the electrode moves relative to the solution with which it is in contact.

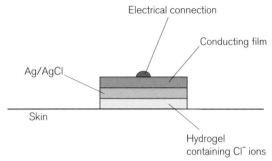

Figure 2.7 Sequence of layers in a typical silver, silver chloride ECG electrode, an example of a system exhibiting low polarization resistance.

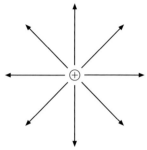

Figure 2.8 Representation of the electric field produced by a positive charge; the arrows show the direction of the force that would be experienced by another positive charge.

THERMISTORS

Thermistors are resistors, the resistance of which changes with temperature. Two types are available: those in which the temperature change is positive as temperature increases and those in which it is negative. Thermistors may be used for temperature measurement.

ELECTRIC AND MAGNETIC FIELDS

The term *field* is used to describe how a physical quantity varies with position; i.e. a particular physical quantity has a definite value throughout a region of interest and this value may vary with position. Static electric charges produce an *electric field* (Fig. 2.8). Moving electric charges produce an additional field of a different kind, known as the *magnetic field*.

Electric current and magnetism are linked. An electric current results in a magnetic field, and a changing magnetic field induces an electric current in any conductor present in the field. The latter principle, known as electromagnetic induction, is the basis of electricity generators, used, for example, to generate the mains electricity supply.

Electromagnetic field and electromagnetic radiation

An alternating current produces changing electric and magnetic fields, changes which move outwards from the conductor carrying the current with a characteristic speed. The combination of the two fields is known as the *electromagnetic field* and the changing field is known as *electromagnetic radiation*. The speed of propagation of this field is the speed of light, light itself being electromagnetic radiation of a particular range of wavelengths.

Electromagnetic induction

The phenomena of displacement currents, mutual inductance and electromagnetic induction can result in a current in one conductor producing a current in another conductor. Although this phenomenon has practical applications, it can also interfere with the monitoring of biological potentials. The magnitude of both electric and magnetic fields decreases as the distance from the current producing them increases, so moving sensitive equipment away from possible sources of interference should reduce the amount of this interference.

The magnitude of the current induced in an electric circuit by a magnetic field is proportional to the area of the circuit perpendicular to the field and to the rate of change of the magnetic field. Thus high frequency fields, such as those produced by electrosurgical equipment, are likely to be an important source of interference. The interference can be reduced by decreasing the area of the loop, ensuring that ECG leads are closer together, for example.

ELECTRONICS AND CONTROL SYSTEMS

Electronics in any more than the broadest of terms is outside the scope of this book. However, some basic points will be elucidated so that the terms used in this book and when discussing modern medical equipment may be understood.

Analogue and digital electronics

Almost every area of medical technology incorporates modern electronic techniques. The reason for this is that logic and computing power of great complexity and reliability is now feasible and economical. Electronic techniques may be subdivided into two broad groupings, namely *analogue* and *digital*, both of which are employed in most equipment.

In analogue circuits, the values of current and voltage are continuously variable; in digital circuits, these values are limited to discrete steps, the total number of which is usually a power of two. The reason for the use of digital circuits and for their dependence on the power of two arises from the fact that it is comparatively easy to store a value of voltage or current as on or off, but much more difficult to store an exact value for any length of time. It is also easier and more accurate to perform arithmetic and logic functions with discrete values than it is with continuously variable values. The resolution of a voltage that takes only the values zero and one is poor, but by the use of many such circuits, the resolution can be improved. With ten such circuits, for example, 2^{10} different integers, i.e. any integer between 0 and 1,023, can be stored, and the resolution improves to better than 0.1%.

Whereas the numbering system that uses the ten digits 0 to 9 is known as the decimal system of arithmetic, the numbering system that uses only the digits 0 and 1 is known as the binary system. The conversion of numbers between the decimal and binary systems is illustrated in Table 2.1. The word *bit* is an abbreviation of binary digit.

Table 2.1								
	Binary							
	MSB							**LSB**
Decimal	2^7	2^6	2^5	2^4	2^3	2^2	2^1	2^0
0	0	0	0	0	0	0	0	0
1	0	0	0	0	0	0	0	1
2	0	0	0	0	0	0	1	0
3	0	0	0	0	0	0	1	1
4	0	0	0	0	0	1	0	0
5	0	0	0	0	0	1	0	1
6	0	0	0	0	0	1	1	0
7	0	0	0	0	0	1	1	1
8	0	0	0	0	1	0	0	0
9	0	0	0	0	1	0	0	1
10	0	0	0	0	1	0	1	0
200	1	1	0	0	1	0	0	0
255	1	1	1	1	1	1	1	1

MSB = Most significant bit
LSB = Least significant bit

Almost all modern electronic instrumentation and control systems use a combination of analogue and digital circuits. The inputs to electronic processing systems are usually analogue voltages. They may be biopotentials such as the ECG or EEG, or a voltage generated by a transducer. An analogue signal is converted into digital form using a circuit known as an *analogue to digital converter* (ADC), which converts an analogue input into the nearest discrete value. The performance of an ADC is determined in part by the number of output bits it generates. A 12 bit ADC, for example, produces a number between 0 and $2^{12} - 1$, i.e. 4095, so its full-scale resolution is approximately 0.025%. A *digital to analogue converter* (DAC) has the reverse function of converting a signal in a digital form into an analogue form.

Microprocessor systems

Microprocessors used in electromedical equipment use similar technology and techniques to personal computers. Several different integrated circuits are used to perform various functions within the complete microprocessor system. The central processing unit (CPU) carries out mathematical and logic functions but requires other circuits to perform additional functions. Input and output (I/O) circuits provide the interface between the microprocessor and external functions. The CPU cannot carry out any functions without a program or software which may be held in *read only memory* (ROM). The contents of ROM cannot be altered by the microprocessor and are retained when power is removed from the system. In much electromedical equipment, software upgrades are normally performed by changing the module that contains the software.

Microprocessors also use memory that can be altered by the CPU. It is said to be volatile because this form of memory, *random access memory* (RAM), is cleared by the disconnection of the power supply. It is used by the CPU for temporarily storing data and for making calculations.

As microprocessor systems use the binary numbering system, it is necessary to use multiple connections between each of the integrated circuits (ICs), and these connections are usually referred to as *buses*. There are three buses in a microprocessor system: a *data bus* which carries the actual data being manipulated, an *address bus* which carries the addresses of the data stored in the memories, and a *control bus* which, as the name implies, carries the control and timing signals. Synchronism is maintained by a crystal controlled clock or oscillator.

Because of the complexity of the interconnections involved in modern electronics, extensive use is made of printed circuits (Fig. 2.9). Once the printed circuit has been designed it has the advantage of ease of economic manufacture without wiring errors and also with high reliability.

Control systems

The term *control system* may be used when the control of anything is more complicated than, for example, the direct manual manipulation of a valve to control gas flow. A simple example of a control system would comprise a control loop consisting of an actuator which operates on a valve, a transducer which senses the flow and an electronic module which generates a feedback signal from the transducer to the actuator (Fig. 2.10). Such systems are found in ventilators, for example. This seemingly complex system is arranged so that any change in pressure which would cause an alteration in flow may be rapidly

and automatically corrected. A separate input, which may be either manual or from some other part of a larger system, may be arranged to alter the value of the required flow.

Transducers

A transducer is a device that converts one form of energy into another. Most transducers convert an input to an electrical signal, which then undergoes further processing for use to display or record some measurement or to form part of a control system. Many different physical, and in some cases chemical, properties are used in transducers; individual transducers will be discussed in the relevant chapters.

Displays

It is now common practice to use various forms of electronic display in anaesthetic delivery machines to indicate gas flow, gas and vapour concentrations, ventilator

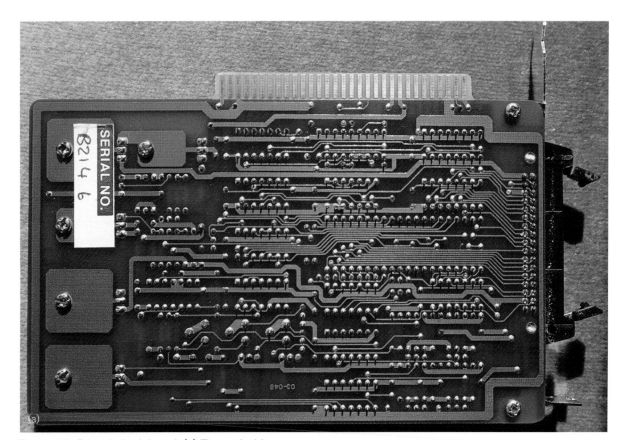

Figure 2.9 Printed circuit board. **(a)** The track side.

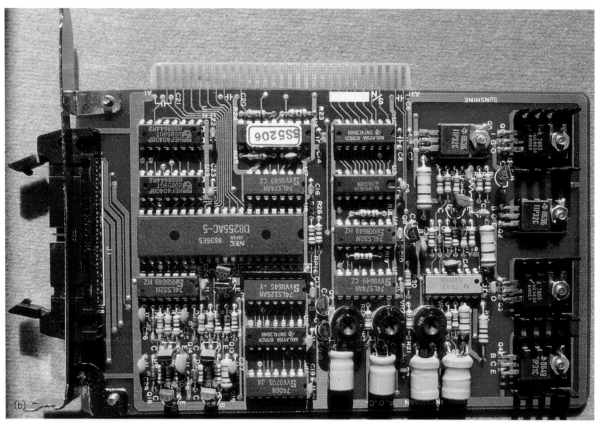

Figure 2.9, cont'd Printed circuit board. **(b)** the component side. Note there are conductive tracks on both sides of the board. The components may be conventionally attached to the board by passing their leads through holes in the board and then soldering the connection to make it permanent. Surface mount components are now also used that have shorter connections which are soldered to the same surface of the board as the component is mounted.

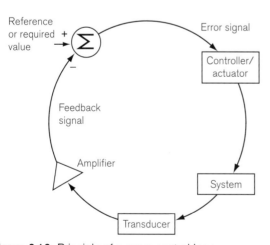

Figure 2.10 Principle of a servo control loop.

parameters, and the safety status of the machine. These displays use various forms *of optoelectronic* technology. Optoelectronic displays of simple alphanumerical data may use light-emitting diode (LED) displays or liquid crystal displays (LCD). More complex displays including graphical representations of dynamic pressure and flow require some form of picture display, which may be provided by a cathode ray tube (CRT) or thin film transistor (TFT) display, the latter being a type of LCD display engineered to produce better performance than the simple LCD display.

Fuzzy logic

In many logical situations, there are just two conditions: on/off, go/no-go, one/zero, yes/no. There are, however, several situations where things are not so clear-cut: for example, at what point is an arterial blood pressure considered as being hypertensive?

Consider a collection of diastolic arterial blood pressure measurements. These can be assigned to two groups (called sets) such as normal (up to 80 mmHg) or abnormal (above 80 mmHg). Using classical logic (Fig. 2.11a), each value belongs in one group only. This logic becomes unreasonable when 80 mmHg is interpreted as normal but 81 mmHg is abnormal (a difference of only 1 mmHg). If the data is now divided into two 'fuzzy sets' (Fig. 2.11b) where the ordinate (vertical axis on the graph) indicates the relative membership of the group as a percentage, then there is an area of overlap. A given diastolic reading (e.g. 85 mmHg) will belong in two groups, 75% in the normotensive group and 25% in the hypertensive group. This information can be incorporated into computer programming where an automated

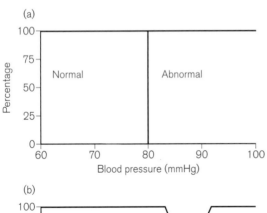

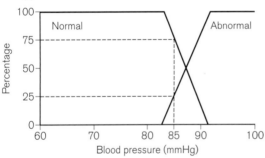

Figure 2.11 Examples of logic sets. **(a)** Subdivision of blood pressure into two groups using classical logic. **(b)** Subdivision of blood pressures into two groups using fuzzy logic.

response is required. For example, consider an inotrope used to control blood pressure in an automated system. With separation into classical sets, if the pressure were either 1 or 50 mmHg above a preset limit, the system would switch off. When the pressure dropped below that limit the system would switch back on at the same delivery rate. The pressures would fluctuate greatly. With 'fuzzy logic sets' the system would adjust according to the degree (%) of change outside a given value. This has been shown to provide much closer control.

Neural computing

The origins of neural computing date back to the 1940s but have been overshadowed by advances in conventional computing, especially with the advent of extremely large-scale integrated circuits. Neural computing is now rapidly expanding but must not be considered as competitive but rather as complementary to conventional digital computing. The main difference between conventional and neural computing is that conventional computers have to be explicitly programmed, whereas neural computers adapt themselves during a period of training based upon examples with solutions presented to them. Neural computing is so called because the basic unit of the system is similar in function to a neurone (Fig 2.12a). During the training period the weight applied to any input is adjusted to vary the strength of any particular input to the neurone where the decision is made. Neural networks (Fig. 2.12) are set up to form a neural computer.

Neural computing has a special role to play in areas of signal processing and data handling involving pattern recognition, for example, in the automatic analysis of the electrocardiogram and electroencephalogram.

ELECTROMAGNETIC COMPATIBILITY

Electrical interference that may affect electromedical equipment is generally of two types: *conducted emissions* that reach the equipment through conductors such as those providing mains power, and *radiated emissions* that reach the equipment through propagated electromagnetic fields. Conducted interference can be reduced by improving the local quality of the mains electricity supply or by removing interference by electronic means. Radiated interference is more difficult to eliminate in the usual hospital environment.

Electronic equipment may, intentionally or otherwise, emit electromagnetic radiation. When this radiation

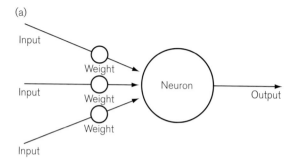

(a)

Input

Weight

Neuron

Input

Weight

Weight

Input

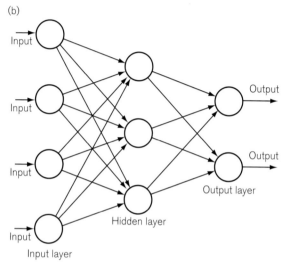

(b)

Input

Input

Input

Output layer

Input

Hidden layer

Input

Input layer

Figure 2.12 Neural networks. **(a)** The structure and function of a single neurone, **(b)** a typical three layer neural network.

interferes with the correct operation of other equipment, it is known as *electromagnetic interference* (EMI). Such interference is capable of causing malfunction of electro-medical equipment, which may be life threatening in such cases as infusion pumps or ventilators. The effect of EMI on a patient monitor might be to produce artefacts in the display, but its effect on an infusion pump might be to alter the contents of the electronic memory holding the infusion rate.

The likelihood of EMI is a function of the strength of the electromagnetic field generated. Communication equipment devices used in hospitals thus have the potential to interfere with the operation of electromedical equipment. These devices, in decreasing order of field strength (and decreasing likelihood of causing EMI) include emergency services (e.g. police and ambulance) radio handsets, security radio handsets as used by portering staff, mobile phones (cellphones) and cordless phones.

Although there are standards that specify the intensity of electromagnetic field that should have no effect on various types of electromedical equipment, communication equipment of all types should not be allowed to come within several metres of medical devices, particularly life support equipment. Users may not realize that cellphones, whilst switched on, emit pulses intermittently, even when they are not being used. It is also helpful to remember that the electromagnetic field generated (e.g. by a cellphone) decreases by an inverse square law as the distance between the telephone and the equipment increases, although reflection within closed spaces such as rooms may diminish the effect of this law.

THE ELECTROMAGNETIC SPECTRUM

Radio waves, heat, light and X-rays are all types of electromagnetic radiation and all travel with the same velocity of 3×10^8 m s^{-1} in a vacuum. The various subdivisions of the spectrum have different properties and different methods of generation, absorption and detection, but may be described by wavelength (λ), wavenumber ($1/\lambda$), frequency (v) or photon energy (hv) (Fig. 2.13). A basic grasp of the electromagnetic spectrum helps the anaesthetist to understand the principles behind the various forms of gas analysis, pulse oximetry and other monitoring techniques as well as those of surgical diathermy, radiology and nuclear medicine with which he or she is likely to come in contact during the course of the working day.

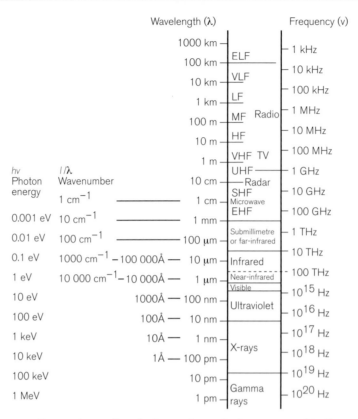

Figure 2.13 The electromagnetic spectrum. eV = electron volt, a unit of energy equal to the work done by an electron accelerated through a potential difference of one volt. Å = angstrom, a unit of length equal to 10^{-8} cm or 10^{-10} m or 0.1 nm. The ground state diameter of a hydrogen atom is about 1 Å.

FURTHER READING

Asbury A J, Tzabar Y (1995) Fuzzy logic: new ways of thinking in anaesthesia. (*Editorial*) British Journal of Anaesthesia 75(1):1–2

Gookin D, Rathbone A (1997) *PCs for Dummies*, 5th edn. New York: Hungry Minds

Horowitz P, Hill W (1989) *The Art of Electronics*, 2nd edn. Cambridge: Cambridge University Press.

Medical Devices Agency (1997) Safety Notice MDA SN 9706 *Mobile Communications: Interference with Medical Devices.* London: Medical Devices Agency.

Medical Devices Agency (2001) Safety Notice SN 2001(06)

Update on Electromagnetic Compatibility of Medical Devices with Mobile Communications: TETRA (Terrestrial Trunked Radio System) and Outside media broadcasts from hospital premises. London: Medical Devices Agency.

Nickalls RWD, Ramasubramanian R (1995) *Interfacing the IBM PC to Medical Equipment.* Cambridge: Cambridge University Press.

Sinclair I (2002) *Electronics Made Simple*, 2nd edn. Oxford: Newnes.

Walters G (2000) *The Essential Guide to Computing.* New Jersey: Prentice Hall.

3

The supply of anaesthetic and other medical gases

Hubert Bland

Medical gases are classified as medicinal products by the Medicines Act 1968 (UK) and more latterly by the European legislation EC 2001/83. This recent legislation requires that the manufacture of medical gases is covered by a Manufacturer's Licence and the marketing and sales are covered by a Marketing Authorisation (previously known as a Product Licence). In the UK, the Medicines and Healthcare products Regulatory Agency (MHRA) issues these licences. Similar legislation exists in most countries, but not all.

Medical gases are an important part of everyday clinical practice. From the discovery and application of oxygen and nitrous oxide to the more recent development of the use of nitric oxide and heliox, the principles of 'first do no harm' have remained constant.

Supplying a pharmaceutical in a highly pressurized metal cylinder, which is returned to the manufacturer for refilling, remains a unique concept in drug delivery. However, manufacturing, packaging, delivery and application are now advancing rapidly.

During the next 10 years, the clinician can expect to see new gases such as Heliox, xenon and carbogen in common use on the ward and in theatre. The use of xenon, a gas possibly offering neuroprotection, will increase in anaesthesia. With this will come the challenges of ventilating with a gas approximately five times more dense than air.

Advances in the manufacturing of gases and materials have been significant in the last 20 years. Extensive and detailed regulatory documentation exists and is referred to throughout this chapter.

Medical gases for use in anaesthesia and critical care are generally supplied either in bulk (oxygen and Synthetic Medical Air) or in cylinders on manifolds: nitrous oxide, medical air, Entonox and in some hospitals, Heliox. In both cases gases are then delivered through a pipeline system to wall or pendant outlets. However, there are some situations such as emergency back-up supplies, patient transfer and where pipelines are not available, when gases must be provided directly from cylinders.

Oxygen can also be supplied by means of an oxygen concentrator, although this would only be considered for military purposes, or where a bulk supply is not available due to geographical constraints.

PROPERTIES OF MEDICAL GASES

The properties of some of the common medical gases are summarized in Table 3.1. The newer gases and possible new therapeutic directions are briefly discussed below.

Details of carbogen (5% CO_2 + 95% O_2), lung function gases, medical gas for laser surgery, and other gases not listed here, are available from the manufacturers. Extensive information on the properties of all gases can be obtained from the BOC Special Gases website *www.bocspecialgases.co.uk*. Data sheets containing detailed up-to-date product information on medical gases are available at *www.bocmedical.com*.

Heliox

Heliox is a mixture of oxygen and helium. Currently this gas has regulatory approval for 21% O_2 and 79% helium premixed, in the UK, as Heliox21. Heliox is licensed for the treatment of respiratory obstruction and, although traditionally this has been confined to emergency use, it is increasingly used in many departments in the hospital and in the emergency services.

The heliox gas mixture is less dense than air (which is sometimes termed nitrox for comparison) and for this reason it behaves differently when used with anaesthetic and respiratory equipment. Its behaviour is governed by an altered flow pattern related to the alterations in turbulent and laminar flow and Reynolds number, and also its thermal conductivity which affects measurement devices. If administered from standard air or oxygen flowmeters, flow readings will need to have a conversion factor applied. Appropriate conversion tables are available from the manufacturer. Flow/volume measurements on ventilators are similarly affected, hence only readings from machines designed for ventilation with helium mixtures can be assumed to be accurate.

Xenon

It should be noted that this gas is around five times denser than air. Ventilation is only possible with equipment specifically designed for use with xenon. It is not a standard medical product, being provided as a 'special' gas. It is filled to a lower pressure than oxygen and heliox, and consequently should be used with compatible low-pressure regulators. Its density will slow down its flow through narrow tubes, including standard flowmeters. A conversion factor of 0.468 should be applied. Until a licence is granted for its use in anaesthesia or other applications, special care should be taken in the use and administration of this gas. Xenon exhibits anaesthetic and neuroprotective activity and its use by anaesthetists will doubtlessly increase over the next 10 years.

Nitric oxide

A toxic gas when given in high concentrations, this gas is used extensively in the intensive care environment in very low concentrations as a pulmonary vasodilator. It is administered with specialized, compatible equipment. It is being investigated as an immunomodulator, in platelet function alteration and for domiciliary use.

Carbon monoxide

Carbon monoxide is being investigated in a number of therapeutic areas (anti-inflammatory, vasodilatory, cytoprotective potential, and optimization of organ transplantation). No chromium-plated equipment should be used in conjunction with CO because there is a risk of formation of highly toxic chromium containing compounds.

MEDICAL GAS CYLINDERS

Gas cylinders produced today can be manufactured from a range of materials. Historically all medical cylinders were produced from low-carbon steel, whilst more recently lighter, stronger, molybdenum steel cylinders have been introduced, allowing cylinders to be filled to higher pressures, up to 300 bar(g) ((g) *denotes gauge pressure; see Chapter 4*).

In areas where portability is not an issue; such as on cylinder manifolds where cylinders can be easily moved on trolleys or where cylinders are filled with liquid gases and weight is less of an issue, then these older types of cylinders are perfectly adequate.

In some applications, such as use of anaesthetic machines in MRI locations, it is not possible to use conventional steel cylinders as the steel in the cylinders would be attracted to the magnetic field and would damage the unit. Pin index aluminium cylinders are available for this application, but it is recommended that where possible, gases should be piped into the unit from outside.

Where portability is a requirement, the demand is for lighter, easier to use cylinders. Recently introduced *composite cylinders* are defined as cylinders having two or more different materials; commonly known as '*hoop wrap*' cylinders they are manufactured from either lightweight steel or aluminium liners and are then strengthened by

Table 3.1 Physical properties of common pressurized gases

	Oxygen	Nitrous oxide	Carbon dioxide	Xenon	Nitric oxide	Carbon monoxide	Helium
Physical state in cylinder	Gas	liquid	liquid	Gas	Gas	Gas	Gas
Molecular weight	32	44	44	131	30	28	4 (He)
Melting point (°C)	N/A	−90.81	−56.6	−112	−164	−205	na
Boiling point (°C)	−183	−88.5	−78.5 *	−108	−152	−192	−269
Critical temperature (°C)	−118.4	36.4	30	16.6	−93	−140	−268
Relative density, gas (air=1)	1.04	1.5	1.52	4.5	1	1	0.14
Relative density, liquid (water=1)	N/A	1.2	0.82	N/A	1.3	N/A	N/A
Vapour pressure at 20°C (bar)	N/A	50.8	57.3	N/A	N/A	N/A	N/A
Solubility water (mg/ml)	N/A	2.2	2000	644	67	30	1.5
Appearance/Colour	Colourless	Colourless gas	Colourless gas	Colourless gas	Colourless gas	Colourless gas	Colourless gas
Odour	None	Sweetish	None	None	Pungent	None	None
Other data		Gas/vapour heavier than air. May accumulate in confined spaces, particularly at or below ground level	Gas/vapour heavier than air. May accumulate in confined spaces, particularly at or below ground level	Gas/vapour heavier than air. May accumulate in confined spaces, particularly at or below ground level. Note that due its density, Xe will flow through standard flowmeters more slowly. A conversion factor of 0.468 should be applied	Currently supplied in N₂ at less than 1000 ppm	Currently only supplied at mixtures of less than 0.3% in air and helium	Use the appropriate conversion chart when using oxygen flowmeters

N/A, not applicable
* Sublimation
Note: all values STP.
Mixed gases, e.g. Heliox, will have different physical properties. For exact values, please contact the manufacturer.

wrapping an Aramid material (Kevlar or Carbon Fibre) in an epoxy resin along the parallel portion of the cylinder. This gives the cylinder enormous strength whilst reducing weight. They can also be filled to high pressures, up to 300 bar(g).

Cylinder sizes

Technically, cylinders are defined by their water capacity and range between 1.2 litres to 47.2 litres and are identified by a size code ranging from C size to J size. Tables 3.2 to 3.7 give details for oxygen, nitrous oxide, Entonox, carbon dioxide, Heliox21, xenon, nitric oxide and carbon monoxide cylinders. The water capacity of the various cylinder sizes is given in Table 3.2.

Cylinder filling and maintenance

Most gases are stored in cylinders as compressed gases such as oxygen, medical air, helium and heliox. Gases such as nitrous oxide and carbon dioxide are liquefied under pressure. The liquid is in equilibrium with the gas and the pressure is dependent on the temperature. These gases are filled by weight to ensure they are not overfilled. The tare weight (weight when empty) of the cylinder is subtracted from the target total weight when full. This "fill ratio" is critical. If there were an insufficient gas space in the cylinder when full, a comparatively small increase in temperature would cause a significant increase in pressure and could, in an extreme situation, cause the cylinder to rupture.

Table 3.2 Relative sizes and specifications of commonly used oxygen cylinders

Cylinder Size	C	CD/DD	D	E	F	HX	G	J	ZX
Nominal cylinder pressure at 15°C (bar)	137	230	137	137	137	230	137	137	300
Valve type	Pin index	Integral	Pin index	Pin index	Bull nose	Integral	Bull nose	Side spindle Pin index	Integral
Contents (litres)	170	460	340	680	1360	2300	3400	6800	3970
Water capacity (litres)	1.2	2	2.32	4.68	9.43	10	23.6	47.2	10
Dimensions (mm)	430×189	520×100	535×102	865×102	930×140	940×140	940×140	1320×178	1520×229	940×143
Empty weight (kg)	2.0	3.0	3.4	5.4	14.5	15	34.5	68.9	10

Table 3.3 Relative sizes and specifications of commonly used nitrous oxide cylinders

Cylinder Size	C	D	E	F	G	J
Nominal cylinder pressure at 15°C (bar)	44	44	44	44	44	44
Valve type	Pin index	Pin index	Pin index	Handwheel 11/16" × 20 tpi	Handwheel 11/16" × 20 tpi	Handwheel 11/16" × 20 tpi
Contents (litres)	450	900	1800	3600	9000	18000
Dimensions (mm)	430×189	535×102	865×102	930×140	1320×178	1520×229
Empty weight	2.0	3.4	5.4	14.5	34.5	68.9

Table 3.4 Relative sizes and specifications of commonly used Entonox cylinders

Cylinder Size	D	CD	ZD	F	HX	G	ZX
Nominal cylinder pressure at 15°C (bar)	137	137	260	137	137	137	260
Valve type	Pin index	Integral	Integral	Side spindle pin index	Integral	Side spindle pin index	Integral
Contents (litres)	500	440	794	2000	2200	5000	3970
Dimensions (mm)	535×102	520×100	465×90	930×140	940×140	1320×178	940×143
Empty weight (kg)	3.4	2.7	3.1	14.5	15.5	34.5	10

Entonox, a mixture of 50% oxygen and 50% nitrous oxide exists as a gas. The pseudo critical temperature of Entonox in pipelines at 4.1 bar is below −30°C. Nitrous oxide in an Entonox cylinder however begins to separate out from Entonox if the temperature falls below −6°C. A homogenous mixture is again obtained when the temperature is raised above 10°C and the cylinder is agitated.

Table 3.5 Relative sizes and specifications of commonly used carbon dioxide cylinders

Cylinder Size	C	E	VF	LF
Nominal cylinder pressure at 15°C (bar)	50	50	50	50
Valve type	Pin index	Pin index	Handwheel 0.86" × 14 tpi	Handwheel 0.86" × 14 tpi
Contents (litres)	450	1800	3600	3600
Dimensions (mm)	430×89	865×102	930×140	930×140
Empty weight (kg)	2.0	5.4	14.5	14.5

Table 3.6 Relative sizes and specifications of commonly used Heliox21 cylinders

Cylinder Size	F	HX
Nominal cylinder pressure at 15°C (bar)	137	200
Valve type	Bullnose	Integral
Contents (litres)	1200	1780
Dimensions (mm)	930×140	940×140
Empty weight (kg)	14.5	15.5

Cylinders of nitrous oxide and carbon dioxide should always be used in the vertical position with the outlet uppermost to prevent liquefied gas from being vented from the valve and causing possible injury in the form of a freeze burn or damage to any associated equipment.

Some applications require carbon dioxide in liquid form. This is supplied using cylinders fitted with a 'dip tube' connected to the cylinder valve, which allows liquid from the bottom of the cylinder to be drawn up through the valve (Fig. 3.1). These cylinders, supplied in F size and known as LF, have a white stripe down the length of the cylinder body. For other CO_2 applications where vapour is required, VF cylinders should be used. It is important to ensure that the correct cylinder is used to prevent damage to equipment.

Table 3.7 Relative sizes and specifications of commonly used xenon, nitric oxide and carbon monoxide cylinders

	Xenon	**Nitric oxide**	**Carbon monoxide**
Cylinder size	No medical standard size currently available	Various – depending on manufacturer	No standard cylinder size currently available for medical use – provided as a special gas
Nominal cylinder pressure at 15°C (bar)	Filled to low pressures of around 30 bar	Filled to a lower pressure than standard medical gas cylinders (around 30 bar)	Relatively low pressure fill – currently available between 8 and 36 bar
Valve type	Low pressure regulator required	Special equipment needed	Note: Will require low pressure compatible regulators

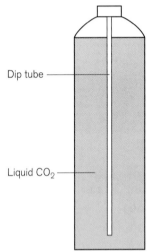

Dip tube

Liquid CO_2

Figure 3.1 LF type CO_2 cylinder with dip tube for delivering liquid CO_2.

When a high flowrate is drawn from small nitrous oxide or carbon dioxide cylinders up to size F, the temperature of the liquid drops and can result in a significant pressure drop which may in turn result in poor performance when using equipment such as a cryogenic probe. To ensure equipment performs correctly the user should consider alternating cylinders. A good indicator of this pheno-menon is the appearance of water vapour condensing on the outer surface of the cylinder, which can freeze.

Checking for cylinder contents falls into two categories. Compressed gases such as oxygen, medical air, helium, Heliox and Entonox (which, although 50% of it's contents are nitrous oxide, remains as a gas in the cylinder under normal ambient temperatures) can be checked by use of a pressure gauge, as the pressure is directly proportionate to the volume. However, the content of cylinders containing nitrous oxide and carbon dioxide can only be determined by weight, as the pressure in the cylinder will remain constant until all the liquid is exhausted and only then will the pressure fall. Subtracting the tare weight (stamped on the neck of the cylinder) from the total weight will give an estimate of contents.

Cylinder identification

The correct method of identifying the contents of a cylinder is to read the label on the cylinder. It is often assumed that the colour of the cylinder or the type of valve fitted indicates the gas inside it. The label (Fig. 3.2) contains all the key information for the user:

- The product name, chemical symbol and pharma-ceutical form of the product;
- The product specification;
- Hazard warning diamonds;
- Product licence number;
- Cylinder contents in litres;
- Maximum cylinder pressure;
- Cylinder size code;
- Directions for use and information for storage and handling.

The cylinder label also has a unique batch label (Fig. 3.3), which contains: the batch number; fill and expiry date; and the size and type of gas. This label is fitted every time the cylinder is filled. It has two important purposes: (a) to provide vital information for a batch recall should the cylinder be involved in an incident; and (b) to provide information for proper cylinder rotation.

Cylinder testing

All cylinders must undergo hydraulic testing and internal inspection at regular intervals, to ensure they remain safe

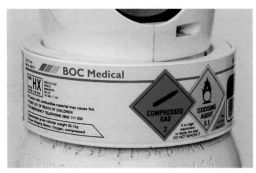

Figure 3.2 Cylinder label.

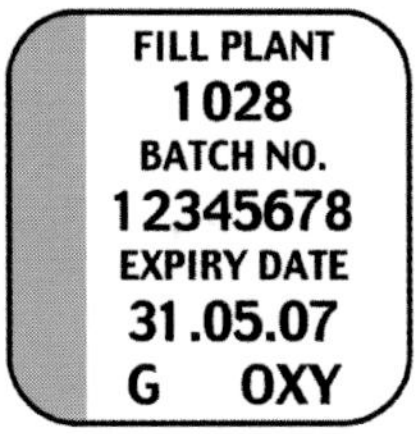

> **FILL PLANT**
> **1 028**
> **BATCH NO.**
> **1 2345678**
> **EXPIRY DATE**
> **31 .05.07**
> **G   OXY**

Figure 3.3 Batch label.

to use. The test is carried out every 10 years for steel cylinders and every 5 years for composite cylinders. A shaped, colour coded plastic ring around the cylinder neck indicates when the next test date is due. Cylinders can last many years and tend to be withdrawn due to new technology rather than deterioration.

Colour coding

Medical cylinders in the UK conform to colour codes specified in ISO 32 and BS EN 1089. The colours relate to the shoulder of the cylinder only. Figure 3.4 shows the colour codes for medical gas cylinders in the UK.

Cylinder valves

Medical cylinder valves can generally be categorized as follows:
- Pin Index and Side Spindle Pin Index valves;
- Bull Nose valves;
- Handwheel valves;
- Integral valves.

Pin Index System

Pin index valves are fitted to small cylinders and are commonly connected directly to medical equipment such as anaesthetic machines (Fig. 3.5).

Side spindle pin index valves (Fig. 3.6) are fitted to large cylinders of medical oxygen, medical air and Entonox for pipeline manifolds and to F size Entonox cylinders.

Both types of pin index valves conform to ISO 407 and adopt an index system which incorporates a combination of holes positioned to correspond to pins located on the equipment, making it impossible to connect the cylinder to a different gas connection. Figure 3.5 shows the different pin positions. The pin index system also prevents filling with incorrect gas, as the gas suppliers use the same non-interchangeable filling connections.

Pin index cylinders require a seal between the face of the cylinder valve outlet and the equipment to which it is fitted. The seal, known as a 'Bodok' washer (Figs 3.7 and 3.8), is a bonded seal and is manufactured from a non-combustible material. As with any sealing joint where high-pressure cylinders, especially oxygen, are concerned, they must be kept clean and in good condition and should never become contaminated with oil or grease. If a gas tight seal cannot be achieved by moderate tightening of the screw clamp, it is recommended that the seal be changed. Never use excessive force.

Bull Nose valve

This type of valve (Fig. 3.9) is fitted to F and G size cylinders including medical oxygen, medical air, helium, and mixed gases such as Carbogen and some Heliox cylinders. The valve is spindle operated and has a 5/8-inch female outlet thread into which a regulator is fitted. The spindle mechanism is assembled in two parts to reduce wear to the nylon seat and to ensure a gas tight seal without the use of excessive force.

All bullnose valves are fitted with an MPR (minimum pressure retention) device, to ensure that a positive pressure of approximately 2 bar is retained in the cylinder to prevent the ingress of moisture (Fig. 3.10). When connecting regulator equipment to the valve, the user should always adopt the proper connecting procedure. Ensure the 'O' ring (Fig. 3.11) fitted to the regulator is in good condition and hand tighten the regulator only. Once fitted, open the spindle valve slowly, to prevent gas surge, at least one full turn and note the position of the regulator gauge needle. A simple test for leaks can be carried out by closing the cylinder spindle valve and noting any drop in pressure shown on the gauge. If a leak does exist, spraying the joints with a leak detection spray will identify it. If a leak is evident at the valve outlet, replace the 'O' ring and repeat the procedure. If the leak persists, fit a replacement regulator. When changing an empty cylinder, close

Gas	Identification markings on cylinder shoulder		BOC product information leaflets[†]
Oxygen		White	MED/004041
Nitrous oxide		Blue	MED/004040
Entonox (50% N_2O/50% O_2)		Blue/white	MED/004042
Air		Black/white	MED/004038
Oxygen/carbon dioxide mixture (95% O_2/5% CO_2)		Grey/white	MED/004035
Helium/oxygen mixture (79% He/21% O_2)		Brown/white	MED/004034
Carbon dioxide	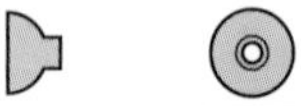	Grey	MED/004039
Helium		Brown	MED/004037

* Note: Cylinder identification colours are those specified in ISO 32 (1977) and BS EN 1089-3 : 2004
† Up-to-date product information leaflets can be downloaded from www.bocmedical.com

Figure 3.4 Cylinder colour codes.

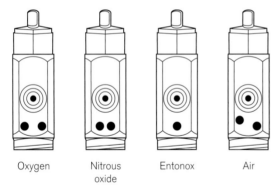

Oxygen   Nitrous oxide   Entonox   Air

Figure 3.5 Pin Index valves.

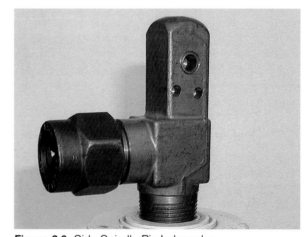

Figure 3.6 Side Spindle Pin Index valve.

the valve spindle and purge the regulator before attempting to remove it.

Handwheel valves

Large nitrous oxide cylinders for use on cylinder manifolds and carbon dioxide cylinders of size F and G are fitted with handwheel valves which are surrounded by a protective guard (Fig. 3.12), and which have a gas specific, side outlet, male thread.

Integral valves

The introduction of integral valves (Fig. 3.13) has revolutionized the industry by removing the need for

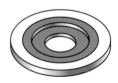

Figure 3.7 Bodok washer.

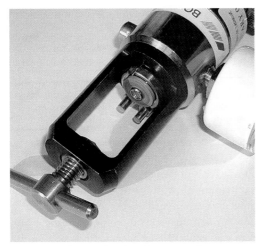

Figure 3.8 Bodok washer fitted to a regulator.

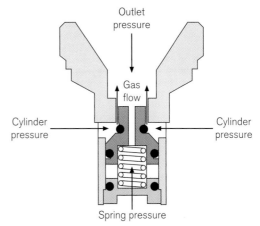

Figure 3.10 Schematic showing MPR device.

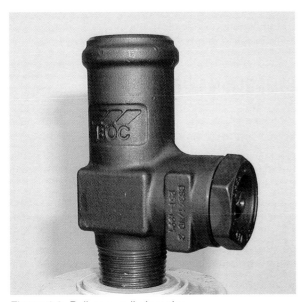

Figure 3.9 Bull nose cylinder valve.

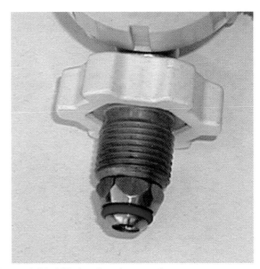

Figure 3.11 'O' ring fitted to regulator.

connecting a regulator. This has greatly improved safety and eliminated the need for regulator maintenance by hospitals. Because it has its own built-in regulator, it can be filled to a much higher pressures as no lower-pressure rated equipment can be fitted to it.

Some integral valves have a combination of a clickstop flowmeter giving 0 to 15 lpm in stepped increments and a female BS Schraeder connection at 4 bar(g) to provide a power source for driving equipment. This type of valve is currently fitted to cylinders up to 10 litres water capacity. Care must be taken with these valves to ensure that the valve is not left between click stops where no gas will flow.

Material compatibility

As materials burn more readily in an oxygen environment, special care is needed when determining materials used in the manufacture of equipment. The elastomer materials used in O rings, seats and seals must be resistant to burning in 100% oxygen and must not generate dangerous gases from the ignition of components. BS EN 15001 provides advice on materials which can be used safely.

Tamper evident seals

All cylinder valves are fitted with tamper evident seals when delivered. These seals are usually shrink wrapped

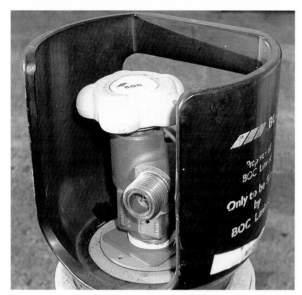

Figure 3.12 CO_2 cylinder with handwheel valve.

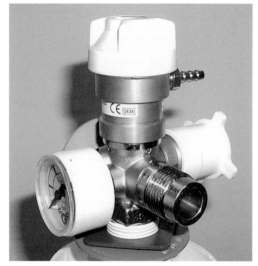

Figure 3.13 An integral valve without its guard.

around the valve or, in the case of integral valves, are in the form of a tear off. They identify cylinders as being full and should only be removed at the point of use. Bull nose valves have a protective cap, which should be replaced after use.

Storage of medical gas cylinders

Cylinders should be stored in accordance with recommendations detailed in HTM 2022. They should not be stored with non-medical cylinders. The store should:

- be under cover preferably inside and not subjected to extremes of heat;
- be kept dry clean and well ventilated;
- have good access for deliveries and a reasonably level floor surface;
- allow segregation of 'Full' and 'Empty' cylinders;
- permit separation of different gases and cylinder sizes;
- allow for strict stock rotation to enable cylinders with the oldest fill date to be used first
- be sited away from storage areas containing combustible materials or sources of heat or ignition;
- have warning notices clearly posted prohibiting smoking or naked lights in the vicinity;
- allow for large cylinders to be stored vertically in concrete pens and small cylinders to be stored horizontally in wooden or plastic racks to prevent damage to the cylinders;
- not allow the temperature to fall below 10°C where full Entonox cylinders are stored;
- be designed to prevent unauthorized entry.

CYLINDER MANIFOLDS

Few hospitals have cylinder manifolds for their main oxygen or medical air supply, but most have nitrous oxide and Entonox manifolds and whilst there are minor differences in operation for each gas, in general they are designed and operate along the same principles.

An average cylinder manifold configuration contains two equal banks of gas cylinders with a centrally located control panel, which provides a nominal output pressure of 4 bar (7 bar for surgical air). The change over from 'duty' to the 'stand-by' bank should be automatic. The installation should also contain a manually operated reserve of at least two cylinders (Fig 3.14).

The total storage capacity of the manifold should be based on one week's supply with a minimum of two days' supply on each bank and a supply of three days' spare cylinders held in the manifold room. Any additional cylinders should be held in the general medical gas store.

Table 3.8 gives nominal and usable capacities of cylinders commonly used on manifolds.

Cylinders are attached to the manifold via a copper tailpipe with a gas specific connection and seal. Each connection has a non-return valve fitted to enable single cylinders to be changed in the event of a leak or tailpipe rupture. The cylinders are held captive by individual chains to a back bar. All cylinders on both the duty and

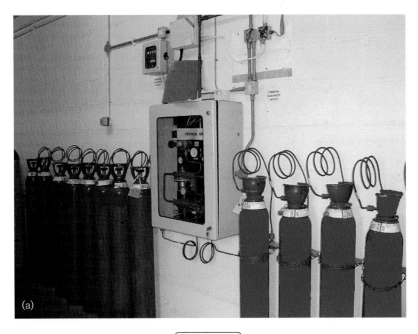

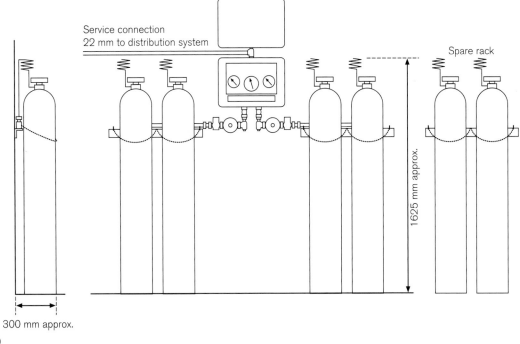

Figure 3.14 A nitrous oxide cylinder manifold **(a)**, with schematic below **(b)**.

Table 3.8 Cylinder capacities

Gas	Cylinder size	Nominal capacity	Usable capacity*
Oxygen	J	6800	6540
Nitrous oxide	G	9000	8900
Entonox	G	5000	4740
Medical air at 400kpa	J	6400	6220
Medical air at 700kpa	J	6400	5540[†]

*The usable figures are based on a residual pressure of 7 bar in the cylinders ([†]15 bar residual pressure).

stand-by bank should be fully open. The central control panel determines which is the duty bank. When this bank falls to a pressure of 8 bar, it switches to the stand-by bank and signals to the alarm panel that the duty bank is empty and the stand-by is running. The responsible person should then change the empty bank of cylinders.

If the empty bank is not changed or should a manifold fault occur, once the stand-by bank (now duty bank) pressure falls to 8 bar, then a pipeline pressure fault registers. The emergency bank should then be manually opened and the main manifold isolated via a shut-off valve, until normal conditions can be restored. The following alarm indications apply:

- a green 'normal' condition;
- a yellow 'duty bank empty, stand by running' condition;
- a yellow 'duty bank empty, stand by low' condition;
- a yellow 'emergency/reserve banks low' condition; and
- a red 'pipeline pressure fault' condition.

Nitrous oxide manifolds have heaters fitted to the supply line to prevent freezing during periods of high demand. It is common throughout mainland Europe for nitrous oxide to be supplied in bulk, although to date there are no liquid installations in the UK.

Safety precautions

The manifold room should:

- be constructed from a fireproof material, either brick or concrete;
- have ventilation to the top and bottom to allow for circulation of air;
- ideally be located to enable a delivery vehicle access to prevent manhandling cylinders long distances;
- be well lit;
- be temperature controlled at 10 to 40°C. This is especially important in the case of an Entonox manifold as nitrous oxide and oxygen can separate out at temperatures below −6°C. It is advisable to let the cylinders stand for 24 hours in a temperature of more than 10°C before fitting them to the manifold.
- contain only cylinders for use on the pipeline(s) located in the manifold room;
- not be used as a general store;
- have sufficient warning signs on the outside and inside of the building.

Only suitably trained persons should be permitted to change cylinders and an activity log should be completed when cylinders are changed.

BULK OXYGEN SUPPLY SYSTEMS

Almost all hospitals in the UK have their piped medical oxygen supplied from an on-site, bulk oxygen supply facility. The rationale for using a bulk system is driven by economics both in terms of gas cost and the removal of labour-intensive distribution associated with compressed cylinders. At 15°C, one volume of liquid oxygen gives 842 times its volume; compare this with a J size cylinder of the type used on a pipeline of 130 times its volume.

The first bulk medical oxygen system was installed in the UK in the mid-1960s and currently almost 400 hospitals have bulk medical oxygen supplied in this way. Oxygen consumption has risen steadily over the years, for a number of reasons. Historically, piped oxygen was confined to critical areas such as operating theatres and ICU's and very few wards had piped oxygen. Today, in most modern hospitals, almost every department will have piped oxygen and most wards will have some degree of piped oxygen services.

Modern operating procedures have resulted in a significant increase in immediate post-operative oxygen treatment. Ventilation techniques have also lead to a growth in oxygen consumption. An average 800-bed teaching hospital will consume around 500 million litres of oxygen in a year. It is difficult to relate to such large numbers, which is why supply companies refer to volume in hundreds of cubic metres (HCMs). So using the above example, the annual usage would be 5000 HCM. In cylinder terms it would relate to around 73 500 J sized cylinders.

Whilst the volumes appear to be enormous, the actual cost per litre is extremely low, at around 0.0008 pence per litre in the UK. As a result of the year-on-year growth, increasingly larger vessels are required, which in itself can lead to problems of location, especially at inner city hospitals where space is at a premium and safety factors may be compromised.

Since the 1960s, the recommended 'on-site' storage capacity has increased from 6 to 14 days and is now based on a risk assessment which is referred to below.

Cryogenic liquid system (CLS)

The CLS system consists of:
- an insulated cryogenic storage vessel to store the bulk liquid oxygen;
- an ambient heated vaporizer to convert the cryogenic liquid oxygen into a gas for supply to patients via a pipeline distribution system;

- a control panel to control the pressure and flow of gas to the pipeline; and
- a telemetry system.

The CLS can comprise:
- a single vessel containing operational stock with a cylinder manifold containing the secondary supply. Figure 3.15 shows a schematic of a single vessel installation.
- a main vessel containing operational stock with a second vessel either along side or remotely located containing reserve stock, and a cylinder manifold containing emergency stock. (Fig. 3.16)

A CLS should comply with recommendations in Chapter 6 of HTM 2022 and take account of the criteria laid down in the European Standard BS-EN 737-3, the British Compressed Gas Association (BCGA) Code of Practice CP 19, Rev.2, 1996 and the relevant UK legislation. HTM 2022 also contains more detailed schematics of all types of CLS installations.

The basic function of a liquid oxygen vessel is to store cryogenic oxygen at −183°C, in what is effectively a vacuum flask, the inner vessel being made from stainless steel, with an outer shell of carbon steel. Between the two vessels is a vacuum, the space being filled with a high-performance insulating material. The vessel is commonly known as a VIE (vacuum insulated evaporator).

Liquid oxygen sits in the bottom of the vessel whilst gas sits at the top at a pressure of 10.5 bar. Because it is impossible to maintain a perfect insulation, the inner container is continually trying to draw heat from the atmosphere, although the effects of this are offset by the evaporation of liquid during use. If there is no demand,

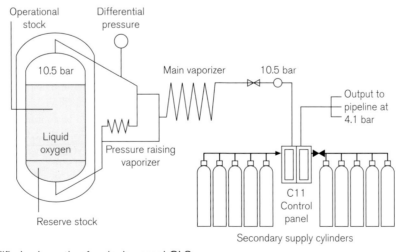

Figure 3.15 Simplified schematic of a single vessel CLS.

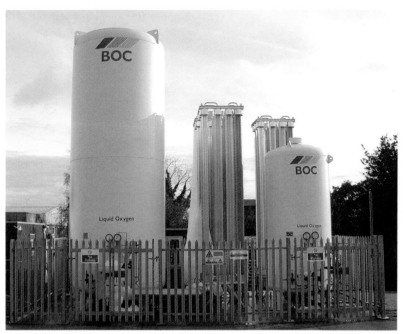

Fig 3.16 A twin vessel CLS installation.

the pressure inside the vessel rises, and to prevent the safety relief valve from blowing gas to atmosphere, a valve opens and allows gas to pass into the pipeline distribution line.

Conversely, if there is high demand, the pressure in the vessel will tend to fall. When this happens, liquid is withdrawn from the bottom liquid valve passing through a pressure-raising coil which raises the pressure to 10.5 bar. During normal operation the liquid converts to a gas as it passes through a process vaporizer, which can be a simple ambient vaporizer, or duplex timed automatic switching vaporizers designed to allow one to operate whilst the second one defrosts. The C11 control panel has duplicate regulators for security. These are designed to control the pressure at 4.1 bar for the main supply and 3.7 bar for the emergency cylinder supply. The control panel is designed to pass flows of 3000 litres per minute from the main VIE supply and 1500 litres per minute through the emergency cylinder manifold.

The control panel relays alarm conditions to a central alarm panel, usually located in the engineering department, with secondary panels located in critical areas throughout the hospital. The conditions can vary, depending upon the type of installation. A simple VIE with a cylinder manifold emergency would give the alarm conditions in Table 3.9.

The VIE has a contents gauge which operates on differential pressure. The pressure at the bottom of the vessel is greater, because of the mass of liquid oxygen, than that at the top and the gauge compares the difference and converts it into an analogue readout.

It is advisable to install a telemetry system to the CLS to provide continuous condition monitoring for both the supplier and the hospital CLS management.

Siting requirements

The installation should be located inside a fenced compound, be accessible to road tankers and be sited in accordance with the British Compressed Gases Association (BCGA) code of practice and safety distance data provided by the installer. In general, all hazardous buildings, flammable materials, public access, vehicles and surface water drains, must be at least 5 metres and in some cases 8 metres from the nearest point of the compound. The compound and the hardstanding area directly in front of the fill connection must be concrete and should be designed to contain any liquid spillage. Tar or asphalt should never be used in the vicinity as they form an explosive mixture when in contact with liquid oxygen.

Sizing

Sizing the installation is based on a Risk Assessment (RA) model, which is detailed in Section 6 of HTM 2022. The RA considers a number of issues amongst which are:

- historic information;

Table 3.9 Alarm conditions for a simple VIE with a cylinder manifold backup (refer to text and Figure 3.15)

Status/Fault Condition	Indication	Legend
Normal operation	Green	Normal
Primary supply system operational stock empty **Primary supply system** reserve stock in use	Yellow	Liquid low Re-fill liquid
Primary supply system reserve stock empty **Secondary supply system** in use	Yellow	Re-fill liquid immediately
Secondary supply system low **Lead secondary supply system** content below 50%	Yellow	Change cylinders
Pipeline pressure fault (high, low)	Red	High pressure Low pressure

- the proximity to the gas supplier;
- potential growth;
- the diversified flow factors (a calculation based on the number of outlet points and their uses);
- vehicular access for delivery tankers;
- the vulnerability of the site to external damage;
- environmental issues;

The CLS is normally owned by the gas supply company and the hospital pay a three element charge;

- a gas price per HCM;
- a service element which includes rental, maintenance and capitalization of the installation; and
- a delivery charge.

Liquid cylinder installations

Where the annual consumption of a hospital is considered too great for a compressed cylinder manifold but is insufficient for a CLS, then a liquid cylinder (LC) installation can be considered. This type of installation is not dissimilar to a compressed manifold, having the same configuration of banks of cylinders and a control panel (Fig. 3.17).

However, the installation has significant advantages in that each LC contains the equivalent gas capacity of 24 J size compressed gas cylinders and on a typical four-cylinder LC manifold, the capacity is equivalent to 72 size J cylinders. Another major advantage over compressed cylinders is that the LCs are a semi-permanent installation, in that they remain static and are filled from a remote fill point, usually on the outside wall of the

compound; this removes the need for manual handling and connecting.

Any pressure build-up in the reserve manifold automatically feeds into the pipeline through the control panel.

The only disadvantage when compared to a CLS is the flowrate limitation. A CLS is capable of $3000\,l\,min^{-1}$ under normal conditions whereas a LC installation is capable of $500\,l\,min^{-1}$ and whilst this is normally sufficient for a mid-range pipeline system, it should be considered when considering options:

- an LC installation will usually have a two cylinder compressed emergency supply;
- an alarm panel linked to the control panel provides for similar conditions to those of a single CLS installation; and
- an LC installation must be sited in the open air with protection from the elements.

OXYGEN CONCENTRATORS (PSA PLANT)

An oxygen concentrator or Pressure Swing Adsorber (PSA) can be considered as an alternative to a traditional supply where no reliable liquid oxygen supply is available, such as an off-shore site or a site where the safety criteria for liquid installations cannot be met.

Operational process

An oxygen concentrator operates on the principle of adsorbing, under pressure, other gases in the atmosphere,

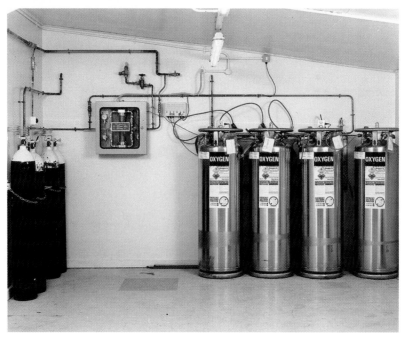

Figure 3.17 A liquid cylinder installation.

onto the surface of an adsorbent material, known as zeolite. Because oxygen is not adsorbed by the zeolite, it is free to pass through into storage for use.

The zeolite is sealed in a vessel known as a sieve bed. The sieve beds operate in pairs, one adsorbing whilst the other regenerates. The waste product, mainly nitrogen, is discharged to atmosphere. The process is capable of producing oxygen concentrations of about 95%. The remainder is made up mainly of argon with a small percentage of nitrogen. During closed circuit anaesthesia it is reported that a build-up of Argon could occur.

The major components of a hospital PSA plant are:

- Duplex compressors;
- Receivers;
- Dryers;
- Duplex molecular sieves;
- Vacuum pumps;
- Filters;
- Line pressure regulators;
- Control system;
- Oxygen performance monitoring system; and
- Back up cylinder manifold.

Figure 3.18 shows a schematic layout for a hospital system.

In addition to the economic considerations, a number of other issues must be considered: The process generates a great deal of heat, hence ventilation and cooling for the product and the compressors are a major consideration.

Should the plant fail, the emergency cylinder manifold will feed into the pipeline at higher concentrations (99.5%) than the plants operating norm of 95%. This may have an effect on downline equipment, particularly in critical care areas.

A more appropriate application for oxygen concentrators is in the home environment where a low-flow, low-pressure, system can provide continuous oxygen to COPD patients. A typical unit (Fig. 3.19) operates on a mains supply and can provide up to 5 l min^{-1} at an oxygen concentration of 94%. It is extremely efficient and needs little maintenance by the patient, who need only wash the inlet filter from time to time. It can be piped around the home to small wall mounted outlets. The concentrator is usually sited in a hallway and needs no special ventilation. The typical noise level when operating normally is around 40 db.

SYNTHETIC AIR SYSTEMS

As an alternative to a conventional compressed air system, synthetic air may be a consideration, especially at the design stage of a new hospital or where purity is an issue.

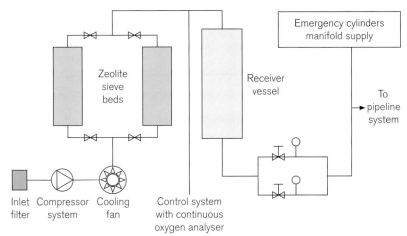

Figure 3.18 A schematic layout for a hospital system.

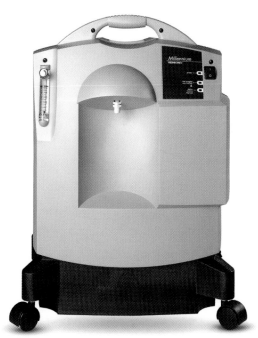

Figure 3.19 A home oxygen concentrator: the Millennium Respironics™ Oxygen Concentrator. Image courtesy of Respironics Inc. and its affiliates, Murrysville, PA USA.

The 1998 European Pharmaceutical monograph for medical air puts greater emphasis on the control of hydrocarbons and moisture and consequently an increased need for monitoring the performance of air systems is required. Synthetic Medical Air (SMA) contains no hydrocarbons or moisture and is produced by mixing liquid oxygen and liquid nitrogen in the gas state. The

installation makes use of the existing liquid supply with a liquid nitrogen vessel alongside. Both vessels would have smaller back-up vessels on the site (Fig. 3.20).

The initial control system is very similar to the conventional CLS mentioned earlier, with the addition of duplex mixing panels and gas analyzers providing continuous monitoring of gas purity. The gas is then stored at 4 bar(g), but could be stored at higher pressures for surgical air and regulated down to 4 bar(g) for medical use.

The benefits of SMA are:

- maintenance free;
- no purity issues;
- no power supply required; and
- availability of nitrogen on site for surgical power tools.

MEDICAL COMPRESSED AIR

Medical compressed air (MA) is classified by the European Pharmacopoeia as a drug, and therefore warrants the same degree of care and cleanliness that any drug demands during its manufacture, storage or transportation to the patient. MA is provided into a pipeline system by three methods:

1. compressors;
2. cylinders connected to a manifold; and
3. by mixing liquid oxygen and liquid nitrogen, also known as Synthetic Air.

This section will deal with the provision of MA by compressors.

The initial components of MA manufacture are the same as any industrial requirement and comprise a

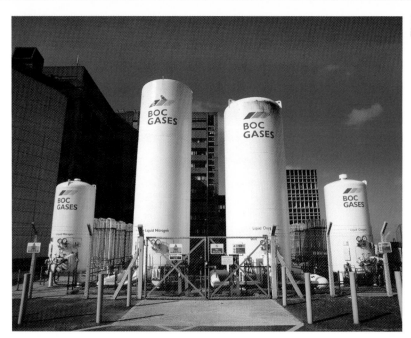

Figure 3.20 A synthetic CLS installation.

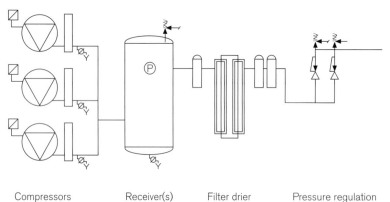

Figure 3.21 Main components of a typical medical compressed air plant.

Compressors   Receiver(s)   Filter drier   Pressure regulation

compressor, a receiver for the storage of gas, and some form of regulation to monitor and control the pressure in the pipeline (Fig. 3.21). Where MA differs from its industrial cousin, is the degree of conditioning that needs to be applied to the raw compressed air, before it can be administered to the patient. Compressors for MA plant can be any of three types: Reciprocating, Screw or Rotary Vane, all having their individual benefits and selection is normally made by the manufacturer based on demand, location and initial cost. Whatever pumps are used they should be identical to each other and capable of maintaining the total demand of the hospital with one

pump off line, for example, where two pumps are used, each pump should have the capacity of the total demand, whereas where four pumps are used, three pumps running would need to be able to cater for the hospital's maximum demand.

One of the by-products of compressing air is water vapour, which then condenses into water and can collect in receivers and pipelines in the system. Another contaminant in normal compressed air is oil, as this is used to lubricate the compressor and can be carried over in the air stream. The third danger in this area would be particulate matter collected from the air or picked up in

Table 3.10 Maximum allowable contaminants for medical air

Contaminant	Maximum allowable amount
Water	60 ppm
Carbon monoxide	5 ppm
Carbon dioxide	500 ppm
Oil	0.1mg m^{-3}
Sulphur dioxide	1 ppm
Nitrogen monoxide	2 ppm
Nitrogen dioxide	2 ppm

the process of compression and storage, such as rust particles picked up from the receiver. For MA, all of these contaminants, as well as others, need to be removed before it can be provided for patient use. See Table 3.10 for the specification required by the European Pharmacopoeia for MA. This degree of cleanliness is achieved by a series of filters and driers installed after compression but before distribution into the pipeline system.

Of equal importance to the quality of the MA are the control of the pressure and the security of the supply. MA is normally distributed at 400 kPa, and is maintained at this pressure by a pressure-reducing valve fitted after the drier/filtration assembly and is further protected by a pressure relief valve designed to protect the system from over-pressurization should a fault occur with the reducing valve. Of main importance is the control system, which is responsible for making all of the individual parts of the unit work in unison, for controlling the safety back-up devices and ensuring that alarms are raised if any component fails to perform in its prescribed manner.

As with all other medical gas supply units, all vital components in the design of the system are provided in at least duplex so that one component (filter/drier/compressor, etc.) can act as a standby for use if any other component fails or needs to be taken out of service for maintenance.

Medical air may be used in patient ventilators, as a carrier for drugs in nebulization or for humidification, and also for some devices such as automatic tourniquets.

In some areas of the hospital, air is also distributed at a higher pressure for use as a power source for medical tools, such as those used for orthopaedic work. Known as Surgical Air (SA), the gas has similar properties as MA but is of a higher pressure (up to 1100 kPa) and, as it is not used for life support, it does not require the same degree of standby/back-up as true medicinal gases.

Where demand for both MA and SA is small, it is acceptable to utilize one compressed air plant to provide the two supplies, and to regulate the gas pressures accordingly. In this instance it is imperative that all regulation and control is in the plant room and that both services are piped away from this point in parallel.

As noted above, MA could also be provided from manifolds or as synthetic air. It is worth noting that the provision of MA and especially SA from cylinder manifolds is not really a practicable option, because of the high consumption rates.

The terminal units will be discussed in detail under pipeline distribution, but it is important to note that those used for both MA and SA are, as with other gases, of different dimensions, ensuring that the risk of cross connection and delivery of the wrong gas is reduced.

It is sometimes practical to run the MA pipeline network to the dental department or similar departments requiring a sterile supply of air. In such instances, the cost of running pipework over long distances can sometimes outweigh those incurred by the use of smaller local compressors.

MEDICAL VACUUM SYSTEMS

Although medical vacuum, by its very nature cannot be termed a gas, let alone a medical gas, medical vacuum (MV) is always installed with the other true gases and with the same types of valving and equipment. This, together with the fact that it is covered by the same standards as medical gases (HTM2022, C11 and EN 737) means that piped vacuum services are invariably considered alongside the provision of medical gases.

The purpose of MV is to assist in the removal of fluids during medical or surgical procedures. The principal of fluid removal is the same in all cases; a drainage tube is passed from the patient into an interceptor collection jar where any solid and liquid waste is trapped. The vacuum is then passed into the piped vacuum system via a regulator and bacterial filter to the terminal unit in the same way as the medical gases (Fig. 3.22, see also Chapter 22).

The pipeline system carrying the MV back to the plant is usually of the same materials and standard as that of the medical gases, with the exceptions that the sizes are normally larger due to the higher percentage pressure drop and that in some instances the larger pipe sizes

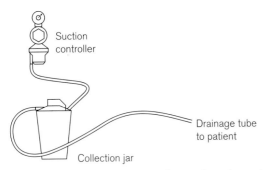

Figure 3.22 Typical components of a ward suction set.

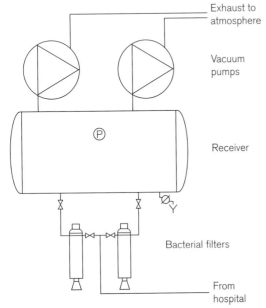

Figure 3.23 Main components of a typical medical vacuum plant.

(over 54 mm) can be of a plastic material to reduce installation costs.

At the vacuum plant (Fig. 3.23), there are additional bacterial traps and collection jars to collect any materials that may have accidentally by-passed the interceptors at the patient level. These components are predominantly provided to protect the plant and thereby maintenance staff from contamination. It is advisable, however, to ensure that infection control procedures are carried out when any maintenance work is being undertaken, especially if this involves changing the bacterial filters.

From the filters the vacuum is drawn in to the receiver. The receiver is designed so that the pumps, operating between 550 and 650 mm Hg subatmospheric, cycle no

more than 6 times per hour. This prevents excessive wear and tear on the system and is good engineering practice.

MV plant can be thought of as a compressor in reverse; air is taken from the MV pipeline and 'compressed' into the atmosphere. As with medical air, it is essential to have pumps sized so that there is at least one pump capable of acting as a standby in case one pump fails. It is permissible to have two, three or four pumps in a set, the rule being that the combined capacity of the plant equates to 75% of the maximum design flowrate of the system with one pump stationary. The exhaust from a vacuum pump may be combined with other vacuum pumps but where this is the case, a non-return valve must be fitted to the exhaust so that it does not 'drive' the standby pump. The exhaust pipeline(s) however *must* be vented to atmosphere at high level, normally at roof level and away from all other air intakes or openings into the building (doors, windows, etc.).

The normal pumps used for MV in the UK are of a rotary vane type, although reciprocating pumps are used in some parts of the world. Both of these types of pump have a capacity to generate a subatmospheric pressure of up to 650 mmHg at sea level and are perfectly adequate for the purposes of medical vacuum. At higher altitudes though, it would be more difficult to achieve the negative pressure required and the settings on the plant control systems would need to be changed to allow for this lower operating range.

Again, as with the compressed air plant, the most important item is the plant management and control system. This operates the cut in and cut out of the pumps, cycles the duty so that each pump has the same amount of use and passes any faults back to the alarm and indication system.

In certain parts of the world (USA, for example) medical vacuum systems are also used to deliver the negative pressure requirements for anaesthetic gas scavenging system (AGSS). In the UK we tend to utilize a totally separate vacuum source for this purpose, a less powerful vacuum but with higher flowrates ($120\,l\,min^{-1}$ per terminal unit). As this vacuum source is of a lower technical requirement, greater savings can be made both in capital terms as well as running costs.

Performance levels and specifications for a medical vacuum service

For the UK, the specifications for a piped vacuum service are laid down in the HTM2022 1997 edition. In brief the guidance states that:

Table 3.11 Main plant alarm

Service Legend	Liquid Oxygen	Manifold Supply	Air Plant	Vacuum Plant
Normal	Normal	Normal	Normal	Normal
Condition 1	Refill liquid oxygen	Standby running	Plant fault	Plant fault
Condition 2	Refill oxygen immediately	Standby low	Plant emergency	Plant emergency
Condition 3	Reserve low	Reserve low	Reserve low	
Condition 4	Pressure fault	Pressure fault	Pressure fault	Pressure fault

- the design and operating pressure should not be any less than 450 mmHg at the plant;
- a pressure drop of 50 mmHg is allowed within the distribution pipework;
- a minimum pressure of 400 mmHg is required at the back of the terminal unit; and
- a pressure drop of 100 mmHg is allowed across the terminal unit to the probe, which has to maintain a minimum pressure of at least 300 mmHg whilst delivering a flow rate of 40 l min^{-1}.

ANAESTHETIC GAS SCAVENGING SYSTEMS

These are considered specifically in Chapter 20. They do however form part of what is termed Medical Gas Piped Services, and common aspects of the piping and distribution are considered further in this chapter.

ALARM AND INDICATION SYSTEMS FOR PIPED GASES

There are two different types of alarm system used within a hospital medical gas system: main plant alarms and local or ward alarms. The former is used to provide indication of the condition of the plant at the source of the system where it is generated or stored. The latter is used to provide an indication of the condition of the gas at the point of use.

The main plant alarm (Table 3.11) consists of a series of panels at strategic positions throughout the hospital. These will usually give the indication that everything is normal; their main function though is to give advance warning that something might be in the process of failure. As an example, if one of the banks on a manifold runs out, it will change over to the standby bank. As soon as this happens, the alarm will be triggered that cylinders need changing on that manifold. The service is not in danger, as the manifold is designed to act in this way but, if no one attends to the manifold and the standby bank runs out also, the second condition alarm will be initiated and in this condition the system is about to become empty. If the pressure does fall below the minimum required then the final condition, pressure fault will commence. At this stage, patients will need to be provided with alternative supplies.

The third condition on the system is used to monitor the failsafe emergency supply source; although this should not be used as a main supply, it may provide the hospital with some essential emergency time to act.

In addition to the indications on the main alarm panels, additional indication will appear on each plant control panel or manifold, which will provide a more detailed but visual-only indication of the nature of the fault or emergency.

A local or area alarm panel has a much different function. The alarm condition on a local or ward-based alarm is used to indicate that something has *already* gone wrong. Each gas in every ward or department is monitored

Table 3.12 Typical local alarm panel legends			
Service Legend	**Oxygen**	**Medical Air 400 kPa**	**Vacuum**
Normal	Normal	Normal	Normal
Condition 1	High pressure	High pressure	High pressure
Condition 2	Low pressure	Low pressure	Low pressure

for fault by a pressure switch mounted in the pipeline, downstream of the final Area Valved Service Unit (AVSU). Typically this is set at ±20% of line pressure for that particular gas so that, if a high- or low-pressure condition exists within the area, the alarm will indicate the fact (Table 3.12).

On both types of alarm panel the indication is both audible and visual. A two-tone sounder and a flashing legend indicates what the fault is and on what service. The audible alarm can be muted but will reinstate itself after 15 minutes if the fault has not been cured. On clearance of the fault, the alarm panel will automatically reset itself to 'Normal'.

DISTRIBUTION SYSTEMS

Medical gases are distributed throughout the hospital at a nominal 400 kPa through pipelines designed to achieve a minimum pressure drop from the source (e.g. compressed air plant) to the point of use at the patient. This is achieved by some quite complicated calculations based on the initial pressure, the flowrate required and the diameter of the pipework. In simple terms, the higher the required flowrate, the larger the diameter of the pipe needed to carry it. So, for example, the pipeline in a plant room could quite conceivably be 54 or even 76 mm diameter, whereas by the time the pipes enter at ward level they would not normally be in excess of 22 mm and by the time they are in the patient bedhead, normally as low as 12 mm.

The 'gases' normally distributed by pipeline in hospitals within the UK are:

- Oxygen O_2 (400 kPa)
- Nitrous Oxide N_2O (400 kPa)
- Entonox   50% O_2/50% N_2O
- Medical Air   MA (400 kPa)
- Surgical Air   SA (700 kPa)
- Vacuum   Vac
- Anaesthetic Gas Scavenging   AGSS

They all carry an individual colour code as, shown in Fig. 3.24.

Other gases, such as helium and hydrogen, are supplied in piped services to pathology laboratories, but are not frequently used in direct connection with patients, so are not therefore considered in this book.

For detailed information concerning the regulations and standards required for fixed distribution pipework, those imposed by the appropriate Government or Health Ministries should be consulted. In the UK, these are quoted in HTM 2022 and its supplement, which refer to the 'permit to work' system laying down the procedures to be adopted when service maintenance, repair or alterations are to be undertaken.

In this chapter, only a brief description can be given of the fixed pipework, because this part of the installation is 'behind the wall'; it is more appropriately the concern of the hospital engineer. The anaesthetist or designated medical officer should, however, be aware of the nature of the installation and should always be informed and consulted before any alterations to it are made.

The pipes used are *half hard* and manufactured from phosphorous de-oxidized non-arsenical copper to BS EN 1412:1996 grade CW024A to prevent degradation of gases. 'Half hard' refers to the heat treatment of copper pipes, which allows them to have a higher pressure rating. Pipes are degreased, purged and filled with nitrogen and have end-caps fitted to maintain cleanliness prior to delivery and installation at site. Pipefittings used for jointing these pipes are made from the same materials. All

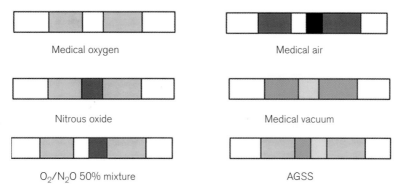

Medical oxygen

Medical air

Nitrous oxide

Medical vacuum

O_2/N_2O 50% mixture

AGSS

Figure 3.24 Colour codes for medical gas pipework.

components should be cleaned to a minimum specification of 2 mg min^{-2}.

To reduce pipe corrosion, jointing of the pipelines on site must only be of copper-to-copper using a silver solder brazing alloy to grade CP4 (5% silver) utilizing a nitrogen purge and no flux. This has become known as the fluxless brazing method. Soft solder or compression fittings should never be used, nor should joints to any other metal, for example, brass, bronze or gun-metal.

Valves will be installed at various points along the route or network: at each department or ward, at the branch of each riser and at the entry to buildings or exit of plant rooms.

Valves within plant rooms should be left unlocked, though all other valves should be locked and only unlocked under a permit to work and supervision of the authorized person.

Valves at ward entrances or departmental isolation valves are normally termed AVSUs (Area Valved Service Units) or ZSU (Zone Service Units) and are specifically designed to provide not only gas isolation but also other functions as described below. Furthermore, an AVSU is housed in a lockable box that has a glass fronted panel, which can be broken by the ward staff to allow isolation of gas flow to areas in case of fire, fracture or other catastrophe (Fig. 3.25).

AVSUs also permit additional connections into the gas stream by the use of a Non-Interchangeable Screw Thread (NIST) system. The NIST union contains a self-sealing valve so that when the blanking nut is removed and the appropriate NIST connection is made, the self-sealing valve is automatically reopened. These branches may be used to purge pipelines or to introduce a local supply during alterations or breakdowns. The AVSU junction also allows the insertion of a 'spade', which is used by

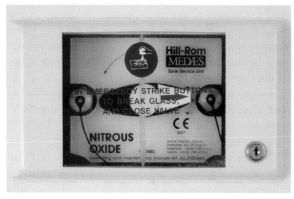

Figure 3.25 A typical AVSU (see text), note blanked off NIST connectors on either side of valve.

service engineers to ensure absolute closure of the pipeline, irrespective of the action of the valves.

AVSUs are installed in such positions as to protect each department or ward. They should be installed on the natural route from a department that would be passed on an emergency exit from the unit.

The pipework itself should be identified by labels placed upon it in regular intervals (Fig. 3.24), in accordance with the identification code described in Section 13 of HTM2022 and further marked as to the direction of flow.

Pipework is normally always concealed in today's installation procedures, though in the past it has been mounted on the surface. The later arrangement is not only aesthetically less attractive, but also less satisfactory from the standpoint of general hygiene and cleanliness.

Terminal outlets

The distribution pipework terminates in outlets that are in the form of self-sealing sockets (Fig 3.26).

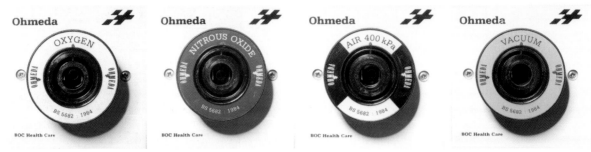

Figure 3.26 Terminal outlets. Note the different diameter recesses (collar indexing system) that match the collar on the relevant probe (see Fig. 3.27).

In 1978 a British Standard was published (BS 5682, upgraded in 1984) that laid down a specification for the design of terminal units. This is now in the process of being superseded by a European Standard BS EN 737, for the dimensioning and construction of the terminal unit and its associated probe. It specifies that the terminal unit should consist of two sections:

1. The first section, a termination assembly, should be permanently attached to the appropriate pipeline.
2. The second, the 'Schrader' socket assembly containing the quick connect probe socket, can be removed by a service engineer, but must be designed so that it cannot be accidentally connected to a different gas service.

A termination assembly for a pressurized gas (but not a vacuum) must have a check valve so that work can be carried out on any terminal unit without shutting down all the terminal units for that gas in that area. It should be designed to operate automatically as soon as the socket assembly is removed.

The design of the components needs to be such that gas specificity is maintained for each element, to such a degree that no terminal unit can be assembled and include parts from different gases. The identity of the gas for each terminal unit should be permanently displayed on all individual components. The socket assembly, when assembled will only accept a probe with the same gas identity, by utilizing a collar indexing system that is unique to that gas service.

Flexible pipelines

The flexible pipeline connects the terminal outlet to the medical equipment; it has three components:

1. a quick connect probe that fits the terminal outlet (Schrader probe);
2. a flexible hosepipe; and

3. a NIST connection that fits the equipment, e.g. the anaesthetic machine.

The actual male part of the probe for the terminal outlet is designed such that it is the same size for all gases. To prevent connection to the wrong gas service, the probe for each gas supply has a protruding indexing collar (Fig. 3.27), This collar has a unique diameter that fits only the matching recess fitted to the socket assembly for that gas.

The British Standard also stipulates the following:

- It must not be possible to twist the probe while it is connected to the unit unless it is connected vertically to a pendant. To this end, the collar is provided with a notch that fits over a rigid pin in the socket assembly.
- It must be possible to insert or remove the probe simply and quickly using one hand only. The socket assembly has a spring-loaded outer ring, which when depressed releases the locking mechanism holding the probe, and causes the probe to be ejected.
- The unit must seal off the flow of gas when the probe is withdrawn.

The flexible hose

This is the section of the system in which damage and wear are most likely to occur. Originally the hose for each gas was constructed of the same black reinforced rubber or neoprene tubing, identified only by a short length of coloured sheath at each end. Several accidents, some resulting in fatalities, have been caused by the attachment of the probe for one gas at the upstream end of such a hose, but with the socket or union for another at the downstream end. The incidence of such accidents should be reduced by the current practice of most manufacturers, which is:

- to produce hoses for the different gas services, complete with the appropriate connections, under

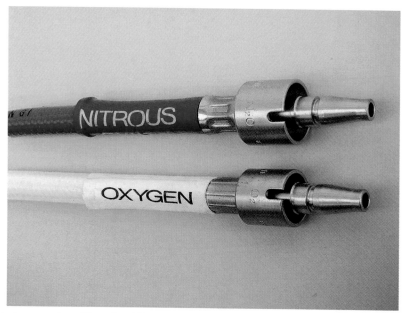

Figure 3.27 Flexible hose probes. Note the difference in size of the indexing collar.

strict quality control systems and with necessary checks to ensure correct application. Furthermore, it is now a recommended practice that a damaged hose should not be repaired on-site but should be returned in its entirety to the manufacturer in exchange for a factory-made service replacement.

- to use characteristically coloured tubing for each gas (Fig. 3.28). The development of such self-identifying tubing was unfortunately delayed by the difficulties involved in manufacturing it with the necessary antistatic (electrically conductive) properties.

The non-interchangeable screw thread (NIST) connector

To ensure that the gas services are attached correctly to the relevant piece of medical equipment, each hose is fitted with a unique connector. This takes the form of a nut and a probe (Fig. 3.29). The probe has a unique profile for each gas supply and fits only the union on the receiving equipment. The profile has two cylindrical shapes which form a unique combination. Note that the first part of the nitrous oxide probe is smaller than that for oxygen, but the second part is larger. Hence the tip would fit into the oxygen receiver but the larger second part would prevent full engagement. The first part of the oxygen probe is too large for the nitrous oxide receiver and so would not fit.

The nut has the same diameter and thread (in the UK)

for all the gas services but can be attached to the anaesthetic machine only when the probe is correctly engaged. The term 'non-interchangeable screw-threaded connection' is ambiguous as it can give the impression that the screw threads are different and cause the unique fit, which is untrue.

The connections between the hose and fittings must be secure and tamper-proof. Both the BS terminal unit and NIST probes have serrated spigots, which are pushed into the ends of the hosepipe. To prevent their working loose, a stainless steel sleeve (ferrule) is placed on the outside of the hosepipe and spigot and compressed (crimped) by a 30-ton press, The ferrule is sufficiently robust to defy all but the most determined attempts at removal as well as compressing the hosepipe onto the spigot with such force that if an attempt were made to pull the two apart, the hose would stretch and break before the components separated.

TESTS AND CHECKS FOR MEDICAL GAS PIPED SERVICES

- Anaesthetists must hold themselves responsible for checking only that part of the Medical Gas Pipeline Services (MGPS) system between the terminal unit and the patient. They should be able to take for granted the quality and unfailing supply of gases.

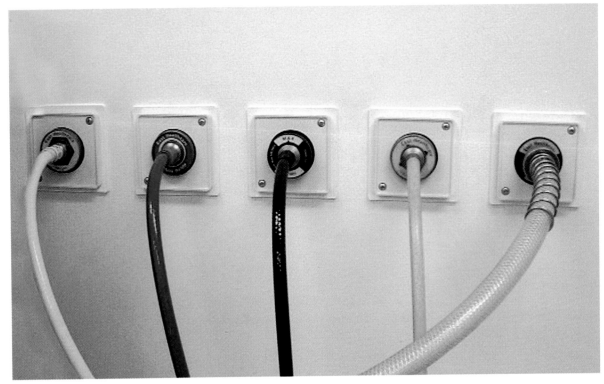

Figure 3.28 Colour coded hoses.

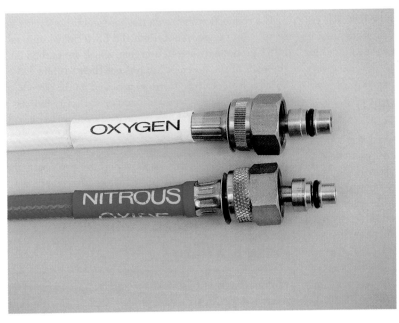

Figure 3.29 NIST connectors with the locking collars manipulated to reveal the different gas specific profiles of the probes.

- Quality control is usually considered to be the province of the hospital pharmacist, who should order, or make, tests to confirm the identity of the gas, its purity and composition, and freedom from contaminants, including solid particulate matter. Compressed air should also be examined for water vapour and oil mist on a quarterly basis to ensure compliance with the European Pharmacopoeia. The pharmacist is usually responsible for maintaining adequate supplies of cylinders.
- The engineering department is responsible for organizing both planned preventive maintenance and emergency repairs, as well as for the design compliance, continuity of supply and indication and warning systems (alarms).
- Designated theatre staff are usually responsible for changing cylinders and holding a store of portable oxygen cylinders with flowmeters and suction equipment for use in emergencies or during shutdown for maintenance and alterations.
- The anaesthetist is responsible for the correct insertion of the pipeline probes and any necessary adjustments. A fuller description of 'cockpit drill' is to be found in Appendix IV of HTM 2022.
- The supplement to HTM 2022, which should be consulted for further details, describes a 'permit to work' system. Essentially, this is a code of practice for repairs and preventive maintenance on the MGPS system in which the engineer discusses with the appropriate people the nature and timings of the work to be done and ensures that independent services for medical gases such as oxygen and vacuum may be made available as required. The 'permit to work' document with no less than six parts to be completed (depending on the degree of hazard) may at first seem to be yet another proliferation of the already burdensome paperwork in hospitals, It does, however, increase safety and improve the relationships between departments.
- Finally, and most importantly, the whole operation and management of the medical gas system is described in Volume 2 of HTM2022 'Operational Management'. This demands a policy on the use and management of Medical gases with defined responsibilities and roles. It is essential that this document is produced for each hospital, specific to the risks and procedures of that particular site. The medical gas supplier should be in a position to assist in its production.

FURTHER READING

BOC Gas (2002) *Safe with Medical Gases*, Guildford, Surrey: BOC Ltd.

British Standards Institute (1998) Part 1 *Medical Gas Pipeline Systems – Terminal Units for Compressed Medical Gases and Vacuum*, BS EN 737. Milton Keynes, UK: British Standards Institution.

British Standards Institute (2004) *Anaesthetic and Respiratory Equipment Compatibility with Oxygen*. BS EN ISO 15001.

British Standards Institute (1998) Part 2 *Medical Gas Pipeline Systems – Anaesthetic Gas Scavenging Systems – Basic Requirement Medical Gas Pipeline Systems*, BS EN 737. Milton Keynes, UK: British Standards Institution.

British Standards Institute (2000) Part 3 *Medical Gas Pipeline Systems – Pipelines for Compressed Medical Gases and Vacuum*, BS EN 737. Milton Keynes, UK: British Standards Institution.

British Standards Institute (1997) Part 1 *Pressure Regulators for use with Medical Gases – Pressure Regulators and Pressure Regulators with Flowmetering Devices*, BS EN 738. Milton Keynes, UK: British Standards Institution.

British Standards Institute (1999) Part 2 *Pressure Regulators for Use with Medical Gases – Manifold and Line Pressure Regulators*, BS EN 738. Milton Keynes, UK: British Standards Institution.

British Standards Institute (1999) Part 3 *Pressure Regulators for use with Medical Gases – Pressure Regulators with Integral Cylinder valves*, BS EN 738. Milton Keynes, UK: British Standards Institution.

British Standards Institute (1998) *Specification for Probes (quick connectors) for use with Medical Gas Pipeline Systems*, BS 5682. Milton Keynes, UK: British Standards Institution.

British Standards Institute (2004) *Transportable Gas Cylinders. Gas Cylinder Identification (Excluding LPG) Colour Coding.* BS EN 1089–3.

HTM 2022 (1997) *Medical Gas Pipeline Systems – Design, Installation, Validity.* London: The Stationery Office.

Grant, WJ (2005) *Medical Gases – Their Properties and Uses.* Aylesbury: HM & M.

International Organization for Standardization (2004) *Small Medical Cylinders, Pin Index Yoke-type valves.* ISO 407. Geneva: International Organization for Standardization.

International Organization for Standardization (2004) *Cylinder Valve Outlets for Gas Mixtures – Selection and Dimensions.* ISO 5145. Geneva: International Organization for Standardization.

International Organization for Standardization (1977) *Gas Cylinders for Medical Use – Marking for Identification of Content.* ISO 32–1.

4

Measurement of pressure and gas flow

Paul Beatty

Any system for delivering anaesthetic gases requires the consistent and accurate measurement of gas flow and pressure. In order to be able to understand the detailed design of modern anaesthetic machines, this chapter will consider how such measurements are obtained and the basic physical principles involved.

FORCE, PRESSURE AND FLOW

Force is that which causes an object to move or, more accurately, to accelerate. Once it is moving, Newton's Laws tell us that it will continue to move in a straight line at a constant rate unless some other force is applied to it. The SI unit of force is the *Newton* (N), which is defined as the force that causes a mass of 1 kg to accelerate by 1 metre per second per second (m s^{-2}). Other units of force occasionally used are the kilogram force (kgf) and the pound force (lbf). These are forces equivalent to the force exerted by the earth's gravity on masses of a kilogram and a pound, respectively.

Pressure is force per unit area over which the force acts, i.e.

Pressure = Force/Area

In any gas or liquid, pressure acts in all directions equally, whereas force acts in a given direction. For example, in a full hypodermic syringe, the liquid can be pressurized by applying a force to the plunger of the syringe. This is applied in the direction of travel of the plunger. However, if there were a leak in the barrel of the syringe, the liquid would squirt out sideways from the leak, as well as from the syringe outlet (Fig. 4.1), due to the pressure created by the force acting in all directions within the barrel of the syringe. The amount of pressure generated depends on the area of cross section of the barrel since it is over this area that the force acts. Thus, for the same applied force, a syringe with a larger bore has a lower pressure than one with a smaller bore.

The SI unit of pressure is the *Pascal* (Pa), which is the pressure that results from the application of 1 N over an area of 1 square metre (m^2). Because a pressure of 1 Pa is rather small, gas pressures in anaesthesia tend to be measured in kPa. Other units of pressure that may be used in anaesthesia are pounds per square inch (psi) and Bar (the pressure exerted by the atmosphere at sea-level, which is the result of the weight of atmospheric gases bearing down on the surface of the earth).

Flow is the result of differences in pressure. If a liquid or gas encounters a region in which one point has a higher

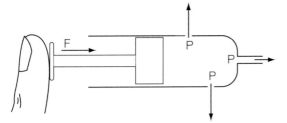

Figure 4.1 When the user exerts a force *F* on the plunger of an intravenous syringe, it is applied in one direction only, but the resulting fluid pressure *P* is exerted in all directions.

pressure than another, then it will move away from the point of higher pressure towards that of lower pressure. That motion is *flow*. The commonest type of unit of flow encountered in anaesthesia considers the volume of flow of a liquid or gas in a given time. The SI unit is metres cubed per second ($m^3 s^{-1}$). As this is very unwieldy, litres per second ($1 s^{-1}$) or litres per minute ($1 min^{-1}$) are normally used. Strictly, these units describe *Volume Flow*. However, there is an alternative type of flow measurement.

All the gas laws, i.e. Boyle's Law, Charles's Law and Gay Lussac's Law, can be summarized using the *Ideal Gas Law* (see Chapter 1), which relates the pressure and volume of a given mass of gas to its temperature:

$PV = nRT$

where P is the pressure of the gas, V its volume, T its temperature, R a constant and n the number of moles of gas present. Volume flow assumes constant pressure and temperature, but a measurement of flow can be independent of pressure, flow or temperature by considering the number of moles of gas passing in a given time. This measurement of flow is *Mass Flow*, and is the basis of mass flow controller or meters used in some types of modern anaesthesia machines.

ATMOSPHERIC PRESSURE AND PARTIAL PRESSURE

The definition of the Bar given above shows that the air exerts a pressure, called *atmospheric pressure*. Atmospheric pressure is measured using a barometer, the simplest form of which is the Fortin barometer (Fig. 4.2). This consists of a long transparent tube, sealed at one end, which is filled with mercury and inverted with its

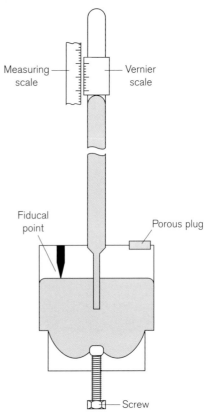

Figure 4.2 Fortin barometer. The level of the surface of mercury in the lower chamber is equilibrated to ambient pressure via the porous plug. The screw is adjusted until the surface of the mercury is touching the fiducal point. The level of the mercury in the column then represents the ambient pressure and is measured using the Vernier scale.

open end in a bath of mercury exposed to atmospheric pressure. The atmospheric pressure acting on the surface of the mercury in the bath will support a column of mercury of about 760 mm above the surface of the mercury in the bath, leaving a virtual vacuum between the surface of the mercury in the tube and the sealed tube end. The height of column of mercury is measured using a Vernier scale at the top of the tube, which can be adjusted using the knob on the side of the barometer tube.

This measurement of atmospheric pressure leads to a further unit for pressure, millimetres of mercury (mmHg or Torr). If the tube of the barometer is 1 cm^2 in diameter, a column of mercury 760 mm high will weigh 1.033 kg, which means that atmospheric pressure is 760 mmHg = 1 Bar = 1000 millibars = 15 psi = 1033 kg cm^{-2} = 1.01 $\times 10^5$ N m^{-2} = 1013 kPa.

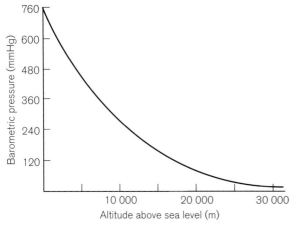

Figure 4.3 The relationship between barometric pressure and altitude above sea level.

Returning to *The Ideal Gas Law* in the form given above, it is clear that it makes no difference whether different gases contribute the moles present. So the expression for two different gases can be rewritten as:

$$PV = (n_1 + n_2)\, RT = n_1 RT + n_2 RT$$

This is *Dalton's Law of Partial Pressures* and shows that each gas exerts its own *partial* pressure independent of its companions. For example, if air is 20% oxygen and 80% nitrogen, then for an atmospheric pressure of 760 mmHg, the partial pressure of oxygen will be 152 mmHg and the partial pressure of nitrogen will be 608 mmHg. However, as Fig. 4.3 shows, barometric pressure falls with altitude. Thus when treating a patient at high altitude, a larger percentage of oxygen is required to supply the same partial pressure of oxygen. It is this partial pressure, not percentage of gas, which is clinically most important. The relationship between altitude and the partial pressure of the components of atmospheric air are shown in Fig. 4.4.

ABSOLUTE, DIFFERENTIAL AND GAUGE PRESSURES

Since the barometer measures pressure with reference to a vacuum, the measurement made is an *absolute pressure measurement*. There are other types of absolute measurements of pressure made with anaesthetic equipment. Mostly these are related to measurements of high pressures such as those encountered in gas cylinders.

Differential pressure measurement is used where the difference in pressure between two points is required.

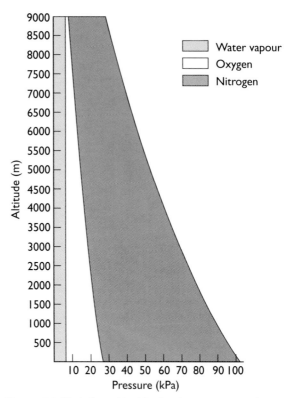

Figure 4.4 Variation with altitude of components of inspired air. Saturation with water vapour by upper airways is assumed.

The simplest differential pressure measurement system is the manometer, as shown in Fig. 4.5. This takes the form of a U-shaped tube, partially filled with liquid such as water. Gas at pressure P is applied to end A, with end B open to the atmosphere (so having atmospheric pressure applied to it). The pressure at A causes water to be pushed to the other limb of the U so that the level in the right-hand limb moves to point b above where it was before the pressure was applied, and the water in the left-hand limb is depressed below its original level. If both move by a distance of 5 cm then the difference in water level created is 10 cm, indicating a pressure difference between the A and B of 10 cmH$_2$O. Since the end B is open to atmosphere, the pressure at A can be thought of as being above atmospheric and is referred to as *gauge pressure* and is sometimes denoted by (g). If the ends A and B are at different points within a closed system, such as between the pleural cavity and the alveoli, then the pressure measured is a true differential pressure.

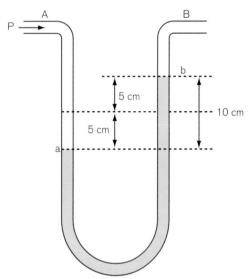

Figure 4.5 A simple manometer. A pressure *P* is applied at A. This causes a depression of the fluid level at *a* and a corresponding rise of the fluid level at *b*. In this case the tube is filled with water and the pressure is 10 cm of water.

METHODS OF MEASURING PRESSURE

Mechanical methods

Bourdon gauge (Fig. 4.6)

The Bourdon gauge is robust, inexpensive and can withstand high pressures. It consists of a curved flattened tube, elliptical in section. When pressure is applied, the tube expands and in doing so attempts to straighten out. Levers, gears or a rack and pinion mechanism translate this movement to a dial pointer. The inlet has a constriction within it to protect the gauge from sudden increases in applied pressure. This gauge is normally used in anaesthesia to indicate cylinder and pipeline pressures. In this application, the pressures measured are much greater than atmospheric pressure. As the response to the applied pressure is determined by the mechanical properties of the Bourdon gauge tube, it effectively measures absolute pressure.

Aneroid gauge

The mechanical principles of an aneroid gauge are shown in Fig. 4.7. It measures absolute pressure and, as with the Bourdon gauge, the movement generated by application of pressure to a chamber is translated into movement of a dial by a mechanical linkage. The amount of movement generated is controlled by the compliance of the aneroid

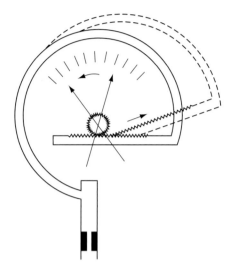

Figure 4.6 The principle of the Bourdon tube pressure gauge. Note the constriction at the inlet.

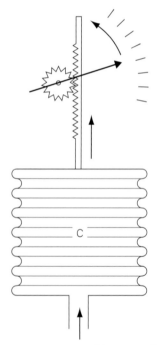

Figure 4.7 Low-pressure aneroid gauge with low-pressure chamber (C).

chamber so that the more rigid the chamber the higher the pressure that the gauge will indicate. The sensitivity of the gauge can be controlled by the gearing ratio of the rack and pinion. Where encountered in anaesthetic devices, aneroid gauges are relatively delicate and sensitive but able to indicate low pressures. They may be used

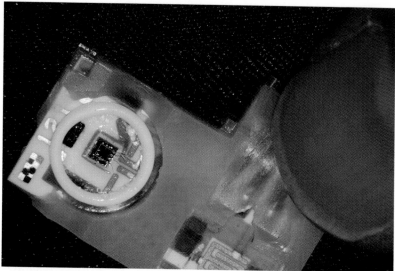

Figure 4.8 A solid state electronic pressure transducer as used in a typical single patient use invasive arterial pressure monitoring set. The coupling gel or 'membrane', which is interposed between the lumen of the monitoring line and the transduction chamber has been removed, remnants of which remain visible. A ceramic plate, onto which is printed the electrical circuit, houses the piezoresistive chip which forms the base of the chamber. An 'O' ring seals the chamber against the housing of the transducer.

to measure airway pressure or blood pressure. If the chamber is sealed and evacuated, the gauge becomes the familiar *aneroid barometer*. Electronic sensors of pressure have largely superseded the aneroid gauge.

Electronic methods
Solid-state electronic pressure transducers

Electronic pressure gauges are now the commonest method for the measurement of pressure and (in modified forms) force, in anaesthetic machines and devices such as blood pressure machines or infusion pumps. They can be used for both absolute measurements and differential measurement, depending on how they are housed and mounted. A typical solid-state electronic pressure transducer is shown in Fig. 4.8.

When used as an absolute pressure monitor, such a transducer is mounted within a chamber, isolated from the medium in which the pressure is to be measured by a flexible membrane such as a colloid gel. Pressure is thus transmitted to the transducer. The sensitivity and pressure measurement range of the transducer is determined by the inherent sensitivity of the *piezoresistive* transducer. If used as a differential pressure transducer, the sensor is mounted so that each side of the transducer is connected to one of the two possible pressure inlets.

Piezoresistivity is the property of a material whereby its electrical resistance changes when subjected to

mechanical stress. Although this is a common property, semiconductor materials show particularly large piezoresistive responses and are therefore used to make very sensitive pressure transducers (strain gauges).

In a solid-state pressure transducer, a single piezoresistive strain gauge is formed on a thin single piece of silicon. The resistance of this strain gauge becomes higher or lower as the silicon slice is flexed by the applied pressure. The resistor is used as one of the four resistors of a Wheatstone Bridge circuit (Fig. 4.9), where four resistances are placed in a diamond formation. The voltage difference across the bridge is zero, that is, the bridge is balanced when

$$\frac{R_1}{R_2} = \frac{R_3}{R_4}$$

When out of balance, the voltage generated across the bridge can be arranged to be proportional for small changes in the resistances, provided the bridge is near to balance. Strain gauges in general, and piezoresistive gauges in particular, are very sensitive to changes in temperature. Provided all the resistances within the Wheatstone Bridge are exposed to the same temperature changes, all the resistances change proportionally and thus the balance condition is unaffected. In solid state pressure transducers, it is relatively simple to ensure that all the resistors in the bridge are exposed to the same temperature changes, by placing them in the same silicon slice that

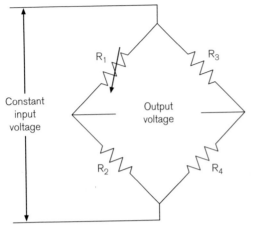

Figure 4.9 A Wheatstone Bridge circuit. In the Wheatstone Bridge the output voltage is balanced and equal to zero when R1/R2 = R3/R4 for a constant input voltage or current.

Table 4.1 Characteristics of flow and volume measurement in anaesthesia

Gas flow *into* breathing system
Continuous flow
Dry gas
Resistance to flow irrelevant
Slow response to change in flow rate
Single or mixed gases

Gas flow and volume *within* breathing system*
Intermittent flow
Wide range of flow rates
Rapid response
Very low resistance to flow
Mixed gas composition
High humidity
Integration of flow, breath by breath

* NB *Exhaled* volumes should *always* be measured rather than inspiratory volumes, as then the anaesthetist always has an indication that *at least this volume* has been exhaled despite any leaks in the system.

contains the strain gauge but in a position where they are not subject to mechanical stress.

MEASUREMENT OF GAS FLOW

The measurement of gas flow is vital to anaesthesia and can be approached using a number of different physical principles. The practical flowmeters include those that respond to gas velocity, volumetric flow, gas momentum and mass flow. All are affected by whether the flow to be measured is laminar, turbulent or reciprocating. In some types of flowmeter, the design of the flowmeter itself ensures that the required flow regime is present, in others the operating flow conditions are set by the application. In addition to being sensitive to the flow regime, they are also affected by changes in gas composition which makes the measurement of respiratory flows, where expiratory and inspiratory gas composition and humidity vary, inherently more difficult than the measurement of flow in dry, single gas composition situations within anaesthetic machines. The correct selection of the type of flowmeter for the chosen application is thus essential. Table 4.1 shows the general characteristics upon which selection of a type of flowmeter depends.

Differential pressure flowmeters
Constant area differential pressure flowmeters
Three types of differential pressure flowmeter are in common use (Fig. 4.10). In all three, some sort of resist-

ance to flow is placed in the flow stream and the pressure drop across the resistance is calibrated as a measurement of flow.

In the case of the *Tubular flowmeter* (Fig. 4.10a), the pressure drop across a tube (or set of tubes) in the stream is measured. Provided the tube is long enough, then even if the flow in the stream is turbulent initially, the tube makes the flow laminar. As a result, the pressure drop P across the tube is proportional to the volumetric flow rate F, and the constant of proportionality is the resistance R:

$$P = RF$$

Resistance is inversely proportional to the area of the tube and proportional to its length. Since length is usually limited by practical considerations and the need to make the flow in the tube laminar, to reduce resistance requires increasing cross-sectional area, which decreases pressure drop and requires that the pressure transducer used is more sensitive. The *Fleish pneumotachograph*, an example of a tubular flowmeter (Fig. 4.11), consists of a set of tubes and is designed to have a very low resistance to respiratory flows and has a very fast response rate. Its construction maximizes the pressure drop, ensures laminar flow measurement conditions with short tubes, whilst minimizing the resistance by using a bundle of small-bore metal tubes. To prevent expiratory gas condensing in these tubes, they are heated. However, a

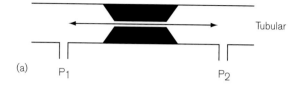

Tubular

(a) P_1 P_2

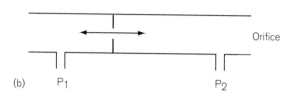

Orifice

(b) P_1 P_2

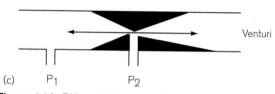

Venturi

(c) P_1 P_2

Figure 4.10 Differential pressure flowmeters. P_1, P_2, differential pressures.

very sensitive and stable pressure transducer is required to make the respiratory flow measurements.

The principle of the Orifice flowmeter is the resistance produced by a simple hole (Fig. 4.10b) in a plate in the flow stream. The orifice causes the flow downstream of itself to be turbulent whether the incoming flow is turbulent or not. The pressure drop achieved is thus proportional to the square of the volumetric flow rate, which makes calibrating an orifice flowmeter difficult, even over a limited range of flow rates. However, orifice flowmeters are cheap to make. Since the flow associated with the orifice flowmeter is essentially turbulent it seems an unlikely candidate for a transducer for respiratory, reciprocating flows. However, wire screen respiratory flow heads, which effectively use multiple orifices in a similar way to the multiple tubes of the Fleisch pneumo-tachograph, have fast responses and low resistances to respiratory flows. The wire mesh in these flowmeters can, as before, be heated to prevent condensation effects.

The final type of differential pressure flowmeter is the *Venturi flowmeter* (Fig. 4.10c). In this type, the gas is forced through a smoothly narrowed portion of tube. The differential pressure is measured between points upstream of the Venturi and its 'throat' (narrowest point). Since the gas is compressed by the restriction it has to accelerate as it passes through the throat. This decreases the pressure in the throat relative to the upstream pressure. Pressure difference is approximately proportional to the square of the flow rate. Venturi flowmeters can be made very accurately but are expensive and are unsuitable for reciprocating respiratory flows.

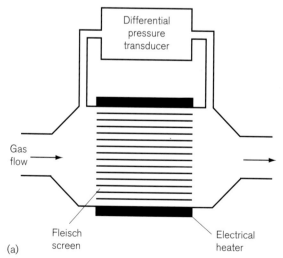

Differential pressure transducer

Gas flow

Fleisch screen

Electrical heater

(a)

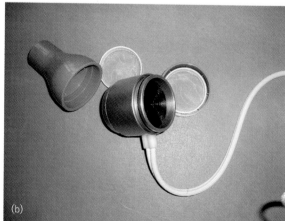

(b)

Figure 4.11 Fleisch pneumotachograph. **(a)** Schematic and **(b)** clinical example.

Variable-area constant differential pressure flowmeters

In the variable-area constant differential pressure flowmeter, the size of the orifice varies with volumetric flow rate to maintain a constant differential pressure. The most familiar design is known as a *rotameter*. Rotameter is actually a trade name of Elliot Automation, but the term is now ubiquitously applied to this type of flowmeter, regardless of detailed design or manufacturer. The rotameter is a development of several other variable-area constant differential pressure flowmeters that have been used in anaesthesia in the past. These include designs by Coxeter, Heidbrink, McKesson and Connel. In the rotameter, a low mass bobbin is suspended by the gas flow in a transparent (usually glass) tube with a tapering internal radius narrowest at the bottom.

During gas flow, an orifice is created by the annulus between the bobbin and the tube. At any given flow within the operating range of the rotameter, the bobbin will find a level at which the differential pressure created by this annulus results in a force upwards equal to the force of gravity downwards on the bobbin. As shown in Fig. 4.12 for a given bobbin and tube design, this equilibrium point will occur at a certain point in the tube for a flow of, say $1.7\,l\,min^{-1}$. If the flow is then increased to $6\,l\,min^{-1}$, the bobbin will rise until the annulus is sufficiently large enough for equilibrium to be re-established. At low flow rates, flow is a function of viscosity because the comparatively longer and narrower annulus behaves like a tube. With higher flow rates, the annulus is shorter and wider and behaves like an orifice

and is therefore density-dependent. Thus rotameters are only calibrated for a particular dry gas. The weight of the bobbin decides the pressure of operation of the rotameter and is thus constant.

The flow rate indicated by the rotameter is normally read from the top of the bobbin against a scale, but the exact reading point from the bobbin must be shown diagrammatically on the apparatus. Calibration of a rotameter can be calculated from physical principles by knowing the weight of the bobbin and the taper of the tube or, more practically, it can have its scale marked on to it when different constant flows of gas are applied. The scale is not normally marked from zero since, at flow rates giving positions near to the bottom of the tube, inaccuracies are more likely to occur. The minimum flow scale mark is the first with reliable accuracy.

The scale on a rotameter need not be linear if a non-linear taper is used. Figure 4.13 shows a rotameter flow tube with a shallow taper for increased sensitivity at low flows, then a deeper taper for higher flow rates to allow a greater range. An alternative arrangement, allowing improved accuracy, is the use of double flowmeter tubes in series (cascade flowmeters), where the first much narrower tube (and lighter bobbin) has a more gentle taper to allow an expanded scale at low flows (typically reading from $0.25\,l\,min^{-1}$ to $1.0\,l\,min^{-1}$).

The accuracy of the rotameter is dependent on the bobbin being consistently in the centre of the tube. Variation away from the centre might lead to a change in effective annulus area or changes in flow pattern around the bobbin, affecting the consistency of the differential pressure generated. Thus rotameter accuracy is dependent on the tube being vertical. Most bobbins used in rotameters in anaesthetic equipment are also spin stabilized to keep them in the centre of the tube. This is done by cutting angled slots in the top flange of the bobbin (Fig. 4.12) to act as windmill vanes. A further design feature is to have a bobbin with a low centre of gravity so that it is more stable in the gas flow.

It is important that the only forces acting on the bobbin are those generated by the differential pressure due to flow and the force of gravity. Static electricity or extra drag, due to dirt on the tube sides, can both lead to under-reading. Static electricity may be neutralized by having earthing wires or springs at the top or bottom of the tube. If the bobbin is not spinning easily, momentarily changing the flow to either zero or maximum, forces the bobbin to touch these wires and can restore normal working. However, in the case of wires at the top of the tube, it is

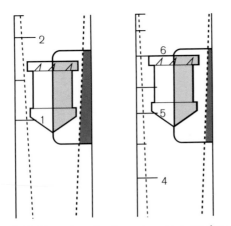

Figure 4.12 The rotameter. In each case, a portion of the tube has been cut away to show that the gap, or annulus, varies with the flow rate. The calibration should be read from the top of the float (e.g. in the right-hand diagram the flow rate is $6\,l\,min^{-1}$).

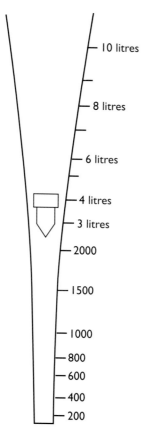

Figure 4.13 A flowmeter tube with varying taper to give an elongated scale at lower flow rates but allowing calibration for high flow rates also.

possible in some older designs for the bobbin to become stuck and apparently indicate an erroneous high flow rate, so caution is recommended. Alternative precautions against the effect of static electricity can be to disperse the static on the tube by spraying it with water or coating the internal surface of the tube with an invisible thin conductive layer of gold.

Erroneous assumptions of zero flow can be made if the bobbin is not easily visible when at the top of its travel in the flowmeter tube. This risk has since been designed out by placing a stop lower down in the tube.

Constant temperature hot-wire anemometry

Until recently, the only type of fresh gas supply flowmeter on the anaesthetic machine would have been the rotameter. However, the desire to integrate the functions of the anaesthetic machine with both patient monitoring and ventilator control, in order to create a single inte-

grated anaesthesia workstation, has produced the need to measure gas flows in ways that can be linked to electrical outputs. Differential pressure flowmeters, when combined with solid-state pressure transducers, can produce an electrical output of fresh gas flow and/or respiratory flows in ventilators. An alternative is the hot-wire anemometer, which can now be used more freely than in the past as flammable anaesthetic agents have been taken out of service.

Anemometry is the measurement of the velocity of gas flow. If that flow is contained in a tube of fixed cross-sectional area, then it is easy to calibrate flow rate in terms of gas velocity. If a wire is heated to a fixed temperature above ambient and placed in a gas flow, the rate that heat is lost from the wire is dependant on the surface area of the wire, the density, viscosity and specific heat of the gas and the velocity of the gas flow across the wire. In fact, the rate of heat loss is proportional to the square root of the velocity of the gas.

In constant temperature hot-wire anemometry, the wire forms part of a Wheatstone Bridge arrangement (Fig. 4.14), which measures the instantaneous resistance of the wire. The resistance will increase as cooling occurs. The output from the Wheatstone Bridge is fed to an electronic amplifier, the output from which is used to control the current going to the hot-wire to keep it at a constant temperature/resistance. Thus, the output from the amplifier becomes a measurement of the heat transfer from the wire and hence the gas velocity.

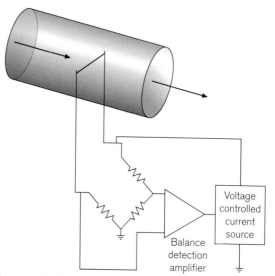

Figure 4.14 Schematic of a hot wire anemometer in a Wheatstone Bridge arrangement.

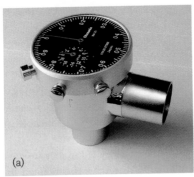
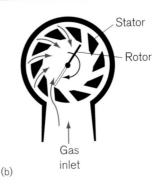

Stator

Rotor

Gas
inlet

(a)   (b)

Figure 4.15 (a) Inferential type flowmeter colloquially referred to as the Wright's respirometer. **(b)** Plan view of the Wright's respirometer.

Hot-wire anemometers (see Fig. 12.7) are very sensitive and have very fast response times. As well as being used as sensors of fresh gas flow, they can also be used as sensors of respiratory gas flows. However, since the heat transfer from the wire is dependant on the physical properties of the gas and hence its chemical composition, some care in calibrating the anemometer for changes in inspiratory/expiratory gas composition and humidity is required.

Mechanical flowmeters

The term 'mechanical flowmeter' can be conveniently adopted to cover all flowmeters where there is a mechanism in the path of the flow that moves continuously at a speed that is proportional to the flow rate. In anaesthesia they have tended to be turbine-based.

The Wright's respirometer

The Wright's respirometer (Fig. 4.15a) is an inferential mechanical flowmeter, or rather integrated volume meter. It is inferential in that the turbine it uses does not rely on sensing the entire flow stream but allows some of the flow to leak past the turbine vane. Its principle is shown in Fig. 4.15b.

Gas flow to be measured is deflected through a tangentially slotted stator that directs the flow onto a turbine, giving the gas a circular motion (Fig. 4.15b). The turbine is of low mass and the gas flow imparts rotation, by giving up some of its momentum. At equilibrium, the rate of rotation of the turbine is proportional to the volume flow rate. Effectively, one rotation of the turbine is equivalent to the passage of a given volume of gas through the respirometer. Thus, it can be thought of as a volume integrator rather than a true flowmeter. In the original form, which is still on sale, the movement of the turbine, is connected to a watch dial-like mechanism via a gearing mechanism and is calibrated in litres.

However, when used to measure exhaled gases containing water vapour, condensation in the gearing mechanism leads to corrosion. Also the mechanical mechanism has a high inertia, which is added to the inherent inertia of the turbine and friction in the bearings of the turbine mounting. When following the flow curve of an expiration, this inertia leads to under-reading of integrated volume at low initial flows, followed by reasonably accurate measurement in the middle part of the breath, followed by over running in the late part of the breath as flow decreases. As a result, in normal adult breathing, the inaccuracies tend to balance out giving reasonably accurate measurements of tidal volume. However, at high and low breathing rates, the inertia affects can lead to poor precision.

To reduce inertia, the mechanical linkage has been replaced with a magnetic coupling of the turbine (Fig. 4.16) to an electronic scale, where a Hall effect transducer is used to count the number of rotations of the turbine. Hall effect transducers are semi-conductor detectors that respond to very small changes in magnetic field.

The axial turbine flowmeter (Fig. 4.17)

In this system the turbine is mounted with its axis at the centre of the tube in which flow occurs. Upstream of the turbine there is a series of vanes which impart rotation to the flow. This rotation, in turn, imparts rotation to the turbine where, as in the Wright's respirometer, the rate of rotation of the turbine is proportional to the volume flow rate. Detection of the rotation is optical, with the turbine blades interrupting a light beam, which shines across the tube.

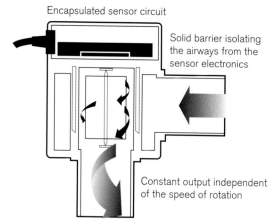

Encapsulated sensor circuit

Solid barrier isolating the airways from the sensor electronics

Constant output independent of the speed of rotation

Figure 4.16 Side view of the electronic version of Wright's respirometer.

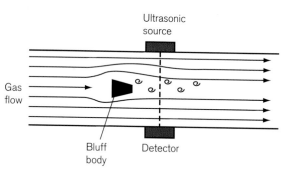

Ultrasonic source

Gas flow

Bluff body   Detector

Figure 4.18 Vortex shedding flow transducer.

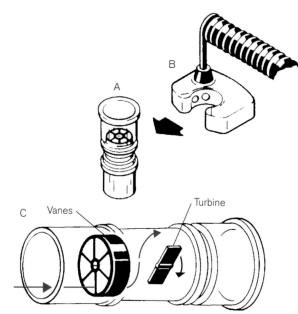

B

A

C   Vanes   Turbine

Figure 4.17 Sensor components for the Ohmeda respiratory volume monitor. This sensor assembly is composed of two parts: A, cartridge; and B, optical sensor clip; C, gas flow through cartridge.

This design of flowmeter has been used in several guises, particularly in ventilators, over a number of years. The anaesthetist will most likely have encountered it as Ohmeda's respiratory volume monitor, which is illustrated in Fig. 4.17. The advantage of the axial arrangement is that the turbine can be made lower mass and thus has less inertia than a vertical turbine, such as the Wright's

respirometer. It thus suffers from less inertia inaccuracies and is accurate over a wider range of flow rates.

Ultrasonic flowmeters

Ultrasonic flowmeters are being increasingly used for anaesthetic gas flow measurement. Two forms have been used: *Vortex shedding* and *Time of Flight*.

The vortex shedding ultrasonic flow transducer

The schematic of a vortex shedding ultrasound flow transducer is shown in Fig. 4.18. It consists of a tube in the middle of which is a bluff body that is designed to create vortices of turbulence downstream in its wake. The number of vortices that are shed is linearly proportional to the flow rate. The vortices are detected by their disruption of a narrow ultrasonic beam placed downstream at right-angles to the flow. By putting a second bluff body, facing the opposite way to the right of the ultrasonic detectors, the transducer can be made bi-directional and can detect reciprocating respiratory flows. Changes in gas composition can affect the rate of vortex shedding but the transducer is relatively insensitive to gas composition change.

The time-of-flight ultrasonic flow transducer

The schematic of the time-of-flight ultrasonic flow transducer is shown in Fig. 4.19. Two ultrasound transmitter/receivers are placed, facing each other, in the middle of the flow. In an alternative design, they are placed facing at each other across the flow steam at an oblique angle. They alternately give ultrasound pulses that each other receive. The time-of-flight of these upstream and downstream pulses is measured. Upstream into the flow, the time-of-flight is increased by the flow velocity, whilst downstream it is reduced by the flow velocity. Given the distance between the transducers, the velocity of flow can be

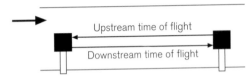

Figure 4.19 Time-of-flight transducer.

calculated from the length and the difference of the reciprocals of the two times of flight.

The measurement is actually a variety of anemometry. The absolute time-of-flight is dependant on the speed of sound in the gas and is therefore affected by gas composition changes.

Spirometers

Spirometer is a term used to describe a device that is used to measure exhaled tidal volumes and flow rates. Vitalograph makes the most common single-breath spirometer used in anaesthesia for preoperative assessment (Fig. 4.20).

Exhaled gas from the patient fills a light-weight bellows and causes a stylus to move across a chart. At the same time, the chart is moved at a constant speed at right-angles to the stylus movement. Thus, a chart of exhaled volume against time is plotted from which volumes and flow rates may be deduced. Gradually this classical design of spirometer is being replaced with electronic versions that use differential pressure flowmeters to

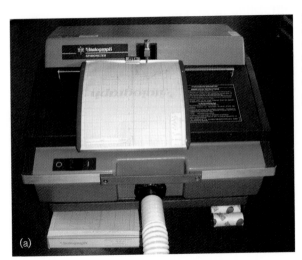

(a)

Figure 4.20 (a) The Vitalograph bellows spirometer. **(b)** Exhaled breath direct from the patient's mouth passes through the inlet causing the bellows to inflate and the stylus to mark the paper proportional to the exhaled volume. As the bellows lift off the switch, the paper carriage is moved horizontally by the motor at a constant rate so that exhaled volume is recorded against time. Typical tracings are shown in **(c)**.

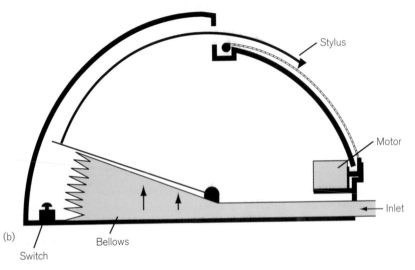

(b)

Switch

Bellows

Stylus

Motor

Inlet

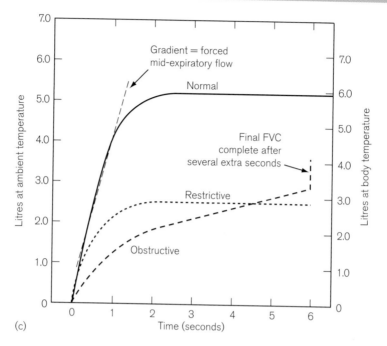

Figure 4.20, *cont'd.*

measure exhaled flow. A microprocessor is then used to integrate the obtained flow to give the characteristics graphs of Fig. 4.20c, or to perform direct calculations of forced expiratory volume (FEV), FEV_1 (forced expiratory volume in 1 s) and vital capacity (VC). This can be done in a hand-held device, such as the Vitalograph Micro shown in Fig. 4.21.

Peak flow meters

Peak expiratory flowmeters are used for the surveillance and management of chronic obstructive airways disease. Anaesthetists come across measurements of peak expiratory flow (PEF) in the preoperative assessment of surgical patients and hence should be aware of some recent developments.

The Mini-Wright peak flowmeter (Fig. 4.22) has long been in use as a low-cost device for the day-to-day measurement of PEF. Several similar designs exist, all of which, in distinction to the Wright's respirometer (see above) and full size peak flowmeter, are of the variable outlet constant pressure type.

These devices carry their own inaccuracies and were calibrated originally according to the very first type of meter that was available. However, improvements in flow

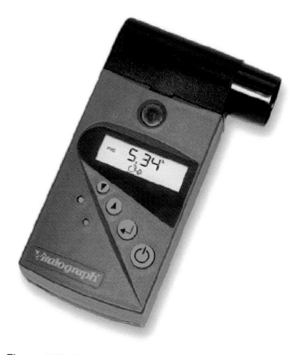

Figure 4.21 Vitalograph Micro.

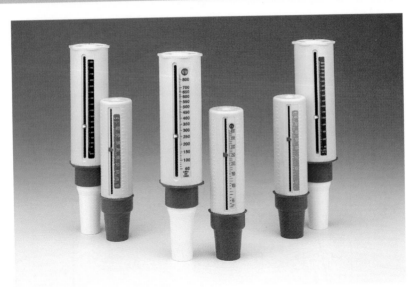

Figure 4.22 The Mini-Wright peak flowmeter – Standard and low range versions with the different calibration scales. (The long-standing Wright scale is now superseded in the EU, see text.) From left to right: Wright-McKerrow (Wright) scale, European Union scale, American Thoracic Society scale. Photo courtesy of Clement Clarke International Ltd.

calibration methods, made possible by computerized pump systems, has led to concern over the last ten years about the inaccuracies of these devices, particularly regarding over-reading in the mid-range of the meters. As a consequence, the European Community has issued a new standard, EN 13826, enforceable from 2004, which will allow only devices meeting these more stringent accuracy requirements to be CE marked. From 2004, Mini-Wright peak flowmeters have a new EU scale and clinicians need to become familiar with revized 'normal' values for PEF in health and disease states.

FURTHER READING

Hemmings HC, Hopkins PM (eds.) (2004) *Foundations of Anesthesia: Basic and Clinical Sciences* 2nd edn. Elsevier Science.

Roberts F (2003) 'Measurement of Volume and Flow in Gases'. In: *Anaesthesia and Intensive Care Medicine* The Medicine Publishing Company Ltd.

Miller MR (2004) Peak expiratory flow meter scale changes: implications for patients and health professionals. *The Airways Journal* **2(2)**: 80–82.

5

Vaporizers

Andrew J Davey

Many inhalational anaesthetic agents are liquids under normal storage conditions and need to be in a vapour form before they can be administered to a patient. In order that they may be administered safely, an understanding of the phenomenon of vaporization is required.

LAWS OF VAPORIZATION

Molecules of a liquid have a mutual attraction for each other (a phenomenon called cohesion), which is sufficiently great for them to remain in close proximity. But they also possess varying degrees of kinetic energy and are in constant motion, colliding with each other. If the liquid has a surface exposed to air or other gases, or to a vacuum, some molecules with a high kinetic energy will escape from this surface, resulting in the process of evaporation or vaporization. The molecules from the liquid, which exist in the gaseous phase, are known collectively as a vapour. This vapour exerts a pressure on its surroundings, which is then known as vapour pressure. If the space above the liquid is enclosed, some of the molecules that have escaped while moving freely in the gaseous state will collide with the surface of the liquid and re-enter it. Eventually, there will occur an equilibrium in which the number of molecules re-entering the liquid equals the number leaving it. At this stage the vapour pressure is at a maximum for the temperature of the liquid and so is called the saturated vapour pressure (SVP).

Factors affecting vaporization of a liquid
Temperature
Vaporization is increased if the temperature of the liquid is raised, since more molecules will have been given sufficient kinetic energy to escape. Figure 5.1 shows the vapour pressure curves of volatile anaesthetic agents (as well as water) and shows how they vary with temperature. If the liquid is heated, a point is reached at which the SVP becomes equal to ambient atmospheric pressure. Vaporization now occurs not only at the surface of the liquid, but also in the bubbles that develop within its substance. The liquid is now boiling and this temperature is its boiling point.

The boiling point of a liquid may therefore vary with atmospheric pressure. At high altitudes (where the air is thinner and has a lower ambient pressure) there is a significant depression of the boiling point. This may render the administration of agents with low boiling

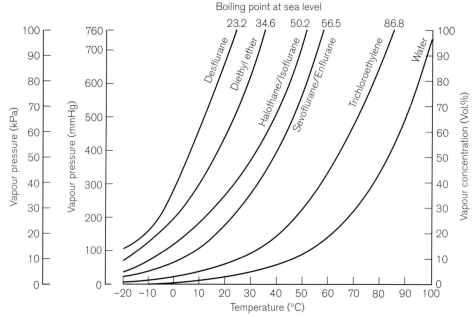

Figure 5.1 Vapour pressure curves for anaesthetic agents.

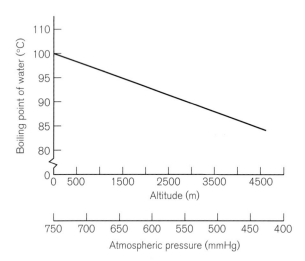

Figure 5.2 Variation of boiling point of water with atmospheric pressure or altitude.

points, such as ether, difficult. Figure 5.2 shows the depression of the boiling point for water with change in atmospheric pressure.

Volatility

The speed at which a liquid vaporizes depends not only on its temperature and ambient pressure, but also on its volatility. A more volatile liquid has weaker cohesive forces between its molecules, such that they require less energy (i.e. a lower temperature) to vaporize (Fig. 5.1).

The surface area of the liquid

The greater the surface area of the liquid, the more space there is for molecules to leave the liquid. Vaporization is therefore proportional to the surface area of the liquid.

Removal of vapour from the vicinity of liquid

If the container holding the liquid is not closed, molecules will still leave the liquid and some will escape into the atmosphere. Some, however, will collide with adjacent vapour molecules and be bounced back into the liquid. If a gas is passed across the surface of the liquid, vapour will be removed more quickly allowing fresh vapour to form. Vaporization is therefore proportional to gas flow (convection) across the surface of the liquid (provided the temperature of the latter remains constant).

A liquid at a given temperature has a mixture of molecules with varying energies. Vapour molecules entering the vapour phase tend to be the ones with the highest energy (the hottest). The remaining liquid molecules have a lower average kinetic energy (and therefore a lower temperature). Fewer molecules remain with sufficient energy to form a vapour and so vaporization decreases.

VAPORIZING SYSTEMS

The various organic liquids that possess anaesthetic properties are too potent to be used as pure vapours and so are diluted in a carrier gas such as air and/or oxygen, or nitrous oxide and oxygen. The device that allows vaporization of the liquid anaesthetic agent and its subsequent admixture with a carrier gas for administration to a patient is called a *vaporizer*. It must be constructed so that it provides a stable and predictable concentration of anaesthetic vapour when used under normal operating conditions (temperature and barometric pressure) and at flows rates of gas used by the rest of the anaesthetic delivery system.

In addition to this, a suitable method of calibrated dilution of the vapour is required as even the least potent of volatile anaesthetic agents is too powerful to be administered as a saturated vapour.

TYPES OF VAPORIZER

Suitable vaporization may be achieved by either:
- splitting the carrier gas flow so that only a portion passes through the vaporizer. This picks up saturated vapour and then leaves to mix with the remainder of the gas that has gone through a bypass. The final concentration may be altered by varying the splitting ratio between bypass gas and vaporizer gas, using an adjustable valve. This type is often referred to as a *variable bypass vaporizer* (Fig. 5.3); or
- alternatively, the vaporizer can be constructed so that it heats the anaesthetic agent to a temperature above its boiling point (in order that it may behave as a gas) and which can then be metered into the fresh gas flow (Fig. 5.4a). Similarly, a vaporizer may contain a fine metal sieve that is submerged in the anaesthetic agent and through which a small independent gas supply (normally oxygen) can be made to pass. The minute bubbles produced have a very large surface area and produce a saturated vapour at ambient pressure, which can then be passed through a flowmeter into the fresh gas flow (Fig. 5.4b). These types of vaporizer are often referred to as *measured flow vaporizers*.

It should also be noted that the various anaesthetic inhalational agents currently available have widely differing potencies and physical properties and hence require devices constructed specifically for each agent. Very potent agents (halothane, enflurane, sevoflurane,

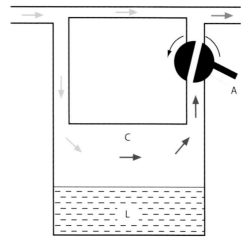

Figure 5.3 A schematic diagram of a variable bypass vaporizer. A, flow splitting valve that can be rotated to alter the relative diameters of the vaporizer and bypass channels and so vary the flows through them; L, Liquid; C, vaporizer chamber.

isoflurane and desflurane) require vaporizers that can accurately control the concentration of vapour leaving the vaporizer. However, agents such as diethyl ether, with a lower potency, may be used safely with simpler apparatus (if necessary), in which the vapour concentration is not accurately known, since there is less risk of over-dosage.

Variable bypass vaporizers
Design features
Surface area of contact between carrier gas and the liquid
Vaporizers, which are required to be very accurate, should always present a saturated vapour to the carrier gas across a wide range of flows. To ensure sufficient vaporization at the highest planned flow, a sufficiently large surface area of liquid should be present. This size is also governed by the volatility of the agent used. A highly volatile liquid will require a smaller surface area The surface area for vaporization of a liquid can be increased by causing it to spread (by capillarity) over a large sheet of porous material which may be folded in such a way that the carrier gas passes across its entire surface (Fig. 5.5).

Temperature
As vaporization progresses, the vaporizing liquid as well as the vaporizer cools and the quantity of vapour produced decreases. In an attempt to retain the performance of the device, the temperature drop is minimized or prevented by the incorporation of a heat source (heat sink). This

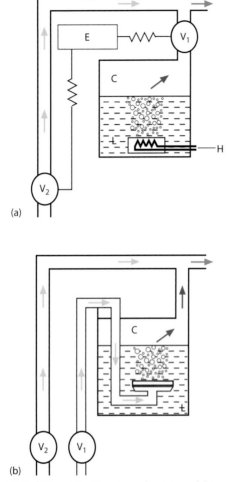

Figure 5.4 Schematic diagrams of measured flow vaporizers. **(a)** H, electric heater; L, liquid anaesthetic agent; C, vaporizer chamber; V_1, V_2, flow control valves; E, electronic valve controller to proportion flows. **(b)** L, liquid anaesthetic agent; C, vaporizer chamber; V_1, V_2, flow control valves.

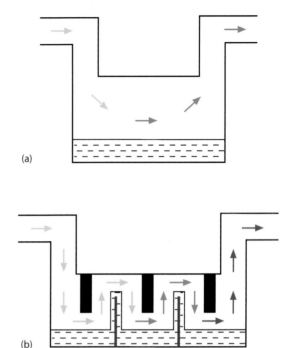

Figure 5.5 Vapour pick-up in vaporizers. **(a)** Carrier gas passing over a small surface area of liquid anaesthetic agent. **(b)** The surface area for vaporization is increased by porous wicks dipped into the liquid. The carrier gas is also made to pass close to the surface of the liquid by the baffles and thus increasing vapour pick-up.

normally takes the form of a water bath or substantial metal jacket or even a heating element surrounding the vaporizing liquid. These devices may also control the temperature of the carrier gas entering the vaporizer. Metal jackets and water baths, however, can only transfer a finite quantity of heat and so only minimize the inevitable fall in temperature.

In order to maintain the expected output of the vaporizer when this occurs, a greater proportion of carrier gas is required to pass through the vaporizing chamber in order to collect sufficient vapour molecules. This is achieved by using devices that sense temperature changes (temperature-compensating devices (Fig. 5.6) and which then alter the flow through the vaporizer.

Two types are commonly used.

1. The first (Fig. 5.6a & b) consists of two dissimilar metals or alloys placed back to back (i.e. a bi-metallic strip). As the two metals have different rates of expansion and contraction with temperature, the device has the ability to 'bend'. It can therefore be used to vary the degree of occlusion in the aperture of a gas channel (usually the bypass) and thus alter the flow of carrier gases through it.

2. In the second arrangement (Fig. 5.6c & d), the bi-metallic device consists of a central rod made of Invar, a metal alloy with a low coefficient of expansion, sitting inside a brass jacket, the top part of which is attached to the roof of the vaporizing chamber. The rod is attached only at the base of the brass jacket, which has a higher coefficient of expansion. The outer surface of the jacket is immersed in liquid anaesthetic agent in the vaporizing chamber. As the aforementioned liquid cools, the brass jacket contracts more than the

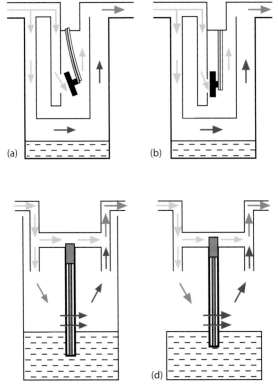

Figure 5.6 Temperature-compensating devices. **(a)** The bi-metallic strip in a vaporizer bypass operating at ambient temperature. **(b)** The same device operating at a cooler temperature; the bi-metallic strip has moved closer to the inflow increasing the resistance in the bypass and increasing the amount of gas passing through the vaporizing chamber and therefore increasing vapour pick-up. **(c)** A bi-metallic arrangement that works on a similar principle. The inner rod is made of Invar, a relatively non-expansile metal. The outer jacket is in contact with the vaporizing liquid and is made of an expansile metal (brass). **(d)** When this contracts (with cooling) it drags the choke on the inner rod into the bypass, increasing the resistance to flow through it.

Invar, which is pushed upwards into the bypass, restricting the flow of gas.

In heated vaporizers, the heating elements are thermostatically controlled. They are therefore automatically temperature compensated and do not require the addition of the devices above.

Potency of anaesthetic agent

As described above, current anaesthetic vapours are too potent to be administered as saturated vapours and require suitable dilution. Therefore, only a proportion of

the gas intended for the patient is diverted in the vaporizer to collect vapour. This amount may be varied to produce the desired concentration by using an adjustable flow-splitting valve (see Fig. 5.3). This is usually a rotary valve incorporated within the vaporizer outlet. It proportions the flow of gas between the vaporizing chamber and the vaporizer bypass system, thus controlling the final vapour composition (i.e. the more gas going through the vaporizer chamber, the greater the amount of vapour leaving the vaporizer). The flow-splitting valve is calibrated in percentage of the vapour in the final gas/vapour composition. However, this valve is accurate only if the vaporizer is temperature-compensated (see above). As both the temperature-compensating mechanism and the flow-splitting valve work by altering resistance through the vaporizer, the devices are dependent on each other. Therefore, each vaporizer for a designated anaesthetic agent is individually calibrated at the factory (see below) for that agent and at a specific temperature and flow rate of carrier gas.

As the potency of anaesthetic agents varies widely, the flow splitting ratios must be individually tailored for each agent and vaporizer design. Agents with high potency will require a wide splitting ratio so that a smaller amount of gas passes through the vaporizer. This produces a lower final concentration when mixed with bypass gas.

Volatility

The flow splitting ratio must also be adjusted to match the volatility of the agent. For example, at any given temperature, a very volatile agent will produce a higher saturated vapour pressure than a less volatile agent, even though they may have similar potencies. The former, however, requires a flow-splitting valve with a wider ratio so as to increase the dilution in order to provide a similar concentration. Table 5.1 shows the relative potency and volatility of some liquid anaesthetic agents that influence vaporizer design.

Types of variable bypass vaporizers
Draw-over vaporizers

The early vaporizers relied on the patient's respiratory effort to draw gas over the vaporizing surface (hence their name). Unfortunately, draw-over systems are subjected to very variable flow rates, i.e. from 0 to $60 \, l \, min^{-1}$ (the peak inspiratory flow in a hyperventilating adult). At these higher flows the carrier gas may fail to pick up a saturated vapour resulting in a reduced concentration leaving the vaporizer. Furthermore, the gas pathways must

Table 5.1 Relative potency and volatility of some liquid anaesthetic agents

Agent	Volatility			Potency
	Boiling point (°C) at 100 kPa	SVP at 20°C (kPa)	SVP at 20°C (mmHg)	MAC (vol%) in 100% O_2
Desflurane	23	88.5	669	6
Diethyl ether	35	57.9	440	19
Isoflurane	48	31.5	240	1.15
Halothane	51	31.9	243	0.76
Enflurane	56	23.1	175	1.68
Sevoflurane	58	21.3	156–170	2

MAC, minimum alveolar concentration
SVP, saturated vapour pressure

offer little resistance to flow so as not to compromise the patient's inspiratory effort. This restricts the design of the vaporizer components, especially the flow splitting valve (see above) which must have sufficiently wide a bore. It is very difficult to design a flow-splitting valve that will work accurately over a wide range of flow rates, i.e. $1–60 \, l \, min^{-1}$. As discussed above, the valve must present a low flow resistance so that at flows of $60 \, l \, min^{-1}$ (the peak flow in a patient breathing spontaneously), no respiratory embarrassment is caused. However, if the flow across this valve drops to about $4 \, l \, min^{-1}$, the resistance through the valve will be so low that carrier gas will preferentially pass across the bypass channel rather than through the vaporizing chamber where it has to mix with and then push the 'heavy' vapour out into the attached breathing system. At this flow and below, there is thus bound to be a marked fall in vaporizer performance.

Plenum vaporizers

A vaporizer could be made more accurate if the carrier gas was pressurized to make it as dense as the vapour, so that at lower flows it would more readily mix with this rather than tend to pass above it in the vaporizing chamber. Furthermore, if a smaller, continuous flow of gas, i.e. $0–15 \, l \, min^{-1}$ were used, there would be a less rapid removal of vapour, ensuring that a saturated vapour was present at all times. This would allow the vaporizer to be calibrated very accurately. This type is usually referred to as a plenum vaporizer (plenum being the term which describes a pressurized chamber). The typical flow resistance ($2 \, kPa$ ($22 \, cm \, H_2O$) at $5 \, l \, min^{-1}$) found in

plenum vaporizers, renders them unsuitable for use as draw-over vaporizers. The high intermittent flow rates in a breathing system, generated by a spontaneously breathing patient or a mechanical ventilator, are accommodated by siting a reservoir (bag or bellows) downstream, which stores gas and vapour during exhalation.

However, flowmeters on an anaesthetic machine are calibrated for use at or around atmospheric pressure. Therefore, the final design of a plenum vaporizer develops from a compromise between the high carrier gas pressures required for accurate vapour delivery, and the low pressures required to maintain the accuracy of the flowmeters.

FACTORS AFFECTING VAPORIZER PERFORMANCE

Extremes of temperature

It is obvious that a temperature-compensating mechanism can operate only within a reasonable temperature range. At too low a temperature, vaporization will be low, and it may be uncontrollably high when it is too hot.

Barometric pressure

Ideally, a vaporizer should also be calibrated at a specific barometric pressure. Strictly speaking, as a saturated vapour is only altered by temperature, one might expect the calibration of a vaporizer to be independent of barometric pressure. However, changes in barometric pressure will affect the carrier gas composition passing through the vaporizer, which in turn will affect the concentration of vapour in the mixture leaving it. For example, when the barometric pressure is reduced (at altitude), the number of molecules of carrier gas flowing through the vaporizer is reduced. However, the number of vapour molecules collected by the gas in the vaporizing chamber remains unchanged, although these now represent a higher percentage of the total number of molecules leaving the vaporizer. This effect, however, is so small under the normal operating conditions, that it is inconsequential. However, extremes of pressure may have a significant effect. For example, at very high altitude (low barometric pressure), a very volatile liquid such as ether may boil at ambient temperature. This may render the use of such agents difficult. Figure 5.2 shows the variation of boiling point with atmospheric pressure.

Pumping effect

When a resistance is applied to the outlet of the anaesthetic machine, such as that which occurs when manually assisted or controlled ventilation is used, or with ventilators that are powered by the fresh gas flow (e.g. Manley ventilators), there is an increase in the anaesthetic gas pressure, which is transmitted back to the vaporizer. This back pressure is intermittent and variable. When it occurs, it causes carrier gas within the vaporizer to be compressed. Gas in the outlet is already saturated and therefore cannot pick up any more vapour. When the back pressure is released, the expanding carrier gas, which is also saturated with vapour, surges out through both the inlet and outlet of the vaporizer chamber. The gas that leaves the inlet enters the bypass and adds to the vaporizer output to increase in the final vapour output. (Fig.5.7 demonstrates the sequence of events.)

This effect can be minimized by the fitting of internal compensating mechanisms. It may be achieved either by:
- increasing the resistance to flow through the vaporizer and bypass so that the carrier gas develops a higher pressure within the vaporizer, so as to reduce the pumping effect. However, the pressure increase due to vaporizer design should be as small as possible as these pressures are transmitted back to the flowmeters, which are calibrated for use at atmospheric pressure.
- building an elongated flow passage into either the inlet or outlet of the vaporizer to minimize the effect of surges in pressure (Fig. 5.8). Some vaporizer designs employ both mechanisms. The former cannot be fitted

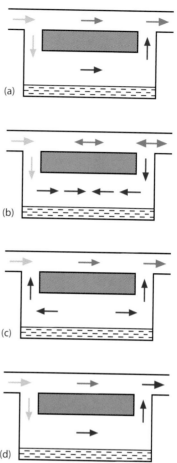

Figure 5.7 (a) Flow through vaporizer with no back pressure. **(b)** Back-up pressure and/or reverse flow causing build-up of carrier gas in the vaporizer chamber. **(c)** Release of back pressure causing gas and saturated vapour to escape through the vaporizer inlet and outlet and into the bypass. **(d)** Anaesthetic vapour in the bypass gas added to that from the vapour outlet so increasing the final vapour concentration.

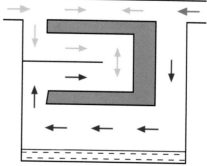

Figure 5.8 Elongation of the inflow channel in a vaporizer preventing saturated vapour reaching the bypass.

to draw over vaporizers as they would produce too great a resistance to flow (see below, Temperature-compensated vaporizers).

Furthermore, where plenum vaporizers are fitted, some anaesthetic machines now incorporate a non-return valve on the end of the back bar, so that the back pressure surges on the vaporizer are reduced. However, pressure still builds up to some extent in the back bar when the non-return valve closes due to higher downstream pressure.

Liquid levels

The liquid level within the vaporizing chamber may affect performance. If the vaporizer is overfilled, insufficient exposed surface area of wick may cause a drop in vapour output. Additionally, over-filling may result in dangerously high concentrations, due to spillage of liquid agent into the bypass.

Anaesthetic agents

The anaesthetic agent halothane contains a stabilizing agent, thymol. This is a waxy substance which, if left in the vaporizer, would clog the felt or cotton wick found in older models, reducing the potential surface area for vaporization. This would then reduce the vaporizer performance. Thymol would also 'gum up' the vaporizer, making the control knob difficult to adjust, as well as compromising the internal mechanism. The manufacturers, therefore, used to advise that the liquid agent be drained off and replenished at intervals. This advice should be tempered by consideration of economy and the frequency with which the vaporizer is employed. Recent models from most manufacturers for use with halothane have wicks made from synthetic materials that do not absorb thymol into the fabric, so many can now recommend a service interval (often with a change of wick) of 5 years. Vaporizers used with other agents often have a 10 year service interval.

Carrier gas composition

Vaporizer output may be affected when the carrier gas composition is changed. This is due to changes in viscosity and density, which alter the performance of the flow-splitting valve. Increasing the concentration of nitrous oxide reduces the vapour concentration. This is of little importance in clinical practice at present. However, the interest in the gas Xenon (which is five times as heavy as air), as a potential anaesthetic, may change this. There is also a further mechanism causing a change in vaporizer output when nitrous oxide concentrations are increased. Nitrous oxide dissolves in volatile agents, so that the effective total gas flow through the vaporizer is temporarily reduced.

Stability

Some vaporizers, if tilted or inverted, may allow the liquid agent to contaminate the bypass. This has caused a fatality in the past when a vaporizer was accidentally overturned prior to attachment to the machine.

Summary of vaporizer performance

Vaporizer performance can thus be affected by:

- temperature (unless the vaporizer includes some compensatory device that minimizes the effect of temperature, such as a heat sink and/or temperature compensator);
- flow, all vaporizers are affected to some degree by flow (performance data are usually available from the manufacturer). Plenum vaporizers perform better than draw-over vaporizers;
- barometric pressure (minimal effect in clinical practice);
- variable vaporizer working pressures (back pressure surges);
- liquid levels within the vaporizer;
- movement and tilting of vaporizers (see below, under Specific vaporizers);
- carrier gas composition;
- stabilizers in the inhalational agent (e.g. thymol).

CALIBRATION OF VAPORIZERS

Vaporizers designed to give an accurate output are individually calibrated prior to leaving the factory. Typically, they are filled with the designated anaesthetic agent and left in a room at a standard temperature (23°C) for 4 hours. A blank control dial (linked to a computer) is attached and rotated at various carrier gas flow rates. The output concentration is measured using a sample that is analyzed by a refractometer (see Fig. 17.3). The dial (which has a unique serial number) is then removed and a calibration scale etched onto it from the information stored on the computer. It is then re-attached to that same vaporizer and the calibration confirmed prior to leaving the factory. Vaporizers may also have the calibration confirmed in a similar manner, following servicing.

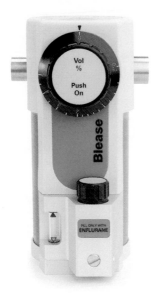

Figure 5.9 Screw fill port on a vaporizer.

FILLING OF VAPORIZERS

In the original plenum vaporizers, a screw-threaded stopper in the filling port was simply unscrewed, liquid agent was added and the stopper reconnected. These systems were criticized and have largely disappeared from use as the vaporizer could easily be filled with the wrong agent. Despite this, they are still supplied by all the major manufacturers for certain countries (Fig. 5.9) and are referred to as 'screw-fill' systems.

Agent-specific filling devices (in the UK) (Fraser Sweatman pin safety system) were introduced by Cyprane (which became Ohmeda and is now part of G.E. Systems) in the early 1980s, in which the distal end was keyed to fit a vaporizer calibrated and labelled for a specific agent and the proximal end keyed to fit only the neck of the bottle for that agent (Fig. 5.10). This is now referred to commonly as the 'key fill' system. Although this device goes some way to reducing the potential for filling vaporizers with the wrong agent, it is by no means foolproof. Some countries take supplies of agent in large bottles and then subsequently decant into smaller bottles. Early supplies of isoflurane into the UK could be fitted (prior to 1984) to enflurane-keyed fillers. The two most recent agents, sevoflurane and desflurane, are presented

in sealed bottles to which the agent specific filling device is already fitted and made tamper proof with a crimped metal seal. The filling devices also have valves, which are only opened when inserted fully into their respective filler ports, so as to prevent spillage (Fig. 5.11a & b). The desflurane system is called Saf-T-Fil and the sevoflurane, Quik-Fil.

EXAMPLES OF VARIABLE BYPASS VAPORIZERS

Temperature-compensated vaporizers
TEC 4 (Datex Ohmeda)
Figure 5.12 shows a TEC 4 (with a keyed filler), its mode of operation and performance charts.

When the vaporizer is attached to the back bar of an anaesthetic workstation, gases destined for the patient pass through it via three channels. In the OFF position, the gases pass through the inlet (1) and into one channel (2) across the top of the vaporizer, without coming into contact with the vaporizing chamber or the temperature compensating device, and leave through the outflow (3).

In the ON position, this pathway closes and the other two channels are open. The vaporizer channel has an elongated passage (4) that funnels carrier gas to the bottom of the vaporization chamber. Inside the latter, two concentric wicks (5) separated by a nickel-plated copper helix (6) are placed so that their bases are immersed in the reservoir of anaesthetic liquid. The latter is drawn up into the wicks, which become saturated with agent and present a very large area from which it evaporates. The gases passing through the chamber become saturated with vapour by the time they have passed between the wicks and have travelled upwards in the gaps made by the helical spacer to the rotary valve in the control knob (7). In the version used with halothane, the wicks are made from cotton and may clog up with the thymol preservative, so need to be changed every year. Vaporizers for use with other agents have a service interval of two years.

The proportion of gases passing the two channels is determined by (a) the resistance to flow in the temperature-compensating device (8) and (b) the calibrated control knob (7) which varies the resistance through both the bypass (9) and the vapour chamber exit (10). The percentage of vapour at the outlet depends on the amount of vapour-laden gases that is mixed with the fresh gases passing through the bypass. As the temperature within the vaporization chamber falls (reducing the

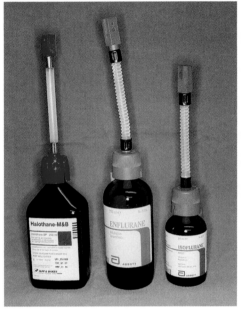

(a)

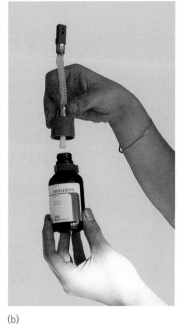

(b)

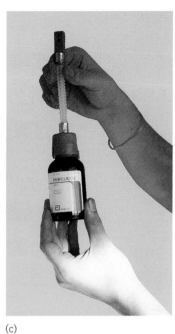

(c)

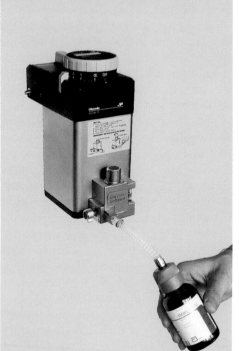

(d)

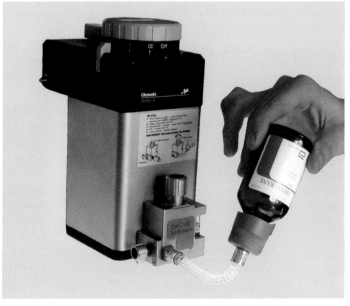

(e)

Figure 5.10 **(a)** Fraser Sweatman pin safety system for (left to right) halothane, enflurane and isoflurane. Note that the tops have unique grooves (shape and position) that fit only the specific filling ports on matching vaporizers. The screw caps for the bottles have unique grooves that fit only the collars on matching bottles. **(b)** and **(c)** A pin safety system being attached to a bottle for isoflurane; **(d)** and **(e)** the connection and filling of a vaporizer.

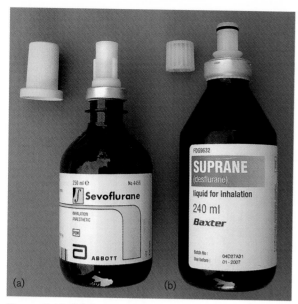

Figure 5.11 (a) A sealed bottle of sevoflurane with its uniquely shaped filler connected. Note that the filler on the bottle is secured by a crimped metal seal.
(b) Similarly, a sealed bottle of desflurane; the filler is attached at manufacture. As the contents are pressurized at ambient temperature, the glass bottle is encased in a plastic coat to prevent it exploding if damaged.

Table 5.2 Comparison of TEC vaporizers (using halothane)

Element	Cyprane TEC 4	Ohmeda TEC 5
Nominal working range		
Flow (l min^{-1})	0.25–15	0.25–15
Ambient temperature (°C)	18–35	18–35
Capacity		
With dry wicks (cm^3)	135	300
With wet wicks (cm^3)	100	225
Dimensions		
Width (mm)	105	114
Depth (mm)	145	197
Height (mm)	225	237
Temperature-compensated (ambient and cooling effect)	Yes	Yes
Pressure-compensated	Yes	Yes
Keyed filler option	Yes	Yes
Selectatec mounting option	Standard	Standard
Non-spill	Yes	Yes
Allowable tilt	180°	180°
Integral interlock	Yes	Yes
Safety 'lock-on' facility	Yes	Yes
Safety 'off/isolation' facility	Yes	Yes
Resistance to gas flow Vaporizer 'on' Carrier gas O$_2$ @ 5 l min^{-1} @ 21°C (kPa) (cmH$_2$O)	2.06–2.84 21–29	1.47–1.96 15–20

vapour concentration produced), the thermostatic valve closes. This causes a greater proportion of the total gas flow to passes through the chamber; by this means the vapour concentration in the output is kept constant.

The vaporizer has some significant design features. If it is accidentally inverted, the liquid agent will not spill into the by-pass. It also incorporates an interlock facility. If two vaporizers with this latter feature are placed on a back bar (see below), the first vaporizer to be switched on extends lateral rods that impinge on the adjacent vaporizer preventing its operation. Also, the vaporizer dial cannot be turned if the vaporizer is improperly mounted on the anaesthetic machine, i.e. not seated correctly and locked on to the back bar.

The TEC 5 and TEC 7

These vaporizers are identical in function to the TEC 4 but have larger filling capacities. The TEC 7 (Fig. 5.13a) also offers a wider selection of filler assemblies and a change in the cosmetic appearance over the TEC 5 (Fig. 5.13b) to match the manufacturer's workstation.

They have a number of design improvements over previous models. The wick assembly comprises a hollow tube of Teflon cloth held open by a steel wire spiral and wound into a helix within the vaporizer. This arrangement greatly increases the surface area for vaporization over previous Tec models. Two additional features are the improved filling action for the key fill system (Fig. 5.13a and d) and an easier mechanism than the TEC 4 for switching on the vaporizer dial and disengaging the dial lock (now a single handed action). Table 5.2 highlights the differences between TECs, 4 and 5/7.

Blease DATUM

This fulfils all the criteria for a temperature compensated vaporizer. It has:

- a heat sink;
- a thermal compensating device;

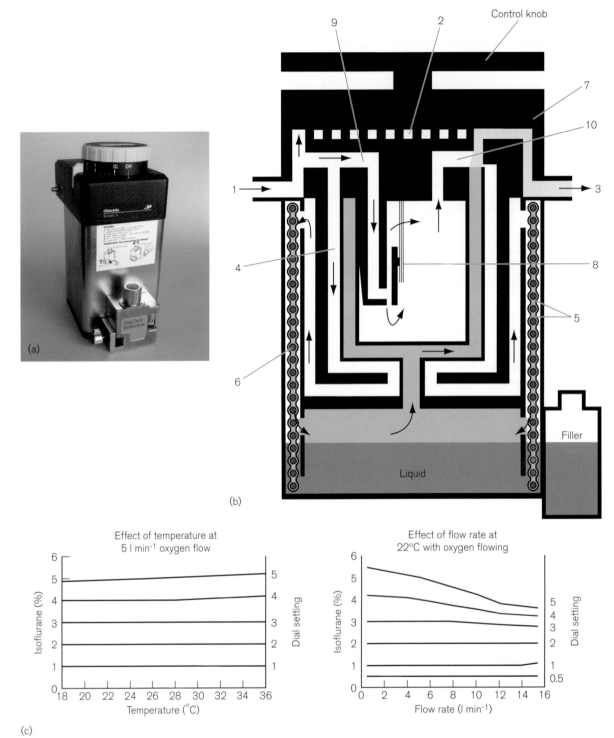

Figure 5.12 (a) The TEC 4 vaporizer. **(b)** working principles. 1 =inlet 2= bypass when off 3 = outlet 4 = vaporizer channel 5 = vaporizer wicks 6= helix wick support 7=rotary valve 8 = temperature compensating device 9 = bypass when on 10 = vapour chamber exit. **(c)** Performance characteristics for variations in temperature and flow.

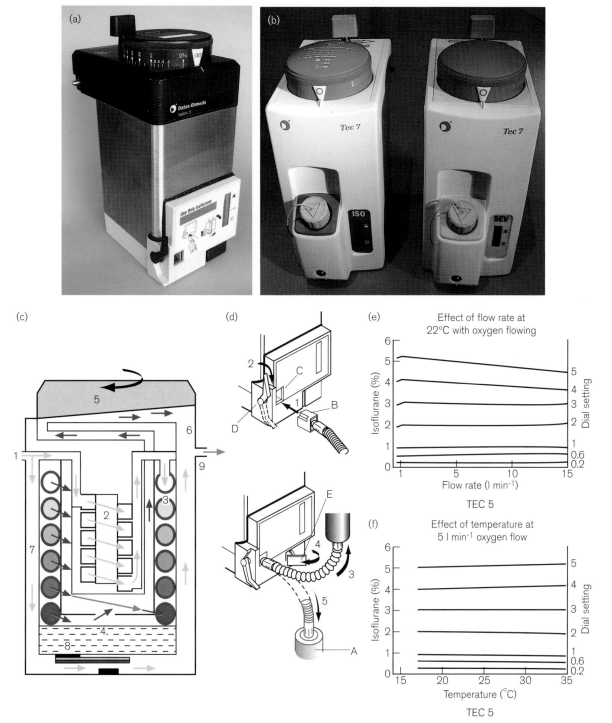

Figure 5.13 (a) The TEC 5 vaporizer. **(b)** TEC 7 vaporizers. **(c)** Working principles of TEC 5 and TEC 7 vaporizers: 1, inlet; 2, elongated passage that prevents 'pumping effect'; 3, helical wick; 4, base of vaporizing chamber; 5, rotary valve for metering vapour saturated carrier gas; 6, mixing chamber; 7, bypass; 8, temperature-compensating device; 9, outlet. **(d)** Filling the vaporizer. 1, insertion of keyed filler B into vaporizer filling port C; 2, applying the lock D to make the filler/vaporizer connection secure; 3, inverting and raising the bottle of agent to create a filling pressure; 4, opening the chamber lock E to fill the chamber; 5, lowering the bottle below the vaporizer to empty the chamber if required. **(e), (f)** Performance of TEC 5, as influenced by changes in flow rate and temperature.

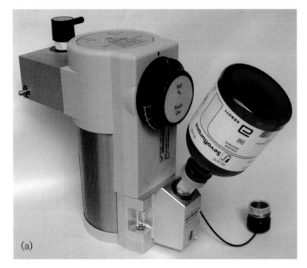

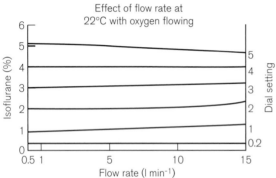

Effect of flow rate at
22°C with oxygen flowing

Effect of temperature at
5 l min⁻¹ oxygen flow

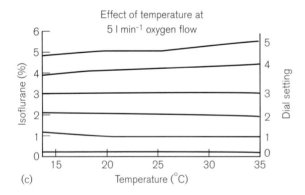

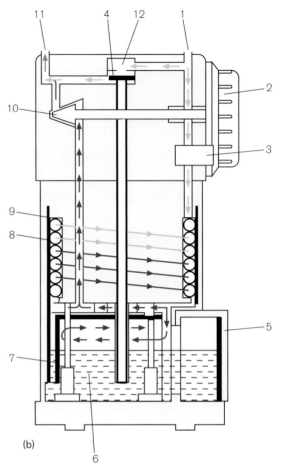

Figure 5.14 (a) The Blease Datum vaporizer with agent-specific filler for sevoflurane. **(b)** Working principles. 1, fresh gas input; 2, control dial; 3, zero lock; 4, thermal compensator rod; 5, filler block for agent-specific device; 6, agent reservoir; 7 and 9, wick extension; 8, elongated Teflon wick; 10, vapour control valve; 11 combined gas and vapour output; 12, variable resistance bypass valve. **(c)** Performance characteristics for variations in temperature and flow.

- a large surface area for vaporization; and
- an elongated inlet to minimize the damping effect.

The earlier version had a very large heat sink made of brass, in order to reduce the cooling effect of vaporization: hence the vaporizer weighed 11 kg. The latest version (Fig. 5.14a) has an improved thermal conductivity and now weighs 7.5 kg. The earlier version had a stainless steel outer covering but was separated from the main body of the vaporizer by a layer of plastic. The latter has been removed to improve the absorption of radiant heat from the surroundings and has enabled less brass to be used. The heavy weight of the vaporizer helps to seat the vaporizer firmly on the back bar when it is connected to the anaesthetic workstation and so reduces the potential for leaks. The working principles of the vaporizer are shown in Fig. 5.14b.

The wick is made from a long tube of PTFE (Teflon) wadding that is supported internally by a wire coil (8). This is wound into a spiral to create a large surface area for contact with carrier gas that passes through the tube. At the base of the spiral, the Teflon is made to drape into the liquid reservoir (7). The material has a high capillarity to ensure that the wick is saturated at all times, even when the reservoir is low (liquid level compensation).

In the OFF position, there is a 'zero lock' (3) on the dial that isolates the vaporization chamber so that all the patient designated gas travels through the bypass. In the ON position this gas is split into two flows. One passes through the elongated wick (8), collecting vapour, the elongated passage behaving as a damping device to counteract the pumping effect. From here, the gas, which is now saturated with anaesthetic vapour, travels through to the vapour control valve (10), operated by the control dial (2). It then joins the remainder of the gas in the bypass. A thermal compensator (4) alters the flow through the bypass (12), to correct for changes in vapour production at lower temperatures. The bi-metallic device consists of a central rod made of Invar, a metal alloy with a low coefficient of expansion, part of which sits inside a brass jacket, the top part of which is attached to the roof of the vaporizing chamber. The rod is attached only at the base of the brass jacket, which has a higher coefficient of expansion. The outer surface of the jacket is immersed in liquid anaesthetic agent in the vaporizing chamber. As the aforementioned liquid cools, the brass jacket contracts more that the Invar, which is pushed upwards into the bypass restricting the flow of gas (see Fig. 5.6 c and d).

Unlike the TEC vaporizers, the control dial may be turned on when it is not connected to a machine and so if this is left on and the vaporizer is inadvertently tipped, there is the potential for liquid anaesthetic agent to enter the bypass. However, the relevant channels are placed towards the front of the vaporization chamber near the filler block. If the vaporizer falls on its side, the filler block prevents these channels from being submerged in liquid agent. Figure 5.14 c shows the performance curves for the vaporizer.

Dräger 'Vapor' 2000 series of vaporizers

Figures 5.15 a, b and c show a vaporizer, a flow diagram and performance curves. Models in the range are all compensated for temperature and pumping effects. In the OFF position, gases destined for the patient are directed through the bypass (12) in the vaporizer without coming into contact with anaesthetic vapour.

When the vaporizer control dial is switched ON, these gases split into two flows with one part initially flowing through a series of baffles (2) that counteract pressure surges (the pumping effect). From here, it is directed through the vaporizing system, where it becomes saturated with vapour. This takes the form of a tubular wick (3) coiled in a spiral, through which the gas passes. The outer surface of the spiral is attached to a sleeve of similar material (4) that dips into the liquid anaesthetic agent in the reservoir (5), so as to keep the spiral wick soaked. The wick is made of a synthetic material with a high capillarity but which does not absorb agent. Therefore, a stabilizing agent, such as thymol that is added to halothane, will not clog the wick and reduce its efficiency. This allows the vaporizer to be used for prolonged periods between services.

From the vaporizing chamber, the saturated gases pass to a conical control valve (6), whose aperture is adjusted by the calibration dial (7). From here they pass to a mixing chamber (9), where they blend with bypass gases prior to leaving the vaporizer. If the operating temperature of the latter drops, a compensating device (8), a bi-metallic device (Fig. 5.6 c,d), proportionately decreases the flow of gases through the bypass so as to maintain the output of the vaporizer.

In the OFF position , the vaporizing chamber has a small connection to atmosphere (11) that allows some gas to escape when liquid agent is added. This makes the filling process easier.

Although the principles of vaporization are identical, the Dräger Vapor 2000 has some modifications over the previous versions that improve efficiency and safety. These are highlighted in Table 5.3.

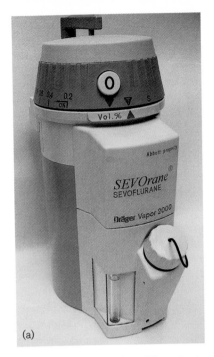

(a)

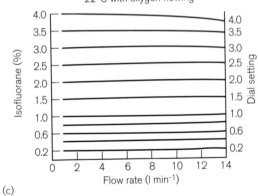

Effect of flow rate at
22°C with oxygen flowing

(c)

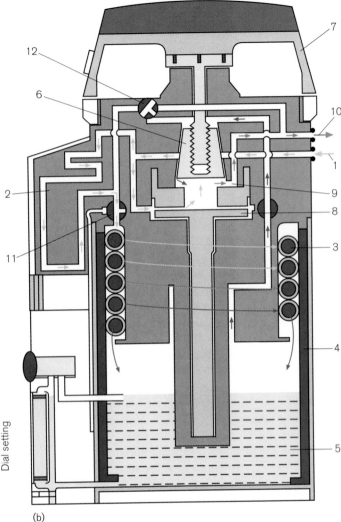

(b)

Figure 5.15 (a) Dräger Vapor 2000 vaporizer. **(b)** Working principles: 1 = gas input, 2 = damping the chamber, 3 = tubular wick, 4 = wick extension, 5 =reservoir chamber, 6 = concentration control valve, 7 = calibration dial, 8 = temperature compensation device, 9 = mixing a chamber, 10 = output, 11 = bypass tap, 12 = bypass tap.
(c) Performance characteristics.

Table 5.3 Comparison of Dräger Vapour 19 and Dräger Vapour 2000		
	Dräger Vapour 19	**Dräger Vapour 2000**
Principle of vaporization	Identical	Identical
Filling volume (ml)	140	280
Safe tilting when transporting vaporizer (degrees)	0–45	Any position
Temperature range (°C)	15–35	10–40
Flow control range	0.2–5.0 Vol. %	0.2–8.0 Vol. % Enf., Sevo 0.2–6.0 Vol. % Hal., Iso
Removal of anaesthetic agent prior to transport	Yes	No
Low flow suitability	Good	Very good
Vapour can be switched on without locking plug-in system to back bar	Possible	Not possible

Penlon Sigma Delta vaporizer

The Penlon Sigma Delta, shown in Figs. 5.16 a and b, includes all the features of a modern Plenum vaporizer.

In the OFF position, gases destined for the patient are directed via the inlet (1) through the bypass (2) to the outlet (3). A closing mechanism prevents any gases without coming into contact with anaesthetic vapour in the vaporizer

When the control knob (4) is turned on, the closing mechanism is released and a second channel is opened that ducts a portion of these gases through the vaporizing system. They pass initially through a helical damping coil (5), that prevents saturated vapour tracking back through the vaporizer and contaminating other gases in the back bar (the 'pumping effect').

From here they pass into the vaporizing chamber (6) and around the wick (7). The latter is novel in that it is made of sintered polyethylene (1 metre long), which is held in close proximity to a copper backing plate. The two are then coiled into a spiral, the top and bottom of which are made gas-tight. The carrier gases, therefore, have to pass around the spiral, coming into contact with the whole surface area of the wick. The wick assembly is designed as a cartridge for ease of removal and cleaning, and has a long service life. The recommended service interval is 5 years for halothane vaporizers and 10 years for all others.

Gases saturated with anaesthetic vapour leave the chamber and pass through an orifice whose aperture is varied by a needle valve (8) attached to the control knob.

The latter, therefore, controls the amount of vapour-laden gases flowing through the device to mix with the bypass gases.

A bi-metallic temperature-compensating element (TCE) (9) is placed in the vaporizing chamber, so that its base is immersed in the vaporizing liquid. When the liquid agent cools, the aperture of the TCE closes and diverts more gas through the vapour chamber pathway, in order to maintain the accuracy of the vaporizer output.

The vaporizer is interesting in that it is relatively light (5 kg), being made of aluminium. Aluminium has a better thermal conductivity than brass and so, despite its weight, it conducts a similar amount of radiant heat as does an equivalent sized brass device. The rotary control can be turned on when the vaporizer is disconnected from an anaesthetic workstation. If this occurs and the vaporizer is tipped on its side or inverted, then liquid vapour could enter the outflow from the vaporizing chamber.

Plenum vaporizers with electronic control

Conventionally, vaporizers have two main parts, a chamber for producing a saturated vapour, and a mechanical system for regulating gas flow through the chamber. The control of accurate vapour output requires precision engineering of expensive materials with each component, contributing a degree of variability in performance. Hence, there is the need to calibrate each vaporizer

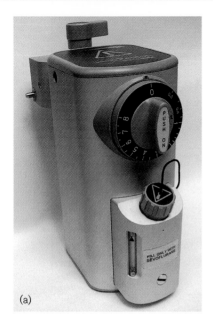

(a)

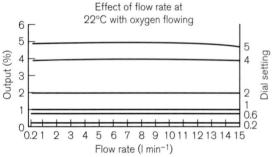

Effect of flow rate at 22°C with oxygen flowing

(c)

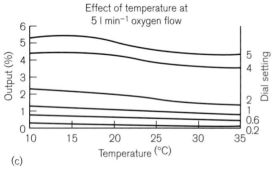

Effect of temperature at 5 l min⁻¹ oxygen flow

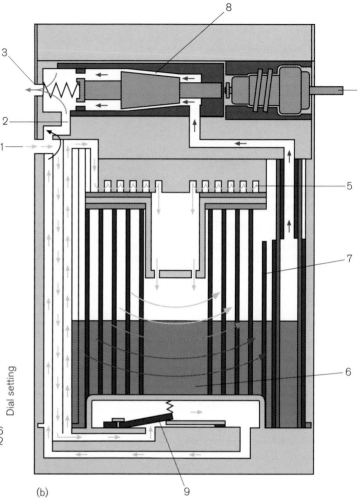

(b)

Figure 5.16 (a) Penlon Sigma Delta vaporizer. **(b)** Working principles: 1 = inlet. 2 = bypass. 3 = outlet. 4 = control knob. 5 = helical damping coil. 6 = vaporizing chamber. 7 = wick. 8 = needle valve 9 = temperature compensating element. **(c)** Performance characteristics.

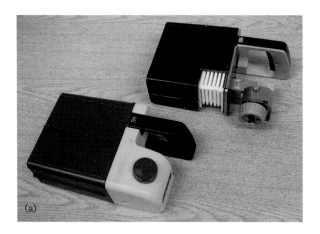

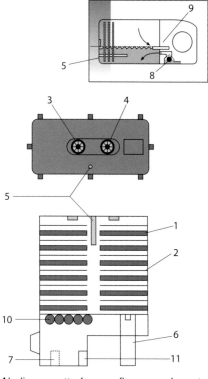

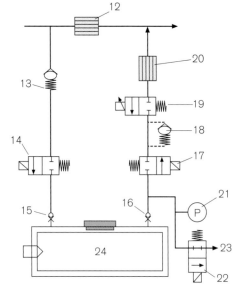

Figure 5.17 **(a)** Aladin cassette for sevoflurane and a cutaway cassette showing the lamellae. **(b)** Diagram of an Aladin cassette: 1 = lamellae, 2 = metal plate, 3 = inflow back valve, 4 = outflow back valve, 5 = temperature sensor, 6 = handle, 7 = filling system, 8 = ball valve, 9 = air channel, 10 = cassette ID magnets, 11 = liquid level window. **(c)** Diagram of the control unit: 12 = bypass flow measurement, 13 = one way valve, 14 = inflow close valve, 15 = inlet check valve, 16 = outlet check valve, 17 = outflow close valve, 18 = liquid flow prevention, 19 = proportional flow valve, 20 = agent flow measurement, 21 = cassette pressure sensor, 22 = cassette pressure relief valve, 23 = flow to scavenging, 24 = Aladin cassette.

individually and to be able to identify each component by serial number to ensure correct reassembly when serviced. With the introduction of electronics into the anaesthesia machine, it is now possible to regulate vapour concentration with electropneumatic proportional flow valves controlled by microprocessors. A single control system may be installed on a workstation and can be used for all volatile anaesthetic agents.

Datex-Ohmeda Aladin vaporizer

This has a conventional vaporizing chamber in the form of a detachable cassette and an electronic vapour control unit built into the anaesthetic workstation (see also Chapter 6, Datex-Ohmeda ADU).

The cassette

The cassette (Fig.5.17a and b) is a metal box that is divided into two sections. The larger rear section is filled with a synthetic material that behaves as a wick. It is formed into lamellae (1) interspersed with metal plates (2) to create a convoluted pathway, so as to maximize vapour pick up. The back panel has inflow (3) and outflow (4) spring loaded mechanical ball valves, to prevent a leak of agent when transported. There is also a contact (5) for the temperature sensor that is placed within the vaporizer to measure the temperature of the liquid. The front section of the unit has a handle (6) and a conventional vapour specific filling system (7) with a clear glass window displaying the liquid level. When this is used, the liquid passes into the rear section through a one-way valve (8). If the cassette is more that 7 degrees off the horizontal, this closes and the filler will not accept any further liquid into the unit. There is also an air vent (9) between the two halves. When the liquid level in the rear half reaches this, it closes and prevents overfilling. The top of the front section houses a row of five magnets (10) arranged in a sequence that provides unique vapour identification for that cassette. The latter is spill proof when transported and is maintenance free for all agents. When the cassette is plugged into the workstation, matching probes engage and open the mechanical ball valves on the back of the unit. If the workstation is in use, the temperature sensor is activated and the reed switches positioned over the magnets on the control unit, identify the agent in use.

The cassette for use with desflurane has a slightly different construction. It has no glass sight that could be damaged by the greater pressures generated by this agent when stored at room temperature.

Capacitor plates, that sense the level of agent, are fitted inside the device and three copper contacts on the top of the unit power the capacitor and transmit the information to the main workstation display, where it is displayed as a bar chart. Also there is a fan in the ADU workstation that is activated when the desflurane cassette is fitted, that directs heat from the workstation electronics onto the vaporizing chamber when this has cooled below a critical level.

The control unit

(Fig. 5.17c) This behaves as an electronic variable bypass. When the user sets an anaesthetic concentration on the front panel of the workstation, the fresh gas flow is split into two. The bulk of the gases pass across the bypass where the flow is measured (12). A smaller portion of the gases pass through a mechanical one way valve (13), through an electronic 'inflow close valve' (14), through the open ball valve (15) in the back of the cassette (that is opened when the cassette in plugged into the workstation) and into the vaporizing chamber. It picks up saturated vapour and leaves the cassette via the other open ball valve (16), an electronic 'outflow close valve' (17) and a liquid flow prevention valve (18) to the proportional flow valve (19), that controls vapour output.

From here it passes to the agent flow measurement device (20) and into the outlet of the control unit, where it joins the bypass gas in a mixing chamber. The electronic inflow and outflow valves are open when the vaporizer is in use. Otherwise they remain closed to prevent a leak of gas destined for the patient when a cassette is not attached.

A microprocessor gathers information regarding the agent used, its temperature in the cassette and the flow of gas in the bypass. It makes a calculation for the amount of agent to add to the bypass gas to provide the desired concentration and instructs the proportional flow valve to open sufficiently to provide this. The calculated vapour concentration is displayed electronically on the workstation. The outflow pathway from the cassette is fitted with an electronic pressure sensor (21). If the outflow pressure exceeds 2.5 bar, a relief valve opens (22) and vents the flow to scavenging (23).

Draw-over vaporizers

All the plenum vaporizers described above offer resistance to the gas flow. For this reason the gases have to be driven through them. However, pressurized gas sources are not always available in some countries or in certain situations. Draw-over vaporizers, with their low-resistance gas pathways can be installed within a breathing system and are, therefore, a useful alternative to plenum systems despite not being as accurate. Figure 5.18 illustrates various breathing systems in which a draw-over vaporizer has been installed. In systems a–d, exhaled gases are vented to the atmosphere, suitably scavenged where appropriate. However, in system e, the patient's exhaled gases are recirculated through the vaporizer. This is of importance, since not only will the concentration of volatile agents be increased by the repeated passage of the gases through the vaporizer, but the latter must be of a type without cloth wicks, since these could become saturated with water condensed from the expired air and so cease to function.

Typical examples of draw-over vaporizers are described below.

The Oxford Miniature Vaporizer (OMV)

This vaporizer (Fig. 5.19a and b) is primarily used with portable anaesthetic equipment with the armed forces and has the advantage that it may be drained of one anaesthetic agent and charged with another. Detachable scales are available for several agents. It is very simple to use and needs little in the way of servicing.

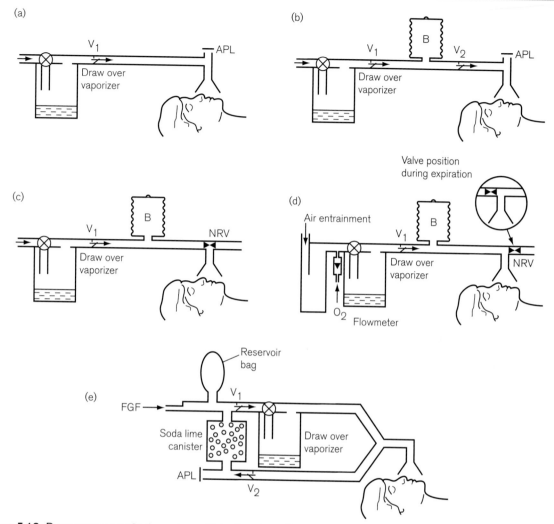

Figure 5.18 Draw-over anaesthetic systems. Note that they all contain non-return valves to prevent reverse flow through the vaporizer. System a is used for spontaneous respiration. System b incorporates a bellows and therefore requires a second non-return valve (V_2). If this is used for controlled ventilation (system c), an additional non-return valve (NRV) is often substituted for the APL valve. If the former is of a design which has a tendency to jam, the second valve V_2 is either removed, or in the case of the Oxford Inflating Bellows, held open by a magnet. In system d an oxygen flowmeter has been added. During the expiratory phase, the continuing supply of oxygen flows into the reservoir and is stored for use in subsequent breaths. In system e the vaporizer has been placed in a circle breathing system. A vaporizer in this position is often referred to as a vaporizer in circle (VIC).

It has a flow splitting valve (1) that separates carrier gas (2) into bypass gas (3) and gas that passes through the vaporizer to pick up vapour (4). It has stainless steel wicks (5). It is not temperature compensated, but there is a sealed compartment (6), filled with water plus antifreeze, which acts as a heat sink to minimize changes of temperature. The 'Triservice' version is described in Chapter 29.

Epstein, Macintosh, Oxford (EMO) ether inhaler

This has been deservedly the most popular draw-over vaporizer (Fig. 5.20) for the administration of ether, and is still widely used throughout the world. For spontaneous respiration, it is often used in conjunction with the OMV (Oxford Miniature Vaporizer). The latter is usually filled with halothane to provide smooth and rapid induction of anaesthesia, which is then continued by ether from the

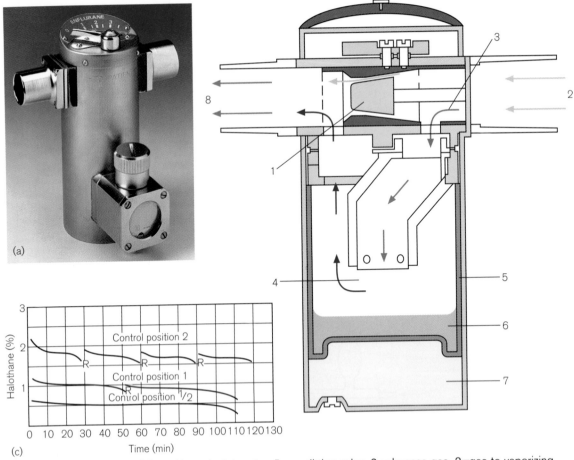

Figure 5.19 OMV vaporizer. **(b)** working principles. 1 = flow splitting valve, 2 = bypass gas, 3=gas to vaporizing chamber, 4=saturated vapour and gas in vaporizing chamber, 5 = stainless steel wick, 6 = liquid agent, 7 = water jacket, 8 = output from vaporizer. Permission granted by Penlon UK Ltd. **(c)** Performance characteristics

EMO. Both vaporizers may be used in conjunction with self-inflating bellows for techniques employing controlled ventilation.

MEASURED FLOW VAPORIZERS

TEC 6 (Plus) (Desflurane)

This vaporizer (Fig. 5.21a and b) has been designed specifically for the volatile agent desflurane. This agent is unusual in that its boiling point is around room temperature and so it would not remain as a liquid in the reservoir of a conventional vaporizer. It, therefore, requires an unusual design, which dispenses with most of the conventional compensating devices mentioned above.

The reservoir of the TEC 6 has two thermostatically controlled electric heating elements (1), which raise the temperature of the desflurane to 39°C. At this temperature, the SVP is 194 kPa (1500 mmHg). When vapour is required, a shut-off valve (2) opens and pure vapour under pressure is allowed to escape from the reservoir (3). It passes to an electronic pressure regulator (4) that reduces the pressure to that normally found in a plenum vaporizer (1–2.5 kPa) and then to a variable flow restrictor linked to the calibrated concentration selection dial (5), from where it is fed into the carrier gas flow leaving the vaporizer (6).

Fresh gas flow into the vaporizer (7) has to pass through a narrow restriction (8) so that its pressure (which increases with flow) matches that normally found in a plenum vaporizer. With increasing flows, two independent

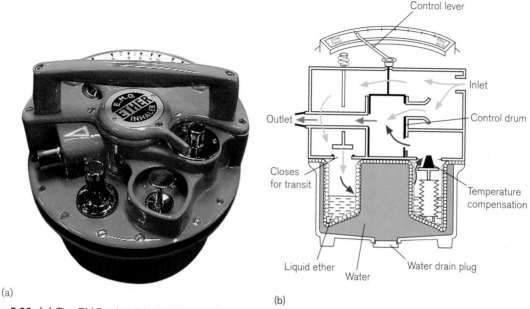

Figure 5.20 (a) The EMO ether inhaler. This is a low-resistance vaporizer which is both temperature and level compensated. **(b)** Working principles. Note that there is a mass of water, which provides a heat sink. When the control lever is put to the 'close for transit' position, the ether chamber is sealed off to prevent spillage.

sensors (9) in the pathway detect the pressure rise and instruct the desflurane pressure regulator to increase proportionately the desflurane pressure (and flow) to the selection dial, so as to maintain the set vapour concentration. If the readings from the two sensors are not similar, the shut-off valve closes and isolates the vaporizing chamber.

The vaporizer has a number of other features:

- The vaporizer heaters are switched on automatically when the unit is connected to the electricity supply. However, a 5–10 min warm-up time is required to reach operating temperature. During this time the concentration dial cannot be turned on.

- There are two more electric heaters in the upper part of the vaporizer to prevent vapour condensation.

- The concentration dial has graduations of 1%, but from 10–18% these are 2% increments. There is an interim stop at 12%, which can be manually overridden to access the higher concentrations.

- The front panel has 5 lights (Light Emitting Diodes (LEDs)). From top to bottom they are: OPERATIONAL LED to indicate that the unit is ready to be used; NO OUTPUT LED for when the agent drops below minimum operating level; LOW AGENT

LED to indicate that refilling is required; WARM UP LED (see below) and ALARM BATTERY LOW LED for when the back-up alarm power is either low or disconnected. The latter consists of a 9-volt alkaline battery which requires changing annually. The front panel also houses an LCD (liquid crystal display of twenty vertically mounted bars) that receives electronically processed signals from a sensor in the reservoir. The bars gradually disappear as the vaporizer empties, at which point the heaters are switched off and the low agent LED flashes. There are three symbols displayed on the side of the LCD. The uppermost (equivalent to all twenty bars showing), indicates that the reservoir is full (390 ml). The middle, a mark indicates that a 240 ml refill is possible (a whole bottle) and the lowest indicates that the reservoir has only 60 ml left.

- At the beginning of the warm-up time, the vaporizer begins a self-testing sequence. The warning alarm sounds for 1 sec and all the LEDs flash. When operating temperature is reached, the warm-up light (amber) extinguishes, the operational light glows (green) and the concentration dial unlocks.

- There is a detector which shuts off the vaporizer if it senses more than a 15-degree tilt off the vertical axis.

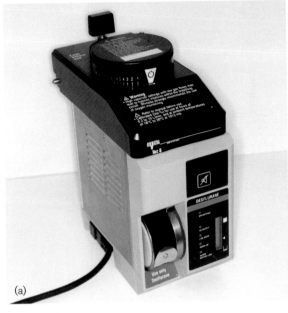

(a)

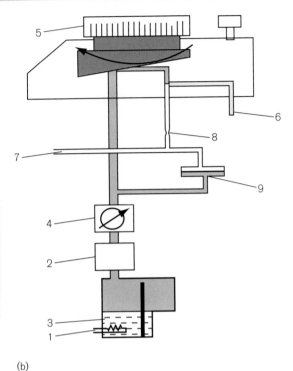

(b)

Figure 5.21 (a) The TEC 6 vaporizer. **(b)** Working principles. 1, Heater in the vapour chamber; 2, shut-off valve; 3, reservoir; 4, electronic pressure regulator; 5, concentration dial; 6, vaporizer outflow; 7, fresh gas inflow; 8, restrictor; 9, differential pressure sensors. **(c)** Performance characteristics of TEC 6 vaporizer.

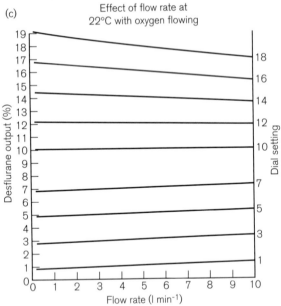

(c)

LCD bars fall below the 240 ml refill mark, then it will accept the whole bottle. When empty, the bottle may be returned to the starting position at which point the spring in the filler port will eject the filler nozzle. The filling process may be carried out even when the vaporizer is in use. As the bottle is pressurized, it is coated in plastic to prevent the glass splintering in the event of damage. Overfilling is prevented in normal circumstances, by placing the outlet from the reservoir above the level attained by the bottle in its filling position. However, should the vaporizer be tilted (and this can only happen if the vaporizer is not in use and not attached to the back bar), overfilling can occur although, liquid will be prevented from leaving the reservoir by the shut-off valve. When the vaporizer is next commissioned, a small amount of liquid might leave the reservoir but would rapidly vaporize.

- The filler port accepts only the specific filler nozzle (SAF-T-FIT), which is crimped onto the supply bottle for desflurane. To fill the vaporizer, the filler nozzle is pushed into a spring-loaded aperture in the filler port, which is then rotated upwards by inverting the bottle. The contents of the bottle will then decant into the vaporizer reservoir. If the latter is filled only when the

FURTHER READING

Pumping effect

Cole JR (1966) The use of ventilators and vaporizer performance. *British Journal of Anaesthesia* 38: 646–651.

Henegan CPH (1986) Vapour output and gas driven ventilators. *British Journal of Anaesthesia.* 58: 932.

Loeb R, Santos B (1995) Pumping effect in Ohmeda Tec 5 vaporizers *Journal of Clinical Monitoring.* 11(5): 348.

Thymol and Halothane

Carter KB, Gray WM, Railton R, Richardson W (1988) Long term performance of TEC vaporizers. *Anaesthesia* 43: 1042–1046.

Gray WM (1988) Dependence of the output of a halothane vaporizer on thymol concentration. *Anaesthesia.* 43(12): 1047–1049.

Vapour output

James MF, White JF (1984) Anesthetic considerations at moderate altitude. *Anesthesia and Analgesia* 63(12): 1097–1105.

Jones CS (1980) Gas viscosity effects in anesthesia. *Anesthesia and Analgesia* 59(3): 92–96.

Leigh JM (1985) Variations on a theme splitting ratio. *Anaesthesia* 40: 7072.

Loeb RG (1992) The output of four modern vaporizers in the presence of helium. *Canadian Journal of Anaesthesia* 39(8): 888–891.

Palayiwa E., Hahn CEW, Sugg BR (1985) Nitrous oxide solubility in halothane and its effect on the output of vaporizers. *Anaesthesia* 40: 415–419.

Palayiwa E, Sanderson MH, Hahn CE (1983) Effects of carrier gas composition on the output of six anaesthetic Vaporizers. *British Journal of Anaesthesia* 55(10): 1025–1038.

Schaefer H.G, Farman IV (1984) Anaesthetic vapour concentrations in the EMO system. *Anaesthesia* 39: 171–180.

Scott DM (1991) Performance of BOC Ohmeda Tec 3 and Tec 4 vaporisers following tipping. *Anaesthesia in Intensive Care* 19(3): 441–443.

White DC (1985) Symposium on anaesthetic equipment. Vaporization and vaporizers. *British Journal of Anaesthesia* (Review) 57(7): 658–71.

Wright D, Brosnan S, Royston B, White D (1998) Controlled ventilation using isoflurane with an in-circle vaporiser. *Anaesthesia* 53(7): 650–653.

Filling devices

Richardson W, Carter KB (1986) Evaluation of keyed fillers on TEC vaporizers. *British Journal of Anaesthesia* 58(3): 353–356.

Sato T, Oda M, Kurashiki T (1988) A new agent-specific filling device for anesthetic vaporizers. *Anesthesiology* 68(6): 957–959.

Uncles DR, Conway NE (1994) Key issues in vaporizer filling. *Canadian Journal of Anaesthesia* 41(9): 878–879.

Wittmann PH, Wittmann FW, Connor J, Connor T (1994) A new keyed vaporizer filler. *Anaesthesia* 49(8): 710–712.

Individual vaporizers

Blease Datum User and Maintenance Manual. Issue 2, December 1999.

Dräger Vapor 2000 Instructions for Use, 10th edn. August 2003.

Graham S (1994) The desflurane Tec 6 vaporizer. *British Journal of Anaesthesia* 72: 470–473

Hendrick JF, De Cooman S, Deloof T, Vandeput D, Coddens J, De Wolf AM (2001) The ADU vaporizing unit: a new vaporizer. *Anesthesia and Analgesia* 93(2): 391–395.

The TEC 6 Operation and Maintenance Manual. *Datex Ohmeda English Language.* Issue 7, March 1994.

The TEC 5 Continuous Flow Vaporizer Operation and Maintenance Manual, *Datex Ohmeda* Issue 1, November 1989.

Penlon Sigma Elite User Instruction Manual Penlon Ltd. February 2001.

Vaporizers in circle systems

Baker AB (1994) Low flow and closed circuits. *Anaesthesia in Intensive Care* 22(4): 341–342.

Brosnan S, Royston B, White D (1998) Isoflurane concentrations using uncompensated vaporisers within circle systems. *Anaesthesia* 53(6): 560–564.

Hazards

Cartwright DP, Freeman MF (1999) Vaporisers (editorial) *Anaesthesia* 54: 519–520

MRHA Medical Device Alert. *Overfilling of Vaporisers* 31, Nov 2003.

Munson WM (1965) Cardiac arrest: hazard of tipping a vaporiser. *Anesthesiology* 26: 235

Palayiwa E, Hahn CEW (1995) Overfill testing of anaesthetic vaporizers. *British Journal of Anaesthesia* 74: 100–103

The anaesthetic workstation

Ali Diba

The anaesthetic workstation (Fig. 6.1) has evolved over the years from the simple inhaler for the admixture of volatile anaesthetics, through anaesthetic machines with calibrated delivery of inspired agents, to reach the modern workstation complete with integral ventilator, breathing system and patient and machine monitoring. Future developments, beyond automated record keeping which is already a reality in many institutions, will undoubtedly be the integration of the machine into institutional information networks and perhaps online access to expert systems for decision support (see Chapter 24, Information Technology and the Anaesthetic Workstation).

Throughout this process, developments have been driven by the need for safety; including fail-safe systems, and by 'designing out' the possibilities of dangerous user errors. This aspect of the workstation may be regarded as having developed with successive generations of improvements and modifications having been incorporated, such that the 'anaesthetic machine' component of a modern workstation is still recognizable as a descendant of the first generation Boyle's trolley. Over time, technological safety features have become enshrined in national and international standards which are largely adhered to. As such, an analysis of critical incidents may help to inform a

logical approach to the understanding of the safety features and design of modern machines, and for this reason such a section is included in this chapter.

FUNCTIONS OF THE MODERN WORKSTATION

Inhalational anaesthesia is still the most commonly used technique worldwide. Recently, the AneoTivas, a much simpler anaesthetic machine designed for the delivery of two intravenous anaesthetic agents only (with integral respiratory support and patient monitoring) failed to get past the prototype stage. The anaesthetic workstation, an elaboration of the continuous flow anaesthetic machine, has thus developed to accurately and continuously deliver a safe mixture of gases and vapours for the administration of anaesthesia. The component parts of the modern workstation represent its various and extended functions:
- safe provision, selection and delivery of anaesthetic gases and vapours together with an appropriate built-in breathing system, usually a circle system;
- provision of back-up supplies of gases in the event of failure of the primary sources;

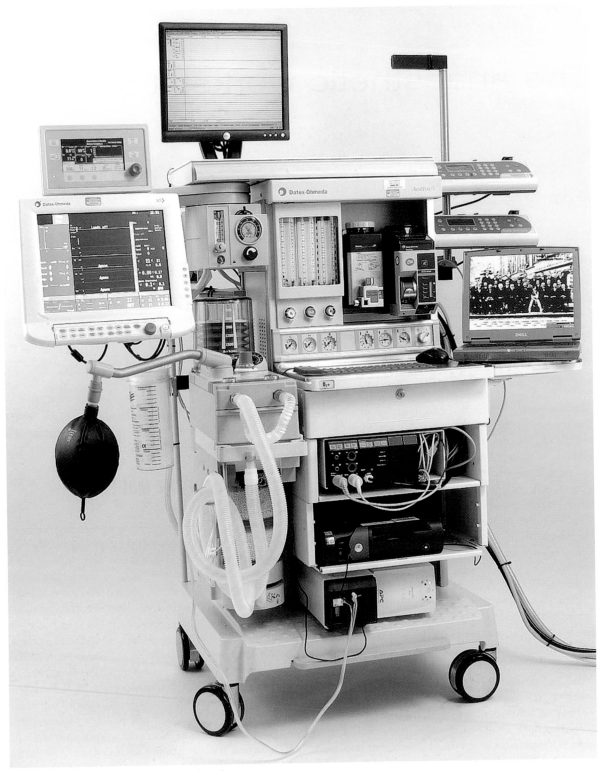

Figure 6.1 A modern anaesthetic workstation.

- respiratory support in the form of sophisticated automatic ventilators capable of managing the full range of patient needs;
- monitoring of machine function and settings;
- monitoring of patient physiological variables;
- automated archived record keeping (or at least the facility to output monitored parameters to other systems) and ideally on-line access to information and administration networks;
- the integration of the display and auditory signalling of monitored modalities;
- provision of appropriate connection to an anaesthetic gas scavenging system;
- provision of medical vacuum via a suction regulator;
- provision of supplemental oxygen using auxilliary O_2 flowmeter (reduced risk of inadvertent anaesthesia);
- work surface and storage facility for 'everyday' items; and
- provision of mains electricity sockets for low consumption items used in association with delivery or monitoring of anaesthesia, e.g. syringe pumps. (International standards preclude the powering of one medical device from another. For the purpose of this standard, the workstation is seen as a resuscitation trolley.)

DEVELOPMENT OF THE ANAESTHETIC WORKSTATION

The overriding principle has been to increase safety in anaesthesia. The invisible and unscented nature of the main gases used has meant that the focus of safety in the machine has had to be prevention of the accidental delivery of incorrect gases and gas mixtures. This commences with gas specific connections to wall and cylinder supplies and continues through non-interchangeable gas specific pipework within the machine to standardized arrangements of flow control valves. Along the way, fail-safe devices prevent delivery of N_2O in the event of failure of the O_2 supply which has the highest alarm priority. CO_2, another ill wind, has been largely eradicated from anaesthetic machines, further reducing potential error sources.

Integrated and modular designs

The first machines were solely for gas delivery. Monitoring was a purely clinical modality and a function of the anaesthetist. As individual monitors became available they were connected to or placed onto the machine.

Since then the design of the anaesthesia workstation has moved away from an integrated single entity towards a modular approach of combining various component parts, perhaps even from different manufacturers, to produce devices adapted for many applications and with less in-built obsolescence. This has been driven by the unforeseen growth in the range of possible monitoring modalities which no manufacturer could hope to encompass in one device, and the expansion of the functions of the anaesthesia workstation.

Even 15 years ago, when the majority of machines consisted of a stainless steel trolley with a number of monitors stacked on top, at least one manufacturer was making an integrated anaesthesia workstation where gas delivery and patient monitoring were one singular entity. The Narkomed 2a by North American Dräger had two CRT screens showing all settings and monitored variables. However, by today's standards, the in-built monitoring was rudimentary. Indeed, it is difficult to imagine how we could once again have a scenario where one in-built monitor can satisfy all requirements unless it has the facility for individual monitoring modalities to be interchanged.

The answer has been to return to a modular approach. The basic pneumatic anaesthetic machine is contained within a chassis or framework to which is added:

- a circle breathing system and 'bag in bottle' arrangement to separate respiratory gases from the usually pneumatically driven ventilator;
- a choice of ventilator, often a single design but software driven and available in a number of configurations;
- one of a choice of back bar vaporizers attachment systems, i.e. Selectatec or Dräger;
- a patient monitor of choice, itself often of a modular design where individual parameters can be 'hot swapped', i.e. exchanged whilst actually in use;
- an archived/networked or stand alone anaesthesia record system if so desired; and
- other bolt on parts as considered necessary.

Patient and machine monitoring

Monitoring of patient physiological variables is often approached separately to the monitoring of machine settings and function. Currently, the favoured arrangement is to have at least two monitors. One monitor is integral as part of the ventilator control area and displays the related parameters such as airway pressure and volume changes (also needed for microprocessor control of the ventilator) together with back bar and/or breathing system oxygen concentration. Beyond FiO_2 and simple flow and volume measurements from the breathing system, patient respiratory gas monitoring is usually a function of a second and separate patient physiological monitor. The patient monitor is most conveniently attached on a swing-out arm, allowing the patient, machine and display to be aligned in a comfortable arc for ease of viewing and access.

Separate patient monitoring also has the advantage of allowing standardization of monitors between the operating theatres and ward areas in hospitals. This, together with modular monitoring systems, means that machines can be designated to a variety of surgical scenarios which may have differing needs in terms of patient physiological monitoring.

Monitors can still be integrated such that information from each of the monitoring systems may be prioritized by a computer before any alarm is sounded, although where patient and machine monitoring are largely separate, so far this has tended not to happen. The data may be displayed in the most convenient fashion for easy and quick assimilation and may then be collated to provide a permanent record. Monitoring, where combined with automatic record keeping, can thus also log and reveal both the equipment and the anaesthetist's performance for the purposes of medical audit.

Electronics: monitoring or control?

The modern anaesthetic workstation has been invaded by electronics. In contradistinction to the direction that may have been predicted a few years ago, the role of electronics has remained largely one of monitoring rather than control. The Engström ELSA and the PhysioFlex – machines that exemplified the 'fly by wire' approach of computer control of the anaesthesia machine, and were presented in the previous edition of this text – are no longer available. Apart from microprocessor control of the sophisticated ICU type anaesthetic ventilators, there has not been a massive expansion in the control role of electronics. This, to be lauded if it is the case, may reflect a desire from anaesthetists for an intrinsic empathy with the principle tool of their metier.

The flow of gases through the workstation has largely remained under pneumatic and direct mechanical control. There are currently only one or two machines offering electronic servo control of gas flow or vapour concentrations. Although needle valves (see below) remain ubiquitous for control of gas flows, many machines do use

electronic monitoring (and display) of the flow rates instead of rotameters (see Chapter 4).

Two electronically controlled machines discussed at the end of this chapter represent only a small proportion of the machines in use currently.

THE ANAESTHETIC DELIVERY SYSTEM

Given that the most popular designs of anaesthesia workstation are now essentially modular (in terms of separate patient monitoring from gas delivery) this part of the chapter will concentrate on the gas delivery aspect of the workstation.

The basic design of delivery systems is common to a wide variety of manufacturers and may be considered under a number of headings. A working knowledge of these parts of the machine should allow rapid assimilation of the salient features of any new device.

A typical machine consists of:

- a rigid metal framework on wheels. Attached to this is a source of compressed gas consisting of a pipeline system and/or metal cylinders containing the relevant gases;
- pressure regulators for reducing the high pressures in the attached cylinders to machine working pressures of approximately 420 kPa (60 psi) or 310 kPa (45 psi) in some countries. (The British Standard stipulates 420 kPa which is 61.3 psi. For convenience this has been rounded off to 60 psi.);
- secondary regulators (see below);
- pressure gauges to show pipeline and cylinder pressures;
- a method of metering (e.g. flowmeters), using adjustable valves for proportioning and mixing the various gases;
- a system for attaching vaporizers to the anaesthetic machine for the addition of volatile anaesthetic agents to the gas mixture;
- a safety mechanism to warn of the failure of the oxygen supply and to prevent hypoxic mixtures of gas/vapour reaching the patient (oxygen failure warning device);
- a safety mechanism for releasing high-pressure build-up of gases (back bar pressure relief valve) should a fault occur in the machine;
- a system that bypasses the flowmeter for the administration of a high flow of pure oxygen in an emergency; and
- in-built connection to a circle breathing system with the facility to switch to a single outlet for delivering

the gases and vapours to any other breathing system (the common gas outlet).

Machine framework

The machine framework consists of box-shaped sections of either welded steel or aluminium, which provides both strength and ease of assembly. The design allows for upgrading from a simple model to one with integral monitoring and a ventilator. The machine is usually mounted on wheels with antistatic tyres. These conduct away any static electricity which may affect flowmeter performance and which also present risk of ignition of flammable anaesthetic agents (in parts of the world where these may still be used).

The compressed gas attachments
Pipelines

Each pipeline source is attached to the machine via a gas-specific connection. The latter consists of:
- a body (attached to the machine);
- a nipple; and
- a screw-threaded nut (attached to the machine end of the pipeline hose).

In the UK this is called a NIST (non-interchangeable screw-threaded) connection and is discussed in greater detail in Chapter 3 (Fig. 3.26).

In the USA, a similar system is employed called DISS (Diameter Indexed Safety System). However, the diameters of the nipples and bodies for the various connections are smaller and not compatible with the NIST system. The pipeline union block usually contains a metal gauze filter and also a one-way spring-loaded check valve to prevent retrograde gas leaks should the relevant system be disconnected.

Cylinders

The cylinders are clamped on to the machine by a yoke arrangement and secured tightly using a wing-nut (Fig. 6.2). To prevent installation of the wrong gas cylinder to a yoke, the cylinder heads are coded with appropriately positioned holes that match pins on the machine yoke. This is called a pin index system, for which there is an internationally agreed standard (ISO 2407) (Fig. 3.4). A thin neoprene and aluminium washer (Bodok seal) is interposed between the cylinder head and yoke to provide a gas-tight seal when the two are clamped together.

Cylinder yokes are also fitted with filters and one-way spring-loaded non-return (check) valves. These one-way valves prevent retrograde leaks where two cylinder yokes are connected in parallel and one does not have a cylinder attached.

A leak of not more than 15 ml min^{-1} through an open yoke is acceptable in new machines. However, in older machines the non-return valve is not as efficient owing either to the design (valve not spring loaded) or to wear and tear, and could result in greater than acceptable back-pressure leaks. These leaks, when occurring unexpectedly, have been shown to alter the composition of the gas leaving the flowmeter block and have resulted in the delivery of a hypoxic gas mixture to an attached breathing system (see section on Flowmeters). Blanking plugs (dummy cylinder heads) are available and should be inserted into all empty yokes to overcome this problem (Fig. 6.3).

Pressure (contents) gauges

The pressure in cylinders and pipelines is measured by Bourdon-type gauges (Fig. 4.6). The gas entry to the pressure gauge has a constriction so as to smooth out surges in pressure that could damage the gauge, as well as to prevent total and rapid loss of gas should a gauge rupture. The gauges are labelled and colour coded for each gas, according to the standards for each country. They are also calibrated for each gas used on the machine. The scale on the gauge extends to a pressure at least 33% greater than either the filling pressure of the cylinder or pipeline pressure as well as the 'full' indicated position (at a temperature of 20°C). Each cylinder yoke may be fitted with a gauge or alternatively a single-cast brass block may be used to house the NIST/DISS pipeline connection, cylinder yoke, pressure regulator and housings for the pressure gauges, in order to minimize the number of connections and potential leaks (Fig. 6.4).

Single block manifold

The single cast brass block has given way in recent years to the single block gas manifold (Fig. 6.5), which is drilled to accommodate as many as possible of the gas pipeline and pneumatic valve interconnections. The small compact manifold (Fig. 6.5a) for reasons of design economy does not carry the cylinder yokes and is hence downstream of the primary pressure regulator which is invariably part of the cylinder yoke assembly (Fig. 6.5b).

Pressure regulators (reducing valves)

Pressure regulators are used on anaesthetic machines for three main reasons:

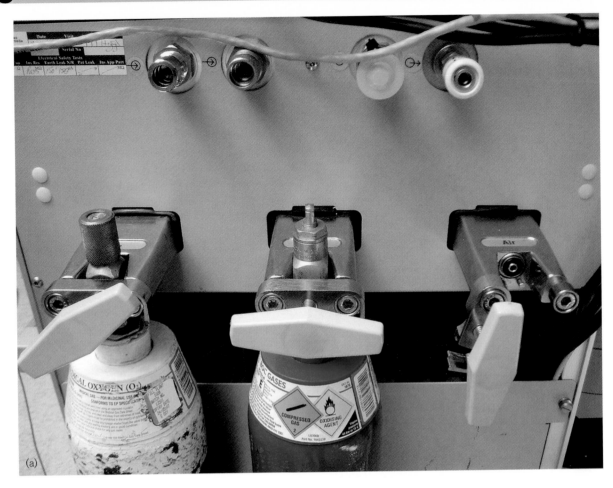

(a)

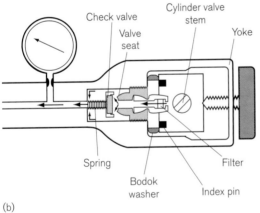

(b)

Check valve
Valve seat
Cylinder valve stem
Yoke
Spring
Bodok washer
Index pin
Filter

Figure 6.2 (a) Cylinder yokes. The empty right-hand yoke shows a Bodok seal and the pins of the pin index system. **(b)** Diagram of cylinder yoke assembly.

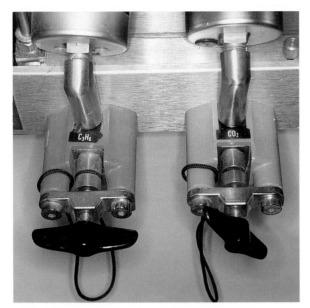

Figure 6.3 Blanking plugs on somewhat ancient cyclopropane and CO_2 cylinder yokes.

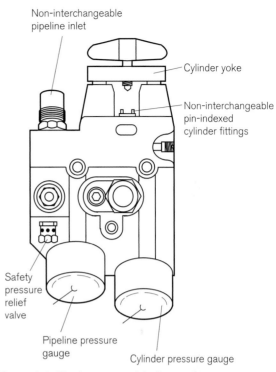

Figure 6.4 Single cast gas block.

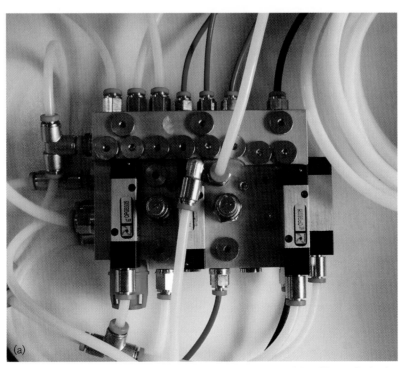

Figure 6.5 **(a)** Single block manifold arrangement of Blease anaesthesia machine. The coil of nylon tubing just visible is an ingenious approach to the need for an O_2 reservoir for operating the Ritchie Whistle. *Continued*

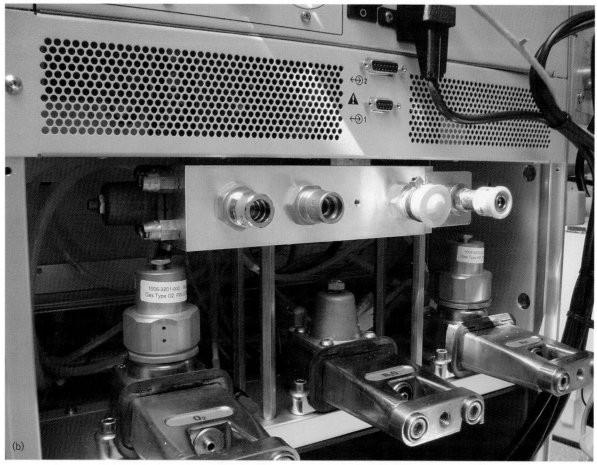

(b)

Figure 6.5, *cont'd* (b) Datex–Ohmeda Aestiva with back plate removed demonstrating cylinder yokes and primary pressure regulators for O_2, N_2O and air together with the aluminium single block manifold above carrying NIST connectors for O_2 and N_2O pipeline supplies (air inlet is blanked off) and auxilliary high-pressure oxygen outlet.

1. The pressure delivered from a cylinder is far too high to be used with safety in apparatus where a sudden surge of pressure might accidentally be delivered to the patient.

2. If the pressure were not reduced, flow-control (fine-adjustment) valves, tubing and various other parts of the apparatus would have to be much more robust, and a fine and accurate control of gas flow would be difficult to achieve. There would also be a danger of pressure building up and damaging other components of the apparatus.

3. As the contents of a cylinder are exhausted, the pressure within the cylinder falls. If there were no regulating mechanism to maintain a constant reduced pressure, continual adjustment would have

to be made of the flow-control valve in order to maintain a given flow rate.

Not only is the pressure reduced, but it is also kept constant, and for this reason the correct term for this type of valve is a *pressure regulator*.

Working principles

In Fig. 6.6, the chamber C is enclosed on one side by the diaphragm D. As gas enters the chamber through the valve V, the pressure in the chamber is increased and the diaphragm is distended against its own elastic recoil plus the tension in the spring S. Eventually the pressure rises high enough to move the diaphragm far enough to close valve V . The pressure at which this occurs may be varied by adjusting the screw X so as to alter the tension in the

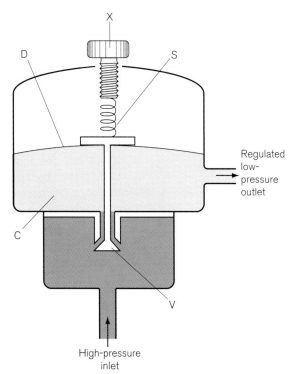

Figure 6.6 A simple pressure regulator. D, diaphragm; S, spring; C, low-pressure chamber; V, valve seating; X, adjustment screw.

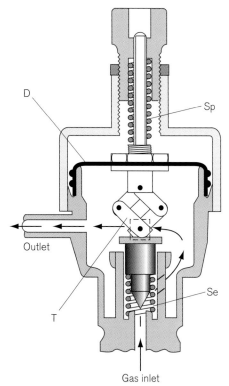

Figure 6.7 The Adams regulator. D, diaphragm; Sp, spring; Se, seat; T, toggle levers.

spring S. If gas is allowed to escape from the outlet of the chamber, the pressure falls and valve V reopens. When the regulator is in use, a steady pressure is maintained in the chamber by the partial opening of valve V.

In another form of regulator (Adams valve), the push-rod is replaced by a 'lazy tongs' toggle arrangement (Fig. 6.7), which reverses the direction of the thrust transmitted from the diaphragm.

The accuracy of regulators

Let us consider that the push-rod is pushed downward by two forces: the tension in the spring and the elastic recoil of the diaphragm (Fig. 6.8). Let these be added together and represented by S. The force that opposes S consists of two parts: the high pressure (P) of the gas pushing on the valve V over an area of a; and the low pressure (p) acting on the diaphragm over an area A, so:

$$S = Pa + pA$$

Thus, if S remains constant, as P falls, p rises so that as the cylinder empties, the regulated pressure increases. In fact, as P falls, the valve V will have to open further

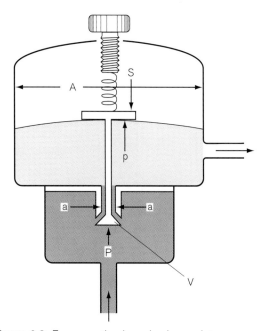

Figure 6.8 Forces acting in a simple regulator.

to permit the same flow rate. The spring expands and therefore its tension is reduced, and in the same way the tension in the diaphragm is reduced. Therefore, as P falls, there is a small reduction in S, which partially reverses the effect illustrated here.

In the Adams valve (Fig. 6.9), it can be seen that the pressure P exerted by the high-pressure gas to open valve V is assisted by the spring and the recoil of the diaphragm S. These forces jointly oppose the force exerted by the low-pressure gas on the diaphragm, so:

$$Pa + S = pA$$

Now as P falls, so does p; therefore the regulated pressure falls slightly as the cylinder pressure drops. At the same time the valve V opens slightly and this, by allowing the spring to expand, reduces S, which slightly accentuates the fall in p. The fall of p can be minimized by making S great compared with Pa.

There are several types of pressure regulator available, the choice being dependent on:
- the maximum flow rate required;
- the regulated pressure to which it is to be set; and
- the maximum input pressure that it is to handle.

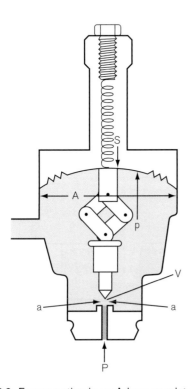

Figure 6.9 Forces acting in an Adams regulator.

For low-pressure regulators, the diaphragms are frequently made of rubber or neoprene, whereas in those for higher pressures the diaphragm is made of metal. Adjustments to alter the regulated pressure should be made only by service engineers. On some anaesthetic machines, 'universal' regulators are used. These operate equally well from an input of 420 kPa (60 psi) from the pipeline, as from a maximum of 14 000 kPa (2000 psi) from cylinders and are of the Adams type. The British Standard stipulates a pressure of 420 kPa (61.3 psi). This has been rounded off in the text to 60 psi. The term 'universal' is also used in a different context (see below).

Interchangeability of regulators
Pressure regulators used to be labelled and coded for specific gases. This is because a special alloy was required in the valve seating for some gases (e.g. nitrous oxide) in order to prevent corrosion. However, modern regulators are designed to be compatible with all anaesthetic gases. This is achieved by using materials such as PTFE coatings on the diaphragms together with nitrile (a hard synthetic rubber) valve seats and chrome-plated brass for the regulator body. These too are described as 'universal' by their manufacturers.

Common faults in regulators
- Damage to the soft seating of valves may occur as a result of the presence of grit or dust, usually from a dirty cylinder. This may cause a steady build-up of pressure in the apparatus when the cylinder is left turned on but with no gas flowing.
- A hissing noise may indicate a leaking or burst diaphragm. The regulator will need replacing or repairing by the manufacturer or service engineer.
- Adams valves sometimes develop a fault that causes continual 'jumping' of the flowmeter bobbin, indicating an intermittent change of pressure and flow rate. This is usually due to the 'lazy tongs' sticking as a result of wear, but it may also be caused by small particles of grit or metal in the lazy tongs or the valve seating.

The older versions of the Adams valves had fins on their nitrous oxide regulators to conduct heat from the surrounding air to prevent excessive cooling of the valves. Prior to this, it was not uncommon for the nitrous oxide to contain a significant quantity of water vapour as an impurity, and this condensed onto the valve seating and then froze, thus jamming the valve. The extra heat conducted by the fins was sufficient to prevent this freezing.

Relief valves on regulators

Safety blow-off valves are often fitted on the downstream side of regulators to allow the escape of gas if, by accident, the regulators fail and allow a high-output pressure. With a regulator designed to give a pressure of 420 kPa (60 psi), the relief valve may be set at 525 kPa (70 psi). These valves may be spring loaded, in which case they close when the pressure falls again, or they may operate by rupture, in which case they remain open until repaired. As a further safety feature, a flow restrictor (usually in the form of a simple pin hole orifice) before the pressure regulator limits maximal flow from the cylinder to about $150 \ l \ min^{-1}$, ensuring that in the event of regulator failure the high-pressure relief valve can dump the maximal flow without further pressure rises.

Primary pressure regulators

Modern anaesthetic machines may have several pressure regulators (primary and secondary) for each gas. Primary regulators are used to reduce high cylinder pressures to lower machine working pressure (typically 420 kPa (60 psi)). The pressures downstream of the primary regulators are not the same in all machines or in all countries.

Some manufacturers adjust their cylinder regulators to just below 420 kPa (60 psi) (i.e. 350 kPa (50 psi)) to give *pipeline preference*. This allows the anaesthetic machine to preferentially use pipeline gas when the reserve cylinders have been accidentally left turned on, so reducing the potential for premature emptying of these cylinders. However, even with this differential, many regulators are known to 'weep', i.e. gradually empty their contents. Reserve cylinders should therefore always be turned off after testing until required again.

Secondary pressure regulators

Several factors cause the machine working pressure (420 kPa in the UK) to fluctuate by up to 20%. For example, at times of peak demand in a hospital, pipeline pressures may well drop by this amount. Similarly, if an auxiliary outlet on the anaesthetic machine is used to drive a ventilator with a very high sudden and intermittent gas demand, a similar pressure drop will occur before the pipeline or cylinder is able to restore the supply. These pressure fluctuations produce parallel fluctuations in flowmeter performance. A second (*secondary*) regulator set below the anticipated pressure drop smoothes out the supply, minimizing these fluctuations. This is important in machines incorporating mechanically linked anti-hypoxia systems attached to the flowmeter bank (see below) as these systems assume that the oxygen supply pressure is constant in order to achieve an accurate flow of gas. A mechanically linked system would not be able to detect altered gas flow rates caused by changing pressures. Furthermore, secondary regulators also prolong the accurate supply of oxygen to the flowmeter if there is a gradual failure of the oxygen supply (i.e. cylinder emptying) prior to the oxygen failure warning device being activated.

Regulators have to meet stringent criteria before being installed. They are required to withstand pressure of 30 mPa (megaPascals) without disruption and their output should not vary more than 10% across a wide flow range ($100 \ ml \ min^{-1}$ to $12 \ l \ min^{-1}$). They should also be fitted with a pressure relief valve that opens at a pressure not exceeding 800 kPa (UK).

Flow restrictors

It was an occasional practice to entirely omit regulators from the pipeline supply (420 kPa (60 psi)) in older anaesthetic machines. Sudden pressure surges at the patient end of the anaesthetic machine were prevented by flow restrictors. These consisted of constrictions in the regulated pressure pipework upstream of the flowmeters. The disadvantage of using flow restrictors without regulators was that changes in pipeline pressure were reflected in changes of flow rate, which made readjustment of the flow control valves necessary. Also, there was a danger that if there was an obstruction at the outlet from the anaesthetic machine, pressure could build up in the vaporizers and cause damage. This was normally prevented by the inclusion of a 'blow-off' safety valve (see section on Back bar below). Flow restrictors do not normally require any maintenance.

Gas-tight connections within the machine

The various components within the anaesthetic machine are joined to each other by a series of pipes. Although now almost entirely made of high density nylon, previously copper piping was standard and hence these components are also briefly described below. Piped medical gas conduits within hospital walls and ducting are still entirely of metal.

Whilst there is no standard for the design of gas piping within the machine, with the advent of nylon tubing, manufacturers tend to use pipes of differing diameters and/or sometimes colour for the different gases to reduce

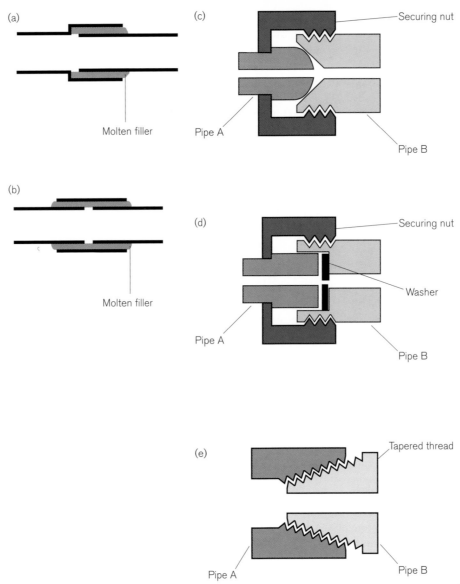

Figure 6.10 Joints in metal tubing. **(a)** Permanent brazed overlapping joint. **(b)** Permanent sleeved joint. **(c)** Ball and cone union. **(d)** Flat seated union. **(e)** Tapered union.

the risk of accidental misconnection during servicing and assembly.

Joints in metal tubing

These may be permanent or detachable. Two metal pipes may be permanently joined by one of two methods:

1. one pipe may have a slightly larger diameter than the other so that they overlap (Fig. 6.10a): and
2. where the diameters are similar, both ends are inserted into a sleeve of metal (Fig. 6.10b).

The adjacent surfaces are then bonded together by brazing (applying a molten filler alloy whose melting temperature is above 430°C) or hard soldering (a similar principle using an alloy with a lower melting point). After making such a joint it is important that all traces of flux are removed. Flux is a material applied to the surfaces to be bonded, allowing the molten filler to spread more evenly. More recently, a system of brazing copper pipes and brass fittings without flux has been evolved. This is used particularly for medical gas pipeline installations.

Where provision has to be made for disconnection and reconnection of a joint, a union is used. This consists of two parts held together in a gas-tight manner, usually by a nut or cap, which screws onto a parallel male thread. Figure 6.10c shows a ball and cone (or cone seated) union, in which the seating is by direct metal-to-metal contact. A flange (or flat seated) union (Fig. 6.10d) requires a washer to complete the seal. With pipes carrying oxygen, this washer should be of non-flammable material.

For some other purposes tapered threads (Fig. 6.10e) may be used and the seal made either by screwing them down extremely tightly or by interposing a sealing compound such as PTFE (polytetrafluoroethylene/Teflon) in the form of a tape. The joint between the valve block and the body of a medical gas cylinder, for example, is sealed by a metal foil between two tapered threads and is designed to melt at high temperatures allowing gradual release of cylinder contents.

Other detachable joints

High-density nylon tubing, connected by metal junctions, is now ubiquitous in anaesthetic machines (Fig. 6.11). It is cheaper, less prone to rupture and simpler to install. Joints are made gas-tight by an 'O'-ring fitted between the components. This consists of a simple ring made to a fine tolerance out of a material such as neoprene. It is housed in a recess in the larger component to stop it becoming dislodged.

In the joint described, the nylon tube is pushed firmly into the junction where it is gripped by an 'O'-ring and a folding spring. The folding spring has backward pointing barbs which grip the tube, preventing its removal. When removal of the tube is required (for maintenance purposes), the barbs of the spring can be retracted by applying pressure to the pushing ring situated on the inlet of the junction. This pushes a bush (leading bush) against the barbs, forcing them away from the nylon tube. Each gas service may have its own unique diameter of tubing and junctions so as to prevent cross-connection.

Valve glands

Where a valve spindle passes from an area of high pressure to one of low pressure, provision must be made to prevent the leak of gases along the line of the spindle. This is achieved by means of a gland. In Fig. 6.12, the nut 'N' must be screwed down sufficiently tightly to ensure that

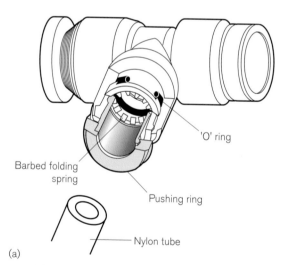

'O' ring

Barbed folding spring

Pushing ring

Nylon tube

(a)

Figure 6.11 (a) Drawing of cut-away of high-density nylon tube and push fit metal 'T' (two-way) junction, showing 'O'-ring and retractable barbed spring. **(b)** Photograph of nylon oxygen pipe inserted into a push fit metal one-way connector.

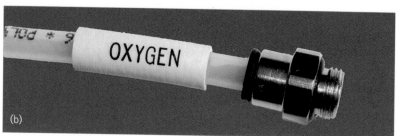

OXYGEN

(b)

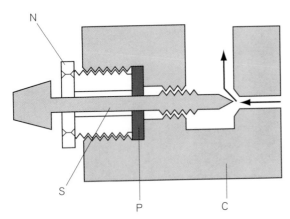

Figure 6.12 A valve gland. The packing (P) is compressed by screwing down the nut (N) until it is applied sufficiently tightly around the spindle (S) to prevent the gas from leaking.

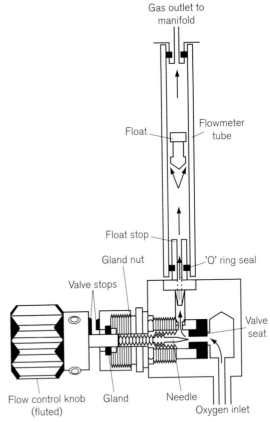

Figure 6.13 The internal mechanics of an oxygen flowmeter and flow control valve.

the packing is applied so closely to the spindle that no gas can escape by this route. There is provision for the nut to be tightened down further to prevent leaks as the packing wears.

The principle can be used for a high-pressure gland, such as that of an oxygen cylinder (see Chapter 3), or in a low-pressure gland such as that in a flowmeter (Fig. 6.13). In the case of high-pressure valves, a special type of leather or long fibre asbestos was at one time used for the packing, but modern glands are filled with specially shaped nylon. Those in low-pressure flow control valves may be filled with rubber, nylon, neoprene or cotton.

'O'-rings

In certain circumstances, the packing of a stuffing box may be replaced by an 'O'-ring (Fig. 6.11a). If the valve spindle S and the casing C are suitably designed, an 'O'-ring is all that is required to prevent leakage at this point. 'O'-rings can withstand remarkably high pressures and yet cause very little friction between the spindle and the casing.

Flowmeters (rotameters)

Gas from either a pipeline supply or cylinder, at a suitably regulated pressure, is passed through a flowmeter, which accurately controls the flow of that gas through the anaesthetic machine. The anaesthetic machine conventionally has a bank of flowmeters for the various gases used (Fig. 6.14). Flowmeters are described briefly here, but more detailed information can be found in Chapter 4.

A typical flowmeter assembly (Fig. 6.13) consists of:
- a needle valve;
- a valve seat; and
- a tapered and calibrated gas sight tube which contains a bobbin.

Gas entering the sight tube pushes the bobbin up it in proportion to the gas flow. The bobbin floats and rotates inside the sight tube, without touching the sides, giving an accurate indication of the gas flow. The sight tube is made leak-proof at the top and bottom of the flowmeter block by 'O'-rings, neoprene sockets or washers. The glass or plastic sight tubes, with their own bobbins, are individually calibrated (in l min^{-1}) for their specific gases at a temperature of 20°C and an ambient pressure of 101.3 kPa and are non-interchangeable. Misconnection is made physically impossible by constructing the glass sight tubes of different diameters and/or lengths or by using a pin index system at each end.

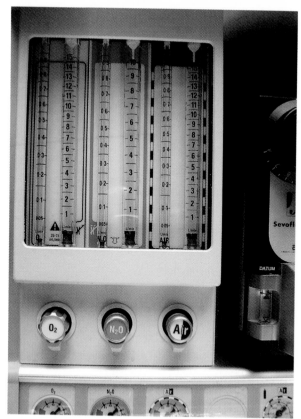

Figure 6.14 A flowmeter bank. Note the 'cascade' flowmeters for all gases and the protrusion of the O_2 control valve.

Flow control valves in the UK have to meet standards set down BS 4272 and EN ISO 60601-2-13 which stipulate that:

1. The torque (twisting force) required to operate them must be high enough to minimize accidental readjustment (this torque can be adjusted by the manufacturer by varying the degree of tightness of the gland nut, although these may work loose during frequent use).

2. Values must be accurate to within 10% of the indicated flow (at flow rates between 10% of full scale or 300 ml min^{-1}, whichever is the greater, and 100% of the maximum indicated flow).

3. When axial push or pull forces are applied to the valve spindle without rotation (at a flow rate 25% of the maximum indicated flow), the maximum flow change must not be greater than 10% or 10 ml min^{-1}, whichever is the greater. (Several older machines have spindles that do not meet this requirement. Axial pressures at a flow rate of

1 l min^{-1} have been shown to change the flow rate by 50% in these machines, with resultant hypoxic mixtures being delivered to the patient, when they are used with a low-flow anaesthetic breathing system.)

4. Each flow control valve must be permanently and legibly marked, indicating the gas it controls (using the name or chemical symbol).

5. As well as conforming to (4), the oxygen flow control knob (Fig. 6.13) must have an individual octagonal profile. When the valve is closed the knob must project at least 2 mm beyond the knobs controlling other gases at all flow rates. Its diameter must also be greater than the maximum diameter of the flow control knobs for other gases.

The flowmeter block

In the UK and many other countries, the flowmeters are traditionally arranged in a block with the oxygen flowmeter on the extreme left, the nitrous oxide on the extreme right and those for compressed air and carbon dioxide (where fitted) in between these. However, some machines, such as those manufactured by Datex–Ohmeda and Blease, incorporate a system that delivers a minimum concentration of oxygen such as 25%, and requires the oxygen and nitrous oxide flow control valves to be adjacent, as they are linked by a sprocket and chain or cogwheel.

The flowmeters are mounted vertically, and usually next to each other, in such a way that their upper (downstream) ends discharge into a manifold. Traditionally, this was unfortunately arranged in such a way that if there were a leak in, say, the central tube, oxygen would be lost rather than nitrous oxide. As a result, a hypoxic mixture could be delivered to the patient (Fig. 6.15a). In most modern machines, oxygen is the last gas to flow into the manifold so that a leak would not lead to such a hypoxic mixture (Fig. 6.15b). As a solution to the same problem, in some countries such as the USA and Canada, the order of the flowmeters in the block has been reversed, with oxygen on the right. However, this too has previously (before the advent of hypoxic guard interlinks) led to patients receiving a hypoxic mixture because anaesthetists have not been made aware of the transposition.

The practice of removing carbon dioxide cylinders (and in the past cyclopropane) from their yokes has exposed a further hazard in older machines. Oxygen can be lost via a retrograde leak through a carbon dioxide (or cyclopropane) flowmeter, even when intact, if the

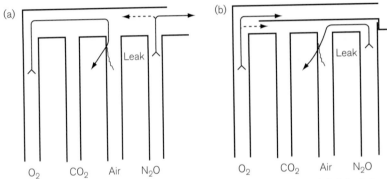

Figure 6.15 Diagram to show the effect of a leak from one of the rotameter tubes. **(a)** A leak from the cyclopropane tube in the traditional form of flowmeter block would result in back-pressure from the nitrous oxide, causing oxygen to escape through the leak. The patient would therefore receive a hypoxic mixture. **(b)** A rearrangement whereby the oxygen is the last gas to enter the mixed gas flow and nitrous oxide rather than oxygen would be expelled through a leak. This would not lead to the patient receiving a hypoxic mixture.

corresponding needle valves are inadvertently left open. Gas can track back from the manifold via the flowmeter and open needle valve to the unblocked cylinder yoke and escape. The one-way (check) valves fitted to cylinder yokes in some machines were never intended to provide a perfect gas-tight seal under all conditions. They were not spring loaded because they were designed to work against high back-pressures rather than the relatively low back-pressures produced in the retrograde leak. This leak may be increased by adding an extra resistance to flow downstream of the flowmeter block (i.e. some types of minute volume divider ventilator or high-resistance vaporizer), which effectively increases the gas pressure in the flowmeter block. All empty cylinder yokes for air, carbon dioxide and cyclopropane (where these still exist) should be fitted with blanking plugs (Fig. 6.3) so as to prevent this problem. Modern standards (EN 740-99) stipulate that a maximum retrograde flow of 100 ml min^{-1} is acceptable, or 10 ml hr^{-1} if the fault condition causing this is not alarmed.

Recent increased interest in low-flow anaesthesia systems has created a demand for flowmeters that can more accurately measure flows below 1 l min^{-1}. This is achieved by the use of two flowmeter tubes for the same gas. The first is a long thin tube accurate for flows from 0 to 1000 ml min^{-1} that complements the second conventional tube calibrated for higher flows (1–10 l min^{-1} or more). Both are activated from the same flow control valve. These 'cascade' flowmeter tubes for each gas are arranged sequentially (Fig. 6.14) so that when the flow control valve is opened the low-flow tube is seen to register first. At flows over 1 l min^{-1}, the bobbin in the low-flow tube is no longer easily visible.

Carbon dioxide flowmeters

The provision of carbon dioxide on anaesthetic machines is somewhat controversial, as several deaths have occurred owing to the inadvertent and excessive use of the gas. Typically, in these accidents, the flowmeter valve had been left fully open, either during a check procedure or at the end of a previous case, and the bobbin was not readily noticed at the top of the flowmeter tube. The next patient then received in excess of 2 l min^{-1} of carbon dioxide. Flowmeters have therefore been introduced that do not have a bezel which can hide the flowmeter bobbin at the top of the tube. Current standards permit a maximum flow of 600 ml min^{-1} from carbon dioxide flowmeters.

Anti-hypoxia devices

Anaesthesia machines in use now must either not be capable of delivering a gas mixture with less than 20% oxygen or have a means to give an alarm at an oxygen concentration of below 20% in the inspiratory gas which must be separate from any 'add on' patient respiratory gas monitoring (EN 740:1999). Of these approaches it has proven ultimately safer and simpler to design a system whereby it is physically impossible to set the nitrous oxide and oxygen flow rates to give hypoxic mixtures. Some approaches taken by manufacturers are discussed below.

Mechanical devices, e.g. 'Link 25' system (Ohmeda)

This device (Fig. 6.16) incorporates a chain that links the flow control valves for nitrous oxide and oxygen. There is a fixed sprocket (cog) on the nitrous oxide spindle that relays its movement to a larger cog on the oxygen flowmeter spindle via a chain. The oxygen cog moves along a static, hollow worm gear, through which the

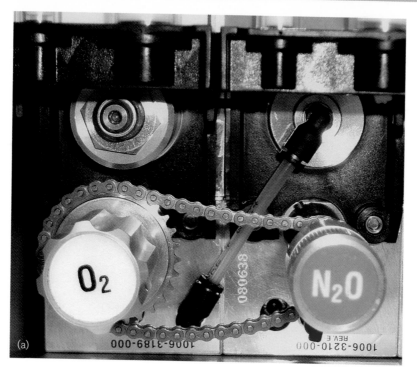

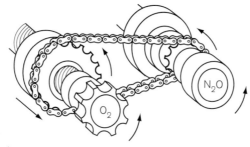

Figure 6.16 'Link 25 system'. **(a)** In place on the Datex–Ohmeda Aestiva/5. **(b)** Schematic of operation.

oxygen flowmeter spindle passes. As the nitrous oxide flowmeter control is turned counter–clockwise (increasing the nitrous oxide flow), the chain link moves this larger cog nearer to the oxygen flowmeter control so that, when a 25% oxygen mixture is reached, it locks on to the oxygen control knob and moves it synchronously with any further increase in nitrous oxide flow. The oxygen flow control can of course be independently opened further but cannot be closed below a setting that if nitrous oxide is flowing, will produce less than 25% oxygen in the mixture. Other manufacturers use inter-linking gears (Fig. 6.17) to achieve the same effect. This type of mechanical link, however, has some limitations:

- It takes no account of other gases in the flowmeter block (air and carbon dioxide) that could potentially dilute the mixture below a 25% oxygen concentration.
- On its own it will not recognize and compensate for variations in gas supply pressure that affect flow-meter performance. However, these systems include secondary pressure regulators (see above) in both the oxygen and nitrous oxide systems, the purpose of which is to prevent variations in gas supply pressure from affecting flowmeter performance.
- At low fresh gas flows into a circle system, a 25% oxygen ratio may be insufficient to prevent the circle patient gas mixture from becoming hypoxic (see Fig. 7.22). Hence a minimum basal flow of oxygen (see below) or a 50% oxygen ratio at low flows is required.

A further safety feature of this system includes a mechanical stop fitted (Fig. 6.17) to the oxygen flow-

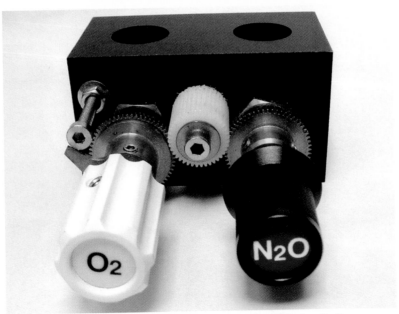

Figure 6.17 Blease mechanical interlink hypoxic guard, showing stop for minimum O_2 flow.

meter control valve, ensuring that a preset minimum standing flow (typically between 25–250 ml min^{-1}) of oxygen is maintained even when the valve is fully closed. This flow, of course, can occur only when the machine master switch for all the gases is switched on.

Pneumatic devices, e.g. pneupac ratio system

This system relies on a ratio mixer valve (Fig. 6.18) to ensure that the oxygen concentration leaving the flowmeter block never drops below 25% of the nitrous oxide concentration. When the machine master switch is turned on, a basal flow rate of 200–300 ml min^{-1} of oxygen is established (Fig. 6.19a). This is independent of, and bypasses, the ratio mixer valve. Nitrous oxide supplied to one side of the valve exerts a pressure on the diaphragm which is opposed by the pressure exerted by oxygen on a separate but coupled larger diaphragm (Fig. 6.19b). Inward movement of the oxygen diaphragm is linked to the opening of a poppet valve that allows more oxygen to flow through the O_2 chamber thus balancing the opposing forces. Any increase in the flow of nitrous oxide results in an increase in pressure on the nitrous oxide side of the diaphragm, causing the latter to move towards the compartment containing oxygen. The ratio of the area of the diaphragms is so constructed that the oxygen flow rate will increase by a ratio of 25% of any increase in the nitrous oxide flow rate. This increased

oxygen flow is independent of the main oxygen flow control valve that bypasses the ratio mixer valve and, of course, can be adjusted independently. The ratio mixer valve does not work in reverse as it takes a single passive N_2O connection from downstream of the N_2O flow control valve whilst taking O_2 from upstream (before) of the O_2 flow control valve; hence, if the nitrous oxide flow rates are reduced, the oxygen flows remain as set before by the O_2 flow control valve. The double diaphragm arrangement also means that rupture of a diaphragm will not result in contamination of the O_2 flow by N_2O.

Electronically controlled anti-hypoxia devices (Penlon Ltd)

In this system, a paramagnetic oxygen analyzer continuously samples the gases mixture leaving the flowmeter bank. If the oxygen concentration falls below 25%, a battery-powered electronic device sounds an audible alarm and the nitrous oxide supply is cut off. This results in an increase in the oxygen concentration and, as a result, the nitrous oxide supply is temporarily restored. If the oxygen flow rate has not been increased, the nitrous oxide disabling system is reactivated and the alarm will again sound. The whole process is repeated, thus providing an intermittent oxygen failure alarm and at the same time assuring a breathing mixture with more than 25% oxygen (although the total flow rate will be lower than intended).

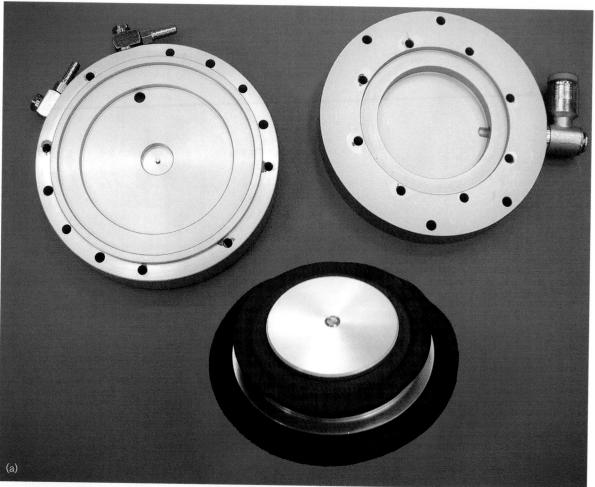

(a)

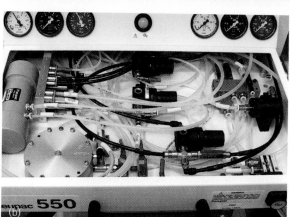

(b)

Figure 6.18 Pneupac oxygen ratio system valve **(a)** opened (and image manipulated) to better demonstrate double diaphragm arrangement and their relative sizes, note that a spacer ring that is interposed between the two valve housings is not shown here **(b)** in place in a Pneupac anaesthesia machine.

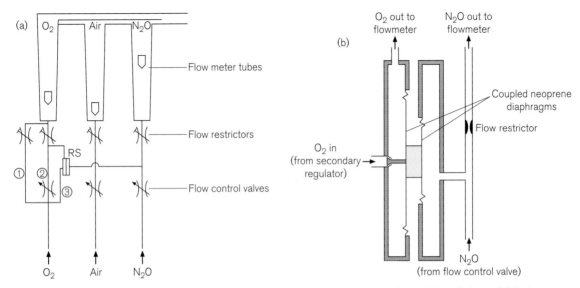

Figure 6.19 Pneupac oxygen ratio system. **(a)** Schematic of pneumatic connections. Abbreviations: (1) independent basal flow set at 250 ml min^{-1}: (2) operator variable flow from flow control valve: (3) flow through oxygen ratio system at 25% of N_2O flow. **(b)** Schematic of oxygen ratio system showing coupled diaphragms.

If the oxygen supply fails completely, there is a continuous audible alarm. The power is provided by a maintenance-free lead-acid battery that is kept charged by the mains electricity supply while the machine is in use and will continue to operate in the absence of a mains supply for 1.5 h. If the audible alarm is activated during this period it will sound for 20 min, after which a visual and audible 'low battery' warning is given. If for some reason the lead-acid battery is not adequately charged at the beginning of an anaesthetic session, the nitrous oxide supply (as well as medical air in US versions) is disabled and cannot be used. However, under no circumstances is the oxygen supply interrupted. This alarm is in addition to the standard oxygen failure warning device (Ritchie Whistle, see below).

Penlon stopped installing this electronic system of hypoxia protection in 2001, largely for reasons of cost, but many of their machines are still currently in use with this technology. Penlon now use a mechanical interlink. (See below, Specific Machines, Dräger Primus for a further example of electronic control of oxygen ratio.)

The back bar

Strictly speaking, the term 'back bar' describes the horizontal part of the frame of the machine, which supports the flowmeter block, the vaporizers and some other components. However, it is often used loosely to also include those components and the gaseous pathways interconnecting them. In fact, in modern machines, the latter are often housed within the framework.

The vaporizers are mounted, either singly or in series, along the back bar, downstream from the flowmeter block. Traditionally, vaporizers were bolted on to the back bar and linked to each other by tapered fittings. The various manufacturers employed different sizes of tapers and mounting positions but these were superseded by the provisions of BS 3849 (UK), which recommended 23 mm 'cagemount' tapers. (The term cagemount originally refers to a type and size of tapered connection for a reservoir or rebreathing bag that has a small wire cage fitted to its inlet to prevent the neck of the bag from being obstructed, when the latter is empty and collapsed. The cagemount taper for vaporizers, though no longer used in the West, is still in use in many parts of the world.)

Modern vaporizers are designed so that they may easily be removed from the back bar and replaced by those for another agent. Systems in which vaporizers may be detached are generally regarded as an advance over the permanent cagemount system. Ease of removal has resulted in a greater flexibility in the choice and use of agents, and also ensures that anaesthetic machines do not have to be taken out of use to allow the servicing of the vaporizers.

Thus, the back bar provides mounting blocks as described below. The Ohmeda 'Selectatec' fitting is perhaps the most popular in the UK but most machine manufacturers now offer their machines with a choice of vaporizer mount.

The Ohmeda 'Selectatec' System (Fig. 6.20)

Each Selectatec station on the back bar has two vertically mounted male valve ports. Between these inlet and outlet ports is an accessory pin and a locking recess. The matching vaporizer assembly has two female ports between which there is a locking assembly and a recess to accommodate the pin. The vaporizer is lowered on to the male valve ports and the locking knob is turned to fix it into the recess on the back bar (Fig. 6.20a). Successive generations of vaporizer are labelled sequentially and although the essential design of the back bar mounting system has not changed, the accessory pin has been added

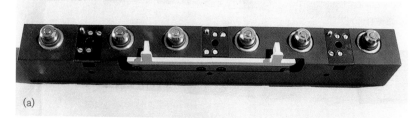

(a)

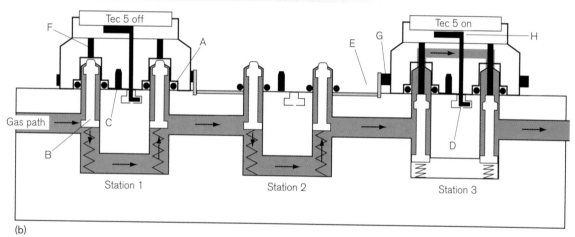

(b)

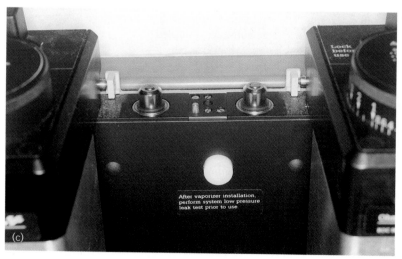

(c)

Figure 6.20 (a) A three-station 'Selectatec' back bar (viewed from behind). **(b)** Schematic diagram showing a TEC 5 vaporizer attached at station 1 and switched OFF, an empty station 2 and a TEC 5 attached at station 3 but switched ON. A, 'O'-ring seal; B, valve; C, TEC 3 lock-out pin; D, recess for vaporizer lock; E, safety interlock; F, recessed spindles in the vaporizer; G, immobilizer rod; H, back bar lock. **(c)** A three-station back bar showing the safety interlock mechanism.

to prevent use of Tec 3 and previous generations on the modern back bar (see below).

'O'-rings on the male valve ports ensure a gas-tight fit. The two female ports on the vaporizer have recessed spindles (TEC 4 and above) that, when the vaporizer is switched on, protrude through the gas-tight seals of the male valve ports on the back bar. The ball valves (which provide the seals) in the male ports are displaced downwards occluding the back bar, and gas from the back bar is diverted into the vaporizer (Fig. 6.20b, station 3). TEC 3 vaporizers had fixed spindles that automatically depressed the ball valves in the male valve ports when the vaporizer was lowered on to the back bar assembly. Gas, therefore, passed through the head of the vaporizer even when it was not switched on or even locked on. This arrangement obviously had a greater potential for gas leaks and has been modified by the retractable spindle assembly on the TEC 4, 5, 6 and 7.

These models also incorporate a 'safety interlock'. This consists of an extension rod that protrudes sideways from a vaporizer as it is turned on, and displaces the equivalent rod on the vaporizer beside it, preventing the latter from being switched on. On a three-station back bar, there is a plastic lever (Fig. 6.20) linking stations 1 and 3. Should station 2 be empty, the lever links the extension rods between vaporizers 1 and 3 to ensure that only one vaporizer can be turned on at any one time. Tec 3 vaporizers had no safety interlock and this is yet another reason for their use being precluded by the fitting of the accessory pin. Presently machines are rarely specified with a three station back bar and this plastic lever is seldom required.

Dräger interlock

The mounting system is similar to the 'Selectatec' version although the dimensions are unique (Fig. 6.21). The mounting system also includes an interlock preventing the administration of more than one vapour. Dräger vaporizers are also available with Selectatec and other fittings.

Problems with detachable vaporizer systems

Removable vaporizer systems generate their own specific problems:

- As mentioned above, there is a greater potential for leaks.
- The vaporizer may be accidentally dropped and damaged in transit to or from the back bar.
- Tipping of older models of vaporizer in transit could result in liquid agent entering the bypass system causing either liquid or high concentrations of vapour to be present in the breathing system.

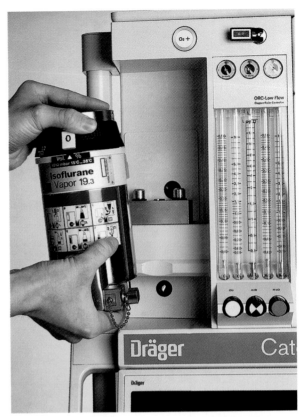

Figure 6.21 Dräger interlock vaporizer and back bar.

- Also, in countries where trichloroethylene is still used, a vaporizer containing this agent may accidentally be attached to a back bar station in a position that results in the vapour being passed into a breathing system containing soda lime. Trichloroethylene is known to react with warm soda lime to produce substances that are neurotoxic if inhaled.

Back bar working pressures

The flowmeter tubes in the flowmeter bank have, as a rule, been calibrated for gas flows assuming no downstream resistance. In a traditional back bar (23 mm internal diameter system) with the vaporizers switched off, the wide bore of the gas passages offers minimal flow resistance and so the back bar pressure developed at conventional flow rates (5–10 l min^{-1}) is marginally above atmospheric pressure. However, many modern back bars have narrow bore (8 mm) gas passages, which increase flow resistance and thus back-pressure on the flowmeters.

The addition of high-resistance vaporizers and minute volume divider ventilators, which cause a build-up of

Table 6.1 Selectatec back bar working pressures

Recorded gas pressures in a two station back bar	Nominal flow rates at atmospheric pressure		*Percentage change in flowmeter sight readings at	
	5 litres	10 litres	5 litres	10 litres
Beginning of back bar (no vaporizers *in situ*) kPa (cmH$_2$O)	1.18 (12)	4.2 (43)	None	Minimal
At 2nd vaporizer station (no vaporizers *in situ*) kPa (cmH$_2$O)	0.78 (8)	2.45 (25)	None	Minimal
Beginning of back bar with TEC 4 vaporizer at 2nd station set to deliver:				
0% kPa (cmH$_2$O)	1.18 (12)	4.2 (43)	None	Minimal
1% kPa (cmH$_2$O)	3.23 (33)	8.5 (87)	None	<5%
5% kPa (cmH$_2$O)	2.74 (28)	7.74 (79)	None	<5%
Total occlusion of common gas outlet kPa (cmH$_2$O)	30.5 (312)		20%	20%

*This column shows the percentage change in sight readings, in a flowmeter initially calibrated at atmospheric pressure caused by the various resistances to flow seen in a 'Selectatec' back bar and TEC 4 vaporizer.

pressure in the fresh gas flow (see Chapter 11, Automatic Ventilators), increases back bar pressures. Table 6.1 shows typical back bar pressures developed and percentage changes in flowmeter settings with the 'Selectatec' back bar with and without a high-resistance vaporizer fitted. It should be noted that the small decreases in the flowmeter indications produced does not mean a decrease in the flow of gas to a patient. It is merely that the gas is compressed at the higher pressures and subsequently re-expands downstream when the various resistances have been overcome. Readjustment of the flowmeters to the original settings following an induced pressure rise would therefore be inappropriate.

Additional safety features

Several safety features are installed either on or downstream of the back bar:

- Intermittent back-pressure surges from certain minute volume divider ventilators can adversely affect vaporizer performance (see Chapter 5), and so most machines employ a spring-loaded non-return valve in the system to prevent these surges reaching the vaporizers.
- Since high-pressure build-up in the back bar can damage flowmeter and vaporizer components, a pressure relief valve (commonly set at 30–40 kPa) is fitted. This is often fitted in the same housing as the non-return valve (Fig. 6.22).

Emergency oxygen

A flowmeter bypass valve for an emergency oxygen supply is now fitted as standard (EN ISO 60601-2-13). The bypass flow joins the pipeline from the back bar just before the common gas outlet such that, when activated, it preferentially supplies oxygen at a rate of not less than 30 l min^{-1} into an attached breathing system. In earlier anaesthetic machines this bypass for oxygen was fitted near the flowmeter block. When it was operated, this resulted in an initial surge of gas and vapour to the patient prior to the pure oxygen being delivered.

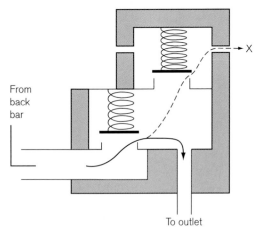

Figure 6.22 Combined non-return and pressure-relief valve at the end of the back bar. If the outlet is obstructed, the gases escape at X, so protecting the back bar from overpressure. A low-pressure relief valve is also available to protect the patient.

The flowmeter bypass valve should no longer have a locking facility since this is regarded as dangerous and has resulted in cases of barotrauma when it has been switched on accidentally.. The valve knob should also be recessed to minimize the chances of its inadvertent operation.

Oxygen failure warning devices
These were first introduced in the 1950s as a response to the problems of unobserved emptying of oxygen cylinders. However, early models could be unreliable as the battery-powered part of the alarm could be switched off or the battery could be exhausted or missing. The gas powered part, which relied on nitrous oxide, could also be switched off or fail simultaneously with the oxygen (in which case the alarm would also not work).

The Ritchie whistle
The Ritchie whistle was introduced in the mid-1960s and forms the basis for most current oxygen failure devices. It was the first device to rely exclusively on the failing oxygen supply for its power. Figure 6.23 shows an oxygen failure warning device incorporating a Ritchie whistle marketed at one time by Ohmeda and still present on older machines in service.

The alarm is powered by an oxygen supply at a pressure of 420 kPa (60 psi) in the UK, which is tapped from the oxygen pipework upstream of the flowmeter block. This enters the alarm inlet valve and pressurizes the rolling diaphragm, opening the anaesthetic cut-off valve, and closing the air inspiratory valve and the port to the

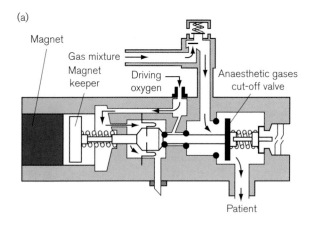

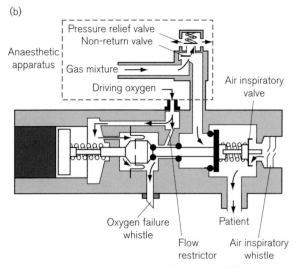

Figure 6.23 Oxygen failure warning device. **(a)** Normal operation. **(b)** Operation during oxygen failure.

oxygen failure whistle. Anaesthetic gases may then pass freely through this device, which is now at standby. The valve is kept in this position by the pressure of the oxygen supply opposing the force of the magnet and the return spring.

Decreasing pressure in the oxygen supply to the flowmeter block activates the valve, permitting a flow of oxygen (via the restrictor) to operate the oxygen failure whistle. The whistle sounds continuously until the oxygen pressure has fallen to approximately 40.5 kPa (6 psi). At a pressure of approximately 200 kPa (30 psi) the force of the magnet keeper return spring and the magnet causes the anaesthetic gases cut-off valve to be closed, cutting off the supply of anaesthetic gases to the patient. At the

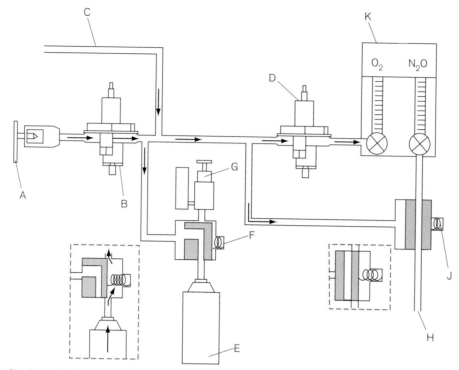

Figure 6.24 A schematic diagram of a current oxygen failure warning device. A, Cylinder yoke for oxygen; B, primary regulator for oxygen (137 000 kPa to 420 kPa); C, pipeline oxygen supply; D, secondary regulator for oxygen (420 kPa to 140 kPa); E, reservoir of oxygen required to power the Ritchie Whistle for a minimum of 7 s; F, spring-loaded regulator. When oxygen supply pressure drops to 200 kPa reservoir E is connected to the Ritchie Whistle; G, Ritchie Whistle; H, nitrous oxide supply; J, spring-loaded shut-off valve to nitrous oxide supply activated when oxygen supply pressure drops below 200 kPa; K, flowmeter bank.

same time the spring load on the air inspiratory valve is released, allowing the patient to inspire room air. Whenever the patient inhales, the inspiratory air whistle sounds.

With the anaesthetic gases cut-off valve closed, the now potentially hypoxic gas from the flowmeter block vents to the atmosphere through the pressure-relief valve on the back bar.

Current oxygen failure warning devices

BS EN 740:1999 and EN ISO 60601-2-13, its replacement, stipulate that anaesthetic workstations in use with gases containing less than 21% premixed oxygen content shall be operated with a gas cut off device. This gas cut off device must either:

- Cut off the supply of all gases other than oxygen, air and premixed gases with an oxygen content above 21%(V/V) to the fresh gas outlet; or
- progressively reduce the flow of all other gases

[except air or premixed gases with an oxygen content above 21% (V/V)] while maintaining the proportion of oxygen until the supply of oxygen finally fails, at which point the supply of all other gases [except air or premixed gases with an oxygen content above 21% (V/V)] shall be cut off.

Also 'the gas cut off device shall not be activated before the oxygen supply failure alarm', and 'the sole means of resetting the gas cut off device shall be restoration of the oxygen supply pressure to a level above that at which the device is activated'.

A gas powered auditory alarm signal for oxygen failure is required to be of at least 7 seconds duration and where the alarm signal is gas powered (as opposed to electrically generated) 'the energy required to operate it shall be derived from the oxygen supply pressure'.

Figure 6.24 shows a schematic diagram of the pneumatic arrangement for an alarm and shut off system that satisfies current standards.

Common gas outlet

The various medical gases and vapours exit the machine via a coaxial 22 mm male/15 mm female conically tapered outlet. Machines must have no more than one common gas outlet, although if there is an integral circle breathing system, gas flow may be switched between this and the common gas outlet (CGO).

This CGO may be fixed, or swivelled through 90° (Cardiff Swivel), and should be strong enough to withstand a bending moment of force of up to 10 Nm applied to its axis, since heavy equipment is often attached.

Previously the CGO was often designed with a metal disk in its base to act as a one-way valve and allow entrainment of room air through a high pitched inspiratory whistle in situations where gas flow was insufficient to meet patient demands during spontaneous ventilation. This facility is now rarely installed as these tilt valves were prone to leaking from impaction of grit on the valve seating. Furthermore, the increased popularity of circle breathing systems for which such a valve serves no function has rendered them obsolete.

Auxiliary gas sockets

Anaesthetic machines may now be fitted with mini-Schrader gas sockets (Fig. 6.25), but only for air or oxygen. These may be used to power devices such as ventilators, gas injection systems for bronchoscopy, and suction units. The sockets should be permanently and legibly marked for their specific gases (air or oxygen) and their working pressure of 400 kPa approximately (in the UK).

VENTILATORS

Automatic ventilators, including their classification and fundamental principles, are discussed specifically in Chapter 11. Ventilators for use in the Intensive Care Unit (ICU) are further considered in Chapter 12.

From the point of view of the anaesthetic workstation, ventilators have developed significantly even in the last decade. Whereas once simple mechanical minute volume dividers placed on the anaesthetic machine were the norm, with a few adventurous manufacturers installing pneumatically driven bag squeezers or intermittent

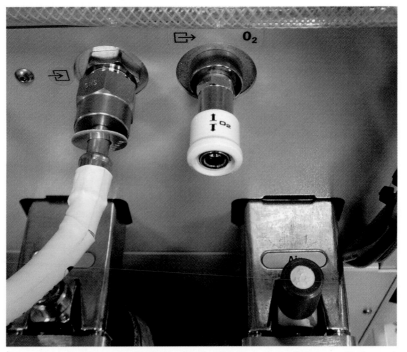

Figure 6.25 An auxiliary oxygen outlet on the back of a Datex–Ohmeda Aestiva/5 anaesthetic workstation.

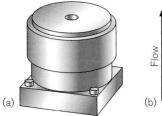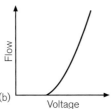

Figure 6.26 (a) Representation of proportional flow valve and **(b)** the relationship between voltage and gas flow. (Figure 11.9a, page 253, shows the mode of operation of a typical proportional flow valve.)

blowers, the modern anaesthetic ventilator is now akin to an ICU ventilator.

Over the past few years, software driven ventilators have become standard, with manufacturers able to offer a variety of ventilatory modes including pressure controlled ventilation, synchronized ventilation and pressure supported spontaneous ventilation as optional extras with the machine's inbuilt ventilator. This flexibility is largely a function of the sophisticated electronic control of the proportional flow valve (see below).

In order to fully separate the pneumatically driven ventilator used by most manufacturers (there are exceptions such as the Dräger Primus below) from the respiratory gases of the patient, the 'bag in bottle' arrangement with a rising bellows is almost ubiquitous.

Proportional flow valves

The heart of the modern ventilator is the proportional flow valve. This type of valve allows extremely accurate and rapid control of the flow of gas from a high-pressure source. Whereas a simple solenoid can oscillate rapidly between on and off positions, the proportional valve is so termed because the excursion of the solenoid (and opening of the attached valve) is proportional to the voltage applied across it (Fig. 6.26). These valves typically allow flow rates between 1 and 120 l min^{-1}. Upstream pressures supplied to the valve of 1.5 to 5 bar require an excursion of only 0.6 to 0.2 mm for a flow rate of 120 l min^{-1}. The rise time for the valve is therefore typically less than 5 milliseconds. Consequently massive flows can be rapidly generated on patient demand, even allowing almost seamless pressure support of spontaneous patient breathing. Downstream flow and pressure sensing permits feedback control of the flow from the valve via a microprocessor control system. Figure 6.27 shows a typical proportional valve.

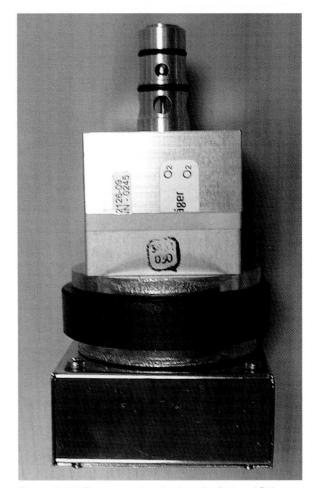

Figure 6.27 The proportional valve of a Dräger ICU type ventilator, here a ruby ball on a sapphire valve seat forms the flow orifice within the narrow steel cylinder at the top of the device.

Control of such valves is accurate enough to permit positive end-expiratory pressure (PEEP) to be applied in some ventilators simply by allowing a bias flow through the valve during expiration. Sufficient flow controlled by a feedback loop is allowed to pressurize the bellows and pop off valve (expiratory valve) in the bellows housing to give the desired level of PEEP.

Some systems, such as the Dräger E series ventilators, use a second or separate proportional valves to control a lower pressure gas flow from which a side arm is used to pressurize the machine side of an expiratory valve for control of inspiration and PEEP or continuous positive airway pressure (CPAP) (Fig. 6.28).

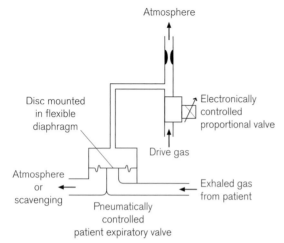

Figure 6.28 Proportional valve control of patient expiratory valve.

INTEGRAL BREATHING SYSTEMS

Concerns about economy in the use of volatile anaesthetic agents and gases, both for reasons of cost and atmospheric pollution coupled with the heat and moisture retaining properties of the circle system, have ensured that the circle has become an integral part of the modern anaesthetic workstation.

The need to both integrate the breathing system into an ergonomic design and allow sterilization of patient gas pathways, can produce a labarynthine system with multiple parts, valves and microswitches to sense the position and function of levers and detachable components (Fig. 6.29). That, in spite of such numerous parts, many of these machines cannot be misassembled and do not leak, is a testament to good engineering design. However the potential for problems to arise in such complex devices must always be borne in mind and it is advocated that a self-inflating bag and alternative source of oxygen is always readily available (see Pre-use check below). A 'top circuit', such as a Mapleson C or D for attachment to the common gas outlet in times of crisis and confusion, is also extremely useful.

ERGONOMICS

Ergonomics is the study of the efficiency of persons in their working environment and *human factors engineering* is the design and development of equipment to improve the ergonomics of a task. This has the effect of making the working environment not only more pleasant but less tiring and less stressful, which should lead to increased safety. The conventional pneumatic anaesthetic machine 'just grew' and there has been little attempt in the past to specifically consider ergonomics. Nonetheless, some design endpoints, reached after a long journey of reducing error and set in current standards, such as those specifying the stand out position and shape of the oxygen flowmeter control knob (together with attendant guards to prevent accidental resetting), exemplify ergonomics in practice.

Given the many demands, detailed above, made of the modern workstation there has to be far greater consideration given to ergonomics at the design stage. Sections of the machine should have clearly defined task orientations with tasks or modalities not divided across different areas of the machine. Modular approaches to the workstation are particularly prone to having various components fighting one another. The execution of multiple linked manoeuvres to achieve a single functional change in the machine settings (e.g. having to alter several switches to go from spontaneous to controlled ventilation) is an example of poor design. This is clearly more error prone, particularly under stressful conditions, than having a single lever and can leave the patient at risk (here apnoeic). The 'Feng Shui,' to misappropriate from Chinese culture, has to be right. A busy-looking machine, where it is not possible to immediately tell where pipes are coming from and going to, is an error prone device.

By contrast, a single item of good ergonomic design sometimes does more to sell a machine than a host of technological advances directed at greater accuracy. In an operating theatre, which may be used for several surgical specialities, the value of features such as a foot operated single break lever which renders the machine easily mobile on its castors should not be underestimated. The ability to have the machine controls and the patient's airway all within an easy arc of reach for the anaesthetist can ultimately affect safety and the ease with which a critical incident is dealt with. For similar reasons, the back of the workstation (in particular, the flexible pipeline and electrical cables) should be treated with equal respect and should not be allowed to resemble an explosion in a souk!

Implicit in the concept of ergonomics is that in a well-designed machine controls and functions are intuitive and it is possible for a new user to quickly learn how to work the device. Militating against this is the desire of manufacturers, particularly where ventilators are concerned, to offer something extra, if only in name.

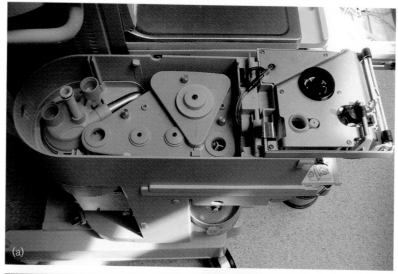

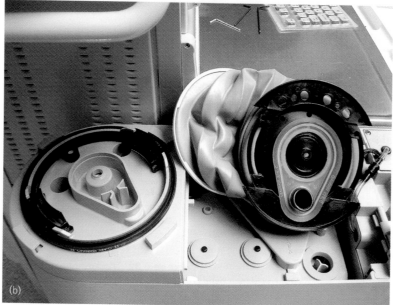

Figure 6.29 Circle system of Datex–Ohmeda Aestiva partially stripped down to show gas pathways, bellows, valves, seals and other autoclaveable parts (including blue silicone rubber parts and 'airbox' in centre of upper photograph). **(b)** Shows the expiratory pop off valve at the base of the bellows.

STANDARDS

A number of standards documents clearly define many aspects of the design of anaesthetic workstations. At the time of writing, BS EN 740:1998 *Anaesthetic Workstations and their modules-Particular Requirements*, which itself superseded BS5724-2-13:1990, is due to be replaced by EN ISO 60601-2-13, *Medical electrical equipment – Part 2-13: Particular requirements for the safety of anaesthetic systems.*

The main standard for all medical devices is IEC 60601-1, *Medical Electrical Equipment General Requirements for Safety*. All medical devices will have some form of Part 2 document: such as 2–13 for anaesthetic machines. All other standards in the series follow this structure, with paragraph numbers relating to

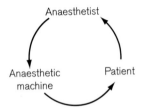

Figure 6.30 Anaesthetic 'control loop'.

the same feature in all documents in that series: paragraph 21 is Mechanical Strength and this will be the same in the 2–13 document. The Part 2 document adds modifications to the basic standard, taking into account the special features and use of the device.

These documents themselves refer to a number of other standards documents. Chapter 30 gives some background explanation regarding standards and their status and purpose.

THE CRITICAL INCIDENT (see also Chapter 31)

The interaction between anaesthetist, anaesthesia machine and patient may be seen as a closed loop control system[2] (Fig. 6.30): with the situation where one or more components of the control loop behave unpredictably described as a *critical incident*.

When an adverse condition begins, the chance of injury to the patient increases with time, as shown in Figure 6.31. There is a time delay before a problem is noticed by the anaesthetist and the cause identified. Another delay occurs before the problem is corrected, after which there should be a recovery to safe conditions if the correction is made early enough. Excessive delay in noticing the problem or in its correction may lead to permanent injury.

The reliability of the human for constant vigilance over long periods of time is questionable and the ability to make decisions when bombarded with multiple sensory inputs is sorely put to the test. Alarm systems should be designed to allow for as much time as possible to correct a problem before injury begins. Examination of Figure 6.31 shows that this may be accomplished by minimizing the pre-alarm period and making it clear to the anaesthetist what the problem is and its level of urgency. Research has shown that *intelligent alarm systems* which integrate and prioritize multiple alarm conditions can lead to a more rapid and consistent rectification of adverse incidents.[3]

The further along the system (e.g. from the gas and electricity supplies to the patient) that a parameter is

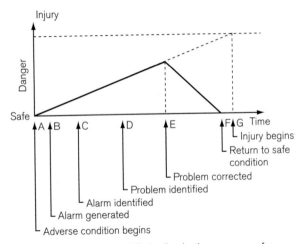

Figure 6.31 Diagram of Schreiber's time course of a critical incident as it would occur in anaesthetic practice.

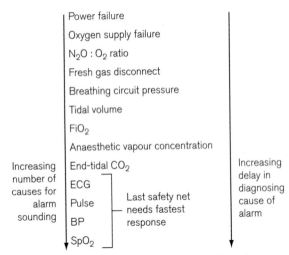

Figure 6.32 The further along the system from the supplies to the patient that a parameter is monitored, the greater the delay before the problem is corrected.

monitored (Fig. 6.32), the greater the delay before the alarm is sounded and the greater the number of possible causes of that particular problem. For example, if the oxygen supply fails, the oxygen supply alarm would sound immediately. Some seconds later, depending on the fresh gas flow into the breathing attachment, the inspired oxygen monitor alarm would become active. However, it may be more than a minute before the saturation, as indicated by a pulse oximeter, would fall below the critical level. Furthermore, the causes of a drop in SpO_2 are numerous compared with the causes of the sounding of the oxygen supply pressure alarm. In this scenario, assuming multiple monitoring points of anaesthesia system and patient, an intelligent alarm system would assimilate the multiple alarm conditions and prioritize the oxygen supply failure, hence leading to the most rapid resolution of the incident.

Alarms

Alarms do not necessarily refer to emergencies but may indicate abnormal situations that may or may not have the potential to become emergencies. Given the number of different parameters surveyed by the workstation monitors, there clearly has to be some system of prioritizing alarms to allow sensible signalling in multiple alarm conditions. Alarm conditions are therefore given a hierarchy from *advisory* (requiring awareness) to *caution* (requiring a prompt response) and *warning* (requiring immediate response). At any time, the condition with the highest priority is preferentially displayed. Ideally an audible warning differentiating between these three levels draws the anaesthetist's attention to a visual indication of what the problem is. *Latching* of alarms means that even if the condition leading to the alarm is resolved, the alarm continues to sound until it is acknowledged and reset. Accepted standards give minimum alarm hierarchies for various parameters and state those that can and cannot be disabled.

Much research has been done on alarms,[4] alarm characteristics and those features that control the perceived urgency, namely: frequency composition, repetition rate, amplitude, and harmonic relation of the frequency components. The urgency of the alarm must be balanced against its liability to distract the target's concentration during critical periods, and the possible nuisance effect from 'false alarms', as well as its effect on non-target audience (e.g. patient or surgeon). This is not an easy task; additionally, an alarm perceived as excessively intrusive may be disabled by the anaesthetist. Although the ISO publish clear standards for alarms (ISO 9703-2), significant latitude is still allowed to manufacturers and even with standards compatible alarm structures it is argued that the current alarms in many popular machines are inappropriate in terms of conveying the correct urgency.[5] Ideally, ultimately alarm signals should be identical across manufacturers for any given modality of monitoring or item of equipment. In any case, it is perhaps time manufacturers revisited this subject.

Nonetheless, the quality of modern monitoring equipment available, as well as the ease and flexibility of operator setting of alarm limits, means that the practice of disabling alarms (rather than setting alarm parameters to prevent inappropriate alarm triggering) is no longer acceptable. By the same token, alarms should not be allowed to continually sound (often a feature of inadequate implied urgency) when there is no perceived problem: this leads to habituation to the alarm sound and ultimately failure to react to appropriate alarms.

PRE-USE CHECK

It is mandatory to check the correct functioning of anaesthetic equipment before use. The Association of Anaesthetists of Great Britain and Ireland (AAGBI) publishes a 'Checklist for Anaesthetic Equipment' to assist in allowing a comprehensive and systematic check of equipment (Table 6.2). The most recent iteration of this, in 2004,[6] recognizes the introduction of microprocessor controlled technology into anaesthetic workstations and attempts not to reduplicate the self-test cycle that modern workstations undergo on start-up. It also stresses the importance of familiarity with these potentially complex pieces of machinery and hence the need for a formal 'induction' onto the machine. Also noteworthy is the requirement that a log should be kept of the completion of a pre-use check according to both the requirements of the manufacturer and the AAGBI checklist.

With all machines and, perhaps even more so with electronically controlled workstations, consideration must be given to the possibility that the machine will fail to deliver any or adequate flows of gas. For this reason it is imperative to check that an alternative oxygen supply and means of ventilation, such as a self-inflating bag, are readily available and functional.

An abbreviated description of the AAGBI checking procedure is produced as a laminated sheet for attachment to each anaesthetic machine. This is reproduced below.

SPECIFIC MACHINES

By considering just a few specific machines, it is possible to get a reasonable idea of the scope of design of the modern workstations currently available. Three machines are therefore considered separately below. When compared with each other it is interesting to observe their differing use of technology and the disparate focus of their

Table 6.2 AAGBI checklist for anaesthetic equipment (with permission from AAGBI).

The Asssociation of Anaesthetists of Great Britain and Ireland
CHECKLIST FOR ANAESTHETIC EQUIPMENT 2004

The following checks should be made prior to each operating session.

In addition, checks 2, 6 and 9 (Monitoring, Breathing System and Ancillary Equipment) should be made prior to each new patient during a session.

1. Check that the anaesthetic machine is connected to the electricity supply (if appropriate) and switched on. Note: Some anaesthetic workstations may enter an integral self-test programme when switched on; those functions tested by such a programme need not be retested.
   - Take note of any information or labelling on the anaesthetic machine referring to the current status of the machine. Particular attention should be paid to recent servicing. Servicing labels should be fixed in the service logbook.

2. Check that all monitoring devices, in particular the oxygen analyser, pulse oximeter and capnograph, are functioning and have appropriate alarm limits.
   - Check that gas sampling lines are properly attached and free of obstructions.
   - Check that an appropriate frequency of recording non-invasive blood pressure is selected.
   (Some monitors need to be in stand-by mode to avoid unnecessary alarms before being connected to the patient)

3. Check with a 'tug test' that each pipeline is correctly inserted into the appropriate gas supply terminal. Note: Carbon dioxide cylinders should not be present on the anaesthetic machine unless requested by the anaesthetist. A blanking plug should be fitted to any empty cylinder yoke.
   - Check that the anaesthetic machine is connected to a supply of oxygen and that an adequate supply of oxygen is available from a reserve oxygen cylinder.
   - Check that adequate supplies of other gases (nitrous oxide, air) are available and connected as appropriate.
   - Check that all pipeline pressure gauges in use on the anaesthetic machine indicate 400–500 kPa.

4. Check the operation of flowmeters (where fitted).
   - Check that each flow valve operates smoothly and that the bobbin moves freely throughout its range.
   - Check the anti-hypoxia device is working correctly.
   - Check the operation of the emergency oxygen bypass control.

5. Check the vaporizer(s):
   - Check that each vaporizer is adequately, but not over, filled.
   - Check that each vaporizer is correctly seated on the back bar and not tilted.
   - Check the vaporizer for leaks (with vaporizer on and off) by temporarily occluding the common gas outlet.
   - Turn the vaporizer(s) off when checks are completed.
   - Repeat the leak test immediately after changing any vaporizer.

6. Check the breathing system to be employed.
   Note: A new single use bacterial/viral filter and angle-piece/catheter mount must be used for each patient. Packaging should not be removed until point of use.
   - Inspect the system for correct configuration. All connections should be secured by 'push and twist'.
   - Perform a pressure leak test on the breathing system by occluding the patient-end and compressing the reservoir bag. Bain-type co-axial systems should have the inner tube compressed for the leak test.
   - Check the correct operation of all valves, including unidirectional valves within a circle, and all exhaust valves.
   - Check for patency and flow of gas through the whole breathing system including the filter and anglepiece/catheter mount.

7. Check that the ventilator is configured appropriately for its intended use.
   - Check that the ventilator tubing is correctly configured and securely attached.
   - Set the controls for use and ensure that an adequate pressure is generated during the inspiratory phase.
   - Check the pressure relief valve functions.
   - Check that the disconnect alarms function correctly.
   - Ensure that an alternative means to ventilate the patient's lungs is available. (see 10. below)

8. Check that the anaesthetic gas scavenging system is switched on and is functioning correctly.
   - Check that the tubing is attached to the appropriate exhaust port of the breathing system, ventilator or workstation.

Continued

Table 6.2, *cont'd.*

**The Asssociation of Anaesthetists of Great Britain and Ireland
CHECKLIST FOR ANAESTHETIC EQUIPMENT 2004**

9. Check that all ancillary equipment which may be needed is present and working.
   - This includes laryngoscopes, intubation aids, intubation forceps, bougies, etc. and appropriately sized facemasks, airways, tracheal tubes and connectors, which must be checked for patency.
   - Check that the suction apparatus is functioning and that all connectors are secure.
   - Check that the patient trolley, bed or operating table can be rapidly tilted head down.
10. Check that an alternative means to ventilate the patient is immediately available. (eg self-inflating bag and oxygen cylinder)
   - Check that the self-inflating bag and cylinder of oxygen are functioning correctly and the cylinder contains an adequate supply of oxygen.
11. Recording
   - Sign and date the logbook kept with the anaesthetic machine to confirm the machine has been checked.
   - Record on each patient's anaesthetic chart that the anaesthetic machine, breathing system and monitoring has been checked.

This check list is an abbreviated version of the Association of Anaesthetists publication 'Checking Anaesthetic Equipment 3 2004'
(Endorsed by the Chief Medical Officer and the Royal College of Anaesthetists)

respective designers. It will be interesting to see, over the next few years, which approach predominates and where the application of technology will prove most effective. Certainly, electronic control of the machine does not dominate now as would perhaps have been predicted ten years ago.

A number of manufacturers still produce simple pneumatic machines with no electronic components or integral breathing systems and there is clearly a role for such equipment. They are reliable, need minimal maintenance and are low cost and admittedly simpler to operate. They predominate in areas where non-anaesthetists may use them for resuscitation and in areas where space may be at a premium or other constraints operate such as anaesthetic induction areas. Their design conforms to the principles outlined above under 'The Anaesthetic Delivery System'; certainly in the UK there should no longer be machines available anywhere capable of delivering an hypoxic mixture.

The following paragraphs are not intended as a critique or assessment of the machines. Features and failures are highlighted purely to make the reader aware of issues that may be pertinent to any device being considered. The purpose of anaesthetic machines is ultimately quite simple – the safe delivery of drugs. Increasing familiarity with a machine can therefore only reveal its inadequacies.

Datex-Ohmeda Aestiva/5

The Aestiva/5 has been a very successful design of anaesthetic workstation (Fig. 6.33). It is, in all respects, a traditional pneumatic machine. There is a built-in circle system and a software driven pneumatically powered ventilator using the 'bag in bottle' arrangement to isolate respiratory and driving gases. The ventilator type is briefly described above and specifically in detail in Chapter 11. Conventional vaporizers are mounted on the back bar. Hypoxic mixture prevention is by use of the Ohmeda Link 25 system (Fig. 6.16). The CGO, as opposed to the integral circle breathing system, is selected by a lever discretely positioned to the side of the absorber.

Its popularity owes more to good ergonomic design than the use of advanced technology. Without doubt, much of this is due to the long-established Datex–Ohmeda AS/3 design of patient monitor. This monitor has hot swappable individual modules for an extensive number of parameters and benefits from a flexible and well laid out display and intuitive operating menu structure. This monitor is neatly housed within the Aestiva with a remote flat panel display which can be mounted on the swing arm of the machine to sit above or below the control panel of the ventilator. Depending on the configuration requested, the machine can offer a significant amount of flat storage or working surfaces and drawers. Use of a single foot operated brake lever renders

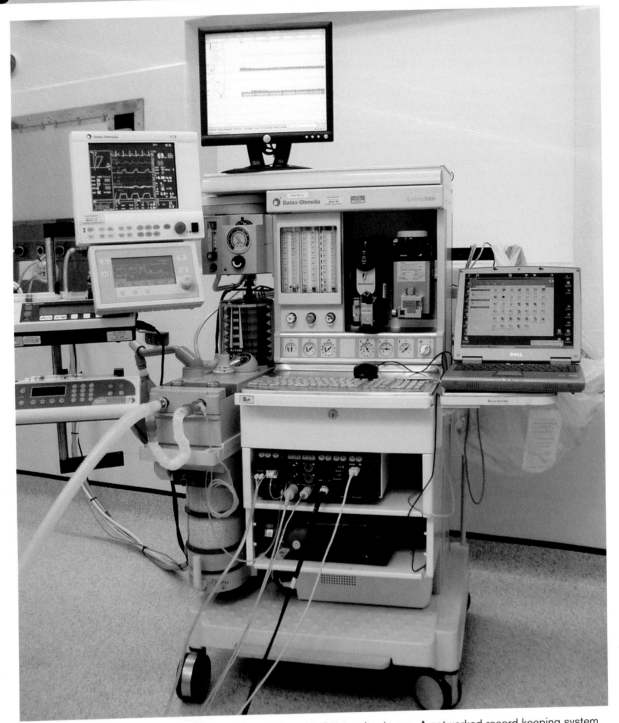

Figure 6.33 The Datex–Ohmeda Aestiva/5 workstation with S/5 monitor in use. A networked record keeping system and a further networked computer are also seen.

the machine freely mobile, allowing easy positioning of machine for access to the patient in any operating room set-up. The overall appearance of the machine is unfussy with clearly defined instrument clusters.

Low urgency ventilator panel alarms, such as the *advisory* alarm for selection of the auxiliary common gas outlet, are too easily ignored. One area where the machine would benefit from a more intelligent alarm structure is in the linking of respiration detected on the sensors of the integral circle system to the position of the auxiliary common gas outlet selection lever. Currently, with no increase in alarm urgency, a patient can breathe spontaneously on the circle system with volumes monitored at the circle displayed on the ventilator panel, whilst anaesthetic gases are delivered elsewhere.

Datex–Ohmeda ADU

First released in 1998, the ADU is still a striking-looking machine by virtue of the absence of traditional rotameters and vaporizers and the presence of twin flat panel displays for patient monitoring and control and monitoring of the pneumatic systems (Fig. 6.34).

The ADU is essentially a modular system and comprises:
- a wall gas unit, taking gas inlets from pipeline supplies and reserve cylinders;
- a fresh gas control unit responsible also for volatile agent admixture;
- an electronic ventilator unit;
- a central electronic unit for integrating control and monitoring; and
- an attached bellows block and compact circle absorber system.

The ventilator and fresh gas control units have their own microprocessor controls which communicate through the central electronic unit. A number of features of the ADU stand out for individual consideration (Fig. 6.35).

In spite of the absence of traditional flowmeters, gas flow is set by the operator using standard needle valves. An electronic switch selects air or N_2O as the 'side gas'. Electronic flow measurement across a laminar flow restrictor for both oxygen and the side gas ensures a minimum 25% oxygen concentration by controlling a proportional valve downstream of the N_2O needle valve when N_2O is selected. Gas flows are shown as pictograms on the user interface which also has a comm wheel for selecting and setting ventilator parameters.

The ventilator is a sophisticated microprocessor controlled pneumatically driven (air or oxygen) design

employing a number of proportional valves for individual control of inspiratory flow, expiratory valve and PEEP valve. Pressure and flow are measured at a number of points in the pneumatic system to allow close control of respiration. A single lever on the bellows block selects between bellows or reservoir bag and APL valve and relays via a sensing microswitch to switch on the ventilator.

Unique amongst machines currently available, is the electronic control of agent concentration. The Aladin cassette system still relies on saturation of a proportion of the fresh gas flow by passage through the vaporizer. Here though, when the desired agent concentration is selected on the machine, a proportional valve controls the flow of gas through the vaporizer. By comparing the bypass flow measurement within the machine with the vaporizer flow measurement, the proportional valve is set to achieve the desired target (Fig. 6.35). Note that feedback control of the agent concentration relies on calculations of flow and does not involve measurement of agent concentration.

The patient monitoring unit of the ADU will be familiar to many as the Datex–Ohmeda AS/3 or S/5 and is a separate modular monitor with no linkage to the control unit of the ADU.

Dräger Primus

The Dräger Primus (Fig. 6.36) represents another departure in design. Its main distinguishing feature is the electronic fresh gas mixer.

Here, unlike the ADU, which utilizes mechanical needle valves set by the operator and subsequent electronic adjustment to the flow of N_2O, fresh gas is mixed entirely by electronically controlled valves according to the desired total flow and oxygen concentration. The operator selects air or N_2O as the carrier gas, and sets a total flow and the desired oxygen concentration (Fig. 6.37). A gas controller unit under feedback control sequentially opens high-speed solenoid valves to allow oxygen and the secondary gas to fill the mixed gas reservoir at the desired concentration. A proportional valve distal to this controls total flow into the pneumatic system. With this form of microprocessor control it is possible to have preset defaults for minimum oxygen concentration and this may be linked to the total set flow such that at total flows below $1.00 \, l \, min^{-1}$ the machine will maintain a minimum oxygen flow of $250 \, ml \, min^{-1}$. Gas flows are shown as virtual flowmeters on the control panel.

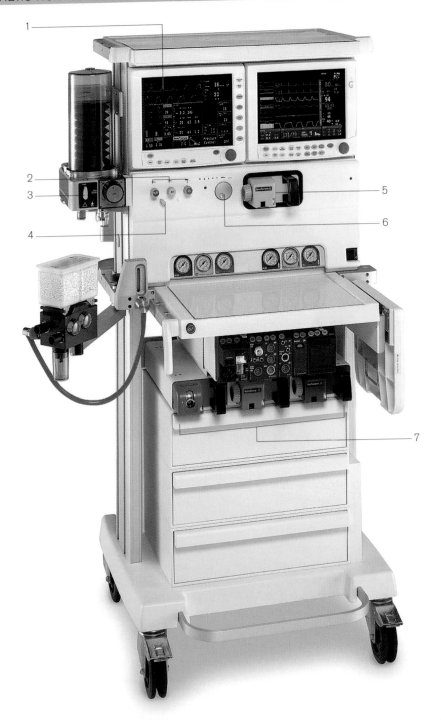

Figure 6.34 The Datex–Ohmeda ADU. Shown here with US standard colour coding for gases. 1) Ventilator user interface. 2) Gas flow needle valve controls. 3) Ventilator selection switch. 4) Side gas selection switch. 5) Aladin™ cassette. 6) Agent concentration selection. 7) Vaporizer storage rack. Photograph courtesy of Datex-Ohmeda.

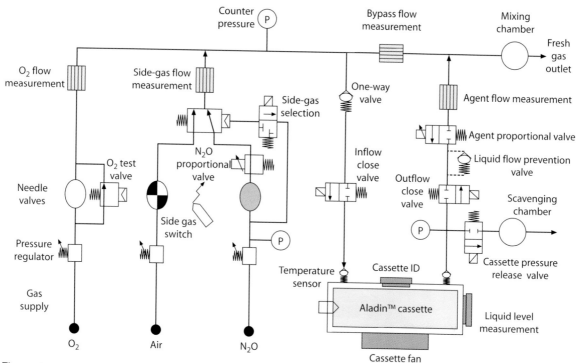

Figure 6.35 Electro-pneumatic system of the ADU.

In case of failure of the gas mixing unit, a graduated oxygen control knob can be deployed delivering gas into the circuit via the traditional calibrated vaporizer.

The Primus, in common with other current machines in the Dräger range, uses an electrically driven piston ventilator (Fig. 6.38) capable of generating flows up to $180 \, l \, min^{-1}$ with a tidal volume up to 1400 ml. The ventilator itself is further discussed in Chapter 11. By arranging fresh gas inflow into the circle on the expiratory side of the ventilator circuit (before the ventilator) and separating them using a non-return valve, the system achieves fresh flow gas decoupling of the delivered tidal volume. An incremental encoder comprising a perforated disk attached to the drive spindle of the piston gives

precise measurement of piston displacement. Measurement of the expired gas flow from the patient allows close matching of the piston's downstroke so as not to generate negative end expiratory pressure whilst also not entraining gas from outside the circuit. This is necessary for the preservation of low fresh gas flows. Gas flow measurement in the patient circuit uses hot wire anemometry. The reservoir bag is in circuit and functional during mechanical ventilation, taking up excess gas flows and also providing a buffer during the downstroke of the piston ventilator (Fig. 6.39). The expiratory control valve uses a proportional valve as discussed above (Fig. 6.28). The software driven 'E Ventilator' is also able to ventilate in pressure control and assisted spontaneous breathing modes.

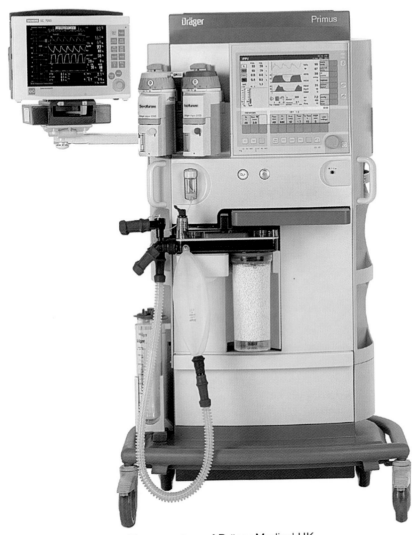

Figure 6.36 The Dräger Primus. Photo courtesy of Dräger Medical UK.

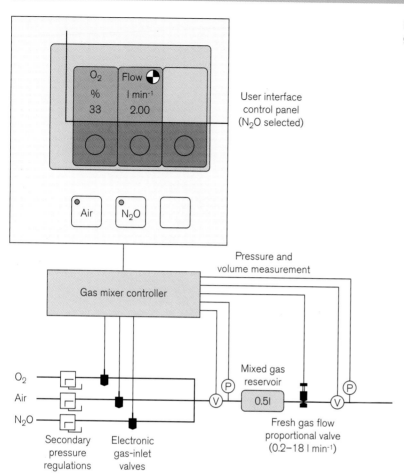

Figure 6.37 Dräger Primus electronic gas mixing unit.

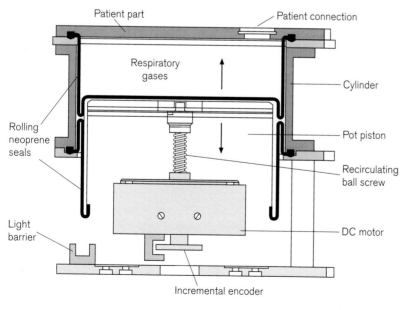

Figure 6.38 Schematic of Dräger E series ventilator.

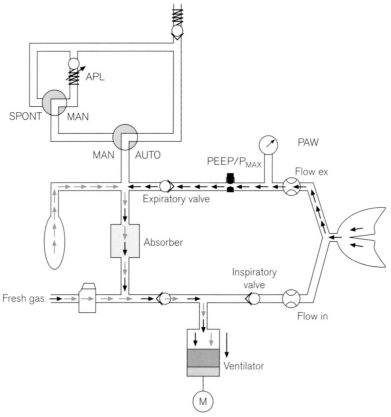

Figure 6.39 Gas flow in the Primus during expiration.

REFERENCES

1. Chawla AV, Newton NI (2002) Machine and monitoring failure from electrical overloading. *Anaesthesia* **57(11):** 1134–1135.
2. Schreiber PJ, Schreiber J (1989) Structured alarm systems for the operating room. *Journal of Clinical Monitoring* **5(3):** 201–204.
3. Westenskow DR, Orr JA, Simon FH, *et al.* (1992) Intelligent alarms reduce anaesthesiologist's response time to critical faults. *Anaesthesiology* **77(6):** 1074–1079.
4. Auditory Alarms in Critical Care Settings: Alarm Bibliography. University of Maryland, Baltimore. http://hfrp.umm.edu/alarms/Alarms_bibliography.htm.
5. Mondor TA, Finley GA (2003) The perceived urgency of auditory warning alarms used in the hospital operating room is inappropriate. *Canadian Journal of Anaesthesia* **50(3):** 221–228.
6. Checking Anaesthetic Equipment 3 (2004) The Association of Anaesthetists of Great Britain and Ireland, London 2004. http://www.aagbi.org/guidelines.html.

FURTHER READING

Dain S (2003) Current equipment alarm sounds: friend or foe? [editorial] *Canadian Journal of Anaesthesia* **50(3):** 209–214.

Mondor TA, Finley GA (2003) The perceived urgency of auditory warning alarms used in the hospital operating room is inappropriate. *Canadian Journal of Anaesthesia* **50(3):** 221–228.

Breathing systems and their components

Andrew J Davey

The definition and classification of methods in which inhalational agents are delivered to a patient have undergone a number of changes since the origins of anaesthesia. Most current anaesthetic literature uses the following definitions and classifications.

DEFINITIONS

- *Breathing systems*. A breathing system (not a circuit) now describes both the apparatus and the mode of operation by which inhalational agents are delivered to the patient, i.e. a Mapleson A type breathing system (mode of operation) would describe the mode of operation of a Magill breathing system (apparatus).
- *Rebreathing*. Rebreathing in anaesthetic systems now conventionally refers to the rebreathing of some or all of the previously exhaled gases, including carbon dioxide and water vapour. Rebreathing apparatus in other spheres, for example, fire fighting and underwater diving, has always referred to the recirculation of expired gas suitably purified and with the oxygen content restored or increased.
- *Apparatus dead space*. This refers to that volume within the apparatus, which may contain exhaled patient gas and which will be rebreathed at the beginning of a subsequent inspiratory breath (Fig. 7.1).

- *Functional dead space*. Some systems may well have a smaller 'functional' dead space, owing to the flushing effect of a continuous fresh gas stream at the end of expiration replacing exhaled gas in the apparatus dead space (Fig. 7.2).

CLASSIFICATION OF BREATHING SYSTEMS

These may be classified according to function:
- non-rebreathing systems, utilizing non-rebreathing valves;
- systems where some rebreathing of previously exhaled gas is possible, but normally prevented by the flow of fresh gas through the system; and

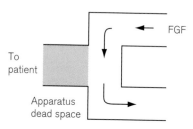

Figure 7.1 Apparatus dead space in a breathing system. FGF, fresh gas flow.

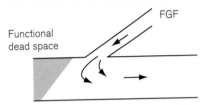

Figure 7.2 Functional dead space in a breathing system with an angled FGF inlet. FGF, fresh gas flow.

- non-rebreathing systems utilizing carbon dioxide absorption:
  (a) unidirectional (circle) systems; and
  (b) bi-directional (to-and-fro) systems.

Non-rebreathing systems

The simplest way to deliver a consistent fresh gas supply to a patient is with a system that includes a non-rebreathing valve (or valves).

Fresh gas enters the system via the inspiratory limb (Fig. 7.3a). This is a length of hosing that has a sufficiently wide bore to minimize any resistance to airflow. It is reinforced so as to prevent collapse, by either manufacturing it with corrugations or by bonding a reinforcing spiral onto the outside of the hose. Both of these methods also allow the tube to be bent without kinking. The fresh gas entering is either sucked in by the patient's inspiratory effort or blown in during controlled ventilation and enters the non-rebreathing valve. This valve is so constructed that when it opens to admit inspiratory gas, it occludes the expiratory limb of the system (see Fig. 7.3a). When the patient exhales, the reverse occurs, i.e. the valve mechanism moves to occlude the inspiratory limb and opens the expiratory limb to allow expired gases to escape (Fig. 7.3b).

The inspiratory limb usually includes a bag (1.5–2-litre capacity), which acts as a reservoir for fresh gas. This reservoir contains enough gas to cope with the intermittent high demand that occurs at inspiration. For example, a patient breathing normally (with a minute volume of 7 litres) may well have a tidal volume of 500 ml inhaled over approximately 1 s. This produces an average inspiratory flow rate (not peak flow rate) of 30 l min^{-1}. Without this reservoir in the system, the FGF rate would have to at least match this figure (probably more, to match the patient's peak inspiratory flow rate) in order to avoid respiratory embarrassment.

The reservoir bag is refilled with fresh gas during the expiratory phase. It can also be compressed manually to provide assisted or controlled respiration, since the non-

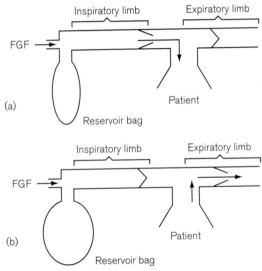

Figure 7.3 Non-rebreathing valve. **(a)** Inspiration. **(b)** Exhalation. FGF, fresh gas flow.

rebreathing valve works equally effectively in this mode as it does for spontaneous respiration. In the non-rebreathing system described, the fresh gas flow (FGF) rate *must not be less than* the minute volume required by the patient.

Systems where rebreathing is possible

A miscellany of breathing systems was developed by early pioneers (largely intuitively) that allowed the to-and-fro movement of inspiratory and expiratory gases within the breathing system. Carbon dioxide elimination was achieved by the flushing action of fresh gas introduced into this breathing system, rather than by the separation of the inspiratory and expiratory gas mixtures by a non-rebreathing valve as described above. As it is mainly the flushing effect of fresh gas that eliminates carbon dioxide, these systems retain the potential for rebreathing of carbon dioxide when FGF rates are reduced

In 1954, Mapleson classified these systems (A to E) according to their efficiency in eliminating carbon dioxide during spontaneous respiration. An F system, the Jackson Rees modification of system E (Ayre's T-piece), was later added to the classification by Willis in 1975 (see below).

Mapleson's classification of breathing systems

Figure 7.4 illustrates a modified Mapleson classification of breathing systems. These all contain similar components but are assembled in different sequences so that they may be used more conveniently in specific circumstances.

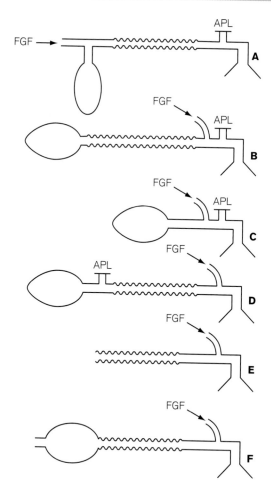

Figure 7.4 A modified Mapleson classification of breathing systems in which there is potential for rebreathing. System **A** houses the gas reservoir in the afferent limb and is alternatively referred to as an afferent reservoir system. The fresh gas flow (FGF) need only be at or just below the patient's minute ventilation without functional rebreathing occurring. Systems **B** and **C** (junctional reservoir systems) require FGF of 1.5 times the minute ventilation to avoid rebreathing. Systems **D, E,** and **F** (efferent reservoir systems) require 2–3 times the minute ventilation to avoid rebreathing.

However, the efficiency of each system is different. They are catalogued in order (A, B, C, D, E, F) of increased requirement of FGF to prevent rebreathing during spontaneous respiration. System A requires .08–1 times the patient's minute ventilation, B and C require 1.5–2 times the patient's minute ventilation and systems D, E and F (functionally similar) require 2–4 times the patient's minute ventilation to prevent rebreathing during spontaneous respiration.

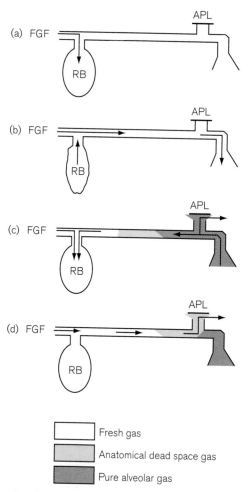

Figure 7.5 The Mapleson A system used with spontaneous breathing (see text). FGF, fresh gas flow; APL, adjustable pressure-limiting valve; RB, reservoir bag.

WORKING PRINCIPLES OF BREATHING SYSTEMS

Mapleson A breathing system (Fig. 7.5)

The Mapleson A system illustrated is the 'Magill attachment', as popularized by Sir Ivan Magill in the 1920s. It consists of the following:

- at one end, an inlet for fresh gas linked to a 2-litre distensible rubber or neoprene reservoir bag. (Not rebreathing bag, as the patient's exhaled gases should never be allowed to pass back into it.) This is attached to:
- a length of corrugated breathing hose (minimum length 110 cm with an internal volume of 550 ml). This

represents slightly more than the average tidal volume in an anaesthetized adult breathing spontaneously. This volume is important as it minimizes the backtracking of exhaled alveolar gas back to the reservoir bag (see below). This is in turn connected to:

- a variable tension, spring-loaded flap valve for venting of exhaled gases. This valve should be attached at the opposite end of the system from the reservoir bag and as close to the patient as possible. It will be subsequently referred to as an APL (adjustable pressure-limiting) valve.

The system makes efficient use of fresh gas during spontaneous breathing. This can be explained by examining its function during a respiratory cycle consisting of three phases: inspiration, expiration, and an end-expiratory pause:

- *The first inspiration.* In Figure 7.5a the reservoir bag and breathing hose have been filled by the FGF and the patient is about to take a breath. The whole system is therefore full of fresh gas. As the patient inspires, the gases are drawn into the lungs at a rate greater than FGF and so the reservoir bag partially empties as shown in Figure 7.5b.

- *Expiration.* In Figure 7.5c the patient has begun to exhale, and because the reservoir bag is not full, the exhaled gases are breathed back along the corrugated hose, pushing the fresh gases in the hose back towards the reservoir bag. However, before the exhaled gases can pass as far as the reservoir bag (hence the importance of the length of the inspiratory hose), the latter has been refilled by the fresh gases from the corrugated hose plus the FGF from the anaesthetic machine.

A point is reached when the reservoir bag is again full and as the patient is still exhaling, the remaining exhaled gases have to pass out through the APL (expiratory) valve, which now opens.

The first portion of exhaled gases to pass along the corrugated hose from the patient was that occupying the patient's anatomical dead space and therefore, apart from being warmed and slightly humidified (a satisfactory state of affairs), they are unaltered, not having taken part in respiratory exchange. This is followed by alveolar gas (with a reduced oxygen content, and containing carbon dioxide), some of which enters the corrugated hose, and some which is expelled through the APL valve when the reservoir bag is full.

- *End-expiratory pause.* The next stage is the end-expiratory pause. The FGF entering the system now drives those exhaled gases, or some of them that had

tracked back along the corrugated hose, out through the APL valve. It can be seen that the expiratory pause is important because it prevents the potential for the rebreathing of exhaled alveolar gases that would otherwise be contained in the hose at the end of expiration (Fig. 7.5d).

During the end-expiratory pause, all the alveolar gases and some of the dead-space gases are expelled from the corrugated hose through the APL valve by the continuing FGF. Thus, during the next inspiratory phase, the gas inspired may well initially contain some of the remaining dead-space gases from the previous breath, along with fresh gas. As explained above, these dead-space gases may be re-inspired without detriment to the patient. The FGF rate may therefore be rather less than the patient's minute volume and rebreathing of alveolar gas is therefore prevented.

In theory, provided there is no mixing of fresh gas, dead-space gas and alveolar gas, and a sufficient end-expiratory pause, the FGF rate need only match alveolar ventilation (approximately 66% of the minute volume), as in this situation alveolar gas only will be vented through the APL valve. In practice, however, a number of factors dictate a higher FGF rate (70–90%), for instance:

- there is mixing of the various gaseous interfaces, which reduces the theoretical efficiency of the system;
- occasionally, larger than expected tidal volumes may well be exhaled and therefore reach the reservoir bag, in which case carbon dioxide will contaminate the reservoir bag and the subsequent inspiratory gases; and
- rapid respiratory rates will reduce or even eliminate an end-expiratory pause and reduce the potential for carbon dioxide elimination that this pause allows.

Mapleson A system and controlled ventilation

The mechanical aspects of the Mapleson A (Fig. 7.6) system (Magill attachment), as described above, relate to its use in spontaneous respiration. However, if controlled or assisted ventilation is used, with the patient's lungs inflated by means of squeezing the reservoir bag, a different state of affairs occurs:

- *Inspiratory phase.* The APL valve has to be kept almost closed so that sufficient pressure can develop in the system to inflate the lungs. During the first inspiratory phase with the anaesthetist squeezing the bag, it is fresh gases that are blown out of the valve.

- *Expiratory phase.* At the end of inspiration, the reservoir bag may be almost empty, and as soon as the anaesthetist relaxes his pressure on it, the patient

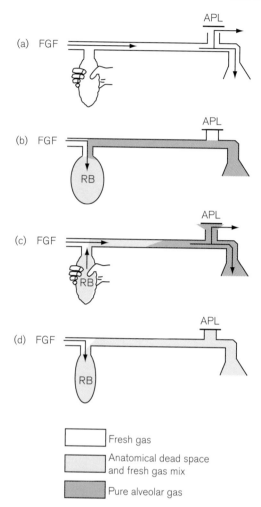

Figure 7.6 Mapleson A system with assisted or controlled ventilation: **(a)** at the end of inspiration; **(b)** at the end of expiration; **(c)** during subsequent inspiration; **(d)** at the end of the subsequent inspiration. Note that much rebreathing takes place (see text). FGF, fresh gas flow; APL, adjustable pressure-limiting valve; RB, reservoir bag.

exhales into the corrugated hose. The exhaled dead space and alveolar gases pass further back along the breathing hose and may even enter the reservoir bag. (The capacity of the standard 110 cm corrugated hose being about 550 ml.) There is usually insufficient pressure within the system to open the APL valve during this phase.

When the anaesthetist squeezes the bag again, the first gases to enter the patient's lungs will be the previously exhaled alveolar gases. The volume of gases escaping via the APL valve during this second inspiratory phase is

initially small (the valve being almost closed) but gradually increases as the pressure in the system rises towards the maximum inspiration. Therefore, the greatest amount of gas will be dumped late in the cycle and will consist mainly of fresh gas. Under these circumstances there is considerable rebreathing (Fig. 7.6c). Furthermore, as alveolar gas will have entered the reservoir bag, there will always be carbon dioxide contamination in any subsequent inspirate. In order to prevent this and thereby minimize the potential for rebreathing alveolar gas, a high FGF rate is required.

This is usually of the order of two times the patient's minute ventilation. This situation is highly wasteful of fresh gas and also increases the potential for pollution.

Other Mapleson A breathing systems

The Lack co-axial breathing system (Fig. 7.7a)

The traditional layout of a Magill system sites the APL valve as close to the patient as possible. However, this:
- reduces the access to the valve in head and neck surgery; and
- increases the drag on the mask or endotracheal tube when the valve is shrouded and connected to scavenging tubing.

The Lack system overcomes these two problems. The original version was constructed with a co-axial arrangement of breathing hoses. Exhaled gases passed through the orifice of the inner hose sited at the patient end of the system and then back towards the APL valve, which is now sited on the reservoir bag mount. The valve is thus conveniently sited for adjustment by the anaesthetist and its weight, and that of any additional scavenging attachment, is now supported by the anaesthetic machine (Fig. 7.7). The system still functions as a Mapleson A system. The co-axial hosing on early models was criticized as being too narrow and having too high a flow resistance. In later models, the inner and outer breathing hose diameters were subsequently both increased, to 15 and 30 mm respectively to overcome this problem. Another problem was that the tubing was heavy and stiff, putting a stress on the connection to the facepiece or endotracheal connection.

Lack parallel breathing system (Fig.7.7b)

Co-axial breathing systems have particular hazards. If the inner hose were to become disconnected or to split, as has been the case, the leak may pass unnoticed. This would drastically alter the efficiency of the system in eliminating carbon dioxide and is therefore potentially

(a)

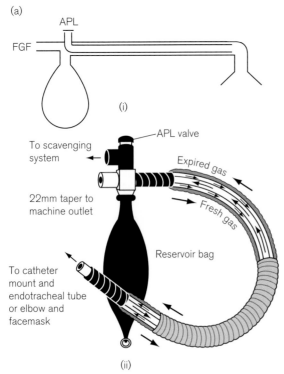

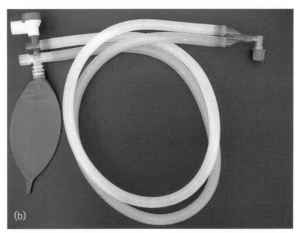

Figure 7.7 (a) The Lack co-axial breathing system. (i) Working principles. (ii) The actual assembly. The outer corrugated hose is partly transparent so that the inner tube may be seen to be intact. The adjustable pressure-limiting valve (APL) is fitted with a shroud having a 30 mm outlet so that it may be attached to a scavenging system. **(b)** The Lack parallel breathing attachment. The inner (expiratory) limb of the co-axial arrangement has been replaced by one that is parallel to the inspiratory limb. FGF, fresh gas flow.

very dangerous. A version of the Lack system with parallel hoses is now available (see Fig. 7.7b).

Mapleson B and C systems

These place both the fresh gas supply, reservoir bag and APL valve closer to the patient, allowing the anaesthetist easy access to the latter two, whilst at the same time allowing the fresh gas source to be sited at a distance if necessary. However, as mentioned above, neither are as economical as the 'A' system for spontaneous respiration. The reasons are outlined below for the 'B' system:

- *The first inspiration.* The system is initially assumed to be full of fresh gas so that during the first inspiration the patient breathes only fresh gas.
- *Expiration.* During expiration, the exhaled gases (initially dead space gas and then the first part of the alveolar gas), mixed with the FGF pass to the reservoir bag. When the latter has been refilled, the remainder of the exhaled gases (the rest of the alveolar gas) and the FGF are voided via the APL valve.
- *End-expiratory pause.* During this phase, it is fresh gas that escapes from the APL valve as this is closer to the valve than the bag.

- *The next inspiration.* This will be supplied by the contents of the bag, which has a mixture of fresh, dead-space and alveolar gas, the proportion of which will be determined by the FGF rate and the rate at which exhalation occurred. If the FGF is high and the exhalation rate was slow, there will be a greater amount of fresh gas in the inspirate.

Mapleson D system

The Mapleson D system with spontaneous respiration

The system is best explained if, again, the three phases of the respiratory cycle are considered: inspiration, expiration and end-expiratory pause:

- *The first inspiration.* The FGF enters as close as possible to the patient end of the breathing system (so as to reduce any apparatus dead space) and the system is filled so that during the first inspiration the patient breathes only fresh gas (Fig. 7.8a).
- *Expiration.* During expiration, the exhaled gases, mixed with the FGF pass down the wide bore hose to the reservoir bag (Fig. 7.8b) and when this has been refilled the remainder of the exhaled gases and the FGF are voided via the APL valve (expiratory valve).

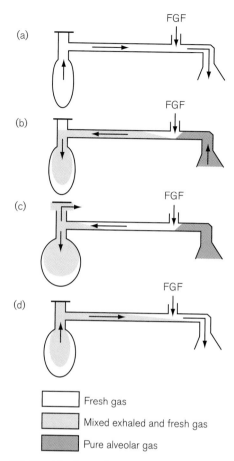

Figure 7.8 The Mapleson D system with spontaneous ventilation (see text). FGF, fresh gas flow; APL, adjustable pressure-limiting valve.

Fresh gas

Mixed exhaled and fresh gas

Pure alveolar gas

Of the expired gases, it is those from the dead space that are voided first, followed by alveolar gases.

- *End-expiratory pause.* During the end-expiratory pause the FGF entering the system passes down the wide bore hose, displacing some of the mixture of exhaled gas and FGF, which is now vented out through the APL valve (Fig. 7.8c). The amount of fresh gas occupying and thus stored in the patient end of the wide-bore hose at the end of expiration, depends on the FGF rate, the duration of the end-expiratory pause, and the degree of mixing (due to turbulence) of the various gaseous interfaces within the corrugated hose.
- At the next inspiration the inhaled gases consist initially of this stored fresh gas followed then by the mixture of exhaled gases and FGF that remain in the tube (Fig. 7.8d).

However, there are practical problems with this concept, since the expiratory pause may be short, particularly during spontaneous breathing (when volatile anaesthetics only are used without opoid supplement). In this case, the FGF needs to be sufficiently high to flush the exhaled gases downstream prior to the next inspiration. In fact, rebreathing of exhaled alveolar gas occurs unless the FGF is at least two times and possibly up to four times the patient's minute ventilation.

It is worthy of note that the Mapleson D system is functionally similar to a T- piece (Mapleson E). However, with a T- piece, the limb through which the ventilation occurs, if used without a reservoir bag, must be of such a length that the volume of gas in it when augmented by the volume of the FGF being delivered during inspiration is no less than that of the patient's tidal volume, otherwise dilution of anaesthetic by entrained air will occur.

Mapleson D system with controlled or assisted ventilation

- *The first inspiration.* As the bag is squeezed, the FGF entering the system as well as fresh gases stored in the wide-bore breathing hose pass to the patient. At the same time, some gases from the reservoir bag are lost through the partially open APL (expiratory) valve (Fig. 7.9a)
- *Expiration.* A mixture of the FGF and exhaled gases passes along the hose, eventually entering the now deflated reservoir bag, causing it to refill (Fig. 7.9b).
- *Expiratory pause.* At this point, provided that there is an expiratory pause, the fresh gas supply continues to flow down the hose to replace and drive the mixed gases out via the APL valve. A longer expiratory pause allows a greater amount of fresh gas to enter the breathing hose (Fig. 7.9c).
- *The next inspiration.* At the next squeeze of the reservoir bag (Fig. 7.9d), the continuing FGF plus the fresh gas now stored in the breathing hose plus any previously expired gases that may remain in the hose, pass to the patient, while some of the mixed gases within the bag escape via the APL valve. The cycle then repeats itself.

Thus to prevent rebreathing in the Mapleson D system, during both spontaneous and controlled ventilation, the FGF must be sufficiently high enough to:
- purge the breathing hose of exhaled gases; and
- supplement the stored fresh gas in this breathing hose so that any mixed gas in the reservoir bag is prevented from reaching the patient. The amount of fresh gas required will always be greater than the patient's minute

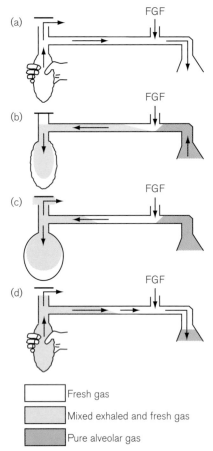

	Fresh gas
	Mixed exhaled and fresh gas
	Pure alveolar gas

Figure 7.9 Mapleson D system with manual ventilation. **(a)** The first inspiration; note that the APL valve is forced open. **(b)** Early exhalation; the APL valve is closed and the partially collapsed reservoir bag is filling. **(c)** Late exhalation/expiratory pause; mixed gas is vented from the system. **(d)** Subsequent inspiration.

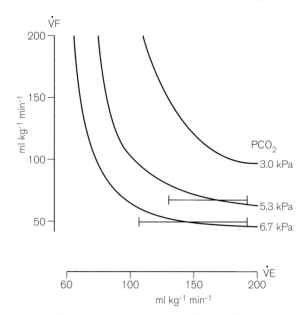

Figure 7.10 Isopleths showing the relationship between fresh gas flow ($\dot{V}_F$), minute ventilation ($\dot{V}_E$) and various alveolar carbon dioxide tensions.

volume and will depend largely on the expiratory pause. The longer the pause, the more effective will be the ability of the fresh gas to purge the breathing hose of expired gas.

However, during controlled ventilation, deliberate use is often made of functional rebreathing. Theoretically, if slow ventilation rates (with long expiratory pauses) and large tidal volumes are chosen, then sufficient expiratory time will elapse to allow a modest FGF to fill the proximal part of the system with sufficient fresh gas to provide alveolar ventilation. This will enter the lungs first, followed by a mixture of previously expired gases, which will then occupy the patient's anatomical dead space. Hence, theoretically, it should he possible to reduce the FGF to the volume required for alveolar ventilation.

In practice, there is turbulent mixing of the various gaseous interfaces so that alveolar gas is widely distributed (and diluted). Even so, provided a sufficiently large controlled minute *ventilation* is delivered so that most of the FGF reaches the alveoli, adequate alveolar ventilation will occur with FGF rates of 70% of the anticipated minute ventilation since, as mentioned above, some re-breathing is acceptable. Figure 7.10 demonstrates this as well as the fact that the arterial carbon dioxide tension remains fairly constant for any given FGF rate, despite alterations in minute ventilation.

Mapleson D systems are thus able to make efficient use of fresh anaesthetic gases during controlled ventilation and could have considerable cost-saving benefits. Figure 7.11 shows how the Mapleson D system may be employed with an automatic ventilator. The reservoir bag is removed and replaced with a standard length of corrugated hose of sufficient capacity to accommodate the air or oxygen that is delivered by the ventilator, and which prevents it reaching the patient in place of the intended anaesthetic gases.

The Bain system

The Bain breathing system (Fig. 7.12) is similar in function to the Mapleson D system. The only difference is that the FGF is carried by a tube within the corrugated

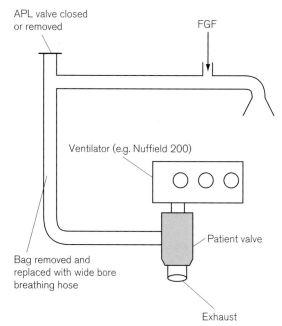

Figure 7.11 Controlled ventilation with a Mapleson D system using a ventilator. Note that with the employment of a ventilator that operates as a 'gas piston', the former must be separated from the breathing system by a suitably long piece of breathing hose (with an internal volume of at least 500 ml). This prevents the driving gas from reaching the patient and diluting the anaesthetic mixture. APL, adjustable pressure-limiting valve; FGF, fresh gas flow.

hose (a co-axial arrangement). In the earlier models in particular, there was a risk that the inner tube could become disconnected at the machine end; if this happened a very large dead space was introduced. It could also become kinked, so cutting off the supply of fresh gases.

Hybrid systems

A number of breathing systems have been described that, by means of a lever switch, can convert the system from a Mapleson A to a Mapleson D or E, allowing a system to be chosen and used in its most efficient mode (i.e. System A, spontaneous respiration, System E, controlled respiration). The Humphrey ADE system (Anaequip UK) seems to be the most popular version (Fig. 7.13a).

With the lever switch in the A mode (Fig. 7.13b), the reservoir bag on the ADE block is connected to the inspiratory pathway, as in a Mapleson A system. The breathing hose connecting the block to the patient is now designated as the inspiratory limb. However, expired gas is carried back along a separate limb to the block and then is vented through an APL valve, which is shrouded to facilitate scavenging. In practice it appears to function more efficiently than a traditional Magill attachment. The improved efficiency is thought to relate to the position and design of the components at the patient end of the system. Towards the end of exhalation in the Magill attachment, the exhaled dead-space gas which has passed up the breathing hose is now returned towards the APL valve by the flushing action of the FGF entering the system. At the APL valve, it meets and mixes with

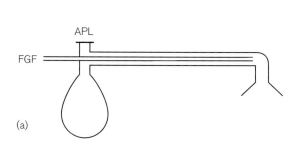

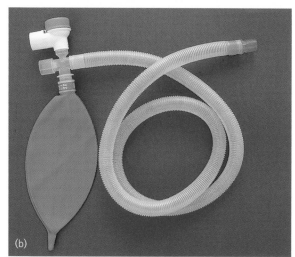

Figure 7.12 The Bain breathing system. **(a)** Working principle. **(b)** Intersurgical disposable. FGF, fresh gas flow; APL, adjustable pressure-limiting (expiratory) valve.

139

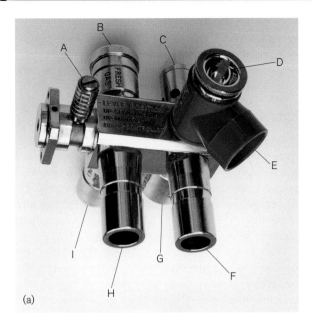

(a)

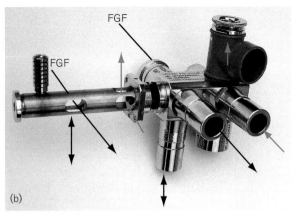

(b)

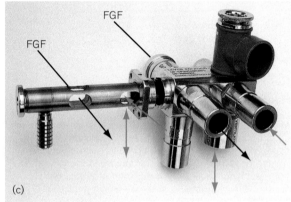

(c)

Figure 7.13 **(a)** The Humphrey ADE system. A, lever; B, fresh gas input; C, overpressure relief valve; D, APL valve with spindle; E, scavenging shroud; F, 22 mm breathing hose port from patient; G, ventilator port; H, 22 mm breathing hose port to patient; I, bag mount. **(b)** An exploded view; with the lever set upright, the system functions in its Mapleson A mode for spontaneous respiration with a recommended fresh gas flow (FGF) of 70 ml kg^{-1} or less if used with capnography. Manual ventilation is easily instituted by pressing on the spindle to close the valve during inspiration and releasing it during exhalation. **(c)** For mechanical ventilation the lever is positioned downwards, converting the breathing system to the Mapleson E mode by isolating the reservoir bag and APL valve but incorporating the ventilator port. The fresh gas flow may be kept the same.

alveolar gas in a turbulent fashion, and a mixture of both is discharged from the valve. However, in the Humphrey (and Lack) systems, alveolar gas is diverted in a more laminar fashion into a physically separate expiratory limb, which minimizes any potential for mixing of the two gas phases in question. This arrangement, and the removal of the APL valve assembly away from the patient end of the system, also reduces apparatus dead space, so that with further modification (see below) it may be suitable for infants and neonates.

With the lever in the D/E mode (Fig.7.13c), the reservoir bag and APL valve are isolated from the breathing system. What was the 'inspiratory' limb in 'A' mode now delivers gas to the patient end of the system as in a T-piece (see

below). The breathing hose returning gas to the ADE block now functions as the reservoir limb of a T-piece. This hose vents to atmosphere via a port adjacent to the bag mount. As this mode does not incorporate a reservoir bag, it is strictly a Mapleson E system. The port described above is usually connected to a ventilator of the 'bag-squeezer' type (see Chapter 11), so that the system can be used in its most efficient mode for controlled ventilation. If a reservoir bag and APL valve were to be attached to this port, it would function as a D system. However, this is not recommended because it may encourage the system to be used uneconomically for spontaneous respiration, as a high FGF is required to prevent rebreathing.

The Anaequip version is supplied with 15 mm smooth-bore non-kinking breathing hose and unique APL valve (see below, the Humphrey APL valve). Interestingly, the use of this smooth-bore hose reduces turbulence in the range of flows seen in quietly breathing adults, so that its performance is little different from that of 22 mm corrugated hose. The narrower-bore hose also reduces the internal volume of the system to an extent that it is now also suitable for use with infants. A low internal volume is important in a paediatric breathing system in order that:

- during controlled ventilation, the small tidal volumes required are delivered more efficiently, and
- during spontaneous respiration, the energy expended by the patient in overcoming the inertia of the gas present in the system is reduced, especially as with high respiratory rates the direction of gas flow is reversed very frequently.

Mapleson E and F systems

The T-piece system

When what are now termed APL valves were first made, they offered a resistance to exhalation, which was deemed unacceptable in certain anaesthetic techniques, such as those used for neonatal and infant anaesthesia. This distinction has become less important (see Chapter 14). To avoid this resistance, the T-piece system was designed by Philip Ayre in 1937. In Figure 7.14 the fresh gases are supplied via a small-bore tube to the side arm of an Ayre's T-piece. The main body of the T-piece is within the breathing system and must, therefore, be of adequate diameter. One end of the body is connected by the shortest possible means to the patient. (The volume of this limb makes up apparatus dead space.) The other end is connected to a length of tubing that acts as a reservoir.

In the case of spontaneous ventilation, the FGF rate must be high. During inspiration the peak inspiratory flow rate is higher than the FGF, so some gases are drawn from the reservoir limb. During expiration both the exhaled air and the fresh gases, which continue to flow, pass into the reservoir limb and are expelled to the atmosphere. During the end-expiratory pause, the FGF flushes out and refills the reservoir limb. The dimensions of the reservoir limb and the FGF rate are governed by the following considerations:

- The diameter of the reservoir limb must be sufficient to present the lowest possible resistance (not more than 0.075 kPa (0.75 cmH$_2$O) for a neonate and not

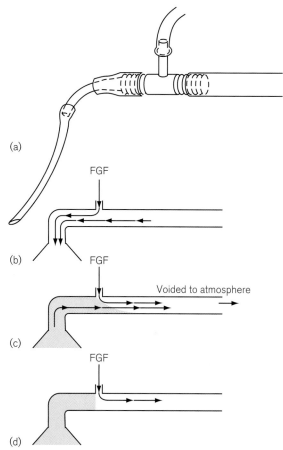

(a)

(b)

(c)

(d)

Figure 7.14 (a) The Ayre's T-piece connected to an endotracheal tube; **(b)** during inspiration; **(c)** during expiration; **(d)** during the expiratory pause. FGF, fresh gas flow.

more than 0.2 kPa (2 cmH$_2$O) for an adult at the appropriate flow rates).

- The volume of the expiratory limb should be not less than the patient's tidal volume. Too great a volume would matter only in that the greater length would lead to increased resistance. Too great a diameter would lead to mixing of the fresh gases with alveolar gas and to inefficiency of the system. For an adult a standard 110 cm length of corrugated hose is satisfactory.
- The optimum FGF rate depends not only on the patient's minute volume and respiratory rate but also on the capacity of the reservoir limb. If the latter is at least that of the patient's tidal volume, then a rate of 2.5 times the patient's minute volume is sufficient. This is the most satisfactory arrangement. However, if the capacity of the reservoir is reduced, the flow rate

must be increased. If the capacity of the reservoir is reduced to zero, the flow rate must be in excess of the peak inspiratory flow rate so as to reduce the possibility of ingress of air.

The shape of the T-piece is also important. Normally the side arm is at right-angles to the body. If it is at an angle pointing towards the patient, there is continuous positive pressure applied which would act as a resistance during expiration. This continuous positive airways pressure is thought to be beneficial in minimizing the fall in functional residual capacity (FRC), especially in neonates. However, if the gases were directed towards the reservoir, a sub-atmospheric pressure would be caused by a venturi effect.

Controlled ventilation with the T-piece

Controlled ventilation may be effected by intermittently occluding the end of the reservoir limb with the thumb. This should be done with care, since when the outlet is occluded the full pressure supplied by the anaesthetic machine is applied to the patient. It would seem prudent to include, in infant systems at least, a blow-off valve set to about 4 kPa (40 cmH$_2$O) pressure, but this is seldom done. A limitation in its use arises from the fact that the peak inspiratory flow rate is limited to that of the FGF. This is overcome in the Rees modification T-piece, described below.

The Rees T-piece (Mapleson F system)

A great improvement to the T-piece was made by Rees, who added a small double-ended bag to the end of the reservoir limb (Fig. 7.15).

However, the tubular portion of the limb should still approximate to the patient's tidal volume, or rebreathing could occur as a result of the mixing of expired and fresh gases. During spontaneous ventilation, small movements of the semi-collapsed bag demonstrate the patient's breathing. During the inspiratory phase of manual ventilation, the bag is squeezed with the open end of the

bag partially or totally occluded by the anaesthetist. During exhalation, the open end is released to allow the gas in the system to escape. This simple method is extremely efficient for infants and small children. Mechanical devices have been placed in the tail of the bag so as to provide a variable restriction similar to that described above. However, these may all be accidentally turned off, occluding the expiratory limb completely, and as the system did not contain an over-pressure safety valve, a dangerously high pressure could build up which could damage the lungs of any infant connected to it. These devices cannot therefore be recommended.

Other paediatric breathing systems are described in Chapter 14.

Alternative classification for Mapleson type systems

An alternative nomenclature has recently been proposed for the systems described above, which relates to the position of the reservoir bag within the breathing system. The Mapleson A system in which the reservoir bag stores fresh gas is described as an *afferent reservoir system*. System D, in which the reservoir bag stores mixed expired gases, is described as an *efferent reservoir system*, and systems B and C, in which the reservoir bag stores mixed inspired and expired gases, are called *junctional reservoir systems*.

The aforementioned Mapleson systems may also be termed by some as 'partial rebreathing systems', owing to their facility for allowing rebreathing of part of the volume of exhaled gases.

Non-rebreathing systems with facility for carbon dioxide absorption

High flows of inhalational anaesthetic agents (i.e. at least approximately equal to the patient's minute ventilation) are regularly used with most breathing systems at the beginning of an anaesthetic for the following reasons:
- both to purge the system of air and to fill it with fresh anaesthetic agents;
- to provide a sufficient amount of inhalational agent for alveolar uptake (which is initially high at the onset of anaesthesia);
- to eliminate exhaled carbon dioxide. (As described previously the efficiency with which this is done depends on the characteristics of the breathing system chosen.); and
- to eliminate body nitrogen.

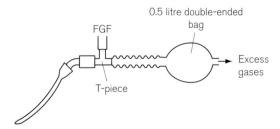

Figure 7.15 The Rees T-piece. FGF, fresh gas flow.

However, when equilibrium between the patient's blood and inspired concentration of anaesthetic has been reached, this inspired concentration is exhaled relatively unchanged, and so the main function of high FGFs in most breathing systems is the elimination of carbon dioxide (whilst at the same time providing oxygen).

Thus, to continue a high FGF after equilibrium has been achieved is both wasteful and expensive and may increase theatre pollution. This exhaled gas at near equilibrium can be re-used in suitable systems if it is purged of exhaled carbon dioxide, and has the oxygen concentration restored (oxygen is always removed from the inspiratory mixture by the lungs at a rate between 120–250 ml min^{-1}). The re-utilization of suitably modified exhaled gases can thus reduce the FGF to very low levels (see below).

Carbon dioxide absorption

Carbon dioxide can be removed from exhaled gases by a chemical reaction with absorbent compounds made from various metallic bases (hydroxides). This reaction requires the presence of water in order that these bases and carbon dioxide (as carbonic acid) can exist in ionic form.

Chemical composition of absorbents

The main constituent of absorbents made by different manufacturers is calcium hydroxide. Other constituents are added to enhance the reactivity. These include;

Sodium/Potassium

Small quantities of sodium hydroxide (1.5–5%) are usually added to enhance the reactivity and the hygroscopic property (ability to bind water) of the mixture, hence the reason that absorbents are often referred to as 'soda lime'. Some manufacturers have added potassium hydroxide for similar reasons, although this has been discontinued (see below).

Barium

Barium lime conventionally is made up of 85% calcium hydroxide, 11% barium hydroxide and 4% potassium hydroxide. The barium hydroxide has its own naturally occurring 'water of crystallization' and, in combination with calcium hydroxide, has never required additional hardeners. However, products containing barium were removed from the market in Autumn 2004.

Water content

The optimal moisture content of the absorbent mixture is between 14–16%. This is essential for the chain reaction set out below:

$$CO_2 + H_2O = H^+ + HCO_3-$$
Carbon dioxide / Water / Carbonic acid

$$2NaOH + H^+ + HCO_3 = Na_2CO_3 + 2H_2O$$
Sodium hydroxide / Carbonic acid / Sodium carbonate / Water

$$Na_2CO_3 + Ca(OH)_2 = CaCO_3 + 2NaOH$$
Sodium carbonate / Calcium hydroxide / Calcium carbonate / Sodium hydroxide

In the second equation, sodium may be substituted by potassium when considering the reaction of absorbents that contained the latter.

The reaction is interesting in that:

- it produces heat energy (it is an exothermic reaction);
- it changes the pH of the soda lime, which allows the use of indicator dyes to show when the soda lime is exhausted; and
- it produces more water than that used up in the reaction. In fact, for each mole of carbon dioxide absorbed one mole of water is produced.

There are other unwanted reactions that take place (associated with dry soda/barium lime), and these are discussed further below.

Other constituents

Zeolite

Zeolites are three-dimensional, microporous crystalline solids that contain aluminium, silica and oxygen in their regular framework; cations and water are located in the pores. Zeolites have void space (cavities or channels) that can host other molecules. They are naturally occurring minerals that are mined in many parts of the world; however most commercial zeolites are produced synthetically. They may be added to soda lime (Spherosorb™) to increase:

- *Porosity of the mixture.* The absorbent becomes more efficient as it becomes more porous, due to the increase in available surface area.
- *Hardness.* The harder the mixture, the less likely it is to form dust. This is carried around the breathing system and is caustic if inhaled. It may also become damp and settle on valves within the breathing system and cause them to become sticky.
- *Water content.* Zeolite also helps to prevent the drying out of the absorbent in adverse conditions. However, should this occur, the zeolite may start to absorb volatile anaesthetic, thereby reducing the concentration in the breathing system especially at the beginning

of an anaesthetic. Up to 80% of the agent may be absorbed in this situation

Silica

Sodium and potassium have traditionally been added to increase the reactivity of absorbents and to provide the hygroscopic (water retaining) properties. However, they are the main cause of degradation by dry soda lime of anaesthetic agents (isoflurane/desflurane) to carbon monoxide and the degradation of sevoflurane to compound A, formaldehyde and methanol. Calcium hydroxide was originally thought to be insufficiently reactive on its own to be a suitable agent. However, new methods of production have led to significantly more porous granules (see above) so that calcium hydroxide alone may now be sufficient as an absorbent. The granules though are much softer as a result and require the addition of silica (LoFloSorb™) to overcome this. The new absorbents have been shown to minimize the production of the unwanted compounds described above, even when dry.

Calcium chloride

The addition of 3% calcium chloride (Amsorb™ Plus) in place of sodium or potassium has a similar but less powerful effect. This product also contains 1% calcium sulphate to improve the hardness of the granule. Unlike absorbents that contain strong bases, there may also be a colour change (similar to the exhausted state) should a sample dry out. Should this occur, the mixture still prevents the formation of carbon monoxide (with isoflurane and desflurane) and compound A (with sevoflurane).

Granule size

The size of the granules is important. Too large a granule size produces large gaps in a canister of stacked granules, leading to poor contact with gases passing through, and consequent inefficient absorption of carbon dioxide. Too small a granule may provide an unacceptably high resistance to gas flow along with the increased possibility of dust formation. The optimum size of granule is thought to be between 1.5 and 5 mm in diameter.

Production

The ingredients are mixed along with added water into a paste. This is treated in a number of ways. Originally the paste was dried and then crushed between rollers so that it formed granules. The product was then sieved through various meshes to retain the sizes quoted above. The dried granules were then sprayed with water to give the right amount of water content to allow optimal reactivity without making the granule soft or sticky. Mesh standards differ between countries due to variations in thickness of the wire used to construct the mesh. In the USA soda lime granules are supplied at between 4 and 8 Mesh USP (2.36–4.75 mm). In the UK the granules are supplied to a BP (British Pharmacopoeia) standard of 1.4–4.75 m (3–10 Mesh). More recently, production methods have been introduced that produce a more uniform size. The paste may be squeezed through a sieve like spaghetti and chopped into little pieces. It may be passed through a mangle that has thousands of dimples on its surface. This produces tiny similar-sized spheres that are blown off the roller by a high-pressure jet of air. The paste may also be placed on a dimpled belt that is passed through a smooth roller. This produces little hemispheres that are removed from the belt in a manner similar to removing an ice cube from its tray.

The dust may be caustic and can produce burns in the respiratory tract if inhaled. This was a problem with the older type of system with 'to-and-fro' absorption (see below, Waters' Canister), where the absorber was placed in close proximity to the patient's airway. However, circle absorbers are usually separated from the patient by at least one metre of breathing hose, which normally hangs in a loop. This allows the dust, if present, to fall out before it can get to the patient. Furthermore, a breathing filter separating the patient from the breathing system would protect against this.

Absorptive capacity of soda lime

Soda lime is capable of absorbing 25 litres of carbon dioxide per 100 g, and barium lime 27 litres of carbon dioxide per 100 g. However, in continuous use, the soda lime appears exhausted (as indicated by the colour change) before these capacities are reached, because the outside of the granule is exhausted before the whole granule is used up. Furthermore, the contact time between the absorbent and carbon dioxide affects the efficiency of the absorbent. Smaller canisters containing 500 g of soda lime appear exhausted at a carbon dioxide load of 10–12 litres per 100 g of absorbent. 'Jumbo' absorbers containing 2 kg of soda lime, which allow a longer contact time between the carbon dioxide and absorbent, appear exhausted at a carbon dioxide load of 17 litres per 100 g.

When the system is allowed to stand for a few hours, the soda lime appears to 'regenerate' as the surface carbonate is diluted by hydroxide ions migrating from within the granule. The colour of fresh soda lime and barium lime depends on which indicator dye is added by the manufacturer. For example if 'titan yellow' is added, the soda lime turns from deep pink when fresh to off-white when exhausted, whereas if 'ethyl violet' is used as the indicator dye, the soda lime changes from white when fresh to purple when exhausted. It is therefore important to know which colour change to expect. Some absorbents (LoFloSorb™) have a green pigment added to the ethyl violet so that it is pale green when fresh but violet when exhausted.

The exothermic reaction

The heat and water produced by the reaction of soda lime on carbon dioxide has been considered to be beneficial in that (at low flows) they warm and partially humidify the inspiratory gas. The temperature and humidity of the inspired gas is related to a number of factors:

- if the FGF rate is high, the dry gas entering the system reduces both the humidity and the temperature of the recirculating gas;
- at low FGFs, if the gas circulation time is high, the humidity and temperature rises;
- the longer the system is in use at low FGFs, the greater are the humidity and temperature of the circulating gas;

The heat produced, however, is not necessarily all beneficial. There is an increased chemical reaction between volatile anaesthetic agents and traditional absorbents in proportion to the temperature within the system:

Trichloroethylene can be decomposed to dichloroacetylene (which is neurotoxic) and further to phosgene, if the temperature within the soda lime exceeds 60°C. Older anaesthetic machines often incorporated a switching system on the back bar that could divert gas directly into a circle system rather than to the common gas outlet. The trichloroethylene vaporizer (where fitted) was always positioned downstream of this switch so that it could never be used with the circle absorber system.

Anaesthetic agents with the CHF_2 moiety (desflurane, enflurane and isoflurane) react with dry, warm soda lime or barium lime (Baralyme™) to produce varying amounts of carbon monoxide (Table 7.1).

Dry barium lime, which contains potassium hydroxide, has a much greater tendency to produce carbon monoxide than does dry soda lime that contains sodium hydroxide. Fresh absorbent, which has approximately a 15% water content appears to prevent carbon monoxide formation.

Table 7.1 Carbon monoxide production by reaction of anaesthetic agents that have the CHF_2 moiety (desflurane, enflurane and isoflurane) with lime

Type of lime		CO (ppm)
Dry soda lime (<2% water)	Potassium hydroxide	50–100
Dry soda lime (<2% water)	Sodium hydroxide	15
Fresh soda lime	Sodium hydroxide	<8

In fact, significant production occurs only when the water content drops below 2%. This problem can occur when the absorbent is allowed to dry out in breathing systems. This happens when the breathing system is left unused for long periods, or when large amounts of dry gas are allowed to pass through it overnight or at weekends. This may occur with some anaesthetic machines, albeit over a long period of time even if the flowmeters are turned off, if:

- they are plugged into the pipeline supply;
- they have a minimal basal flow of oxygen through the machine; and
- the absorber is so constructed that fresh gas is made to flow through the absorbent prior to entering the inspiratory limb.

Carbon monoxide is not easily measured as an exhaled gas as it binds to haemoglobin in the blood first. Its production in a system using absorbents may be difficult to detect. There is not necessarily a colour change in absorbents containing strong bases (potassium/sodium) if they dry out. Suspicion should be raised if there appears to be excessive heat production from the absorbent:

This phenomenon can easily be avoided by using:

- smaller absorbers (so that the contents have to be changed regularly);
- disconnecting them when possible; and
- ensuring that only designs that allow the fresh gas to bypass the absorber are used and unplugging machines from the pipelines when not in use for extended periods.

Sevoflurane may undergo degradation within the absorber, to non-toxic fluorinated products (mainly a sevo-olefin called 'compound A'). Levels rise, as would be expected, with increased concentration of the agent, prolonged anaesthesia, low FGFs and increased operating temperature within the absorber. However, there is no evidence of any danger to patients. In the presence of dried absorbent (especially barium lime) there may be an extreme temperature rise and a number of other breakdown products are produced including formaldehyde and methanol, as well as carbon monoxide. There have been isolated reports of fire or extreme heat in circle systems harming at least one patient. This has prompted the manufacturer to issue a letter to health care professionals in the USA warning of the danger. In the cases investigated the following signs were noted:

- failed induction or inadequate anaesthetic depth;
- clinical sign of airway irritation;
- oxygen desaturation, increased airway pressures;
- severe airway oedema and erythema; and
- elevated carboxyhaemoglobin levels.

In summary the recommendations for preventing the problem are:

- if there is any suspicion that the absorbent has not been in use for an extended period of time it should be replaced;
- the machine should be turned off when not in use so that there is no flow of gas through the absorber;
- the vaporizers should be turned off when not in use;
- the sevoflurane concentrations dialed up on the vaporizer and that measured by an analyzer should be compared and any major disparity should be investigated; and
- a check for excessive heat production from the absorbent should be performed periodically.

Classification of breathing systems utilizing carbon dioxide absorption

Carbon dioxide absorption can be used in two types of system:

1. a 'to-and-fro' absorption system; and
2. a circle absorption system.

'To-and-fro' absorption systems

The Waters' canister (Fig. 7.16)

Here the patient breathes in and out of a closed bag, which is connected to the facemask or endotracheal tube via a canister containing soda lime. The part of the system between the patient and the soda lime is dead space and therefore its volume must be kept to a minimum. This means that the soda lime canister must be close to the patient's head, and this leads to practical difficulties. A length of wide-bore tubing may, however, be interposed between the canister and rebreathing bag without detriment. The fresh gases are introduced at the patient end of the system, and the expiratory valve is usually mounted close by, though it may equally well be put at the

bag end. The canister is usually placed in the horizontal position for convenience, and it is most important that it is well packed, since if there were a space above the soda lime, 'channelling' would occur and absorption would be incomplete (Fig. 7.17).

Furthermore, the soda lime at the patient end of the system becomes exhausted first and so increases the functional dead space of the system.

Canisters are available as pre-packed, disposable units. In those intended for re-use, the soda lime may conveniently be compressed to prevent gaps by the insertion of a spongy 'spacer' at one end. When the canister is closed, the sealing washer should be checked to ensure that it is in the correct position and any soda lime on the threads of the canister or the sealing washer should be carefully removed as these may cause leaks. The whole system should be tested before use.

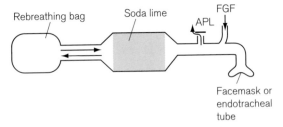

Figure 7.16 A 'to-and-fro' system incorporating a Waters' canister. FGF, fresh gas flow.

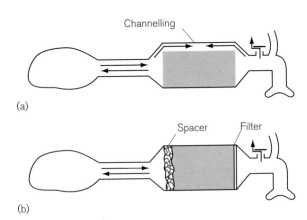

Figure 7.17 (a) Channelling in a Waters' canister. If the canister is not completely filled with soda lime and is placed in a horizontal position, the gases can pass through the void at the top and therefore fail to come into adequate contact with the soda lime. **(b)** The prevention of channelling by the insertion of a spacer to compress the soda lime. Note also the filter at the patient end that prevents particles of soda lime reaching the patient.

Apart from being cumbersome, the 'to-and-fro' system has the disadvantage that the patient could inhale soda lime dust. A breathing filter may be inserted in the patient end of the canister to prevent this.

Circle absorption systems

Here the disadvantages of the soda lime canister being so close to the patient are avoided. The patient is connected to the absorber by two corrugated hoses, one inspiratory and the other expiratory, as shown in Figure 7.18a. The one way or 'circle' flow of gases through the system is determined by two unidirectional valves, V1 and V2, which are accommodated in transparent domes so that their correct action may be observed.

The fresh gas port and the reservoir bag are usually sited in the inspiratory pathway close to the inspiratory valve V_1. This may reduce the resistance to inspiratory effort. Some circle systems position the fresh gas port and

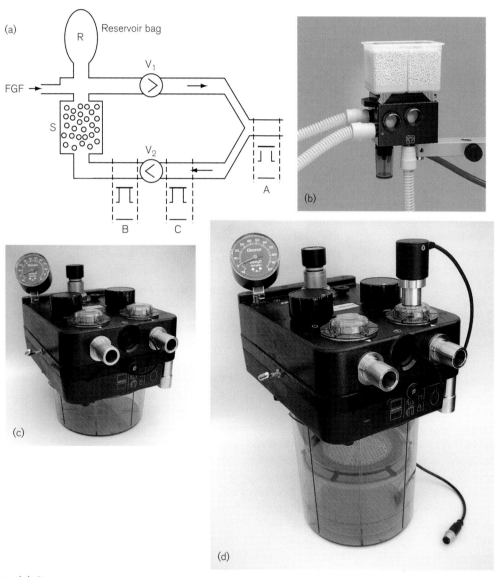

Figure 7.18 **(a)** Schematic diagram of a circle breathing system with absorber. FGF, fresh gas flow; V_1 and V_2, one-way valves; R, reservoir bag; S, soda-lime canister. The diagram highlights the alternative siting of the adjustable pressure-limiting (APL) valve at points A, B or C. **(b)** ADU circle system, Datex-Ohmeda. **(c)** Blease 1 Kg absorber. **(d)** 2 kg absorber fitted with an electronic PEEP valve.

reservoir bag in the expiratory limb of the system downstream of the valve V2. This may require some added inspiratory effort to draw the gas through the absorber. It appears also to have the added disadvantage that if the FGF is left on for long periods when not in use, the dry gas desiccates the soda lime. This has implications for the efficiency of the soda lime and its potential for producing unusual breakdown products (see above). The APL valve is usually mounted downstream of the valve V_2 in the expiratory limb, but before gas entry into the absorber. Here, it can dump excess exhaled gas prior to entry of gas into the absorber. At one time it was considered that an APL valve was best positioned in the breathing system at position 'A' for use with spontaneous respiration (Fig. 7.18a). This would preferentially dump aveolar gas during exhalation, thus increasing carbon dioxide elimination upstream of the absorber and conserving soda lime. However, as scavenging assumed a greater importance, the inconvenience of connecting a cumbersome scavenging hose to a valve in this position has limited its usefulness.

Circle breathing systems are manufactured in many different designs and sizes. Most are two-part systems with one part comprising a fixed body containing the gas pathways, switches and valves; and the other a detachable canister that contains the absorbent. Figures 7.18b, c and d show commercial versions of the system described. Figure 7.18b (ADU circle system, Datex-Ohmeda) has a container for 1 kg of absorbent that may be either disposable or one that can be refilled. During replacement, self-sealing valves on the body of the unit close to prevent escape of patient gas from the rest of the absorber. Figures 7.18c and d show other types of 1 kg and 2 kg absorber, respectively. The rationale for larger absorbers is discussed below. The 2 kg absorber shown is fitted with an electronic PEEP valve (see Chapter 11), which is the requirement in certain countries.

The system shown in Figures 7.19a and b is a disposable version. The valve V_1 is sited in the breathing hose and as close to the patient as possible. In this position it should have a faster response to pressure changes caused by exhalation and closes earlier, although, as it is exhaled dead-space gas that enters the system first, it is immaterial as to which limb this enters initially. Unlike many circle systems that are now an integral part of the anaesthetic workstation, the APL valve is not automatically excluded from the system in mechanical ventilation mode. Therefore, when a ventilator is attached to the reservoir bag port and is in use, the APL valve must be closed fully or gas will be lost from the system.

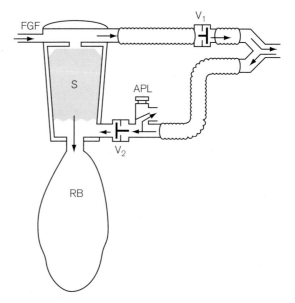

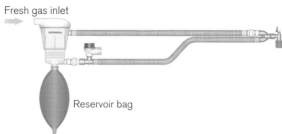

Figure 7.19 The Intersurgical disposable circle system. FGF, fresh gas flow; V_1 and V_2, one-way valves; APL, adjustable pressure-limiting valve; RB, reservoir bag; S, soda-lime canister.

Apparatus dead space

The apparatus dead space is low in circle systems. It consists only of that volume inside the male taper at the end of the Y-piece, which joins the inspiratory and expiratory breathing hoses to the patient. However, the functional dead space of this system may vary if a fault develops in it. For example, if the unidirectional valves malfunction and do not fully close, rebreathing can occur from the expiratory limb. Furthermore, some circle systems used to position the APL valve just upstream of the expiratory unidirectional valve (position C, Fig. 7.18). If this APL valve was mounted horizontally, and the valve screw opened fully, the valve disc occasionally would not seat correctly (although it was supposed to do so) and would cause rebreathing due to ingress of air or exhaust gases through this valve during spontaneous respiration.

Flow resistance

Circle systems impose a greater resistance to breathing than other commonly used breathing systems (Mapleson A–F systems), although less than co-axial arrangements of D systems (Bain system). This is due largely to the fact that there are two extra valves and soda lime in the system (see above). Other causes include:

- A high FGF rate will assist flow in the inspiratory side of the system, thus decreasing any inspiratory resistance, but will increase expiratory resistance through the unidirectional and APL (expiratory) valves.
- The reverse occurs with low gas flows. Low FGF rates will also increase the relative humidity and thus increase the 'stickiness' of the unidirectional valves owing to water vapour condensation, therefore further increasing flow resistance.
- The flow rates developed by rapid respiratory excursion (tidal volume and rate) produce the greatest swings in flow resistance (Table 7.2). These factors may not matter in healthy adults, but they can be unacceptable in young children.

Efficiency of soda lime absorbers

The efficiency of carbon dioxide absorption in a canister depends on the freshness, composition and the available surface area of the soda lime (see above), and the length of time the gas to be treated is in contact with the granules.

Early canister designs contained approximately 480 g of soda lime. These required frequent changes (after approximately 2–2.5 h of continuous use at low FGFs). Many presently used absorbers are of the 'Jumbo' type

which contain 2 kg of soda lime and, since this has a large volume and surface area of granules, the expired gas is in contact with them for a relatively long period of time, so increasing the efficiency of absorption. It has been shown that a 2 kg canister lasts five times longer than a 0.5 kg canister. When a 2 kg canister is employed it usually has two chambers, one above the other. When one half appears exhausted it is refilled and the canister positions reversed so that the previously unused half now bears the brunt of absorption. Not only is the absorption more efficient in the larger absorbers, but also less frequent recharging is necessary.

With the recent introduction of routine expired carbon dioxide monitoring these last two considerations appear to be less of a problem in clinical practice, and the reintroduction of smaller absorbers may well have advantages. These are easier to maintain, to use, to keep clean and have fewer leaks. The soda lime can also be supplied in disposable cartridges (Fig. 7.18b).

However, efficiency must also be compatible with safety and the recent concern that carbon monoxide and compound A may be formed in dry stale soda lime (see above) has prompted some anaesthetists to advocate the use of smaller absorbers requiring more frequent changes of absorbent.

Absorber switch

Traditionally, an absorber bypass switch has been included in a circle system. This allows expiratory gas to be channelled either through the absorption chamber or across a bypass directly into the inspiratory limb.

Some European and American models omit this switch. The rationale for excluding this switch involves safety considerations. Rebreathing of carbon dioxide is rendered impossible under normal operating conditions. However, the routine use of carbon dioxide monitoring in any case lessens this danger.

Ventilator switch

Older absorber systems had a single outlet for connecting either a reservoir bag or the ventilator hose. Switching from one to the other was achieved by manually removing one and substituting the other. It was also necessary to remember that when switching to the ventilator mode, the APL valve (which was often part of the absorber assembly) had also to be closed, otherwise this would cause part of the intended tidal volume to be leaked during controlled or assisted ventilation. Many current absorber models now have two outlets, one for the

Table 7.2 Flow resistance in circle breathing systems		
Frequency (min)	Tidal volume (ml)	Pressure swing (cmH$_2$O)
12	500	$-1 + 1/2$
12	1000	$-1 + 1$
12	1600	$-2 + 1 1/2$
24	500	$-1 + 1$
24	1000	$-3 + 1 1/2$
44	500	$-4 + 3$

Reproduced from Young, TM (1971) Carbon dioxide absorber *Anaesthesia* **26:** 78. With permission.

reservoir bag and the other for the ventilator hose. Either may now be included in the breathing system by operating a switch housed on the absorber assembly. The APL valve is so positioned that it is connected only to the reservoir bag and not included in the ventilator pathway. It, therefore, does not need adjusting when switching from one mode to the other and should be leak free when using the ventilator.

The use of ventilators with circle systems

Any ventilator deemed suitable for use with a circle system must have the following features:

- It must be able to reproduce the effect of manual compression and refilling of the reservoir bag, i.e. it must have a single breathing hose inlet /outlet to allow to and fro movement of gas.
- It must have a valve to vent excess gas in the circle system during the exhalation phase.

- It must have a power source that is independent of the fresh gas entering the circle system, so that a minute ventilation can be delivered that is larger that the FGF (especially when this is set at low flows).
- If the ventilator is gas powered, this driving gas should not be able to contaminate the respirable gas reaching the patient.

There are two types of ventilator that are used to drive circle systems: 'bag squeezer' and pneumatic piston.

'Bag squeezer' Here, the reservoir bag is replaced by a bellows (Fig. 7.20), which may be compressed mechanically or pneumatically. In the latter, the bellows is enclosed in a gas-tight container and the driving gas that enters the container then compresses the bellows but does not mix with the patient gas contained within it.

Pneumatic piston Here, the reservoir bag is replaced by a suitably long length of breathing hose. The driving gas from the ventilator is passed through a special valve (Figs 7.21a and b) into the breathing hose. The latter is sufficiently long so that its internal volume is at least 1.5–2 times greater than the patient's tidal volume and

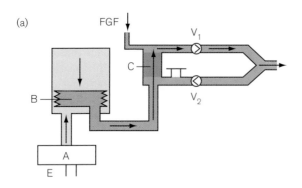

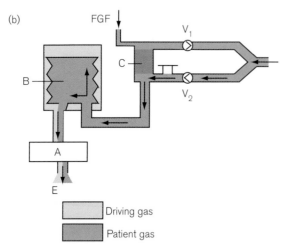

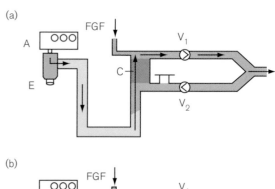

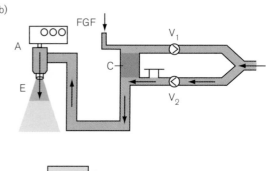

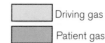

Figure 7.20 'Bag squeezer' ventilator and circle system. **(a)** Inspiratory phase; **(b)** expiratory phase. A, ventilator; B, bellows; C, absorber; V_1 & V_2, one-way valves; E, exhaust; FGF, fresh gas flow.

Figure 7.21 Pneumatic piston ventilator and circle system. **(a)** Inspiratory phase; **(b)** expiratory phase. A, ventilator; C, absorber; V_1 & V_2, one-way valves; E, exhaust; FGF, fresh gas flow.

prevents the driving gas from entering the circle and contaminating the patient gas. This is especially important in many circle systems where the reservoir limb is sited in the inspiratory pathway. Here, driving gas could dilute the inspiratory anaesthetic gas sufficiently to cause an inadequate level of anaesthesia to be maintained.

Mechanical ventilation in circle systems
Control of minute ventilation

The ventilator and circle breathing systems in modern workstations are integrated. The tidal volume that is intended is entered on the ventilator control panel and is delivered to the patient. Transducers monitor the flow to the patient and make adjustments for changes in compliance, resistance and changes in FGF so that the tidal volume remains the same. In older designs, the circle and ventilator function are separate and the tidal volume delivered during mechanical ventilation may be altered by adjusting the ventilator as well as the FGF. Here, although the ventilator may be set to give a known tidal volume, when this reaches the circle it is supplemented by the fresh gas entering the system and which may significantly alter the final tidal volume.

Consider the following FGF entering the circle system:

$$\text{FGF 6 l min}^{-1} = 6000\text{ml/60sec}$$
$$= 100\text{ml/sec}$$
$$\text{If ventilator rate 10/min} = 1 \text{ cycle every 6secs}$$
$$\text{If the Insp./Exp. ratio is 1/2} = 2 \text{ sec insp. /4sec exp.}$$
$$\text{Then inspiratory FGF in 2sec} = 200\text{ml FGF}$$
$$\text{If ventilator setting} = \text{tidal vol. 400ml}$$
$$\text{Total tidal vol.} = \text{Vent tidal vol.} \times \text{Insp.FGF}$$
$$= 400 + 200$$
$$= 600\text{ml}$$

As FGF is reduced, its contribution to the total tidal volume (and therefore minute ventilation) is reduced and that fraction of exhaled carbon dioxide is increased.

Maintenance of circle absorber systems

During prolonged administration at low FGF rates, water vapour condenses in the expiratory hose and circle system canister and this needs to be emptied from time to time. Condensation also occurs in the expiratory unidirectional valve. Not only may this obscure the glass dome so that the correct operation of the valve cannot be observed, but also a drop of water on the cage retaining the valve disc may cause the latter to adhere to it by surface tension. This can hold the valve permanently open, causing the

patient to rebreathe exhaled gas from the expiratory pathway in the system. The tendency of the valve discs to stick is a result of their being made of increasingly lightweight materials in order to reduce the resistance to gas flow.

This complication may be reduced by placing a low resistance bacterial/hydrophobic filter at the end of the expiratory limb of the breathing system. This will protect the valve and absorber system from both bacterial and excess water contamination. Alternatively, the breathing hoses should be changed between cases.

In locations where the cost of the above exercise would be prohibitive, the tubing should be washed and hung out to dry between cases. Secondly, the expiratory valve should be dismantled and wiped clean with isopropyl alcohol. When, after dismantling, the glass dome of the expiratory valve is screwed back on, it is important to ensure that the sealing washer is correctly in place, otherwise a serious leak may occur. If a low-resistance bacterial filter is not used, then the circle absorber housing should be autoclaved (where possible) on a regular basis. Some circle absorbers cannot be autoclaved, but may be cleaned by chemical means.

The soda lime should be changed at regular intervals either when:

- the dye indicates that the majority of the granules are exhausted;
- when using an analyzer, carbon dioxide appears in the inspiratory mixture; or
- when the absorber is unlikely to be used for some time (e.g. over a weekend).

The soda lime container usually has a mark above which it should not be filled. Overfilling may result in granules of soda lime clogging the threads of canisters that screw into position, or may prevent the correct seating of the sealing washer, thus causing a leak or bypassing of the soda lime. Furthermore, leaving this space at the top reduces the preferential 'channelling' effect of the gas stream along the sides, and ensures a more even flow through the container. Since the canister is held in the vertical position, channelling is less of a problem than in the Waters' canister, although some does occur between the granules and sides of the canister as the air spaces are larger here than those between granules within the canister.

Gas and vapour concentration in a circle system

Circle systems are unique in that they function effectively (when a steady state of anaesthesia has been reached) using a wide variety of FGF rates. However, the fate of the various gases within the system needs to be understood in order that it may be used safely and effectively. For example, the internal volume of the apparatus (when using a 2 kg absorber, which consists of the intergranular air space in the absorber (1 litre), the breathing hoses (1 litre) and pathways within the absorber (1 litre), totalling 3 litres, along with the functional residual capacity of a patient of 1.25 litres, provides a large reservoir into which the anaesthetic gas is diluted at the beginning of anaesthesia.

In order to minimize this dilution and provide adequate concentrations of anaesthetic agent, high flows of fresh gas and vapour are required initially in order to flush the residual gas out of the circle system; the higher the flow, the faster this 'wash out' occurs. Lung 'wash out' will of course depend on the patient's minute ventilation. The greater this is, the less time the process takes.

Secondly, the alveolar uptake of anaesthetic agent is greatest at the beginning of anaesthesia. Therefore, the higher the initial FGF rate (up to a value equal to the patient's minute ventilation), the greater is the delivery of anaesthetic agent into the system. This in turn minimizes any reduction in concentration of agent caused by uptake by the patient. When near equilibrium of anaesthetic agents has occurred between the alveoli and blood, exhaled agent concentration almost equals that in the inspiratory mixture, and therefore the high initial FGFs may safely be greatly reduced.

In practice, the FGF is usually reduced in stages:

- *First stage*: the initial flow for patient and breathing system washout, as well as supply of adequate anaesthetic agent to match alveolar uptake, usually takes approximately 5–10 minutes. (The shorter time is suited to the insoluble anaesthetic agents desflurane and sevoflurane, which reach alveolar equilibrium more quickly.) If this flow rate is at or greater than the patient's minute ventilation, then most or all of the exhaled gas will leave the system via the APL (expiratory) valve without passing through the absorber. When used in this mode, it may often be referred to as a high-flow system.
- *Second stage*: an intermediate flow rate of 70% of the minute ventilation for a further 5 minutes will allow purging of the soda lime canister without major changes in anaesthetic concentrations.
- *Third stage*: a lower flow may be selected, the value of which will depend on the availability of gas and vapour monitoring within the system, the efficiency of the

vaporizer (in or out of circle) and personal preference. Flows of the order of 0.5–2 l min^{-1} are commonly used and when the circle is used in this mode it may often be referred to as a low-flow system. A closed flow system is defined as that which has no gas exit (i.e. APL valve fully closed) and in which the FGF equals the uptake by the patient. In practice, however, few if any commercial anaesthetic circle breathing systems are sufficiently leak-proof to be used at such flows.

Oxygen concentrations in circle systems at low FGF

As the FGF in a circle is decreased, exhaled gas that is allowed to recirculate exerts an increasing influence on the subsequent inspired gas mixture. The oxygen concentration of this exhaled gas depends on:

- its original inspired concentration; and
- the alveolar oxygen extraction, which may be unpredictable.

Figure 7.22 shows the decrease in alveolar oxygen concentrations of a 50% nitrous oxide and 50% oxygen mixture under controlled conditions. It can be seen that at a FGF of 1 l min^{-1} the oxygen concentration has dropped to 27% and drops even further at a FGF of 0.5 l min^{-1}. Therefore, in clinical practice the oxygen concentration in a circle at low flows is most unpredictable and monitoring of inspired oxygen with an analyzer is essential. In fact, monitoring of all gases and anaesthetic vapours should be considered mandatory for circle systems at low flows.

The use of volatile agents in the circle system

Volatile inhalational agents can be introduced into the system either by being added to the FGF (vaporizer outside circle/VOC) or by incorporating the vaporizer within the circle (vaporizer in circle/VIC).

Vaporizer outside circle

This is probably the most common method of introducing inhalational agents into the breathing system. At high FGFs, the vapour concentration in the circle is reliably represented by the dial setting of the vaporizer. However, as the FGF is reduced, two phenomena occur:

- Expired gas, which is recycled (and which has a reduced concentration of inhalational agent due to uptake), dilutes the FGF within the system. This reduces the delivered concentration of inhalational

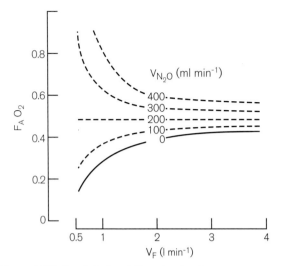

Figure 7.22 Predicted variations in alveolar oxygen concentrations (F_AO_2) produced by decreasing fresh gas flow (V_F) and assuming different levels of nitrous oxide uptake in a 50 : 50 mixture of oxygen in nitrous oxide. A constant oxygen consumption of 200 ml min^{-1} and a constant ventilation required to produce an alveolar CO_2 concentration of 5% have been assumed. The heavy line shows the fall in alveolar oxygen concentration with decreasing fresh gas flow when the inspired and body levels of nitrous oxide have reached equilibrium (zero uptake). (Reproduced with kind permission from *Scientific Foundations of Anaesthesia*, Butterworth/Heinemann.)

agent to below that anticipated by the dial setting on the vaporizer.

- At low FGF, vaporizer efficiency may well be altered, providing a lower or higher than expected concentration of inhalational agent. This is not seen as a problem in modern vaporizer performance but was seen as a problem with models that are now obsolete (e.g. TEC 2 vaporizer).

At low FGFs, and in the absence of a vapour analyzer therefore, the anaesthetist would need to know:

- the performance of the vaporizer in use at that given FGF;
- the expired concentration of inhalational agent; and
- the degree of dilution of the FGF with expired gas (which in turn depends on the patient's minute ventilation).

The lower the FGF, the more difficult it is to predict the inspired concentration of agent. At flows below 2 l min^{-1} it is essential to incorporate a vapour analyzer into the system, especially during controlled ventilation when signs of light anaesthesia may be more difficult to

determine, to ensure that adequate amounts of agent reach the patient.

Vaporizer in circle

If the vaporizer is incorporated into the circle system, it must have a low resistance to gas flow so as to minimize the respiratory work required of a spontaneously breathing patient. High-resistance plenum vaporizers are unsuitable.

With a vaporizer incorporated in the circle, recirculating gas picks up vapour to add to the vapour already being carried, and therefore the vapour concentration may well be greater than intended. Calibration of vaporizers in this system is therefore impossible. The vapour concentration in this type of system depends on a number of factors when equilibrium has been reached:

- *the fresh gas flow*. The lower the FGF, the greater will be the recirculation of gas already carrying vapour and the higher will be the concentration of inspired agent.
- *the efficiency of the vaporizer*. The more efficient the vaporize, the higher will be the inspired concentration of agent. This has important implications with potent inhalational agents. At a low FGF and a large assisted or controlled minute ventilation, the anaesthetic gas may well become saturated with agent at that temperature. For halothane, this will represent a concentration of 33% at 21°C (the saturated vapour pressure for halothane).

Therefore, for potent agents, an inefficient vaporizer is preferable. The presence of a wick in a vaporizer in the circle is also unsuitable, since water vapour will condense on the wick, reducing its efficiency and possibly increasing the resistance to gas flow.

Ether, for which much higher concentrations are appropriate has, however, been widely and safely used with a VIC. Adequate vaporization may be assisted by the use of baffles within the vaporizer that cause the gases to impinge repeatedly on the surface of the ether, or even by bubbling the FGF through the liquid ether. It may also be increased to some extent by the heat from the recirculating expired gases.

Breathing systems with assisted circulation

It has long been appreciated that part of the energy required to propel the gases along the passages of a breathing system must be derived from the patient's respiratory effort. The latter, prejudiced by the depressant effects of narcosis, can become inefficient, and any form of resistance would further impair respiratory function. On the other hand, any form of assistance to flow or of reduction of resistance would be beneficial. To this end, various 'circulators' were devised and expiratory valves that were not spring-loaded were advocated. None are in current use.

Inspiratory assistance

Some of the more sophisticated anaesthetic machines, with integral ventilators and circle systems, may have sensors in the breathing system which detect a patient's inspiratory effort and trigger the ventilator to supplement it (a pressure support mode). This is discussed further in Chapter 11.

PROCEDURES FOR CHECKING BREATHING SYSTEMS

All the breathing systems described above will only function correctly if the components are free of any fault, assembled in the correct order and the connections made gas-tight. A good working knowledge of the apparatus is essential prior to its use by a practitioner. Fatalities have unfortunately occurred where the user:

- was either unfamiliar with the equipment;
- included a non-standard item;
- had not noticed that it had been assembled incorrectly;
- had not noticed that it had developed a fault; or
- the lumen of the system at some point had become occluded by a foreign body.

Therefore breathing systems should be checked prior to each use according to the manufacturer's instructions or against a checklist approved by a hospital department or a national association (e.g. The Association of Anaesthetists of Great Britain and Ireland). A suitable inspection should ensure that:

- the components of the system chosen for use (especially if they are not from the same manufacturer) should always conform to the same national or international standard;
- they are assembled appropriately;
- all connections are secure using a push and twist technique;
- with the APL valve closed, and the patient end occluded, the system is gas-tight when filled and that gas subsequently escapes when the occlusion is removed; and
- when the patient end is occluded for a second time and the APL valve is opened, the gas escapes easily through it.

In addition to this, any co-axial breathing system should have the integrity of the inner limb confirmed. This can be done on a Mapleson D system by occluding the inner limb only (e.g. with a pencil or a 1ml syringe), observing that the bag remains deflated and that the anaesthetic machine safety valve protecting the back bar gives an alarm signal. With a Mapleson A system (Lack co-axial), occluding the inner limb only should cause the reservoir bag to distend (with the APL valve closed).

THE COMPONENTS OF A BREATHING SYSTEM

Rebreathing and reservoir bags

Rebreathing and reservoir bags (Fig. 7.23) are identical, the distinction being solely in the use to which they are put, as explained previously. The commonly-used size in adult breathing systems is 2 litres (i.e. that which when fully but not forcibly distended has a capacity of 2 litres; in clinical practice it is seldom filled beyond this capacity). They are also available in 1 litre and 0.5 litre sizes for paediatric anaesthesia. Larger bags are sometimes used as reservoir bags in ventilators.

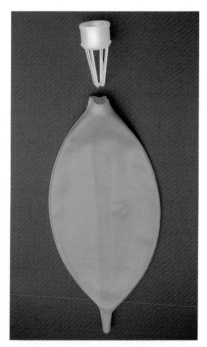

Figure 7.23 2-litre reservoir bag showing the cagemount connector.

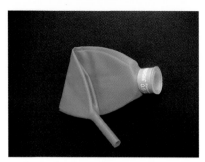

Figure 7.24 Double-ended bag for paediatric anaesthesia.

In adult breathing systems, the capacity to which the bag may easily be distended must exceed the patient's tidal volume. A larger capacity bag (2 litres), however, is safer as it more easily absorbs pressure increases. The neck of the bag is stretched over a female 22 mm metal or plastic tapered connector. A metal or plastic cage is often attached to the part of the connector that fits inside the bag. This prevents the inlet from being occluded if the bag were folded.

'Double-ended' bags

In the Rees T-piece paediatric attachment, a double-ended bag is added to the expiratory limb (Fig. 7.24) and the smaller end acts as an expiratory port the aperture of which can be controlled by the anaesthetist.

The material of which the bag is constructed is important. Where ventilation is spontaneous, the opening pressure of the expiratory valve must exceed that required to prevent the bag from emptying spontaneously owing to its weight or resistance to distension. Therefore, to maintain a low expiratory pressure, the bag must be 'soft'. This was achieved easily when natural latex rubber bags were in common use. The increase in latex allergy in the general population and in healthcare workers has had a major impact on the provision of equipment that had previously contained natural latex rubber. All anaesthetic equipment in the UK is now supplied with natural latex-free parts. These include ventilator bellows and reservoir bags. The latter are made from synthetic compounds such as polychloroprene (neoprene) that is synthetic latex rubber.

Some manufacturers make their bags sufficiently pliant to mimic the elasticity of natural latex. These will distend well beyond their normal filling capacity until they burst but the pressure in the bags will stay below 60 cm H_2O. This is thought to be a safety feature that prevents barotrauma to a patient's lungs should the exhalation pathway in a breathing system containing this bag become occluded. This would be caused most commonly by an APL valve inadvertently screwed shut. Some, however, are made from less compliant material and the pressure may rise to over 60 cm H_2O. These bags should be fitted only to breathing systems that have a pressure relief valve attached either as a separate feature or built into the APL valve (see below).

The observed movement of the bag depends on several factors, such as its shape, size, degree of filling, the tension of the expiratory valve and the FGF rate, as well as on the patient's tidal volume. An accurate estimate of the patient's tidal volume cannot be made simply by watching the bag.

Adjustable Pressure Limiting (APL) valves

The purpose of this valve is to allow the escape of exhaled (expired) and surplus gases from a breathing system, but without permitting entry of the outside air, even during a negative phase. Usually it is desirable that the pressure required to open the valve should be as low as possible, in order to minimize resistance to expiration. It must, however, present sufficient resistance to prevent the reservoir bag from emptying spontaneously, particularly when a scavenging system is employed that exerts a slight sub-atmospheric pressure upon it.

The operating principles of APL valves are based on the Heidbrink valve (Fig. 7.25). The valve disc is as light as possible, and rests on a 'knife-edge' seating that presents a small area of contact. This lessens the tendency to adhesion between the disc and seating due to the surface tension of condensed water from the expired air, or after washing or sterilizing. The disc has a stem that is located in a guide, in order to ensure that it is correctly positioned on the seating, and a lightweight coiled spring, which promotes closure of the valve.

The spring is a delicate coil and is of such dimensions that when the valve top is screwed fully 'open' there is minimal pressure on the disc when seated. However, during the 'blow-off' phase, the disc rises and shortens the spring so that the pressure it exerts on the disc is greater and will close it at the appropriate time. Screwing down the valve top produces progressively increasing tension in the spring. When the top is screwed fully down, the valve is completely closed. If, owing to damage or fatigue, the spring is shortened, the top may have to be screwed down a little in order to ensure closure at the

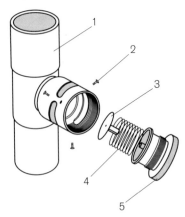

Figure 7.25 The Heidbrink valve: 1, male tapers at both ends; 2, retaining screws; 3, disc; 4, spring; 5, valve top.

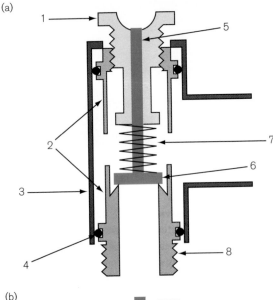

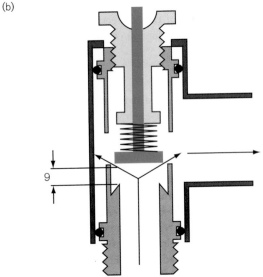

Figure 7.26 'Humphrey' APL valve. **(a)** Inspiration (with valve disc closed); **(b)** beginning of exhalation (valve disc just clearing small funnel). 1, Valve top; 2, valve body; 3, exhaled gas scavenging shroud; 4, 'O'-ring seal between the valve body and shroud; 5, valve spindle; 6, valve disc; 7, valve spring; 8, screw thread to secure valve to the breathing system; 9, 5 mm funnel which accentuates movement of the spindle.

start of inspiration. If it has been elongated, the pressure at which it opens may be excessive. Small screws in the body of the valve, and a groove in the skirt of the top, prevent it from being unscrewed so far that it falls apart.

The Humphrey APL valve

An interesting addition to the standard APL valve is the modification seen on the Humphrey version (Figs 7.13a and 7.26), which is part of the current Humphrey ADE system. Here, the valve disc is attached to a red coloured spindle, which extends through the valve top. When the valve is fully open, the spindle is seen to bob up and down as the disc is lifted up and down during respiration. The valve top is made concave and shiny so that it reflects and magnifies the spindle colour so as to detect even the smallest movement when used in paediatric anaesthesia. The inside of the valve body has a small funnel through which the disc has to move before significant gas can escape. This initial movement of 5 mm accentuates the bobbing action of the spindle, which again is useful when used in paediatric anaesthesia.

When the ADE system is used in the Mapleson A mode, the valve spindle may be held down with a finger if switching from spontaneous to manual ventilation is required. This has a number of advantages:

- As there is no leak from the valve during inspiration, the patient's lung compliance may be more accurately assessed.
- It becomes as efficient as the Mapleson A mode in spontaneous respiration (i.e. the valve is shut during inspiration and open during expiration).
- The valve top may be kept in the 'open' position at all times and does not require repeated adjustment when switching between spontaneous and manual ventilation.

It was originally thought that the increased respiratory work produced by the expiratory resistance of APL valves was detrimental to anaesthetized patients. This is without doubt true when the valve resistance is high (due to sticky valves, narrow valve apertures) or where the respiratory effort is severely compromised (e.g. in neonates). However, modern valve design (with wider valve apertures, lighter valve discs, more delicate springs, better screw threads) minimizes this resistance. Furthermore, a small positive end expiratory pressure (PEEP) effect that these valves may produce is now thought to be positively beneficial, reducing the potential for the functional residual capacity of the lungs to fall below the closing volume in supine anaesthetized patients.

APL valves with in-built overpressure safety devices

Any unexpected pressure rise in a breathing system was made relatively safe by the compliance of the latex rubber of the reservoir bag. This could still fail, for instance if the bag were to be trapped under the wheel of an anaesthetic machine, a dangerously high pressure could develop within the breathing system and be passed on to the patient. Now that latex rubber is no longer used owing to the increase in latex allergy, new materials are used that may not have the same elasticity and so are not as compliant. This safety feature can no longer be relied on. APL valves are now available in which an overpressure safety device has been incorporated.

An example, is shown in Figures 7.27 a, b, c; it has two valves:

1. the inner (3) which is tensioned with a weak spring (4); and
2. the outer (5) which is tensioned with a more powerful one (2).

When the valve top (1) is unscrewed fully (Fig. 7.27a), the outer valve is permanently open but the inner one is closed until exhaled gas forces it open. The pressure required to do this is small (0.15 kPa/1.5 cm H_2O). However. when the valve top is screwed down fully, both valves are closed and in this position the outer one is pushed against the inner so that is has no movement of its own (Fig. 7.27b). An excess pressure is now required to move the more powerful spring on the outer valve which will begin to open at 3 Kpa (30 cm H_2O) and be fully open at 6 Kpa (60 cm H_2O) when the gas flow is 50 l min^{-1} (Fig. 7.27c).

Alternative APL valve design

Many breathing systems are now supplied as single use items. This includes the APL valve (Fig. 7.28a). It is now possible to simplify the design so that the spring and the valve disc are replaced by a neoprene flap valve (1)

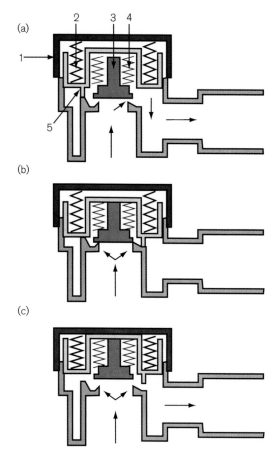

Figure 7.27 An APL valve with an overpressure safety device. 1, Valve control knob; 2, high-pressure spring; 3, valve spindle; 4, light-pressure spring; 5, the part of the asymmetric valve body that rotates during valve closure and occludes the expiratory limb. The figure shows **(a)** the valve open during exhalation; **(b)** the valve closed; and **(c)** the valve closed with the overpressure safety device in action.

(Fig. 7.28b). This opens and shuts in the normal manner during spontaneous respiration. When positive pressure is required, the valve top (2) operates a screw threaded insert (3) that lowers an overpressure relief valve (4). As the valve top is screwed shut, the insert lowers the second valve (4) onto the flap valve housing, gradually occluding the expiratory pathway until complete occlusion occurs (ii). The second valve is fitted with a spring (5), which is strong enough to maintain the occlusion up to a pressure of 60 cm H_2O, but weak enough to cause the valve to lift (iii) and allow gases at a higher pressure to escape.

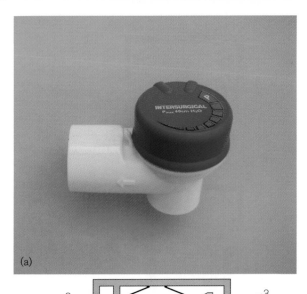

(a)

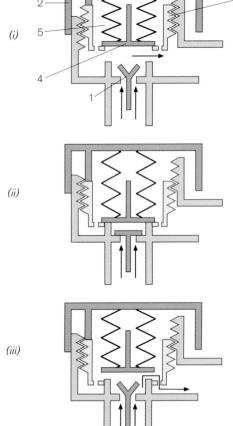

(b)

Figure 7.28 (a) A single use APL valve (Intersurgical™). **(b)** Operation of an Intersurgical™ single use APL valve. 1, Neoprene flap valve; 2, Valve top; 3, Screw threaded insert; 4, Overpressure relief valve; 5, Spring. (i) Valve in open position. (ii) Valve shut. (iii) Overpressure relief valve operated.

Breathing hoses

The hoses connecting the components of a breathing system must be of such a diameter as to present a low resistance to gas flow. Its cross-section must be uniform to promote laminar flow where possible, and although it should be flexible, kinking should not occur.

The most commonly-used hose for a long time was corrugated rubber or polychloroprene (neoprene). The corrugations allow acute angulations of the hose without kinking. The advantage of these materials is that the ends are more easily stretched, and will make a good union with other components of different diameters. They may be sterilized by steam autoclaving and be re-used in countries where single-use alternatives are impractical. The disadvantages are that the irregular wall must cause turbulence and being opaque may harbour dirt and infection unseen. They are also heavy and if unsupported, may drag on a facemask or endotracheal tube.

Various other materials, such as silicone rubber and plastics (polyethylene) are in use, both in corrugated and smooth form (Fig. 7.29). A smooth-bore breathing hose produces less turbulence than the corrugated variety at similar gas flows. It can also be produced so that it resists kinking (by the attachment of a reinforcing spiral of a similar material to its external surface). With smooth-bore hosing, a smaller diameter (e.g. 15 mm) may well be acceptable for use with adult breathing systems (see Humphrey ADE breathing system).

Plastic hosing has become very popular because it is lightweight, cheap to manufacture, and therefore disposable. Some are supplied as complete breathing systems (Figs. 7.12 and 7.19) or in long coils, the appropriate length of which may be cut off at one of the frequent intervals where the corrugations (Fig. 7.30) give way to a shaped connector. More recently, the addition of small quantities of silver mixed with the plastic (Intersurgical Silver Knight™) has been used to make breathing systems bactericidal, both on the inside and the outside of the hosing.

Silicone rubber hosing is autoclavable, unlike many plastics which would melt if so treated. Plastic apparatus intended for single use only is normally sterilized at manufacture by gamma irradiation.

There are several standard sizes of corrugated hose, both ends of which have smooth walls for about 2–3 cm. These ends are designed to fit either tapered connectors (see below) or tapered components of a breathing system. Breathing hose for adult use is normally 22 mm wide so as to reduce the resistance to breathing to a minimum. Paediatric breathing hose has a narrower bore (15 mm) to

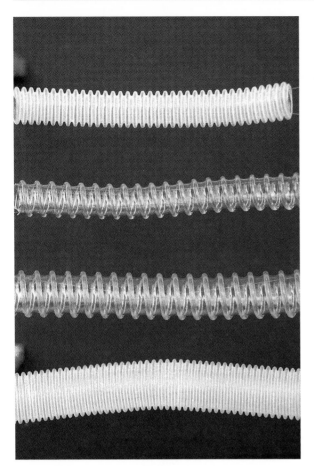

Figure 7.29 From top to bottom: 15 mm corrugated plastic breathing hose; 15 mm smooth-bore hose; 22 mm smooth-bore hose; 22 mm corrugated hose.

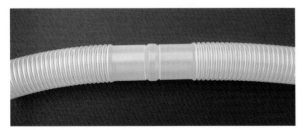

Figure 7.30 Plastic hosing showing a section that may be cut to produce a suitable length.

reduce its internal volume (see Chapter 15) and to make it less cumbersome.

Tapered connections (adapters)

Tapered connections (adapters) provide a useful way of joining rigid tubes or other components together in such a

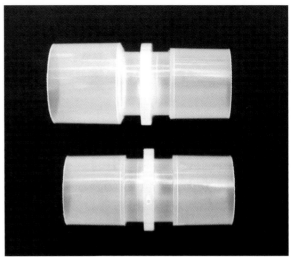

Figure 7.31 Plastic (disposable) 22 mm tapered adaptors. (Top) Female to male; the male part is normally inserted into each end of a breathing hose. (Bottom) Male to male; this is inserted into the distal end of a piece of corrugated tubing when used as an extension for a reservoir bag (Fig. 7.32c).

manner that the joint will not leak. The joint is described as having a male half and a female half, which are pushed together with a slight twist to form a gas-tight fit. The joint may be easily dismantled and reassembled, a feature that makes it useful for the interconnection of breathing systems, catheter mounts and endotracheal connectors.

A leak-proof joint relies on its components being completely circular and having the same angle of taper so that the maximum contact between the components of the joint will occur. The standard also requires that male tapers for breathing systems be fitted with a recess behind the taper so that when rubber and plastic hosing is pushed on to a male connector, its leading edge can contract into this recess to provide a more secure fitting. Examples of tapers are shown in Figure 7.31.

The current ISO and BS recommendations on the sequence of tapers in various breathing systems are set out in Figure 7.32.

Prior to the introduction of any standards, manufacturers were free to decide the size and angle of tapers used with their equipment. However, there is now an internationally agreed size for tapered connections for use with anaesthetic breathing systems and endotracheal tubes so that there is compatibility between equipment from different manufacturers.

The International Organization for Standardization (150.5356, 1987) and the British Standard (BS 3849) specifies the use of:

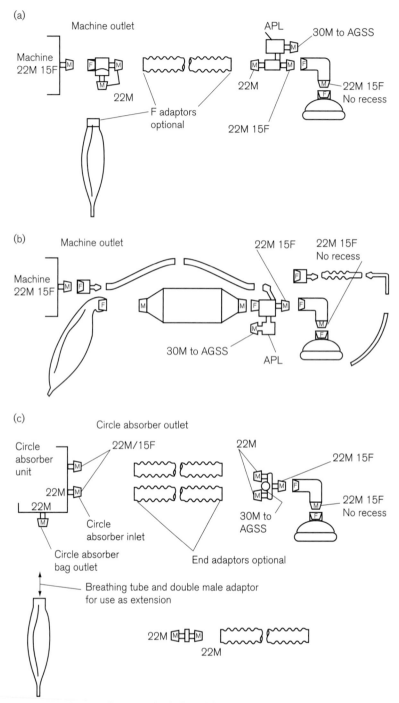

Figure 7.32 Current sequence of tapers in anaesthetic breathing systems as recommended by the ISO and BSI (BS 3849) as from 1988. Typical layout of **(a)** Mapleson A system; **(b)** to-and-fro absorption system; and **(c)** circle absorption system. M, male conical fitting; F, female conical fitting; APL, adjustable pressure-limiting valve.

- 30 mm tapered connections for the attachment of scavenging hose to breathing systems;
- 22 mm tapers for connections within a breathing system; and
- 15 mm connections for the attachment of a breathing system to an endotracheal tube.

Some 22 mm male breathing hose connections are so manufactured that they incorporate a 15 mm female taper for direct connection to an endotracheal tube.

It is worthy of note that the current British Standard requires that a reservoir bag should have a female inlet to fit the male outlet for bag mounts on all breathing systems. However, should a length of breathing hose be required between the bag mount and reservoir bag, a problem arises. The breathing hose is manufactured with two female ends. One will fit the bag mount (male to female) but the other will not fit the bag (female to female). A male-to-male 22 mm tapered adapter is required (Fig. 7.31b).

Problems with tapered connections

Many accidents have occurred as a result of the accidental and unobserved disconnection of tapered joints, especially between the breathing hose and other components of the breathing system such as catheter mounts. The material used in the construction may either wear with frequent use (most plastics and rubber), or become distorted by damage (metal connectors). All taper fit connections must be assumed to be prone to accidental disconnection. Disconnection can be minimized by giving the components of the joint a slight twist following their insertion.

Conversely, some metal connectors made from aluminium alloys may stick together by the phenomenon of cold welding produced by the recommended twist above, and may be very difficult to separate.

Re-use of breathing system components

Items that are intended for *re-use* (i.e. to be used on different patients) are normally made from materials (rubber, neoprene, silicone and metal) that withstand repeated autoclaving.

Some items are designated as *single use* (i.e. to be used on one person only) if they are made from materials such as plastics which are not easily sterilized. Also, if the tapers (see above) are made from materials which are easily distorted with repeated connection, they will be designated for single use only.

A third category has been described. Some items that might be designated as single use because they are not easily sterilized may be acceptable for *limited use*. Provided that these items are protected by a high-quality bacterial filter, some manufacturers will accept product liability if the item is used on a number of patients provided that the item is thoroughly checked between uses.

FURTHER READING

Breathing systems
Boulton TB (1979) Breathing systems. (Editorial) *Anaesthesia* **34**: 605–607.

Classification of breathing systems
Cook LB (1996) Mapleson breathing systems. The importance of the expiratory pause. *Anaesthesia* **51**: 453–460.
Dorrington KL (1996) The Mapleson breathing systems. *Anaesthesia* **51**(10): 988.
Mapleson WW (1998) The elimination of rebreathing in various semi-closed anaesthetic systems. *British Journal of Anaesthesia* **80**(2): 263–269.
Mapleson WW (2004) Editorial I: Fifty years after – reflections on 'The elimination of rebreathing in various semi-closed anaesthetic systems'. *British Journal of Anaesthesia* **93**(3): 319–321.
Miller DM (1995) Breathing systems reclassified. *Anaesthesia in Intensive Care* **23**(3): 281–283.

Mapleson A systems
Chan AS, Bruce WE, Soni N (1989) A comparison of anaesthetic breathing systems during spontaneous ventilation. An *in-vitro* study using a lung model. *Anaesthesia* **44**(3): 194–199.
Ooi R, Lack A, Soni N, Whittle J, Pattison J (1993) The parallel Lack anaesthetic breathing system. *Anaesthesia* **48**: 409–414.
Ooi R, Pattison J, Soni N (1993) The additional work of breathing imposed by Mapleson A systems. *Anaesthesia* **48**(7): 599–603.

Mapleson D, E and F systems
Adams AP (1977) The Bain circuit. Prevention of anaesthetic mixture dilution when using mechanical ventilators delivering non-anaesthetic gases. *Anaesthesia* **32**(1): 46–49.
Henville ID, Adams AP (1976) The Bain Anaesthetic System. *Anaesthesia* **31**: 247–256.
Spoerel WE, Bain JA (1986) Anaesthetic breathing systems. *British Journal of Anaesthesia* **58**(7): 819–821.

Rebreathing with Mapleson systems

Barrie JR, Beatty PC (1993) Rebreathing and semiclosed anaesthetic breathing systems. *Anaesthesia* **48(1)**: 86–87.

Cook LB (1996) Respiratory pattern and rebreathing in the Mapleson A, C and D breathing systems with spontaneous ventilation. A theory. *Anaesthesia* **51(4)**: 371–385.

Cook LB (1997) Rebreathing in the Mapleson A, C and D breathing systems with sinusoidal and exponential flow waveforms. *Anaesthesia* **52(12)**: 1182–1194.

Dorrington KL, Lehane JR (1989) Rebreathing during spontaneous and controlled ventilation with 'T' piece breathing systems: a general solution. *Anaesthesia* **44**: 300–302.

Dorrington KL, Lehane JR (1987) Minimum fresh gas flow requirements of anaesthetic breathing systems during spontaneous ventilation: a graphical approach. *Anaesthesia* **42(7)**: 732–737.

Resistance to flow with Mapleson systems

Kay B, Beatty PC, Healy TE, Accoush ME, Calpin M (1983) Change in the work of breathing imposed by five anaesthetic breathing systems. *British Journal of Anaesthesia* **55(12)**: 1239–1247.

Martin DG, Kong KL, Lewis GT (1989) Resistance to airflow in anaesthetic breathing systems. *British Journal of Anaesthesia* **62(4)**: 456–461.

Hybrid systems

Humphrey D (1983) A new anaesthetic breathing system combining Mapleson A, D & E principles. *Anaesthesia* **38**: 361–372.

Humphrey D (1984) The ADE anaesthetic breathing system. *Anaesthesia* **39**: 715–716.

Humphrey D, Brock-Utne JG, Downing JW (1986) Single lever Humphrey ADE lowflow universal anaesthetic breathing system. Part II: Comparison with Bain system in anaesthesized adults during controlled ventilation. *Canadian Anaesthesia Society Journal* **33(6)**: 710–718.

Orlikowski CEP, Ewart MC, Bingham RM (1991) The Humphrey ADE system: Evaluation in paediatric use. *British Journal of Anaesthesia* **66**: 253–7.

Carbon dioxide absorption
To-and-Fro systems

Shaw M, Scott DH (1998) Performance characteristics of a 'to-and-fro' disposable soda lime canister. *Anaesthesia* **53(5)**: 454–460.

Circle systems

Bracken A, Cox LA (1968) Apparatus for carbon dioxide absorption. *British Journal of Anaesthesia* **40**: 660–665.

Levels of anaesthetic agents in circle systems

Conway CM (1986) Gaseous homeostasis and the circle system. Validation of a model. *British Journal of Anaesthesia* **58(3)**: 337–344.

Cook LB, Chakrabarti MK (1996) Circle systems with a coaxial inspiratory limb. Investigation with a lung model. *Anaesthesia* **51(3)**: 247–254.

Mapleson WW (1960) The concentration of anaesthetics in closed circuits, with special reference to halothane. *British Journal of Anaesthesia* **32**: 298–309.

Mapleson WW (1998) The theoretical ideal fresh-gas flow sequence at the start of low-flow anaesthesia. *Anaesthesia* **53(3)**: 264–272.

Sobolev I, Sellers WF (2001) Rate of change in gas concentrations in a charged circle system with absorber. *Anaesthesia* **56(4)**: 380–381.

Sobreira DP, Jreige MM, Saraiva R (2001) The fresh-gas flow sequence at the start of low-flow anaesthesia. *Anaesthesia* **56(4)**: 379–380.

Wright D, Brosnan S, Royston B, White D (1998) Controlled ventilation using isoflurane with an in-circle vaporiser. *Anaesthesia* **53(7)**: 650–653.

Absorbers and absorbents

Coetzee JF, Stewart LJ (2002) Fresh gas flow is not the only determinant of volatile agent consumption: a multi-centre study of low-flow anaesthesia. *British Journal of Anaesthesia* **88(1)**: 46–55.

Cossham PS (1992) Obstruction to wet soda lime granules. *Anaesthesia* **47**: 10–11.

Knolle E, Linert W, Gilly H (2003) The color change in CO2 absorbents on drying: an in vitro study using moisture analysis. *Anesthesia and Analgesia* **97(1)**: 151–155.

Murray JM, Renfrew CW, Bedi A, McCrystal CB, Jones DS, Fee JP (1999) Amsorb: a new carbon dioxide absorbent for use in anesthetic breathing systems. *Anesthesiology* **91(5)**: 1342–1348.

Carbon monoxide and compound A formation

Baxter PJ, Garton K, Kharasch ED (1998) Mechanistic aspects of carbon monoxide formation from volatile anesthetics. *Anesthesiology.* **89(4)**: 929–941.

Cunningham DD, Huang S, Webster J, Mayoral J, Grabenkort RW (1996) Sevoflurane degradation to compound A in anaesthesia breathing systems. *British Journal of Anaesthesia* **77(4)**: 537–543.

References Medicines Control Agency Drug Alert (1995) EL(95) (ALERT) A/17] Important precautions required when using halogenated anaesthetic agents **78**: 340–348.

Fang ZX, Eger EI 11 (1995) USCF Research shows that CO comes from CO_2 absorbent. *Anaesthesia Patient safety Foundation Newsletter* **9**: 26–29.

Fang ZX, Eger EI II, Laster MJ, Chortkoff BS, Kandel L, Ionescu P (1995) Carbon monoxide production from degradation of desflurane, enflurane, isoflurane, halothane, and sevoflurane by soda lime and Baralyme. *Anesthesia and Analgesia* **80(6)**: 1187–1193.

Funk W, Gruber M, Wild K, Hobbhahn J (1999) Dry soda lime markedly degrades sevoflurane during simulated inhalation induction. *British Journal of Anaesthesia* **82(2)**: 193–198.

Harrison N, Knowles AC, Welchew EA (1996) Carbon monoxide within circle systems *Anaesthesia* **51(11)**: 1037–1040.

Knolle E, Heinze G, Hermann G (2002) Small Carbon Monoxide Formation in Absorbents Does Not Correlate with Small Carbon Dioxide Absorption. *Anesthesia and Analgesia* **95**: 650–655.

Knolle E, Linert W, Gilly H. (2003) The color change in CO_2 absorbents on drying: an *in vitro* study using moisture analysis. *Anesthesia and Analgesia* **97(1)**: 151–155.

Stabernack CR, Brown R, Laster MJ, Dudziak R, Eger EI II (2000) Absorbents differ enormously in their capacity to produce compound A and carbon monoxide *Anesthesia and Analgesia* **90(6)**: 1428–1435.

Strum DP, Eger EI 11 (1994) Degradation , absorption and solubility of volatile anaesthetics in Soda-lime depend on water content. *Anesthesia and Analgesia* **78(2)**: 340–348.

Struys MM, Bouche MP, Rolly G, *et al.* (2004) Production of compound A and carbon monoxide in circle systems: an in vitro comparison of two carbon dioxide absorbents. *Anaesthesia* **59(6)**: 584–589.

Woehlck HJ, Dunning MB III, Kulier AH, Sasse FJ,

Nithipataikom K, Henry DW (1997) The response of anesthetic agent monitors to trifluoromethane warns of the presence of carbon monoxide from anesthetic breakdown. *Journal of Clinical Monitoring* **13(3)**: 149–155.

Yamakage M, Kimura A, Chen X, Tsujiguchi N, Kamada Y, Namiki A (2001) Production of compound A under low-flow anesthesia is affected by type of anesthetic machine. *Canadian Journal of Anaesthesia* **48(5)**: 435–438.

Abnormal heat generation in circle systems

Castro BA, Freedman L, Allen MD, Craig WL, Lynch C III (2003) Explosion within an Anesthesia Machine: Baralyme(R), High Fresh Gas Flows and Sevoflurane Concentration.. *Anesthesiology* **101**: 537–539.

Fatheree RS, Leighton BL (2004) Respiratory Distress Syndrome after an Exothermic Baralyme(R)-Sevoflurane Reaction, *Anesthesiology* **101**: 531 –533.

Laster M, Roth P, Eger EI II (2004) Fires from the interaction of anesthetics with desiccated absorbent. *Anesthesia and Analgesia* **99(3)**: 769–774.

Wu J, Previte JP, Adler E, Myers T, Ball J, Gunter JB (2004) Spontaneous ignition, explosion, and fire with sevoflurane and barium hydroxide lime. *Anesthesiology* **101(2)**: 534–537.

Apparatus

Blanshard HJ, Milne MR (2004) Latex-free reservoir bags: exchanging one potential hazard for another. *Anaesthesia* **59(2)**: 177–179.

Department of Health (1989) *Anaesthetic and respiratory equipment: the use of 22 mm breathing system connections.* Safety Action Bulletin no. 52. Department of Health.

Medical Devices Agency (MDA DB 9501 (1995) *Re-use of Medical devices supplies for single use only.* Medical Devices Agency.

Re-use of Equipment. Intersurgical Technical Bulletin TB 5.4.95.

Airway management devices

Ali Diba

Since the earlier editions of this book, there have been a number of significant changes in the approach to airway management by UK anaesthetists. Foremost in these must be the current predominance of the use of the laryngeal mask airway. Prior to the introduction of this device, there existed a usually clear choice simply between tracheal intubation and facemask application, each with its own distinct attendant problems and advantages. The laryngeal mask as a 'third way' of airway management appears also to have stimulated the development of a number of other devices of varying success, sitting outside the trachea but providing a hands-free and gas-tight airway to the lungs. The use of the flexible fibreoptic endoscope for intubation has finally moved from being seen as a 'minority sport' to a mainstream activity at which anaesthetic trainees rightly feel they must be adept. The corollary to this has been the shift in emphasis from the development of adjuncts to assist intubation by other means to a focus on paraphernalia for fibreoptic intubation. At the same time, concerns about the transmission of infective agents, most recently those responsible for New Variant Creutzfeldt-Jakob disease (nvCJD), have led to increasing reliance on single use airway devices, such that re-usable endotracheal tubes are now a rarity and many hospitals use disposable face masks. Production and material costs and hence price, as well as storage and stocking issues, are more significant considerations in single use items and ultimately this is likely to affect the range and quality of equipment available in hospitals.

Whereas once it was possible for this textbook to aim to be a complete and up-to-date inventory of all equipment that the anaesthetist was likely to come across in his professional life, our aim must now more modestly be to represent examples and classes of devices that are currently in popular use. This is particularly so for this chapter on airway devices, where the field has seen a massive proliferation of equipment.

Three of the fundamental principles of modern general anaesthesia are:

1. the establishment and maintenance of a patent airway to the patient's lungs, especially as this can almost always become obstructed by the collapse of pharyngeal structures, as a result of the administration of the anaesthetic. Failure to re-establish patency within a few minutes can result in brain damage or death.

2. the provision of a leak-free connection between the patient and the breathing system, so as to provide a known and precise concentration of the powerful anaesthetic agents currently used, as well as to apply controlled or assisted ventilation if required.

3. the protection of the respiratory system against contamination from refluxed gastric contents or pharyngeal debris.

These principles have been crucial to the development of the various devices listed below.

MATERIALS USED IN AIRWAY DEVICES

The devices described here are made from materials that either best suit the purpose for which they are intended or, in addition, take into consideration the safety of the patient and the cost of production and use.

Rubber

Although historically used to describe the product extracted from the rubber plant, rubber is now used as a generic term to describe any elastic solid and may be prefixed by a more specific adjective to describe the material used in its production. For example, *natural latex rubber* is extracted from the bark sap of rubber plants as the monomer (C_5H_8). It is washed and then polymerized using acetic acid into its final form for the manufacture of gloves and other highly elastic products. Although cheap and very useful, it degrades easily and is contaminated by plant proteins that are the cause of allergic reactions in susceptible individuals. This problem may be reduced by vigorous washing in the early stages of production to remove the contaminant. Natural latex may be converted to red/black rubber by the process known as vulcanization, where high temperatures destroy the allergenic proteins. *Synthetic latex* materials (nitrile, butyl rubber, and polychloroprene, more commonly known as neoprene) are similar to natural latex, but being synthetic do not have allergenic potential. Silicone rubber is another synthetic compound not related to latex polymers. All these materials can withstand sufficiently high temperatures to be steam sterilized.

Plastics

The most common plastics are polyethylene and polyvinyl chloride (PVC). The former is cheap, fairly pliant, non-allergenic and can be molded easily. It is ideal for breathing hoses, connectors and hypodermic syringes.

However, it is unsuitable for the manufacture of re-usable items as it cannot be autoclaved and components such the tapers on connectors deform with repeated use. It is unsuitable for endotracheal tubes (see below) as other materials cannot be easily welded or glued to its surface (e.g. cuffs). For this purpose, PVC is more suitable. This material is brittle on its own but can be made in varying degrees of softness by the addition of plasticizers. Other materials are described below.

ARTIFICIAL AIRWAYS

Terminology

The term *airway* (or *anatomical airway*) will be used to describe the air passages within the subject, including and beyond the nasal and oral openings. The term *distal* will refer to the part of the airway or device furthest into the subject's airway and the term *proximal* to the part emerging or closest to the mouth or nose. *Artificial airway* then is any device that aims to maintain patency of any of the air passages. Artificial airways may be *simple supraglottic* devices, such as the oropharyngeal and the nasopharyngeal airways. These may not be sufficient to maintain the patency of the airway on their own and may require the patient's jaw to be supported as well. They may be *augmented supraglottic* devices such as the laryngeal mask airway (LMA) and the Airway Management Device (AMD) (see below), which aim to maintain patency of the airway on their own. *Infraglottic devices* are known as endotracheal tubes when inserted via the anatomical airway and intended as the conduit for 'to and fro' respiration. Other examples are jet ventilation catheters, inserted percutaneously, and tracheostomy tubes. The term extratracheal airway[1] has also been used to refer to any artificial airway sited outside the trachea, such as the LMA.

The maintenance of a clear airway in an anaesthetized patient may be achieved by simple elevation of the jaw and/or extension of the head on the cervical spine, which tend to separate the tongue, epiglottis and soft palate away from the posterior pharyngeal wall (Fig. 8.1). Where this is not sufficient (usually in those patients where this space is already reduced by a large tongue, small lower jaw, large tonsils or large diameter neck), the obstruction can often be relieved by inserting a device that separates these structures and thus creates an artificial airway. This may be inserted via the mouth (oropharyngeal airway) or via the nose (nasopharyngeal airway) (Fig. 8.2).

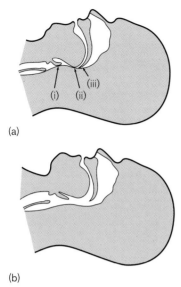

(a)

(b)

Figure 8.1 (a) The obstructed airway following the administration of a general anaesthetic if the jaw is unsupported. The airway may be obstructed by (i) epiglottis and/or (ii) tongue pressing on the posterior pharyngeal wall, or by (iii) the soft palate, occluding the oral or nasal airways. **(b)** The effect of simple elevation of the jaw in a patient with normal anatomy.

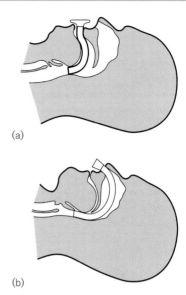

(a)

(b)

Figure 8.2 (a) An unobstructed air passage produced with an oropharyngeal airway. **(b)** An unobstructed air passage produced with a nasopharyngeal airway.

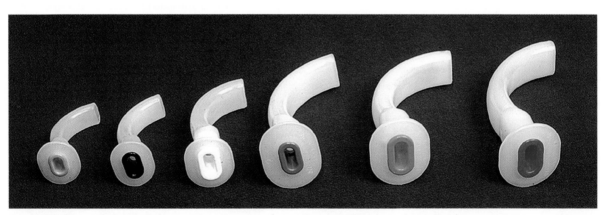

Figure 8.3 Guedel airways in sizes 00, 0, 1, 2, 3, 4 (a smaller size 000 is not shown here).

Oropharyngeal airway

These devices are shaped to emulate and so restore the space present in the pharynx during consciousness by pushing the tongue and epiglottis away from the posterior pharyngeal wall. They are usually circular or oval-shaped in cross-section and are produced in varying lengths and diameters to suit different sizes of patient, from premature neonate to large adult. The proximal end has a flange to limit the depth of insertion and prevent it disappearing into the pharynx. It is also sufficiently rigid or reinforced to prevent collapse should the patient bite on it. When inserted, the distal end should lie just above the epiglottis so as not to irritate the laryngeal inlet. There is a standard colour and number coding for size. The most popular oropharyngeal airway type is the Guedel pattern (Fig. 8.3). To select the correct size of Guedel airway, the distance from the flange to the distal tip of the airway should be about the same as from the patient's lips to the tregus of the ear.

Inserting the airway

The head is extended, the patient's mouth is opened wide and the lubricated device is inserted so that its curvature follows that of the tongue. It often appears to snag about three quarters of the way in. This is usually overcome by lifting the angles of the lower jaw forward with the middle fingers of both hands and gently pushing in the flange with both thumbs. Because of the tendency of the tongue to collapse posteriorly in the unconscious subject, leaving a relatively large space above in the oral cavity, the airway can alternatively be inserted with its curvature initially facing in the opposite direction. When halfway in, it is then rotated to its normal position and inserted fully. However, even correct insertion alone may not be totally sufficient to maintain the airway in a deeply anaesthetized patient. It is often partially pushed out if the patients jaw is left unsupported and allowed to fall backwards. It may also become dislodged with jaw thrust in patients with marked overbite of the upper teeth. Because of the overbite, the lower teeth act as a fulcrum so that downward pressure from the upper teeth on the bite section tends to push the airway out of the mouth, causing partial or complete airway obstruction.

Complications

Gagging, retching or laryngospasm can occur if the airway is inserted into a patient whose pharyngeal reflexes have not been sufficiently depressed by topical or general anaesthesia.

The airway may damage the front teeth, especially if there is:
- a porcelain bridge;
- a crowned tooth or teeth;
- excessive pressure on the above due to postoperative masseter span; or
- overenthusiastic jaw support.

It must be noted however that teeth, crowns and dental bridgework may also be damaged by biting on other teeth and the plastic of an oral airway may be a more forgiving opponent. The best approach is to insert a rubber dental prop (see below) between the patient's molar teeth.

Airways for flexible fibreoptic oral intubation

A number of airways have been designed to assist with fibreoptic oral intubation. Their purpose is to deliver the fibrescope around the back of the tongue and as close to the larynx as possible, ideally having bypassed any secretions. To permit intubation they are either a 'split' pattern to allow the fibrescope to be separated off the airway, as in the Berman and Ovassapian airways, or else of large enough diameter to allow an endotracheal tube and its connector to be delivered through the airway, as in the Optosafe (Fig. 8.4). The airways also act as a 'bite block' to prevent the patient biting and damaging expensive fibreoptic equipment.

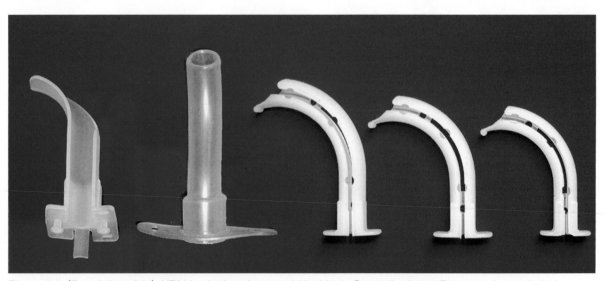

Figure 8.4 (From left to right): VBM intubating airway and bite block, Optosafe airway, Bermann airways in 3 sizes.

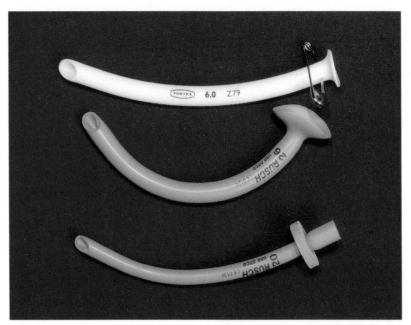

Figure 8.5 Nasopharyngeal airways (from top to bottom) Portex and Rusch designs, the lower with an adjustable flange.

Nasopharyngeal airway

Where a patient has limited jaw opening, awkward or fragile dentition or where the oral airway is frequently displaced by a marked overlapping bite, an alternative artificial airway may be inserted via the nose. This is achieved by inserting a soft plastic, polyurethane or latex rubber tube through the nares and passing it along the floor of the nose down into the oropharynx to a point just above the epiglottis.

The tubes have either a fixed or an adjustable flange (Fig. 8.5) at the proximal end to prevent loss of the device into the nose and to limit insertion of an excessive length, so that the distal end can be made to lie in the correct position above the epiglottis. The tip is bevelled to make its passage through the nose less traumatic. It may also have a hole cut in the wall opposite this so that should the bevel become blocked with mucus during the insertion some patency is maintained. Nasopharyngeal airways are well tolerated by patients during relatively light levels of anaesthesia, for example, during emergence. They are produced in a range of sizes with the length of the airway governed by the internal diameter of the tube. Smaller, more easily inserted and better-tolerated airways can be too short to be effective. The use of nasopharyngeal airways has almost disappeared from UK anaesthetic practice, with the rising popularity of the LMA.

Complications

Complications do occur with the use of nasopharyngeal airways. They may traumatize the nasal mucosa, nasal polyps or adenoidal tissue, producing an epistaxis that compromises the airway further. They should not be used where there is evidence of coagulopathy or other potential causes of epistaxis.

FACEMASKS

Facemasks are designed to fit over the patient's nose and mouth perfectly, without any leaks and yet to exert the minimum of pressure, which might either depress the jaw and cause respiratory obstruction or cause pressure sores. The facemask (Fig. 8.6) consists of three parts: the mount, the body and the edge. A snug fit is achieved by incorporating one or more of the following features into the design: by anatomically shaping the body, by the use of an air-filled cuff at the edge (Figs 8.7b, d and e) that has a soft cushioning effect or by a soft pliable flap (Figs 8.7a and c) that takes up the contour of the face.

The mount normally has a 22 mm female taper if made to ISO (International Organization for Standardization) or BS (British Standards). It is usually constructed of hard synthetic rubber but may be plastic or metal. The former

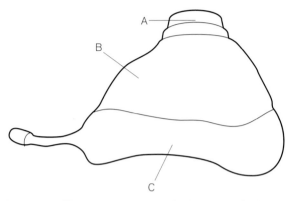

Figure 8.6 The parts of an anaesthetic facemask: A, the mount; B, the body; C, the edge.

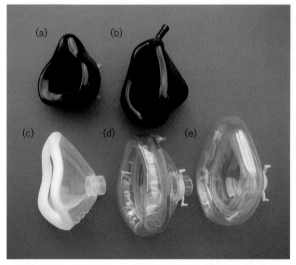

Figure 8.7 A selection of facemasks: **(a)** black rubber 'Everseal' mask with soft pliable flap; **(b)** 'anatomical' facemask in black rubber with air filled cushion; **(c)** single use facemask with flap; **(d)** single use facemask with adjustable air filled cushion; **(e)** single use facemask with pre-filled air cushion. Note: a, d and e carry attachments for use with a harness (see text).

two wear more easily with repeated use and eventually produce a leak or potential for accidental disconnection.

The body may be made from black rubber, neoprene, plastic, polycarbonate or silicone rubber. In some cases, a malleable wire stiffener or wire gauze is incorporated in the body so that the shape may be altered to fit the patient's face. The transparent body of a polycarbonate or plastic facemask permits respiration to be detected by the appearance of condensation during exhalation this is particularly useful during resuscitation. It also theoretically allows earlier detection of regurgitation or vomitus and may be less threatening to anxious adults and small children. (Figs 8.7c, d and e).

The internal volume (apparatus dead space) within the body of the facemask is relatively insignificant in adults but may assume significance in neonates and infants where it could constitute 30% or more of their tidal volume. Hence this part of a paediatric facemask is filled in to minimize the effective apparatus dead space (Fig. 8.8). The use of a larger mask in paediatrics, particularly of the Rendell–Baker or Laerdal pattern, can give a better fit and sometimes paradoxically reduce the effective apparatus dead space by allowing the face to fit further into the mask.

The edge may be anatomically shaped and fitted with a cuff or flap. A good fit is essential to prevent dilution of inhaled gases by room air during spontaneous respiration and to allow positive pressure ventilation to be administered without leakage. It is necessary to stock a variety of types and sizes of facemask, since none will be a good fit for every type of face. Edentulous or bearded patients may be especially difficult. The former are best managed by leaving any dentures in place to prevent the cheeks from falling away from the mask and by using a smaller mask. Beards often prevent a good seal around the edge of the mask and a leak-free fit may sometimes be achieved

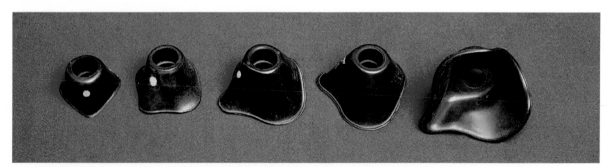

Figure 8.8 The full range of Rendell–Baker paediatric facemasks, sizes 00, 0, 1, 2, 3.

with a bigger mask held firmly with two hands. Anaesthetists have often had to go to bizarre lengths to achieve a useful seal in heavily bearded patients (e.g. using a pierced defibrillator gel pad on the face[2] or even wrapping the entire head in clingfilm[3]). Masks with a cuff have a small filling tube fitted with a plug to enable the degree of inflation to be regulated. The plug must be removed to allow the cuff to deflate if the mask is to be autoclaved.

Whereas some facemasks withstand the high temperatures of autoclaving, others do not. Since these are not easily distinguished, many have adopted uniform policies of disinfection. Care must be taken if chemical disinfection is used as some chemicals, e.g. chloroxylenol (Dettol) are known to have been absorbed by the material of the facemask and have resulted in injury to the patient's skin.

The shift towards disposable single-use items instead of expensive sterilization procedures which may be performed off-site for many hospitals, combined with the even more costly packaging, tracking and logging of this, may soon make re-usable rubber anaesthetic facemasks a thing of the past. The same principles of design nonetheless apply to plastic disposable facemasks (Figs 8.7c, d and e). Materials and components are cheaper and of lower quality, but more importantly, concerning facemasks, there is a much more limited range of designs and sizes. Most, even those for paediatric use, are essentially based on the one design of air-filled cuff and cone-shaped body. They are reproduced with differing quality and materials, by various manufacturers. Models offered for sale have often not stood the test of time, such that problems may only be manifested after a particular supplier's model has been in use for a while. Nominal sizes do not equate between manufacturers. Some cheaper masks do not have a valve to allow adjustment of the volume of the air-filled cuffs which tend to be underfilled and can be of a less pliable nature with the fit suffering as a consequence. Poor design or poor fit, even in the absence of a leak, can cause areas of high pressure on the skin which, if unchecked, may lead to ulceration. It would not be tenable to switch wholesale to disposable masks without keeping a range of more traditional re-usable masks, most notably paediatric designs and large adult sizes. Single-use masks may, however, have a number of advantages beyond their sterility. Plastics are more inert than rubber compounds and the use of natural latex may be dispensed with entirely. Materials are usually see-through and more modern-looking, which may be less

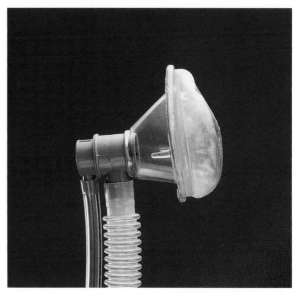

Figure 8.9 A McKesson comfort cushion inhaler.

threatening to anxious patients. Furthermore, the plastic may be scented at manufacture: this, if nothing else, produces an interesting diversion for all concerned.

Masks for some dental anaesthetic techniques are designed to fit the nose only so that the dentist has unimpeded access to the mouth (Fig. 8.9). They are also known as nasal inhalers.

Facemasks are also used for non-invasive ventilation or CPAP in differing scenarios, both in and out of hospital (see Chapter 9, Fig. 9.13). These may be full anaesthetic-type facemasks covering the mouth and nose or just nasal masks. They tend to be single patient use devices comprising plastics and soft silicone rubber, usually of a high quality as comfort and tolerability are key to the success of the treatment. They often incorporate additional ports for valves and airway manometry and will have attachments for retention harnesses to keep the mask comfortably on the patient's face. This is really the only use now for head harnesses, although many disposable anaesthetic masks are still produced with the corresponding ring for attachment of a harness (see Figs 8.7a, d and e).

Angle pieces

This is a right-angled connector (Fig. 8.10) which is commonly used to neatly join a facemask to a breathing system. The downstream end has an external 22 mm male taper that fits the facemask. The upstream end has an

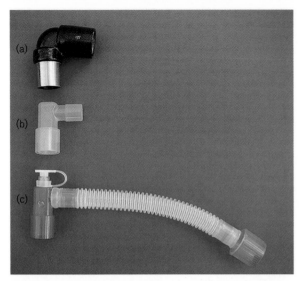

Figure 8.10 Angle pieces: **(a)** older version with 22mm tapers; **(b)** newer design (here single use) with proximal 15 mm external taper and distal dual mode taper (external 22 mm male and internal 15 mm female); **(c)** combined angle piece and catheter mount arrangement (see text).

internal 22 mm female taper which fits the breathing system (Fig. 8.10a).

In some more recent designs (Fig. 8.10b), the downstream end has also been fitted with an additional internal 15 mm female taper so that the angle piece may fit an endotracheal tube as well (see below). The upstream (breathing system) end has also been changed. It now has an external 15 mm male taper instead of the 22 mm female one. This does not cause any incompatibility problems, however, as the breathing systems are made to end in a 22 mm male external taper with a 15 mm female internal taper.

Many institutions now utilize single-use combined angle piece and catheter mount arrangements (Fig. 8.10c). Catheter mounts are discussed below.

AUGMENTED SUPRAGLOTTIC AIRWAYS

Until the advent of the laryngeal mask airway (LMA), first described in 1983,[4] maintaining a clear airway in an anaesthetized patient, unless intubating the subject, might well have involved elevating and protruding the lower jaw, supporting it in this position with a Guedel airway, placing a facemask over the nose and mouth and securing this with a Clausen's Harness to provide a gas tight fit, all

essentially dextrous tasks requiring practised performance. It soon became obvious that the LMA, introduced commercially in 1988, allowed all this to be done with a single device requiring virtually no training in its use but with an astonishing success rate in achieving a clear leak-free airway. Since then a number of other manufacturers have designed airway devices that attempt to effect an airtight seal using an inflatable cuff that lies outside the trachea above the level of the larynx. None has so far been as popular as the LMA, in spite of the occasional publications claiming similar or better performance than the LMA.[5,6]

These devices have several features in common:
- a proximal inflatable cuff that sits over or above the level of the larynx, hence a reliance on an absence of laryngeal inlet closure or spasm;
- 'blind' insertion is possible, obviating the need for laryngeal visualization;
- reliance for correct positioning on a distal soft tip that lodges in the upper oesophagus behind the cricoid ring;
- an inability to guarantee tracheal isolation from gastric contents in the event of reflux or vomiting; and
- use of wide bore tubing not limited by the size of the glottic aditus, therefore the facility for the device to be used as a conduit for other instruments such as a flexible fibreoptic scope.

The laryngeal mask airway

This device is passed through the mouth and into the pharynx so that its distal end lies over the laryngeal inlet.

The distal end consists of a hollow bowl resembling a small facemask, which is surrounded by an inflatable tubular cuff. The latter, when inflated, fits around the laryngeal inlet and supports it in a position away from the posterior pharyngeal wall. The back of the bowl leads into a tube which passes out of the pharynx and mouth. The proximal end of this tube has a 15 mm ISO male connection so that it can be attached to a breathing system. The tube, at its point of entry into the mask, is fenestrated by two thick silicone rubber strands to prevent the epiglottis falling into it and occluding its lumen. A small tube with a built-in self-sealing valve supplies the cuff, so that it remains inflated when injected with air.

LMAs are made from silicone rubber so that they can be autoclaved and re-used to the manufacturer's maximum of 40 times. Originally produced in 4 sizes, two mid-range sizes and two further larger sizes were added later (Fig. 8.11). Experience with sizes $1\frac{1}{2}$, 5 and 6 is

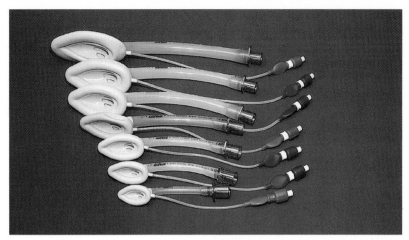

Figure 8.11 The laryngeal mask airway in sizes 1, 1.5, 2, 2.5, 3, 4, 5. A size 6 is now also available which is not shown here.

comparatively limited. It should be noted that although originally developed from plaster casts of cadaveric adult larynxes, subsequent sizes are only scale recreations of the originals with particularly the smallest sizes not providing such a reliable airway. The manufacturers recommendations are as shown in Table 8.1. Note that the term LMA® is a registered trademark of Intavent Ltd, UK. Where the predicted size does not fit well an alternative size may provide a better airway.

An alternative version of the LMA is available in sizes 2–6, in which the tube is made thinner, narrower and longer and is reinforced with a spiral of steel wire to add flexibility without the risk of kinking (Fig. 8.12). This provides better access to the head and neck area as the tube and breathing system connection can be positioned away from the operative site. The reinforced tube is also resistant to crushing if used in conjunction with a Boyle–Davis mouth gag for intra-oral access.

Inserting the LMA

Because the LMA, when correctly placed, would elicit a gag reflex in a patient that is awake, it should only be inserted in a patient whose pharyngeal reflexes have been sufficiently depressed by general anaesthesia or adequate local anaesthesia and/or analgesia. As the device is re-usable and is subject to wear and tear, prior to use it should be checked for damage, particularly leaks, eccentric inflation of the cuff or failure of the self sealing valve on the pilot balloon. The airway tube should also be checked to see that it does not occlude when kinked.

The manufacturer's recommended insertion technique requires that the cuff is deflated fully with the concave

Table 8.1 Manufacturers recommendations for LMA® selection and cuff inflation

LMA size	Patient size (kg)	Maximum cuff volume (ml)
size 1	neonates up to 5	4
size 1½	infants 5 –10	7
size 2	children 10 –20	10
size 2½	children 20 – 30	14
size 3	patients 30 – 50	20
size 4	patients 50 – 70	30
size 5	patients 70 – 100	40
size 6	patients over 100	50

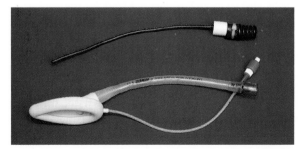

Figure 8.12 The reinforced laryngeal mask airway shown here with a sterilizable insertion aid (design P Andrews, East Grinstead).

part of the mask pressed against a hard surface. This causes the cuff to fold backwards behind the bowl. The back of the mask is lubricated with a water-based gel and the tubular section is grasped like a pen, with the tip of the operator's gloved index finger placed at the junction of the tube and mask. The operator's other hand extends the patient's neck by cradling the occiput so that the patient's mouth falls open. The mask is inserted into the mouth and the bowl is kept pressed against the hard palate as the mask is advanced in one smooth movement into the hypopharynx. The upward pressure against the palate flattens the cuff of the mask to give a smooth thin leading edge. The hard and then the soft palate and finally posterior pharyngeal wall act as a scoop to guide the mask into place and prevent snagging on the tongue or epiglottis. The index finger is withdrawn and the mask advanced further until resistance is felt. Without holding the tube the cuff is then inflated with air. Although the manufacturer gives maximum volumes for cuff inflation it is recommended that the volume used be that which is sufficient to effect a seal. Normally the mask rises a little on inflation of the cuff and it is best to stop inflating when the rise of the mask appears to come to an abrupt halt. Further inflation can sometimes raise the airway leak pressure (the airway pressure at which there is leakage of air around the mask) but usually not enough to qualitatively alter the fit of the mask.

From personal observation, most users do not use the recommended insertion technique and yet find that the device seats well and provides a reliable airway. It is perhaps this feature that accounts for the success of this device.

Alternative methods of insertion

Many users simply grasp the airway near its proximal connector and slide the device down the back of the tongue, relying on the elasticity of the epiglottis to return it to its normal position and not remain downfolded over the larynx. This method does not work for the reinforced version of the LMA, which is too flexible to allow the device to be steered in this manner. Instead it may be grasped near the bowl with Magill's forceps, or a malleable stiffener or stylet may be inserted into the airway tube to give the lacking rigidity. The authors preferred technique uses a home-made device with a 15 mm ISO female connector at its proximal end to firmly connect to the LMA, preventing rotation of the tube on the stylet (Fig. 8.12). In such instances, the introducer should be lubricated to allow ease of extraction when the LMA is positioned.

Elevating and protruding the jaw by placing a thumb into the mouth and pulling on the jaw from behind the front teeth (instead of cradling the occiput) or traction on the tongue, also aids insertion by giving a greater space for passage of the LMA. A longitudinal black line is marked along the full extent of the dorsal aspect of the tube. This should lie in the midline when the tube is *in situ*; if not it will indicate a degree of rotation or misplacement.

Confirmation of correct placement

Remarkably for a device that is inserted blindly, the mask almost always adopts the correct position and provides a patent airway with a success rate in excess of 95%.[7] In a spontaneously breathing patient, the sound of breathing should be non-stridorous and the reservoir of the breathing system should show a normal excursion. In an apnoeic patient, squeezing the reservoir bag should produce normal chest movements with an applied pressure no greater than 2 kPa (20 cm H_2O). A small leak is permissible; a large leak or a higher inflation pressure will usually indicate the possibility of a misplacement (frequently downfolding of the epiglottis or inadequate depth of insertion of LMA), or of breath-holding by the patient.

Indications for using the LMA

- It may replace the use of a facemask and pharyngeal airway in a spontaneously breathing patient, with the added benefit of:
  1. releasing the anaesthetist's hands to deal with other matters, and removing them from proximity to the operative site;
  2. providing a more reliable airway, particularly in patients placed in positions other than supine or where a facemask does not seal well against the face as in bearded patients;
- It may, with certain provisos, replace an endotracheal tube, for example:
  1. in elective procedures involving spontaneous or controlled ventilation, where tracheal intubation would have been used only to give a hands-free and gas tight airway;
  2. in elective procedures where intubation and the prerequisite drugs may elicit particularly undesirable cardiovascular or respiratory responses;
  3. in patients not at risk of aspiration of gastric contents where a difficult intubation (but not difficult airway or mask ventilation) is predicted, as in those with cervical spine problems or limited mouth opening;

4. as an alternative airway following failed intubation or failed mask ventilation. There is now considerable evidence to support the use of the LMA in these scenarios, some even suggesting that the LMA is more likely to be an effective airway in those where intubation has failed than it is in the general population. The device is consequently recommended in many airway management algorithms.

5. as a first choice airway for use in emergencies by non-anaesthetic staff[8] on the basis that success rate at establishing ventilation for non-specialist staff is greater with the LMA than with facemask ventilation or endotracheal intubation;

- It may be used as an aid in difficult intubation. A gum elastic bougie or small diameter long endotracheal tube passed blindly through the LMA has a high chance of entering the trachea (assuming glottic relaxation). A very useful technique is to insert a flexible fibreoptic laryngoscope carrying an Aintree catheter (see below) through the LMA. The fibrescope is delivered to the glottis and the trachea can then be entered under direct vision and requiring an absolute minimum of endoscopy skills. The Aintree catheter is left in the trachea while the fibreoptic scope and LMA are removed, allowing the endotracheal tube of choice to be railroaded into place over the Aintree catheter (Fig. 8.73). This technique has the added advantage of by-passing any debris or bleeding in the oropharynx.

- The LMA can be used as an aid to extubation and recovery, even after pre-operative tracheal intubation. The LMA is less stimulating than an endotracheal tube and less likely to elicit coughing and straining during recovery. It also protects the larynx from blood and secretions arising from the nasopharynx and oropharynx. An example of such use would be insertion of the LMA post tonsillectomy (placement is easier if the endotracheal tube is still *in situ*) in a patient who is still experiencing some oozing to allow 'deep extubation' whilst at the same time maintaining the airway and protecting the larynx from soiling whilst the patient quietly rouses.

- It may be used where a patient needs resuscitation in a position in which a laryngoscope cannot easily be employed.

Contraindications

The LMA does not protect the lungs against aspiration of vomitus or refluxed gastric contents. It should therefore not be used electively in patients with a full stomach or untreated hiatus hernia.

The device is also contraindicated in patients who are difficult to ventilate by virtue of size or chest disease, given that the masks tend not to give a seal at airway pressures in excess of 2.5 kPa (25 cm H_2O).

The LMA is much more susceptible to dislodgment than an endotracheal tube. Also, by nature of being a supraglottic device, airway patency is at the mercy of laryngeal reflexes which themselves may be provoked by dislodgement of the device. It should, therefore, not be used during procedures where access to the airway for repositioning is likely to be problematic. As such, its use for ear, nose and throat surgery and intraoral procedures, such as tonsillectomy, requires careful consideration.

Further designs

A single-use version of the standard model is available. Two further modifications of the LMA have been marketed:

The Intubating Laryngeal Mask (iLMA®, Intavent Ltd, UK). This device is designed specifically to capitalize and improve on the LMA's high success rate at guiding instruments within its lumen into the larynx (see above). It is significantly different from the standard LMA, being primarily aimed at blindly intubating the trachea with large-size cuffed adult endotracheal tubes (Fig. 8.13). The bowl of the device is rigid as is the wide and short-right angled airway tube, which is constructed of stainless steel. This necessitates a novel insertion technique. A handle is provided to allow manipulation of the position of the bowl. The device is supplied with a dedicated endotracheal tube made with a soft rounded silicone rubber tip to better negotiate the curve of the tube and which is less

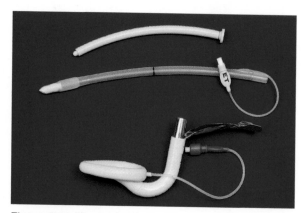

Figure 8.13 The intubating laryngeal mask airway (Intavent Ltd, UK) The LMA can be used with dedicated endotracheal tube and 'pusher'.

traumatic when impacting the larynx. Although compared to the ordinary LMA, the success rate of blind intubation is improved by the use of this version to about 75%,[9] the exact role for this device is still questionable, given that it cannot be relied upon as a blind technique in the difficult intubation scenario and if used as a conduit for a fibrescope (see above), the view may be better through an ordinary LMA.[10,11] Experience with the device as an airway is still comparatively limited and it cannot be recommended for routine use.[12] As with design modifications in general, one must be careful when making inferences based on prior models.

LMA with oesophageal drain (LMA–ProSeal®, Intavent Ltd, UK). In essence, here a second lumen has been added which opens at the distal tip of the cuff of the LMA in order to give access to the oesophagus (Fig. 8.14). The second lumen allows blind placement of a gastric tube and possibly drainage of any refluxed material directly out of the mouth. The design has a number of other modifications (including a communicating second cuff behind the bowl) which result in a better airway seal at normal intracuff pressures.[13] However, there is as yet no indication that this device protects against aspiration of gastric contents, and some evidence that it fails to perform as well as an ordinary LMA for airway maintenance.[14]

Other (augmented) supraglottic airways

Even excluding single-use instruments (and various designs of the simple supraglottic airways), there are currently nine different varieties of augmented supraglottic airway available in the UK. At least one further model is under development at the time of writing[15] and one model – the Cuffed Oropharyngeal Airway (COPA) – has recently ceased production. Their developments must be considered as having been spurred by the success of the LMA. They do not have clearly demarcated applications and a comparison of their merits and demerits is beyond the remit of this chapter. Many of the issues touched upon in the section on the LMA are at least equally pertinent to these other products. Some of these devices are briefly discussed here.

Oesophageal Tracheal Combitube™

This device is conceptually different from the others in that it is designed to allow for blind placement in either the trachea or oesophagus (Fig. 8.15) and is a development of the oesophageal obturator airway. The Combitube™ (Kendall, USA) is produced as a single-use device in only two adult sizes: 37Fr and 41Fr, targeted primarily now at emergency airway management and non-anaesthetic use. The double lumen tube has one lumen that opens beyond the distal cuff, whilst the other lumen ends between the two cuffs and has only side openings. It is inserted blindly into the mouth and advanced until the teeth reach between the timing marks. The proximal high-volume pharyngeal cuff is first inflated with 100 ml of air to fix the device in place then the lower cuff is inflated with about 15 ml. When inserted blindly, the Combitube™ most often enters the oesophagus. The

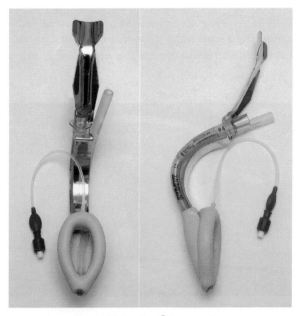

Figure 8.14 The LMA-ProSeal® (see text).

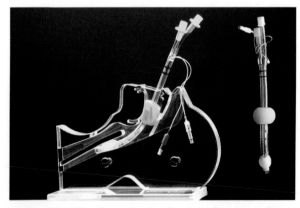

Figure 8.15 The Oesophageal Tracheal Combitube™, Kendall, USA.

proximally longer tube, marked '1', has the lumen ending between the cuffs and ventilation is first attempted through this lumen. If this fails then the second lumen is tried. If oesophageal insertion is confirmed, tube '2' can be used to insert a gastric drain with the smaller balloon acting as an oesophageal obturator. Note that an oesophageal detector device, such as Wee's device, if used prior to ventilation to confirm placement of the tube, may serve to prevent inflation of the stomach in those cases where the Combitube™ enters the trachea. Where ventilation with the Combitube™ is unsuccessful, this may be due to obstruction of the larynx by the oropharyngeal balloon; the device should therefore be withdrawn by 1–2 cm and ventilation attempted again.[16] Oesophageal rupture must be considered an inherent risk with this device;[17,18] the mechanism may involve raised oesophageal intraluminal pressure as a result of the obstruction rather than simply direct trauma.

If endotracheal intubation is attempted at any time after insertion, the proximal cuff is deflated, the tube pushed to the left-hand side of the mouth and conventional laryngoscopy performed. The oesophageal seal effected by the distal cuff should prevent soiling of the pharynx by gastric contents during the procedure.

The difference in design between this and other supraglottic devices perhaps merits the inclusion of the Combitube™ in emergency airway equipment as an alternative 'supra glottic' device.

Laryngeal Tube

This device is composed of a short silicone tube, slightly 'S'-shaped, opening distally between two inflatable cuffs (Fig. 8.16). It is a re-usable device produced in 6 sizes, numbered from 0 to 5, to accommodate neonates to adults. First made in 1999 by VBM Medizintechnik, Germany, the device has since been redesigned such that both cuffs are inflated by the same pilot tube and the insertion tip which enters the oesophagus is a much softer compound. Ventilation is effected by sealing the oropharynx above and the oesophagus below, by the two cuffs. It appears to have a reasonable rate of success at establishing ventilation and may give a better airway seal pressure than the laryngeal mask.[19]

A further model (LTS) has since been produced with a second lumen that opens distally to the oesophageal cuff, for the blind insertion of gastric tubes.

Airway Management Device (AMD)

The AMD™ (Nagor Ltd, UK) is similar in principle to the Laryngeal Tube, the key design features being that the airway tube lumen extends through to beyond the distal cuff and the presence of an integral sterilization tag (Fig. 8.17). Inflation of the distal cuff occludes this segment of the tube, which can otherwise be used to allow passage of a gastric drain. Early experiences with the device have not been good,[20,21] although it has since been redesigned to give a different profile on inflation of the pharyngeal cuff and the original one size has been increased to three sizes.

PA$_{Xpress}$™

The PA$_{Xpress}$™ (Vital Signs, USA), is a single-sized single-use supraglottic airway designed for use in adults (Fig. 8.18) as an alternative to the LMA. It dispenses with the lower cuff in favour of a series of corrugated plastic gills that sit in the hypopharynx. Initial experiences suggest

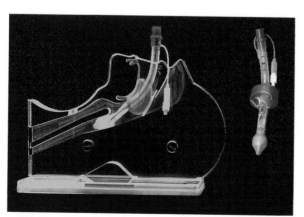

Figure 8.16 The Laryngeal Tube, VBM Medizintechnik, Germany.

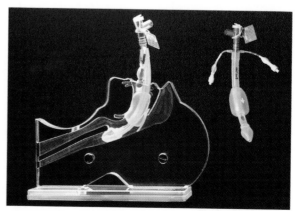

Figure 8.17 The Airway Management Device with integral sterilization tag.

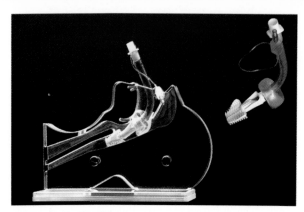

Figure 8.18 The PA$_{Xpress}$.

greater difficulty with positioning the device and a higher incidence of sore throat than the LMA.[22,23]

ENDOTRACHEAL TUBES

The 'gold standard' for securing the airway is still tracheal intubation. A cuffed endotracheal tube provides the best protection for the lungs from inhalation of foreign material, the tube is the least likely device to be dislodged, glottic reflexes are by-passed and for intra-oral and head and neck surgery, only a tracheostomy can potentially give better surgical access (see section above entitled 'Indications for using the LMA', for comparison).

History

Curiously, endotracheal intubation in the form of tracheostomy predates anaesthesia by a number of centuries.[24] As early as 1542, Vesalius[25] recorded intermittently blowing into a reed that was passed into the *aspera arteria* of an animal whose thorax had been opened. He found that this caused the lungs to expand, and the heart to recover its normal pulsations. In 1667, Robert Hook before the Royal Society of London, similarly kept a dog alive for over an hour by ventilating its lungs with a pair of bellows tied into the trachea which had been severed below the epiglottis. Thereafter, artificial respiration by intubation of the trachea became fairly common by the end of the eighteenth century, for treatment of asphyxia and drowning.

A number of milestones are worth mentioning. In 1871, Friedrich Trendelenburg[26] developed a cuffed catheter for insertion through a tracheostomy to prevent soiling of the lungs during operations on the upper airway. This tube with its inflatable rubber cuff would look familiar to any

modern day anaesthetist and was widely used for the next thirty years.[27] In 1878, the Glasgow surgeon William MacEwen[28] placed a metal tube by manual palpation through the mouth into the trachea of a 55-year-old plasterer and, following the administration of chloroform, packed off the laryngeal opening to successfully resect a tumour at the base of the patient's tongue. Endotracheal anaesthesia was born; the term is, however, no longer in common usage. Eisenmenger's tube of 1893 was a wide-bore semi-rigid orotracheal tube carrying an inflatable cuff and a pilot balloon to reflect pressure in the cuff.

The development of tubes and anaesthetic techniques was not a linear progression. In spite of Dorrance's description of the cuffed rubber orotracheal tube in 1910 – Guedel and Waters in 1928 described a similar tube for use with a carbon dioxide absorption technique – it was not until after the polio epidemic of the 1950s that the use of cuffed endotracheal tubes became standard anaesthetic practice. I.W. Magill and E.S. Rowbotham, anaesthetists to the British Army Plastic Unit in Sidcup during and after the Great War of 1914–1918, found that they could provide a superior unimpeded surgical field for the head and neck surgery of Sir Harold Gillies by having the patient breathing to and fro through an uncuffed rubber tube passed blindly through the nose into the trachea. Prior to this, 'insufflation anaesthesia' (as opposed to 'inhalation anaesthesia'), whereby chloroform or ether laden air was pumped into the trachea as advocated by Meltzer and Auer in New York[29], had achieved rapid and widespread acceptance, partly owing to the different needs of thoracic surgery. This technique, when used for head and neck surgery, had necessitated a second tube being inserted for egress of gases in order that the pharynx may be packed to prevent soiling of the trachea. It was this second wide-bore rubber tube that Magill and Rowbotham had found they could 'blindly' insert into the larynx, which subsequently became the singular airway and spawned the dominant technique in the UK for many years. It must be remembered that at this stage the technique of laryngoscopy was still in its infancy. In 1941, Gillespie, writing in Endotracheal Anaesthesia[24,] states: 'An experienced worker should be able to intubate all but the most difficult cases in ten minutes. The beginner will often require thirty.'

Design

An orotracheal tube (Fig. 8.19) usually has a preformed curve that approximates to the anatomical shape of the

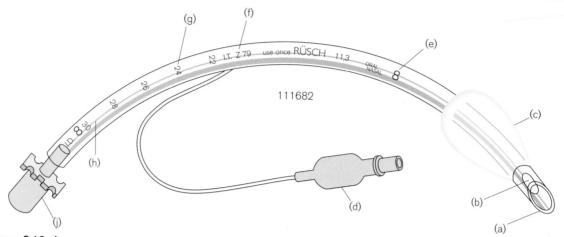

Figure 8.19 An uncut orotracheal tube. **(a)** Bevel; **(b)** Murphy eye; **(c)** tracheal cuff; **(d)** self-sealing valve which keeps gas in the cuff; **(e)** marking to show the internal diameter of the tube in millimetres; **(f)** marking (I.T.Z 79) to show that the plastic has been tested for tissue toxicity; **(g)** the length of the tube in millimetres; **(h)** longitudinal line of radio-opaque material; **(j)** 15 mm connector.

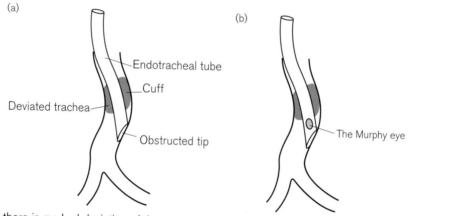

Figure 8.20 (a) If there is marked deviation of the trachea, the end of the tube may be obstructed. **(b)** The distal end of an endotracheal tube with a 'Murphy eye'.

pharynx. This aids insertion and ensures that when the tube is further flexed when *in situ*, it is unlikely to kink. The distal end is cut obliquely (bevelled) so that the aperture faces to the left when held in the operator's right hand. The bevel facilitates insertion and allows the tip of the tube to be seen passing between the vocal cords. There may be a hole (a Murphy eye) in the wall opposite the bevel. This is designed to provide a secondary port for gas movement in and out of the tube should the bevel become blocked or wedged against the tracheal wall (Fig. 8.20). Part of the distal end of the tube may be surrounded by an inflatable cuff which, when inflated, fills to seal the space between the tube and the tracheal wall. The tube carries several markings, one of which is a

longitudinal line of radio-opaque material so that the correct placement can be verified from an X-ray if required. The transverse black mark on some tubes, made several centimetres proximal to the cuff, is designed so as to be visible above the larynx, indicating that the tube has not been inserted too far. The distance from the tip of the bevel is also marked in centimetres on the wall, along with the internal diameter.

Construction materials

Traditionally, endotracheal tubes have been made of red rubber or natural latex, which can be cleaned and sterilized for re-use. However, these materials are opaque and inadequate cleaning is not always apparent from a superficial examination. Occlusion of the lumen occurs occasionally with foreign objects and dried mucus. Perishing may cause the wall of the tube to weaken, increasing the possibility of kinking. The material itself (red rubber) is potentially an irritant when used for long periods and has been blamed for producing laryngeal granulomata.

Currently, plastics (polyvinyl chloride (PVC) and more recently polyurethane) and to a lesser extent, silicone rubber, have replaced red rubber and natural latex as primary materials for the following reasons:

- they are non-irritant and are now inexpensive enough to allow single patient use;
- they can be sterilized more reliably during manufacture;
- blockages may be visible as the material is usually clear;
- the manufacturing tolerances are much closer with plastics, so that there is much less variation in the size of the lumen (important in neonatal endotracheal tubes);
- the cuffs of rubber tubes are usually thick and require high pneumatic pressures to inflate them: inadvertent overdistension of the cuff may result in these pressures being transmitted to the tracheal mucosa with resultant mucosal ischaemia and necrosis if the tubes are used for prolonged periods.

However, plastic tubes do not have the elasticity (springiness) of rubber and may be more difficult to insert in difficult situations. Also, plastic (PVC) tubes, because of their relative rigidity at room temperature compared with rubber ones, appear to cause more trauma when they are inserted via the nasal route. Plastic tubes may be softened pre-insertion by immersing them in warm water; or, particularly for nasal intubation, tubes utilizing softer compound materials may be used, such as the Portex Ivory range of plastic tubes. Here, the use of a greater amount of the plasticizer dioctyl phthalate during manufacture of the PVC results in a softer compound more akin to red rubber. Polyurethane compounds also tend to be softer and more springy but are more expensive to manufacture. Silicone rubber (polymethylsiloxane) is an entirely synthetic material containing no latex derivatives, it is both soft and has the advantage that it will withstand autoclaving and hence can be re-used. It is, however, significantly more expensive and is not generally used for disposable airway products. Siliconized plastic refers to a PVC material incorporating a very small amount of silicone oil to form a surface monolayer with the aim of altering the surface characteristics of the product, for example, to decrease surface adhesion. These tubes tend to be pearlescent or opaque.

The type of plastic used in the construction of endotracheal tubes is tested to make sure that it is non-irritant. Tubes were at one stage marked with a test number, which could be seen on the body of the tube as 'Z79-IT'. This denoted Implant Testing according to the Z79 Toxicity Subcommittee of the ANSI (American National Standards Institute) set up in 1968 in the USA, which established the test method. The test consisted of implanting four samples of the plastic, under sterile conditions, into the paravertebral muscle of anaesthetized rabbits along with two samples of Reference Standard Negative Control plastic for 70–144 h. The implant sites were then examined for signs of inflammation. CE marking now denotes compliance with the essential requirements of the Medical Devices Directive (see Chapter 30).

Size

Conventional wisdom dictated that the widest diameter tube that would pass *easily* through the narrowest part of the airway should always be used in order to minimize the resistance to gas flow within it, and so reduce the work of breathing. In children, the narrowest part of the airway is the cricoid ring, which being conveniently circular can accept a snug fit from a tube (see below). In adults, the narrowest part is the larynx, which is oblong in shape. A subglottic inflatable cuff is therefore needed to achieve a seal. Again, conventionally, the tube should be as short as possible so as to further reduce the work of breathing and to prevent the tube from entering a main (usually the right) bronchus and ventilating one lung only. In adults, selection of the largest tube was also a consequence of early cuff design in seeking to avoid excess distension of the cuffs. More recent approaches however, particularly in adult anaesthetic practice, consider a number of other factors with a consequent trend towards smaller diameter tubes:

- Where a patient is ventilated, the ventilator does the work of breathing. The diameter of the tube does not dictate airway pressures distal to it unless, of course, the tube is so narrow as not to allow sufficient time for passive exhalation. Tube sizes of 6.5 and 6.0 mm ID (internal diameter) do not cause a rise in intratracheal pressures when used for ventilating adult males and females.[30,31]
- Small tubes are easier to insert and reduce the trauma of intubation. The larger the tube, the greater the area

of contact between it and the vocal cords and the greater the likelihood of injury. Hoarseness and the incidence of sore throat is increased dramatically with tubes of greater than 7 mm ID.[32] Abnormalities on CT scans of the larynx are visible at 6 months in a high proportion of patients after, even short periods of intubation.[33] Patients extubated following the use of small soft tubes are immediately able to phonate.

- Even in spontaneously breathing patients, the use of now mandatory continuous capnography, by virtue of being able to demonstrate failing ventilation, allows greater latitude in the selection of tube size. The work of breathing through 6 mm ID tubes is not greatly increased[34] and ventilation is only marginally reduced with no change in functional residual capacity.[35]

Although shorter endotracheal tubes are less likely to migrate into a main bronchus, this must be tempered by the possibility that a tube placed with great difficulty may turn out to be too short or that as the patient's condition changes the tube becomes too short, e.g. in burns patients following the development of massive oedema.

Currently the move towards smaller tubes is somewhat limited, particularly where fixed length or preformed endotracheal tubes (e.g. armoured tubes, RAE tube or Polar tubes (see below)) are used. This is due to the fact that these tubes were designed with the 'largest size' maxim and hence the lengths of the various sections and the cuff sizes are linked to the internal diameter of the tube. Smaller diameter tubes can be too short or have cuffs that are too small to achieve a seal without overinflation. Table 8.2 gives the classical view of tubes and lengths.

Endotracheal tube cuffs

Originally cuffs were made of relatively thick rubber, which could withstand cleaning and autoclaving so that the endotracheal tubes could be re-used. If a small tube

Table 8.2 Lengths of endotracheal tubes

Internal diameter (mm)		Age (years)	Length (cm)	
Oral	Nasal		Oral	Nasal
2.5	2.5	PREMATURE	10.5	13.0
3.0	3.0	0–1	10.5	13.0
3.5	3.5		11.0	14.0
4.0	4.0		12.0	14.5
4.5	4.5	1–2	13.5	15.0
5.0	5.0	2–4	14.0	16.6
5.5	5.5		14.5	17.0
6.0	6.0	5–12	15.0	17.5
6.5	6.5		16.0	18.5
7.0	7.0	13–16	17.5	19.0
8.0	8.0		18.5	19.5
–	6.0	ADULTS (Small women → Large men)	–	24.0
–	6.5		–	24.0
7.0	7.0		–	24.0
7.5	7.5		–	25.0
8.0	8.0		23.0	26.0
8.5	–		24.0	–
9.0	–		25.0	–

A widely used formula for selecting the diameter of an endotracheal tube suitable for children over the age of 1 year is:

$$\frac{\text{Age in years}}{4} + 4.5 \text{ mm}$$

The exact length to which a new tube should be shortened cannot be categorically specified. In some operations it is necessary to pass the tube further down the trachea than in others. Cuffed tubes are generally trimmed to a centimetre or so longer than plain ones.

were repeatedly used in a large trachea, the cuff would become stretched and baggy, developing weak spots which could 'herniate' over the tip of the tube and occlude it (Fig. 8.21). This was another reason for using large tubes. This type of cuff requires a *high pressure* to distend it and may also be referred to as a *low volume* cuff. It tends to inflate in a circular shape and when a seal is just achieved only the widest circumference touches the tracheal wall (Fig. 8.22), with little transmission of cuff pressure. Over-distension increases the area of contact but causes the high pressure within the cuff to be transmitted to the tracheal wall. This cuts off the blood flow to the under-lying mucosa (capillary perfusion pressure is usually about 35 mmHg), which then suffers ischaemic damage.

Medium pressure cuffs are made from a much thinner elastic material such as latex rubber which fits snugly to the tube in its deflated state without appearing too bulky. This type of cuff requires some degree of pressure for inflation, although a seal can be achieved with an intracuff pressure below that in the capillaries supplying the tracheal mucosa. Due to the greater compliance of the material, over-inflation causes less pressure rise than with the high-pressure variety. These materials though are less resistant to tearing and cuffs are more easily damaged by snagging on teeth and instruments or passage through the nose.

Low pressure or *high volume* cuffs are made from a thin inelastic material (PVC) which when fully inflated would have a larger volume than that required to effect a seal. *In situ* there is a large area of contact between the cuff and tracheal wall before full inflation of the cuff. The pressure can therefore be kept low enough to not occlude mucosal blood flow. Low-pressure designs now predominate. This is particularly so in tubes such as tracheostomy tubes used for long-term ventilation on Intensive Care Units. One drawback of this approach to cuff design is graphically demonstrated in Figure 8.23. Here, because the material is not fully unfolded when a seal is achieved, a number of small channels may form running the length of the cuff. These channels may contribute to the causation of ventilator-associated pneumonia by allowing transmission of potentially infective pharyngeal contents past the cuff.

Cuffs are inflated via a small-bore inflation tube either welded onto the outside of the endotracheal tube or more commonly now built into its wall. The inflation tube is

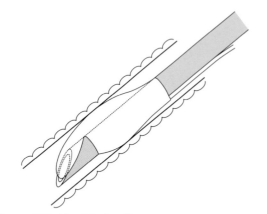

Figure 8.21 Herniated cuff.

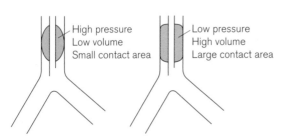

High pressure
Low volume
Small contact area

Low pressure
High volume
Large contact area

Figure 8.22 High and low pressure tracheal cuffs. Medium pressure cuffs have a profile between these extremes.

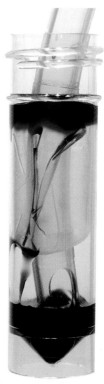

Figure 8.23 Large volume cuff inflated in a model trachea shows formation of numerous folds and channels. After Latto 1997.[36]

connected, at its proximal end to a small pilot balloon to give an indication of the distension of the cuff, and often finally a self-sealing valve mechanism to obviate the need for clamping the pilot tubes.

All cuff types should only be inflated to the pressure necessary to achieve sufficient seal to prevent gas leak at the airway pressures generated by positive pressure ventilation. This has the added advantage that it permits leakage (often audibly) if there is overpressure in the breathing system.

Nitrous oxide and the endotracheal tube cuff

Nitrous oxide (N_2O) diffuses into a cuff-filled with air. This discussion, of course, also applies to the cuffs on augmented supraglottic airways. The rate at which diffusion occurs depends on:
- the permeability of the material from which the cuff is constructed (rubber being more permeable than plastic);
- the surface area of the cuff exposed to N_2O; and
- the partial pressure of N_2O.

The rise in pressure caused by this diffusion into the cuff depends on the compliance of the cuff. Low-volume high-pressure cuffs suffer the greatest pressure rise and may well transmit this rise in pressure to the tracheal mucosa. High-volume low-pressure cuffs expand with only a slight increase in pressure until full inflation; at this point, owing to the inelasticity of the material, the pressure may rise rapidly to up to 12 kPa/90 mmHg. This can damage the tracheal mucosa.

This phenomenon can be avoided if the cuff is filled with either sterile saline or a gas mixture identical to that of the inspired gas, or else by regular monitoring of the cuff pressure and volume.

Alternatively, there are several devices that limit the pressure rise:
- The Mallinckrodt Brandt™ device has a large pilot balloon made from a material that allows the nitrous oxide which has diffused into the cuff to escape (Fig. 8.24)
- The Mallinckrodt Lanz™ (Fig. 8.25) device consists of a special control valve and pilot balloon arrangement. A compliant latex balloon protected within an open larger plastic covering connects to the cuff via a flow restrictor. Insertion of a syringe into the valve bypasses this restriction allowing rapid inflation of the cuff. Thereafter, gradual volume changes in the cuff are buffered by the pilot balloon. When filled with a preset volume the device regulates the cuff pressure to between 20 and 25 mmHg.

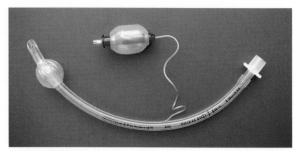

Figure 8.24 The Mallinckrodt Brandt device on a size 8 tracheal tube.

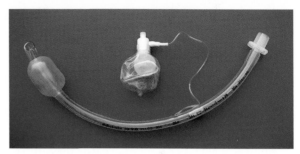

Figure 8.25 The Mallinckrodt Lanz™ device on a size 9 tracheal tube.

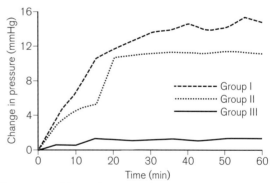

Figure 8.26 Mean changes in intracuff pressure every 5 min in three groups: group I, Mallinckrodt Lo-Contour tube; group II, Portex Profile tube; group III, Portex Soft Seal tube. From Al-Shaikh *et al* 1999,[37] with permission of Oxford University Press.

- Portex Soft Seal cuffs are made of a PVC material using a higher molecular weight plasticizer, which results in a five-fold lower permeability to N_2O. Figure 8.26 compares rises in intracuff pressure between a Soft Seal and two other cuffs during one hour of anaesthesia using 66% N_2O.
- The Bivona 'Fome-Cuf®' is an interesting approach both to the problems of cuff pressure and N_2O

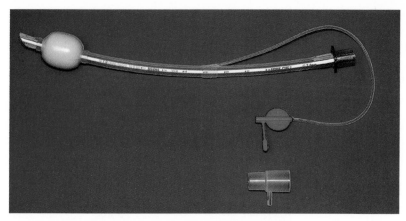

Figure 8.27 Bivona 'Fome Cuf®' endotracheal tube. The pilot tube for deflating the cuff can be connected into the ventilation circuit to equilibrate intracuff pressure during IPPV.

diffusion. Here a piece of shaped foam replaces the air that is used to inflate the cuff; instead the soft cuff here is evacuated to collapse the foam for insertion of the tube and the pilot tube is opened to the atmosphere to allow the foam to expand, to 'inflate' the cuff (Fig. 8.27). Because the pilot tube is left open, diffusion of N_2O does not further inflate the cuff. The pilot tube may also be connected to the ventilation circuit to equilibrate intracuff pressure with proximal airway pressure during positive pressure ventilation.

Nasotracheal intubation

The diameter of tubes inserted through the nose is clearly limited by the size of the nares and the air passages of the nasal cavity. The nasal septum and turbinates may result in a fairly convoluted passageway for the tube. Smaller diameter, softer and thinner walled tubes are therefore needed for ease of insertion and to diminish the chances of causing epistaxis. Similarly, the cuff would ideally be streamlined to the tube as large folds of harsh plastic may themselves cause epistaxis when the cuff is evacuated for insertion. Because of concerns regarding high-pressure cuffs, in modern plastic tubes a compromise has to be made. The inflation line is incorporated as far as possible in the body of the tube.

Uncuffed nasal tubes are popular for use in adults in spontaneously breathing techniques, particularly for short dental cases. The larynx is packed to protect the lungs for the period of the surgical procedure, but afterwards the small soft tubes cause a minimum of irritation and can be removed once the patient has woken. In spite of the now uniform use of disposable tubes, the ideal connector for this purpose remains the metal Magill nasal connector, which creates the least obtrusive setup. This does,

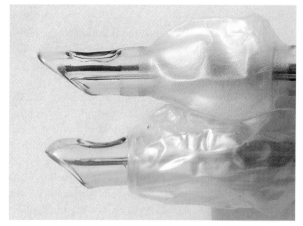

Figure 8.28 A blunt cupped tracheal tube bevel, compared with a standard bevel.

however, require the use of a purpose-built catheter mount (still available from manufacturers such as Intersurgical Ltd).

The design of the bevel is also important; sharp long bevels have tended to be replaced by short bevels with rounded tips (Fig. 8.28) which are less likely to snag on obstructions. Some manufacturers even use a different softer compound for the leading edge of the endotracheal tube.

Common problems with the use of endotracheal tubes

Many of the problems, particularly relating to tube kinking or obstruction by external compression, are rarely seen now with the use of PVC tubes. These soften with warming when in use, appearing more often to remould rather than kink abruptly: so much so that specially

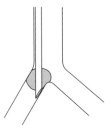

Figure 8.29 Occlusion of the tip of a long endotracheal tube is more likely with more flexible smaller diameter tubes.

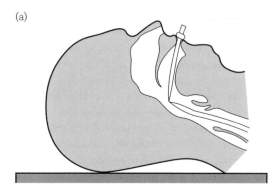

designed non-kinking tubes, such as the Oxford tube and even perhaps many uses of the 'armoured tube', are largely obsolete (see below). Some of the common problems are:

- A tube may be passed too far down the trachea and may enter the right main bronchus.
- There may be a leak between the cuff and the trachea, either because the cuff was not sufficiently inflated in the first place, or because it has subsequently deflated. The latter may be due to damage, overinflation or a fault in manufacture and is demonstrable by inflating the cuff following immersion in water.
- The tube may be obstructed in one or more of several ways. The opening may be occluded if the larynx or trachea is deviated to one side as in Figure 8.20. This may for example happen during thyroidectomy if the gland and trachea are being pulled aside by the surgeon. This pattern of obstruction may be more evident in expiration and is also seen if the tube is advanced too far into the right main bronchus (Fig. 8.29). The Murphy eye counteracts such problems.
- Endotracheal tubes may become kinked in the mouth (Fig. 8.30) or nasopharynx. Modern PVC tubes are more resistant to this form of obstruction. If they must be bent acutely when *in situ*, a reinforced tube or one that is specially shaped should be used (see below, Tubes for special purposes).
- Tubes may become obstructed if bitten by patients awaking from anaesthesia. Red rubber tubes were prone, especially after repeated autoclaving to obstruction by a tightly inserted throat pack or even by inward herniation of the tube wall underneath the high-pressure cuff.
- Tubes are prone to being kinked by the position of the breathing system, e.g. an uncut tube emerging from the mouth or as in Figure 8.31, due to rotational forces being applied by a breathing system.
- All manner of foreign bodies, including the tops of

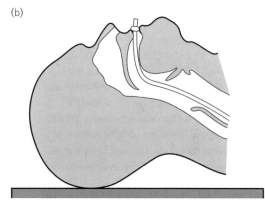

Figure 8.30 (a) Kinking of an endotracheal tube inside the mouth due to excessive neck flexion and softening of the tube owing to its becoming warmer during anaesthesia, all having seemed well at induction. **(b)** Head in correct position.

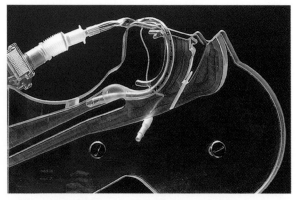

Figure 8.31 Occlusion of the endotracheal tube due to rotational forces by the breathing system.

ampoules, has been found causing blockage within airway devices. This emphasizes the fact that tubes, airways, etc. should not be placed in the same dish as Luer–Lok caps, needles and ampoules, even after use. Diaphragms of dried mucous and even K-Y jelly, which may be virtually invisible, have also been found blocking tubes. In single-use devices, this danger has been superceded by diaphragms of clear plastic being formed across the openings of tubes and other airway equipment when, for unwrapping, they are pushed through their plastic packaging. The invisible film is then kept firmly in place by the connector when the next item in the sequence is attached.

ISO connectors

The endotracheal tube is attached to the other components of the breathing system by a male 15 mm ISO (International Organisation for Standardization) tapered connector (Fig. 8.19j). This connector itself fits into the endotracheal tube via a tapered cone producing a secure connection. In PVC tubes with nylon/PVC connectors, because of the surface characteristics (stiction) of the materials, the seal often can only be broken by cutting the tube. Tubes are therefore supplied from the manufacturer with the connector only lightly inserted so that the tube may be cut to length.

Either the breathing system or 'catheter mount' (see below) houses a matching female 15–mm tapered connector. This two-part design permits a rapid disconnection and reconnection. However, the connection should be made secure with a 'push and twist' movement.

Other connectors

The early pioneers in anaesthesia produced connectors in a variety of shapes and sizes with any of a number of goals in mind, for example:

- streamline the fit in order to improve surgical access around the head and neck of a patient;
- minimize resistance to gas flow; or to
- allow insertion of suction catheters.

Many of these functions have been incorporated into the design of specialist tubes and a more limited range is now available, although the Magill nasal connectors still have a loyal following.

The female part of the 15 mm ISO connector at the proximal end of the tracheal tube allows some variety of functionality (Fig. 8.32), for example:

- swivel connectors to reduce torsion on the tube;
- suction port; or
- bronchoscopy through a gas tight seal.

A smaller standard of 8.5 mm is available for paediatric tubes to reduce component weight (see Chapter 14).

Catheter mounts

The term 'catheter mount' does not appear in BS 6015 (ISO 4135), which is the official glossary of the terms used in anaesthesiology. Its modern equivalent, 'tracheal tube adaptor', is yet to gain common usage. Some historical explanation of the term is appropriate.

Before the introduction of the Boyle's machine with the Magill breathing attachment, the mixed gases, with added vapour of volatile agents, were fed via a narrow bore tube (*catheter mount*) to the patient, with no reservoir bag or expiratory valve in the positions in which we now know them. The end of the tube could be attached to the Boyle–Davis gag or to a catheter that was passed through the larynx into the trachea. In the latter case, the gases and/or vapours were blown constantly down the catheter and were exhausted to the atmosphere by passing through the trachea but outside the catheter (see above, under History).

Currently, a catheter mount usually consists of a short piece of flexible kink resistant 15 mm tubing with a

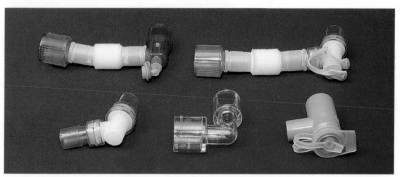

Figure 8.32 A variety of tracheal tube connectors. Clockwise from top left: Intersurgical flexible corrugated models for gas sampling, and with 'Seal-Around' cap on swivel mount for bronchoscopy or suction; Mainz Universal Adaptor (blue-coloured) for endoscopy/intubation via endotracheal tube or facemask; plain angle piece; swivel mount.

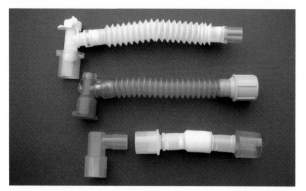

Figure 8.33 A selection of catheter mounts, showing the 15 and 22 mm ISO connections described in the text.

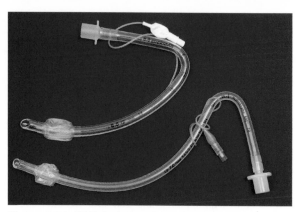

Figure 8.34 RAE design endotracheal tubes for orotracheal intubation (top) and nasotracheal intubation.

15 mm ISO female tapered connector for attachment to the endotracheal tube (Fig. 8.33). The other end of the catheter mount may have either a 15 mm ISO male taper or a 22 mm ISO female taper connector for coupling with the breathing system. Although the device increases the apparatus dead space of the breathing system, the flexibility it imparts makes this an insignificant consideration except in the very young.

ENDOTRACHEAL TUBES FOR SPECIAL PURPOSES

Many 'special' tubes have been devised of which only a few examples are described below. It should be borne in mind that different manufacturers may be able to offer some tubes with a selection of features, be it tip designs (e.g. Murphy or Magill type); cuff and pilot balloon design; or even construction material or additional lumens. Manufacturers' designs of the same type of tube may vary considerably; even small variations can have significant effects on the practicality of devices. Some designs, however, are 'branded' and available only from one company, although others may have a similar design under a generic description. For a full range of tubes or for particular requirements, it is best to consult the manufacturers directly, usually one or other is likely to have the right combination of features. In any case, anaesthetists should be more proactive in demanding particular product specifications to reflect their needs. A feature of anaesthetic equipment that is reflected in their high unit cost is the low production numbers; the corollary to this should be the relative ease of making small variances to a design for a given customer or application.

RAE preformed tubes

There are two separate versions of these tubes, named after their inventors: Ring, Adair and Elwin (Fig. 8.34). The tube for orotracheal intubation has a preformed bend on the part of the tube where it exits the mouth, so that the part housing the ISO connector passes down the chin and away from the face, thus improving surgical access to the mouth, nose and head of the patient. The nasotracheal version is bent where it exits the nose so that the part housing the ISO connector passes upwards to the forehead. It is used to improve surgical access in intraoral procedures.

The main disadvantage of both designs is in the fixed length of the intraoral section. With the trend towards using smaller calibre tubes (because tube dimensions have not been reformulated), this may be too short to reach comfortably below the glottis (see above, under Endotracheal Tubes, Size).

Reinforced tubes

Most endotracheal tubes will kink if bent into an acute enough angle or if compressed by an external force such as from a surgical instrument. There are situations where either or both can occur during the course of an operation. Tubes may be made kink-resistant by embedding a reinforcing spiral of steel or nylon wire into the wall of the tube, which can then be made of a more elastic material than usual (i.e. silicone rubber, latex rubber or soft plastic). This makes the tube very flexible with little preformed shape so that it also becomes more difficult to insert into the trachea. Reinforced tubes have a thicker wall and therefore a smaller internal diameter (ID) for a given outer diameter. The tubes may be inserted over

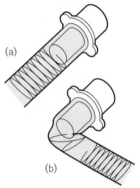

Figure 8.35 Obstruction at the 'soft spot' between the connector and the spiral of an armoured tube. **(a)** With the connector placed correctly; **(b)** with incorrect placement leaving an unarmoured segment of tube.

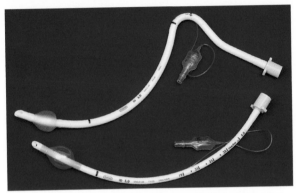

Figure 8.36 Portex Ivory endotracheal tubes: Upper: north facing Polar nasotracheal tube. Lower: Microlaryngeal tube with greater length and larger cuff relative to tube diameter.

a bougie, which has first been passed into the trachea. Alternatively, a malleable stylet can be inserted into its lumen to shape it.

These tubes are usually supplied at a length of 30 cm or greater for an ID of 5.0 mm and above. The steel-reinforcing spiral will not stretch to accommodate a connector so the tubes cannot be cut to a shorter length than supplied. The ISO connectors are therefore usually bonded at production to a non-reinforced part of the tube. Special care must be taken not to insert these tubes too far. Re-usable tubes may be prone to kinking at the 'soft spot' between the end of the connector and the start of the spiral reinforcement (Fig. 8.35).

The greater kink resistance of PVC tubes and the availability of Polar tubes has diminished the need for using these devices.

Polar tubes

Portex, in their Ivory range of tubes, manufacture a Polar tube for nasotracheal intubation in a soft PVC material (see Endotracheal Tubes, Materials) with a preformed curve that takes the proximal end of the tube snugly along the nose and over the forehead (Fig. 8.36). These tubes are well-suited to maxillofacial surgery as they impinge relatively little on the surgical field. If access is also needed to the forehead, as in some cosmetic or reconstructive plastic procedures, the proximal end can be swung down without the tube kinking, to descend over the cheek or chin. The soft plastic of the Ivory range is relatively atraumatic in the nose, which in combination with the springiness of these tubes makes them ideal for 'blind nasal intubation'. Interestingly, the material,

originally called 'Vinyl Portex Tubing,' was actually first developed in 1944[36] as a substitute for the red rubber tubes whose primary materials were in short supply.

These tubes, in sizes 6.0 and 6.5 mm ID, are a good choice for nasal fibreoptic intubation, in spite of the reservations previously mentioned regarding cuff sizes and small tubes (the length in this case is adequate, even for the largest adults).

Microlaryngeal tube

This tube (Fig. 8.36, lower) has a small external diameter (ID usually around 5 mm) but an adult-sized high-volume low-pressure cuff. The tubes are designed to be unobtrusive in the larynx so as to allow surgery around the vocal cords and are long enough for nasal intubation. The high resistance to gas flow in these tubes virtually obligates controlled ventilation with adequate provisions for a long expiratory phase. They can be difficult to insert unless Magill intubating forceps are used. Standard adult-sized bougies and stylets are usually too large to pass through these tubes which, it must be remembered, are not laser resistant.

Carden tube

This tube was developed to facilitate microsurgery of the larynx. It is rarely used now but may perhaps enjoy a resurgence for jet ventilation. It is essentially a shortened cuffed endotracheal tube that sits wholly below the glottis served by a long catheter for insufflation of gas and a long pilot tube for the cuff (Fig. 8.37). It is inserted by grasping it with Magill's endotracheal forceps or as follows. The Carden tube and an uncut plain tube, just

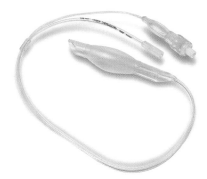

Figure 8.37 Carden tube for laryngeal surgery. Photo courtesy of Portex UK Ltd.

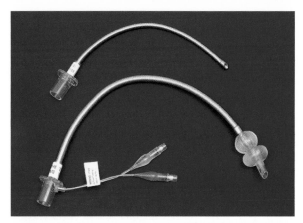

Figure 8.38 Mallinckrodt 'Laser-Flex™' endotracheal tubes. Uncuffed and cuffed showing water filled double cuff arrangement.

wide enough to fit inside it, are threaded onto a stylet. This assembly is introduced through the larynx so that the Carden tube and a centimetre or so of the plain tube pass into the trachea. The cuff of the Carden tube is inflated, the stylet is withdrawn and anaesthesia is maintained in the usual manner through the plain tube. For laryngoscopy, the plain tube is removed as is the breathing system, and gases are delivered directly to the Carden tube through a feed mount. The expired gases escape via the lumen of the Carden tube.

Tubes for laser surgery

Conventional endotracheal tubes of either plastic, silicone or rubber may be damaged by the carbon dioxide, KTP or Nd-YAG laser beam. These materials burn more fiercely in the presence of oxygen or N_2O than in air and are easily ignited by direct impingement of the laser beam. The resultant fire can produce serious upper airways burns. Some examples of tubes that can be used in the presence of a laser beam are described below. They must not be assumed to be laser *proof* and are only indicated for CO_2 and KTP lasers. Figures are provided for maximum power and duration of energy before ignition for different lasers according to standardized tests (e.g. 1 sec at 55 watts or 7 sec at 30 Watts from CO_2 laser for the Laser-Flex).

Mallinckrodt 'Laser-Flex™' *endotracheal* *tubes* (Fig. 8.38). These single-use tubes for oral intubation are made from a gas-tight metal helix with the pilot tubes for the double cuff carried within the lumen of the airway. It is advised that the cuffs, which are not laser resistant, are inflated with saline, ideally dyed with some methylene blue, to prevent ignition of the cuff and so that puncture is obvious. The function of the proximal cuff is to protect the distal cuff and the tube must be replaced if either

cuff is defective. The surface of the tube shaft reflects a defocused laser beam with a lower potential for causing tissue destruction. The tip of the tube is made of a soft plastic for a more atraumatic insertion. The tubes have a markedly reduced inner diameter when compared to PVC tubes of the same outer diameter and care must be taken to allow adequate expiratory time in ventilated patients.

Foil Wrapped (Fig. 8.39). An alternative approach used by some manufacturers is to spirally wrap a suitably small rubber tube with a narrow strip of silver or copper foil (this may be stippled or corrugated to disperse an incident beam). The tube is then overwrapped to give a smooth outer coating. The Rusch Lasertubus is covered in Merocel foam (a porous sponge), which is soaked in saline to help absorb laser energy. This tube is provided with a double cuff arrangement.

Jet Ventilation. If surgical access is going to be significantly impaired by a laser resistant tube, the laryngoscope that is used to suspend the larynx for surgery can be fitted with a metal cannula (Fig. 9.40) that ends above the glottis and can be used for jetting with high-pressure gas. Anaesthesia can then be maintained intravenously. Alternatively, a sub-glottic jet ventilation cannula can be inserted percutaneously or a Hunsaker tube can be used.

Hunsaker tube

The Hunsaker Mon-Jet Ventilation tube (Fig. 8.41) by Medtronic Xomed is a narrow-bore dual lumen tube designed for subglottic jet ventilation of the lungs that allows concomitant airway pressure monitoring or gas sampling from the narrower second lumen. The 33 cm-long device (4.5 mm at its widest diameter) is made of a laser-resistant fluoroplastic and ends in a moulded plastic cage which aims to centralize the discharged jet stream and prevent direct impingement on the tracheal wall mucosa. In combination with a dedicated jet ventilator, such as the Accutronic Medical Systems Monsoon or Mistral models (see Chapter 11), this device allows improved surgical access for unhurried instrumentation

and laser surgery of the major airways. Although the material will not melt and drip or produce a self-sustaining flame, protracted impact of sufficient laser energy will penetrate the tube. An internal stainless steel wire is designed to retain the distal fragment in the event of the tube being severed. Other manufacturers do produce similar designs.

Laryngectomy tube

Conventional endotracheal tubes placed through a tracheotomy following laryngectomy are difficult to fix

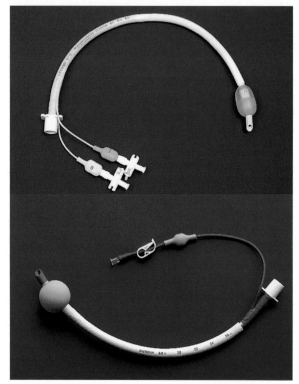

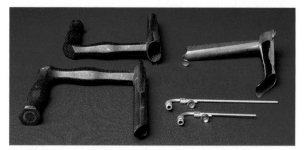

Figure 8.40 Different patterns of laryngoscopes for suspension surgery and examination of the larynx; and alongside jet ventilation cannulae for use with these devices.

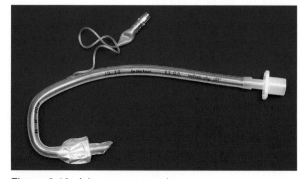

Figure 8.39 The Rusch Lasertubus (above) and Sheridan Laser-Trach® (below, photo courtesy of Hudson RCI) laser resistant single use endotracheal tubes. The embossed copper foil of the Sheridan tube is just visible under the outer covering.

Figure 8.42 A laryngectomy tube.

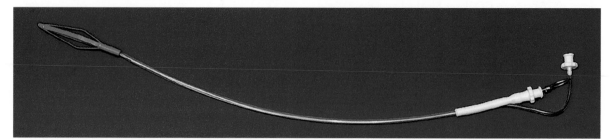

Figure 8.41 The Hunsaker Mon-Jet Ventilation tube.

in place and prone to kinking or slipping down into a bronchus. The 'U' shape of the laryngectomy tube (Fig. 8.42) means it sits nicely on the chest wall with the long straight proximal portion allowing direct connection to a breathing system away from the operative site. The tip is usually cut close to the cuff to minimize the risk of endobronchial intubation.

Tubes for thoracic surgery

Operations within the thoracic cavity may require the collapse of a lung to improve access to other organs, to isolate that lung for its removal or repair, or to prevent contamination from a diseased lung spreading to the other side. This may be achieved in one of three ways.

Endobronchial tubes

Firstly a long tube may be passed, often under endoscopic control, beyond the carina and into the unaffected lung so that the cuff can be inflated within a main bronchus. The other lung is not ventilated and collapses, especially when the pleura is opened. This technique is normally applicable only to the left lung. This is because the right upper lobe bronchus enters its main bronchus very close to the carina and it would be obstructed by the cuff of the tube described. The endobronchial tube may be placed in the trachea initially so as to use both lungs for as long as possible and then advanced when required to isolate the appropriate lung.

Tubes with endobronchial blockers

The second method of isolating a lung is to use a special endotracheal tube through which a fine balloon catheter can be passed either through the lumen of the tube or

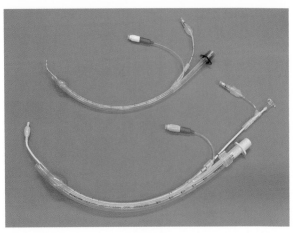

Figure 8.43 Univent tracheal tubes with endobronchial blockers. The lower device allows access to the lung distal to the blocker. Photo courtesy of Fuji Systems Corporation.

through a channel in the wall. The balloon tip is then passed, usually with the aid of a fibreoptic endoscope, into the intended main bronchus, which becomes isolated when the balloon is inflated (Fig. 8.43). Foley catheters and Fogarty embolectomy catheters can be used with care to extemporize in conjunction with ordinary tracheal or tracheostomy tubes.

Double-lumen tubes

The third and most popular method is to use a combination or double lumen tube (DLT) (Fig. 8.44). These are formed by bonding together two tubes of similar diameters but different lengths. The shorter tube ends in the trachea and seals this with one cuff, whilst the longer

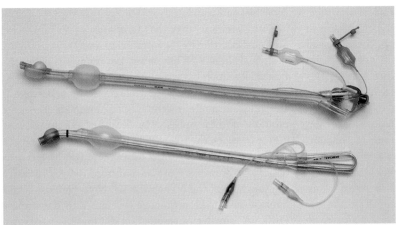

Figure 8.44 Double lumen tubes (both with malleable tracheal introducers in place). Portex right-sided tube (above) and Mallinckrodt Broncocath left-sided tube (below). The scalloping of the distal cuff is just visible on the right-sided tube (see text).

(a)

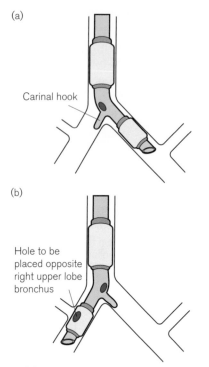

Carinal hook

(b)

Hole to be
placed opposite
right upper lobe
bronchus

Figure 8.45 (a) The endobronchial section of the tube in the left main bronchus with the carinal hook limiting the depth of insertion. **(b)** The endobronchial section of the tube in the right main bronchus with the carinal hook limiting the depth of insertion and the side hole opposite the right upper lobe bronchus surrounded by the adapted bronchial cuff.

tube is designed to fit a main bronchus and seal this with a separate cuff. The cuffs are supplied by separate inflation tubes and pilot balloons, which are marked and colour-coded to aid identification. DLTs are produced in left and right-sided versions. Some designs have a small soft carinal hook to prevent over-insertion of the tube. Because the opening of the right upper lobe bronchus is so close to the origin of the main bronchus, the bronchial lumen on right-sided versions also has a side hole and a cuff that is designed so that it does not occlude this (Fig. 8.45). The bronchial cuff and inflation tube is blue by convention.

Sizes The combined size of the two lumens makes the device sufficiently bulky to prevent its use in children. Because the external shape of the device is circular in cross-section, the lumens of the two tubes are each 'D'-shaped and the size cannot be quoted in terms of an internal diameter. Sizes are quoted in French gauge (Fr). This scale is constructed from the external diameter of

the widest part of the device, measured in millimetres, multiplied by a factor of 3 (corresponding roughly to the circumference). Usual sizes are 28, 35, 37, 39 and 41 Fr; many designs offer only one or two sizes.

Insertion Left-sided tubes are technically easier to insert at laryngoscopy. Also, because the left upper lobe bronchus is not as close to the carina as its right counterpart, depth of insertion of the device is far less critical. Wherever possible the largest possible left-sided DLT is selected and the cuffs are checked for leaks. Left-sided tubes are appropriate for most procedures except for left pneumonectomy. The device is held so that the bronchial tube curves forwards, resembling the Magill curve of an endotracheal tube. It is inserted under direct vision and once through the larynx it is rotated counterclockwise so that the tip enters the left main bronchus. Carinal hooks, if present, may snag on the glottis but should ultimately rest on the carina, confirming that full insertion has been achieved. The two connectors are then joined on to those on a twin tube adapter (catheter mount), which links the tubes to the breathing system. The tracheal cuff is then inflated and manual ventilation is commenced via both lumens. This should produce equal visible bilateral chest movement confirmed by auscultation. The tracheal adapter on the catheter mount is then occluded with a hose clamp so that all ventilation is directed down the bronchial lumen. The left bronchial cuff is then slowly inflated whilst auscultating the right lung until a seal is achieved, at which point no gas entry will be heard. The tracheal lumen is then released so that the tube can be used as intended.

Insertion of right-sided tubes involves clockwise rotation of the DLT and similar checking of left lung inflation with the added proviso that gas entry should also be confirmed over the right upper zone when the bronchial cuff is inflated.

Both versions may be temporarily reshaped for laryngeal insertion by the insertion of a stiff stylet into the bronchial lumen. This must be removed once the bronchial section has passed through the larynx.

Visual confirmation with a fibreoptic bronchoscope is the most accurate method of determining the true position of these tubes. The bronchial cuff should be visible (through the tracheal lumen) at or just beyond the carina, and with right-sided tubes the origin of the right upper lobe bronchus must be confirmed to lie adjacent to the side hole of the bronchial tube. Note that a standard 5 mm diameter bronchoscope will not pass down most DLTs. A smaller diameter intubating or paediatric bronchoscope should be used. Alternatively, the broncho-scope can be inserted through the bronchial lumen of the tube and into the correct bronchus with the DLT being railroaded into place over this guide. With right-sided tubes, the position should be checked every time the patient is moved.

Tubes to assist intubation

The Endotrol endotracheal tube (Mallinckrodt) has a control wire connected to the distal tip running in the wall of the tube on the inner aspect of the curvature. Traction on this wire increases the curvature at the tip of the tube to facilitate intubation. This tube is no longer available in Europe.

Tubes with additional ports/lumens

Endotracheal tubes may have an additional narrow-bore tube fitted to the wall for sampling, pressure monitoring or drug instillation. Sheridan produce a full range of sizes including uncuffed paediatric tubes with an extra lumen ending at the tracheal tip for airway gas sampling or drug instillation.

LITA tube. The extra lumen in this tube has ten small side holes, 8 above and 2 below the cuff for the 'Laryngo-tracheal Instillation of Topical Anaesthetic'. There is evidence demonstrating better tolerance of intubation in sedated patients[37] and conflicting evidence regarding suppression of response to extubation,[38,39] (Fig. 8.46).

Tubes for jet ventilation. Two additional smaller tubes may be incorporated into the tracheal tube lumen to allow jet ventilation and simultaneous monitoring of tracheal pressure. The much wider main lumen of the endo-tracheal tube then permits entrainment of gases and passive exhalation at low pressures. Such tubes are avail-able in cuffed and uncuffed versions depending on the need for airway protection and control of entrained gases.

SUBGLOTTIC DEVICES

Tracheostomy tubes

The distance between the tracheal stoma and the carina in patients is short and variable. Tubes placed in the trachea via a tracheostomy are therefore designed to be non-bevelled, short in length and with the cuff bonded closer to the tip of the tube to prevent accidental endobronchial intubation. They are usually preformed into a right-angle to prevent kinking during neck flexion.

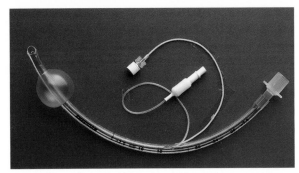

Figure 8.46 Sheridan LITA (Laryngo-tracheal Instillation of Topical Anaesthetic) tube. Black horizontal line indicates uppermost opening. Photo courtesy of Hudson RCI.

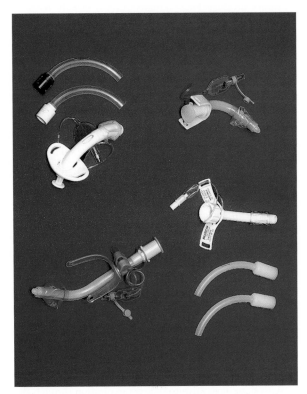

Figure 8.47 Just a few of an immense range of tracheostomy tubes (see text). The bottom left hand device is a tracheostomy tube with an adjustable flange allowing correct positioning of the distal portion of the tube in patients with bigger or oedematous necks.

There are an almost endless variety of tracheostomy tubes when one considers all the variations and options available on the standard design (Fig. 8.47); some are discussed below. At least one manufacturer, Rüsch, will tailor single tubes for individual requirements.

- *Cuffed/uncuffed.* In children and in adults, where positive pressure ventilation is not required, a plain uncuffed tube may be used to maintain the stoma.
- *Fenestrated/non-fenestrated.* Fenestration of the tube allows exhalation through the glottis for the purpose of vocalization. Use of a non-fenestrated inner tube in conjunction permits positive pressure ventilation where required. Care must be taken to ensure the fenestrated part of the tube lies within the trachea and not in the pretracheal tissues *vi.*
- *Long stem/armoured.* In patients with significant swelling or pathology about the head and neck (e.g. patients with burns) ordinary tracheostomy tubes are often too short to reach the trachea. Many manufacturers produce long-stemmed tubes, usually with an adjustable flange and sometimes in conjunction with an armoured tube wall design, allowing the tube to bend where required rather than having a fixed preformed curve.
- *With/without inner-tube.* Inner-tubes may be removed for cleaning to prevent build-up of encrustations; however they are a source of accidental disconnection and do significantly decrease the effective size of the lumen.
- *Foam cuff/Lanz device/Brandt Device.* These are available as with normal tracheal tubes as strategies to deal with the problems of cuff seal pressure within the trachea. (see above, Endotracheal tube cuffs).
- *Above cuff suction/vocalization.* A soft catheter ending above the tracheal cuff may be bonded to the tube to permit suction toilet of the secretions that tend to pool in the larynx and which may contribute to ventilator associated pneumonias. A similar design can be used to insufflate air to permit vocalization even during positive pressure ventilation.
- *Distal pressure monitoring.* A narrow bore tube ending distal to the cuff allows direct measurement of tracheal pressures.
- *Speaking valves.* Tracheostomy tubes may be capped with a one-way valve to redirect expiration through the larynx.

Percutaneous tracheostomy kits

Although a number of different techniques are currently available for percutaneous tracheostomy, the popularization of the approach, as opposed to an open surgical technique, dates from Ciaglia's description of a guide wire and serial dilator method in 1985.[40] The Ciaglia Blue Rhino (Cook Critical Care) (Fig. 8.48) has since super-

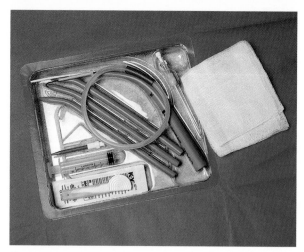

Figure 8.48 Cook Blue Rhino single step percutaneous dilatational tracheostomy kit. Photo courtesy of Cook UK.

seded the serial dilators with a simpler one-step tapered dilator and this alteration has been taken on board by other manufacturers. Ciaglia's percutaneous dilatational tracheostomy (PDT) is currently the most popular technique in the UK.[41] PDT appears to carry a perioperative complication rate comparable or superior to standard tracheostomy but concerns do still exist regarding the overall advantages, which appear to centre mostly on organizational issues in intensive care units.[42] For the guide wire based techniques, bronchoscopy has become accepted good practice to ensure that the tracheal puncture is central and well-positioned and that the posterior tracheal wall is not breached. Paratracheal insertion of the tracheostomy tube is hence prevented. Peroperative bleeding during percutaneous techniques is usually tamponaded by the tracheostomy tube but can be troublesome and occasionally major. PDT is essentially an elective procedure with reported operative times of 5 to 15 mins. Other approaches to percutaneous tracheostomy are briefly described below.

Dilatation of the tracheal puncture following insertion of a guide wire may be accomplished by other means:
- The Rapitrac uses sharp forceps that are held open to admit the tracheostomy tube but are prone to damaging the tube cuff and tracheal wall, it has been largely abandoned.
- By comparison, the Portex guide wire dilating forceps (GWDF) technique (Fig. 8.49) described by Griggs in 1990[43] uses blunt curved forceps to dilate the stoma, which are then removed. GWDF is applicable

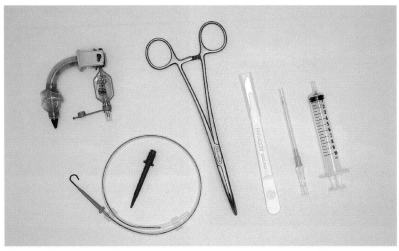

Figure 8.49 Griggs Guide Wire Dilating Forceps percutaneous tracheostomy set. The forceps are recessed on the inner surface of the prongs along the distal curve to follow the guide wire.

in emergencies as it is quicker to perform than PDT but may carry a higher complication rate.[44]

- Another design, Percutwist from Rusch, uses a screw-type dilator to follow the guide wire.
- A differing approach from Mallinckrodt is the trans-laryngeal technique of Fantoni[45] where a specially designed dilator tipped tracheostomy tube is inserted through the larynx and pulled out through the tracheal wall.

Ravussin catheter

Smaller diameter cannulae are simpler, safer and quicker to insert percutaneously into the trachea than formal tracheostomy tubes, particularly if the cricothyroid membrane is used for access. Ventilation (as opposed to oxygenation) however is only possible if high-pressure gas is jetted through the device; with exhalation occurring passively through the larynx. Transtracheal jet ventilation (TTJV) is thus the 'bottom line' in algorithms for the management of failed ventilation and is used electively in other scenarios such as for laryngeal surgery or in the management of the difficult airway, where it may provide ventilation during fibreoptic intubation or tracheostomy under general anaesthesia.[46]

The device of choice is developed from the intravenous cannulae which were originally used and advocated for TTJV.[47,48] Intravenous catheters if used, tend to kink and are difficult to fix at the neck. The Ravussin Jet Ventilation Catheter (VBM Medizintechnik) is available in 13G for adults and smaller 14G and 18G versions for children and babies. The kink-resistant catheter is made of Teflon and is curved with an angled flange on the connector so that it points axially down the trachea when it is fully inserted. The proximal end has a Luer–Lok for connection to a high-pressure gas supply (see below) housed within a 15 mm ISO male connector which allows very temporary low-pressure oxygen insufflation from a conventional anaesthetic system. The distal tip of the catheter has three small lateral holes to centre the device in the trachea during jetting and prevent 'whipping'. Peak airway pressures generated at the carina during TTJV are of the order of 5–13 mm Hg.[49]

The device (Fig. 8.50) with a syringe attached is inserted through the cricothyroid membrane, with aspiration of air confirming intratracheal placement, and the syringe assembly is held still whilst the catheter is advanced off the cannula. Such a device, together with a high-pressure oxygen source, should be available in all areas where anaesthetics are given and where unconscious patients may be admitted. Assembly of a suitable system from disparate items during an emergency is not practicable.

A variety of larger-bore devices for emergency tracheal access, some utilizing guide wire techniques for insertion, are made by several manufacturers. They tend to be an unhappy compromise between allowing low pressure 'to and fro' ventilation and ease of insertion; with no proven

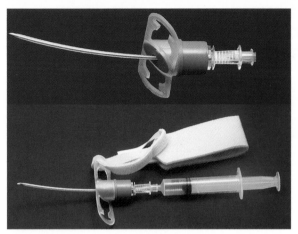

Figure 8.50 Ravussin transtracheal jet ventilation catheter.

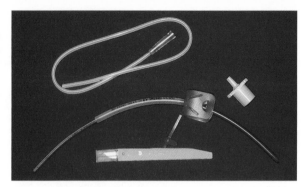

Figure 8.51 Portex Mini-Trach kit.

advantages over more formal percutaneous tracheostomy (see above). They may have a role for 'out of hospital' use but little is known of the long-term effects of attempting to put larger devices through the cricothyroid membrane.[50] The Portex Mini-Trach kit (Fig. 8.51) was originally designed for tracheal toilet.

Manujet

This is a modern version of the manually operated Sanders high-pressure injector for jet ventilation (Fig. 8.52). By squeezing the trigger, oxygen from a standard 4 bar Schrader socket can be intermittently discharged through a suitable cannula or catheter. The Manujet (VBM Medizintechnik) incorporates a pressure regulator that allows jetting pressure to be varied down to below 0.5 bar for use in infants.

LARYNGOSCOPES

These may be considered under two broad categories:
1. Retractor type, like the Macintosh laryngoscope, reliant on retracting tissues to create an uninterrupted sight line between the operator and the objective. Fibreoptics may be used in the light source of these types.
2. Fibreoptic laryngoscopes, where a fibreoptic channel transmits the image from the tip of the device to an eyepiece or camera, thus allowing the observer to effectively view around an obstruction. Fibreoptics are hence also necessitated for light

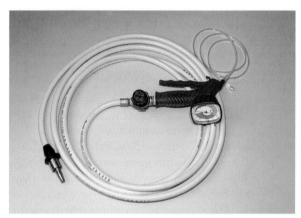

Figure 8.52 Manujet, variable pressure manual injector, VBM Medizintechnik, Germany.

transmission to the objective. Two types of fibre-optic laryngoscope can be categorized:
(i) Rigid fibreoptic laryngoscopes, such as the Upsher and Bonfils, where the fibreoptic-viewing channel is rigid and usually encased in metal. This type of device can also force tissues aside and act as a retractor. Accepted wisdom has it that such instruments require less dexterity and expertise to use than their flexible counterpart.
(ii) Flexible fibreoptic laryngoscopes. The viewing bundle (plus light transmission bundles and an optional instrument channel) is wrapped in a flexible casing. The instrument can thus be made to follow anatomical spaces and will bend as necessary to negotiate almost any route. The term 'flexible fibreoptic broncho-scope' is synonymous in use.

History

Visualization of the vocal cords for intubation was popularized by Sir Robert Macintosh and Sir Ivan Magill in the early 1940s. It was during the insertion of a Boyle–Davis gag that Macintosh conceived the idea of his laryngoscope, which is still the most popular design in use today and has spawned a wide variety of modifications. It consists of a blade that elevates the lower jaw and tongue, a light source near the tip of the blade to illuminate the larynx and a handle to apply force to the blade. The handle also contains the power supply (battery) for the light source. The light comes on when the blade, which is hinged on the handle, is opened to the right-angle position.

Macintosh designed a slightly curved blade (Fig. 8.53) with a small bulbous tip that was designed to be inserted anterior to the base of the epiglottis in an adult. The child and infant blades were not designed by him and he condemned them as being anatomically wrong and unnecessary. Most blades for infants and children and some of those for adults tend to be either straight or with a small shallow curve at the tip only. These are designed to be inserted deeper into the pharynx and posterior to the epiglottis and hence the blades are correspondingly longer.

In UK practice, the term 'laryngoscope' when not further described, is still largely synonymous with the rigid retractor type and more specifically the Macintosh designed laryngoscope. The term 'difficult laryngoscopy' therefore is largely used to describe any situation where only a suboptimal view of the larynx can be obtained with these default devices. For practical usefulness, given the variety of devices now routinely available, this term should always be further defined to describe the circumstances.

Retractor type laryngoscopes

Figure 8.54 shows some of the wide variety of blades currently available. The choice of blade for routine use is probably largely a matter of personal preference. It must be borne in mind that the technique for laryngoscopy is different for the various designs of blade and differing designs may offer better views of the larynx in a given patient. Most blades are detachable from the handle for ease of cleaning and change of blade size where appropriate. The 'hook on' connection for the blade, which allows easy detachment, is very convenient and was developed by Welch Alleyn Ltd in the early 1950s.

Two new standards: ISO 7376/3 (green system) and ISO 7376/1 (red system), have now been developed which allow blades from different manufacturers to be interchangeable, but they have not been universally adopted. In both the bulb is housed within the handle and light is transmitted through an optical 'bundle' to the tip of the blade. Their difference lies in the dimensions of the hinges and the relative positions of the light sources.

Prisms and mirrors are sometimes added to these devices to overcome the principle shortcoming of this class of device, namely that the operator's eye and patient's larynx must be in a straight line with no interposed tissue. So far, such modifications have not proven popular or lasting.

Features of modern laryngoscopes

Figure 8.55 shows a typical instrument with a hook on type Macintosh blade. Some specific points are highlighted below:

* Detachable blade for interchangeable blade designs and ease of cleaning and sterilization;

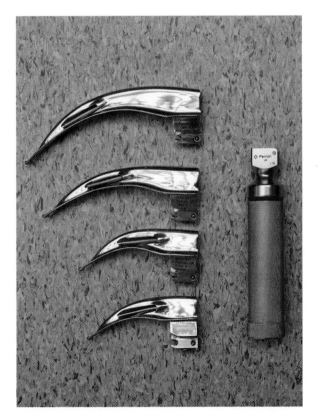

Figure 8.53 Macintosh laryngoscope with 4 sizes of interchangeable blade.

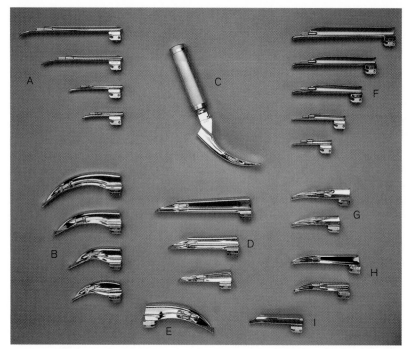

Figure 8.54 Laryngoscope blades. A, Miller pattern: 3, large; 2, adult; 1, infant; 0, premature. B, Macintosh pattern: 4, large; 3, adult; 2, child; 1, baby. C, Macintosh polio blade. D, Soper pattern: adult; child; baby. E, Macintosh pattern left-handed version. F, Wisconsin: large, adult, child, baby, infant. G, Robertshaw's: infant and neonatal. H, Seward: child and baby. I, Oxford: infant.

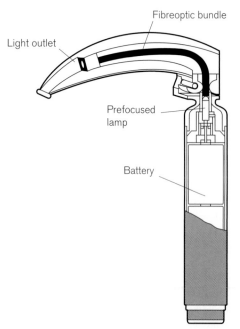

Figure 8.55 The Heine fibreoptic laryngoscope. Note that the lamp is within the handle, thus avoiding unreliable electrical contacts between the handle and the blade.

- Light source sited within the handle. Much brighter xenon gas-filled bulbs are used to compensate for light loss during transmission;
- Light projection via a shaped bundle of glass fibres. The bundle may be manufactured as an integral part of the blade, or may be detachable so that should it become damaged or opaque it may be replaced separately. Fibreoptic bundles are prone to degradation resulting in poor illumination[51] and difficult laryngoscopy;
- Disposable single-use blades are gaining popularity as an alternative to the costly and damaging process of sterilization of laryngoscope blades. These may be of plastic or even metal design but must not be assumed to perform as well as traditional instruments.[52,53]

Laryngoscopy

Figure 8.56 shows how correct positioning of the patient's head with craniocervical extension and lower cervical flexion, the position known as 'sniffing the morning air', allows the laryngoscope to retract the tongue and associated soft tissues into the elastic and distensible area of the floor of the mouth, providing an uninterrupted sight line through to the larynx. Poor views of the larynx can be predicted from this model where there is:

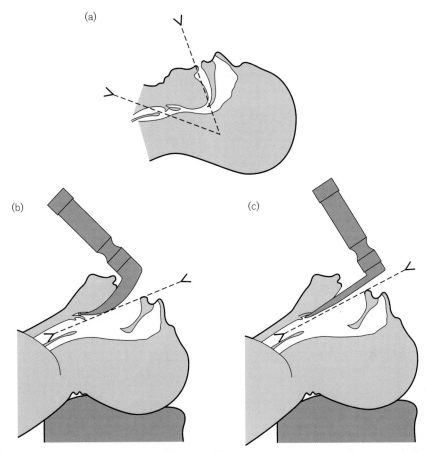

Figure 8.56 **(a)** The 'V' shape of the normal upper airway. The larynx cannot be seen from outside the mouth. **(b)** With the neck extended at the upper cervical spine and the jaw protruded forward by the laryngoscope blade, the 'V' extends into a straight line bringing the larynx into view. The curved blade fits between the base of the tongue and the epiglottis. **(c)** The straight blade passes behind the epiglottis.

- inadequate craniocervical movement or jaw opening;
- reduction in volume of distensible area below floor of mouth as with small receding mandible or following scarring or distortion of the anatomy as from head and neck surgery or radiotherapy;
- tumours of tongue base or larynx; or
- swelling of the posterior pharyngeal wall.

The handle of the laryngoscope is used to lift, i.e. force is applied in the direction of the handle rather than using the handle as a lever. Curved blades are designed for the tip to be inserted into the vallecula with the standard Macintosh blade being inserted to the right of the tongue and hence forcing it to the left side, whereas the straight blade may be inserted posterior to the epiglottis and is particularly useful for small children and adults with a large floppy epiglottis.

Different laryngoscope blades require different techniques for viewing the larynx, which must be learnt to exploit that device. For example, the Henderson blade (Karl Storz, Germany), a modification of the Miller blade, is a long straight-bladed design with a 'C'-shaped cross section (Fig. 8.57) and is intended to be inserted to the right of the tongue with the head turned aside in effectively a 'retro-molar' fashion. A poor view obtained with one design does not predict a poor view with a different design: ENT surgeons using a cone-shaped operating laryngoscope may, often to the annoyance of the anaesthetist who has struggled to intubate the patient, proceed to operate on that very glottis that the anaesthetist could not visualize.

Polio laryngoscope

This variation (Fig. 8.54c) alters the angle between the blade and the handle and is developed to allow the

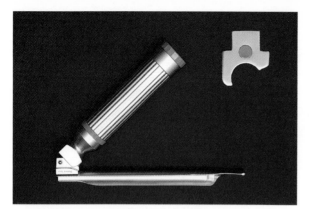

Figure 8.57 The Henderson blade attached to a laryngoscope handle (here in 'ISO Green system' fitting). Inset shows the blade from the rear to demonstrate the profile in cross section.

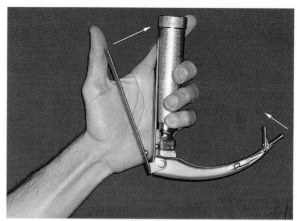

Figure 8.58 The McCoy laryngoscope with the lever deployed to show flexion of the tip.

laryngoscope blade to be more easily inserted into the mouth in patients with abnormal anatomy, e.g. limited neck extension or large breasts, or who are in unusual situations e.g. in a cabinet ventilator for polio. Another device, the Patil–Syracuse handle allows multiple-locking positions for the blade attachment point.

McCoy blade

This is based on a standard Macintosh blade modified by the insertion of a hinge to give an adjustable tip that is operated by a lever on the handle (Fig. 8.58). The blade is inserted in the normal way, and if the view is obscured, the tip can be flexed so that it further elevates the vallecula and epiglottis. Opinion is divided as to its usefulness: although the design has been commercially successful and it is included in many algorithms for airway management there is little evidence to support its widespread use. The effect on laryngeal view is variable depending on whether the base of tongue and vallecula is already optimally elevated.[54] In difficult direct laryngoscopy, activation of the tip may improve the laryngeal view where there is a grade 3 Cormack and Lehane view but is unlikely to do so where the epiglottis cannot be seen (grade 4 view),[55] additionally the incidence of grade 2 or worse views may be increased compared with a standard Macintosh blade even without activation of the tip.[56,57]

Rigid fibreoptic laryngoscopes
Bullard laryngoscope and Upsherscope

These two devices have a broadly similar curve to the blade and use fibreoptics to transmit the image from the tip to the eyepiece. They are designed to elevate the

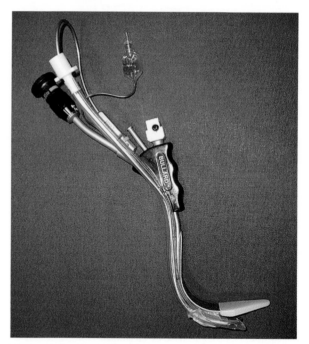

Figure 8.59 The Bullard laryngoscope here with light handle not connected.

jaw without the need for neck extension and for use in patients with limited mouth opening. Whereas the Bullard (Fig. 8.59) uses a fixed stylet to carry the tracheal tube, the Upsherscope (Fig. 8.60) has a 'C'-shaped cross-section which will transmit a tube of the correct diameter to emerge in the field-of-view of the device.

Unlike the flexible fibreoptic bronchoscopes, which have become the 'gold standard' for management of the

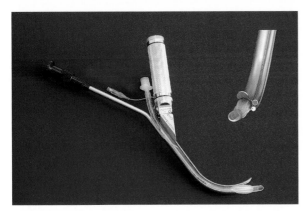

Figure 8.60 The Upsherscope, inset shows the tip of the device with endotracheal tube emerging. The larger light transmission fibreoptic bundle, lies above the much smaller coherent bundle for image transmission. The size of the distal viewing lens explains why fibreoptic devices are so easily foiled by secretions.

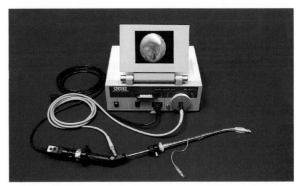

Figure 8.61 The Bonfils laryngoscope with endotracheal tube loaded and connected to a compact combination light source and image-processing unit (both by Karl Storz, Germany).

difficult intubation, this class of device in addition to 'viewing around corners', allows tissues to be retracted to create a view of the larynx. Intubation is, of course, limited to the oral route and applications are far more limited than for flexible fibreoptic intubation. However, there may be a particular indication in the difficult flexible fibreoptic intubation where lack of intraoral space and collapsed overlying tissues are the cause of difficulty as in patients with Obstructive Sleep Apnoea. It must be added this is usually only a problem in anaesthetized patients, but awake intubation is not always possible; for example in children.

The WuScope is a further example of this type. This class of devices appears to enjoy greater popularity in the USA[58] but their exact role is not obvious given their expense, the need for training and that they do not obviate the need for flexible fibreoptic intubation.[59,60]

Bonfils intubating fibrescope

The thin, stylet-like, Bonfils (Fig. 8.61), with a gentle anterior curve at its distal third is designed to be introduced from the side of the mouth in a 'retromolar approach' using the non-dominant hand to elevate the jaw and tongue.[61] The preloaded tracheal tube is advanced off the device once it has been manipulated into the larynx. The design of this device and technique of intubation really dictate that a camera and monitor is used on the eyepiece.

There exists limited published experience to advocate a role for this device.[62] It does, however, herald the arrival of a number of devices that may be seen as crossover category of 'seeing stylet' falling between laryngoscope and intubation aid.[63]

Flexible fibreoptic laryngoscopes

The first use of flexible fibreoptic technology in airway management can be credited to Dr P Murphy[64] who, in 1967, reported using the newly invented choledochoscope for intubation of the trachea.[65] Although initially ignored by fellow anaesthetists, the approach now forms the mainstay of managing difficult intubations. The terms flexible intubating fibrescope, endoscope, scope, bronchoscope, laryngoscope, and even tracheoscope are used interchangeably with varying degrees of precision. For anaesthetic purposes it is more important that the device has the correct length, insertion tube diameter and operating channel for the intended task.

The flexibility of these devices means that they can be made to follow virtually any anatomical space to return an image of the objective. Because they presume no particular anatomical arrangement (i.e. unlike rigid devices there is no preshaped curve) and can work around most obstructions, the technique of flexible fibreoptic intubation has become a 'gold standard' for management of the difficult laryngoscopy. This has tended to create the impression that the technique is the solution to all difficulties with the airway, but this is patently not so. These devices are simply for seeing around corners. For example, where the tracheal additus, however small, can be seen directly by the naked eye (with a simple retractor type laryngoscope), use of a fibreoptic scope can only make the situation more difficult. Additionally, the very small objective lens with its wide angle of view is easily obscured by blood and secretions.

Principles and design

The pathways through which the illumination and the image pass consist of thousands of very fine glass fibres, each typically of the order of 10 μm in diameter. Each fibre consists of a central glass core surrounded by a thin cladding of another type of glass with a different refractive index to that of the core glass. As a result of the difference in refractive indices at the interface of the two materials, light entering the glass fibre undergoes total internal reflection along the length of the fibre to emerge at the other end (Fig. 8.62).

For the purpose of transmitting illumination, the arrangement of the fibres is unimportant. For image transmission, however, the arrangement of the fibres relative to one another must be identical at either end of the bundle, as each fibre carries a tiny portion of the overall image (in the same way that many small dots make up the printed image in a newspaper). This is called a coherent bundle.

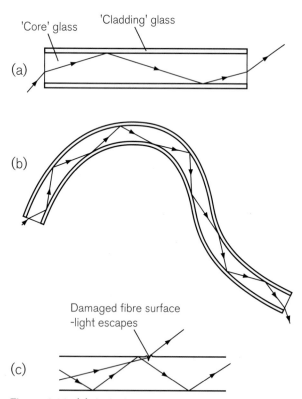

Figure 8.62 (a) A single optical fibre. Note that the light ray is repeatedly internally reflected from the interface between the core and cladding glass. **(b)** If the fibre is curved, the ray is still internally reflected within it. **(c)** If the surface of the fibre is damaged, the light ray may not be totally internally reflected and some light may escape from the bundle.

The fibres are so fine that they are easily flexible and they are lubricated so that they can move relative to each other. The whole bundle may therefore be flexed.

The insertion tube of the typical flexible fibreoptic scope (Fig. 8.63) carries:

- two light bundles, running from the umbilical cord to the tip of the scope;
- one image bundle, running from the eyepiece and its lens system to the objective lens at the tip of the scope;
- one 'working' or 'biopsy' channel of a width dictated by the primary purpose of the endoscope; and
- two angulation wires, which control the more flexible tip of the device.

These are then held together with a stainless steel spiral wrap followed by a stainless steel braid before being covered in a waterproof material to give a rigid cross-section whilst allowing overall flexibility (Fig. 8.64). The fibrescope, whilst able to bend in any plane, is axially rigid to twisting forces, thus rotation of the control handle results in similar rotation of the tip of the device. This forms the basis for control of the tip, which can be rotated so that angulation of the tip, which occurs in only one plane relative to the scope, can be made to take place in any direction.

The fibrescope uses a powerful external cold light source so that the tissues are not damaged by radiant heat. Modern scopes have a detachable light cable which can be replaced by a miniature battery operated light source (Fig. 8.65). These are not normally powerful enough for use with the video camera.

The working channel is used to inject drugs or for suction via the valved port which may be connected to an external high vacuum source.

Usage

Intubating fibrescopes are available with insertion tubes ranging in size from 2.5 mm external diameter for use in infants (this smallest size usually has no working channel) through to over 6 mm with proportionately larger working channels. Only the channels on the largest sizes (primarily bronchoscopes with working channels over 2 mm) are wide enough for aspirating secretions or blood with any effectiveness; oropharyngeal secretions are best tackled with a handheld Yankauer sucker. A device with an external diameter of about 3.5 mm is optimal for use in adults (and non-specialist paediatric practice) giving the best combination of:

- stiffness for ease of insertion; and
- bore, for access and endotracheal tube compatibility.

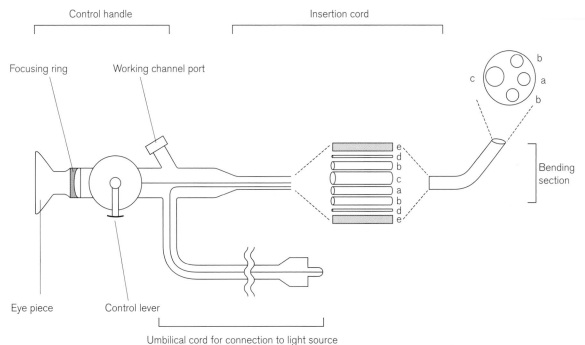

Figure 8.63 Schematic diagram of flexible intubating fibrescope. a, coherent fibreoptic bundle for image transmission; b, light transmission bundles for illumination; c, working channel; d, angulation wires; e, outer casing with spiral wrap and flexible steel braid.

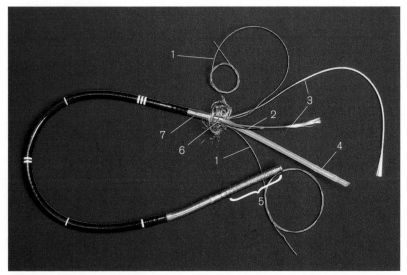

Figure 8.64 Cut away photograph of Olympus intubating fibrescope to show constituent parts. 1, Angulation wire; 2, coherent bundle; 3, light transmission bundle; 4, working channel; 5, bending section; 6, spiral steel wrap; 7, flexible steel braid.

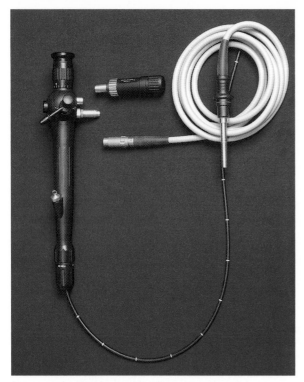

Figure 8.65 Storz 'portable' flexible intubating fibrescope with choice of battery operated and remote light sources.

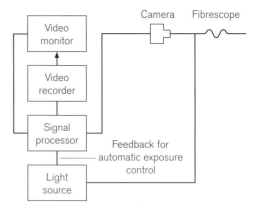

Figure 8.66 Arrangement and interconnection of components for a fibreoptic intubation trolley. The video monitor can toggle between a live image from the camera or playback recorded images.

The advent of the miniature video camera has revolutionized fibreoptic endoscopy. Without doubt these devices should be used with a video monitor rather than with the operator's eye at the eyepiece. The advantages in anaesthetic practice are:

- improvements in teaching techniques;
- more useful assistance from the anaesthetic team, e.g. jaw lift is better maintained by someone who can see the effect it has on the laryngeal view enjoyed by the endoscopist;
- more holistic view of patient's condition if not squinting through an eyepiece and hence less goal obsessed approach to endoscopy/intubation;
- facility to record images for review and documentation; and
- operator comfort.

Figure 8.66 shows the arrangement of components on a typical fibreoptic intubation trolley (Fig. 8.67). Ideally a printer able to capture still images from the outputs of the signal processor or video recorder should also be incorporated.

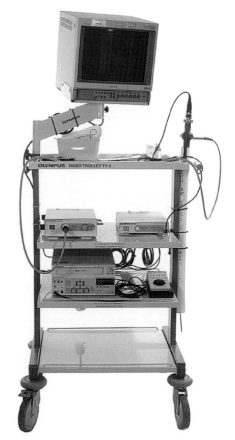

Figure 8.67 A fibreoptic intubation trolley.

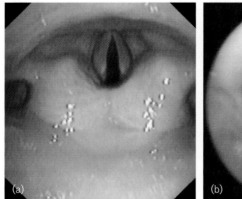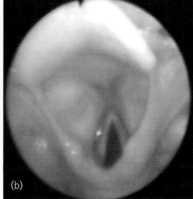

Figure 8.68 **(a)** Image from an Olympus digital video intubating fibrescope; **(b)** image from optical system for comparison of image quality.

The advent of the miniaturized CCD (Charge Coupling Device, effectively the 'retina' of modern electronic cameras), has allowed a new generation of flexible fibre-optic endoscopes where the CCD is placed at the distal tip of the instrument and hence the image suffers no loss from transmission along a length of glass fibres whilst also dispensing with the expense of the coherent fibre image transmission bundle (Fig. 8.68). Such instruments obviously do not have an eyepiece and must be used with a monitor. They are not yet commonplace for airway applications.

Care of the fibrescope

The fibrescope must be cleaned and disinfected following use. Modern devices are fully immersible, this being denoted on Olympus equipment by a blue ring around the control handle (a red ring denotes an item such as the light cable which may be autoclaved). This is best done immediately following use by gentle scrubbing with a nailbrush and soapy water to remove adherent material followed by immersion in a proprietary sterilizing solution and final rinsing in sterile water. Automated machines exist which can even produce a printed paper trail to document completion of the process. The working channel also should be cleaned with a dedicated brush and subsequently flushed with appropriate solutions. Some manufacturers produce immersible and even autocleaveable cameras.

Fibreoptic intubation

Fibreoptic laryngoscopy via the oral or nasotracheal route may be performed on both the awake or asleep patient.

In a patient who is awake following suitable topical anaesthesia or nerve block, the fibrescope may be inserted, advanced behind the tongue and into the larynx. Once in the trachea, a tracheal tube which has been previously loaded onto the fibrescope, is advanced off the scope to lie within the trachea, and the fibrescope is then removed. The patient may be encouraged to protrude the tongue and or lower jaw to create the space in the pharynx necessary for the fibrescope to be able to view, identify and advance through the airway. Deep respiration assists the identification of the larynx if needed. Intubation of the awake rather than anaesthetized patient is often easier for these reasons. Sedation may be used for additional patient comfort but must not render the patient un-cooperative or unconscious. For this reason 'sedation' based on the titration of short acting opiates is preferable in that the antitussive and analgesic properties are useful whilst the patient retains the ability to obey commands and pharmacological antagonism is easy in case of overdosage.

Training. Competent fibreoptic intubation requires a modicum of training and the maintenance of skills by regular deployment. 'Hand-eye coordination' and the control of the fibrescope may be learnt by most with only brief practice on an obstacle course, which may be made in minutes from items found in any anaesthetic room. Thereafter, familiarization with airway anatomy as seen through the fibrescope is necessary. This is simplest and safest on the apnoeic anaesthetized, paralyzed and pre-oxygenated patient.[66] If necessary an assistant provides jaw thrust or tongue traction.

Associated equipment

Endotracheal tubes. The ideal tube for intubation over a fibrescope would have a narrow kink resistant wall with a blunt tapered tip that fits the fibrescope closely so that it may follow the scope easily without snagging on nasal or laryngeal structures[67] although this, of course, would severely restrict the size of endotracheal tube orifice. Dedicated tubes are not yet available in spite of several prototype designs,[68] but Rüsch produce a centring aid designed to bridge the gap from scope to tube. Tubes with soft short bevels, such as the Portex Ivory and the Mallinckrodt reinforced ranges with an internal diameter of 6–7 mm, are generally preferred by specialists.

Bite Blocks. For oral intubation, a dental prop or bite block (Fig. 8.69) ensures that expensive fibrescopes are not inadvertently bitten and is comfortable for the patient.

Conduit airways aim to make oral intubation easier by centring the insertion point in the mouth and delivering the fibrescope closer to the larynx as well as acting as a supraglottic airway (Fig. 8.4). A number of open or split designs are available which allow the fibrescope to be separated from the airway after tracheal insertion so as not to limit the size of tracheal tube that may be used for intubation. They also function as a bite block; but they make tongue protrusion, which is a helpful manoeuvre, quite difficult. They are not necessary for awake intubation and for the trainee endoscopist they remove too much of the learning that may be gained from an oral intubation. The LMA, as a conduit, is discussed separately below.

Tongue Forceps with atraumatic broad-ridged rubber inserts at the tip (Fig. 8.70) allow tongue retraction to create space in the pharynx for fibreoptic intubation and for injection of local anaesthesia.

Ventilation/intubation masks. Where anaesthesia is maintained with an inhalational anaesthetic, endoscopy

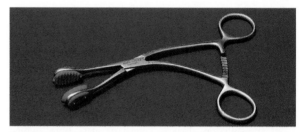

Figure 8.70 Tongue forceps, surprisingly tolerable!

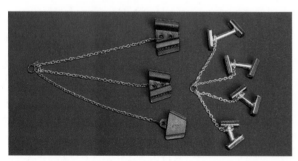

Figure 8.69 Dental props are ideal bite blocks for awake oral intubation as they allow tongue protrusion. The all rubber McKesson pattern on the left are more comfortable.

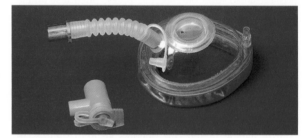

Figure 8.71 Facemask with perforated silicone membrane allowing fibreoptic intubation on the anaesthetized patient, the tube can be forced through the membrane, which is replaceable. The same effect can be achieved using the Mainz Universal Adapter (pictured alongside) and an ordinary facemask.

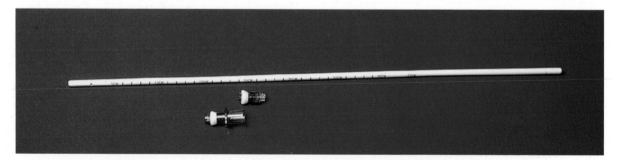

Figure 8.72 The Aintree Intubation Catheter, with Rapi-fit® Luer–Lok and ISO 15 mm adaptors.

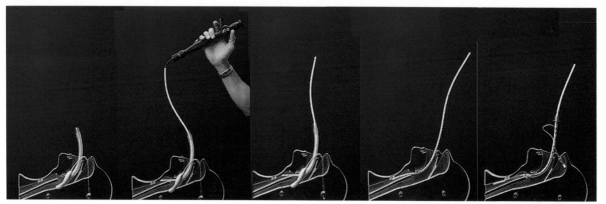

Figure 8.73 Photographic sequence to show fibreoptic intubation through the LMA using the Aintree Intubation Catheter.

may be performed through a mask or anglepiece with a silicone rubber diaphragm with an orifice that stretches to accommodate an endotracheal tube (Fig. 8.71). Such arrangements are difficult to use.

Aintree Intubation Catheter (AIC) (Fig. 8.72). Developed in Liverpool as 'a ventilation-exchange bougie' and first described in 1996,[69] the AIC allows fibreoptic intubation through the LMA or other supraglottic airway. Produced as a single use device by Cook, it is a 56 cm-long hollow plastic catheter that will fit over fibrecopes of 4.0 mm or less diameter, leaving the bending section of the scope free. The assembly is easily passed through the LMA and into the trachea (Fig. 8.73). The fibrescope is then removed followed by the LMA to leave the AIC in the trachea. Tracheal tubes of 7 mm or greater may then be railroaded into place over this. For rescue oxygenation a 15 mm male ISO adapter and female Luer–Lok adapter are both supplied in the package. Great care must be taken if jetting through wide-bore catheters placed close to the carina, for which a much lower driving pressure should be used. The combination of LMA, AIC and fibrescope constitutes a powerful technique for airway management because:

- the standard LMA is a familiar device with a proven track record for establishing an airway;
- the cuff of the LMA seals off the larynx from any blood or debris emanating from above, thus the conduit protects the fibrescope from its greatest adversaries; and
- an absolute minimum of fibreoptic skills are needed to rapidly manipulate the scope into the trachea, the technique is thus within reach of almost all anaesthetists.

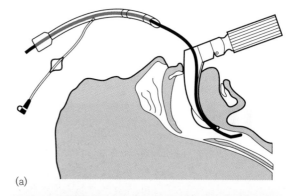

(a)

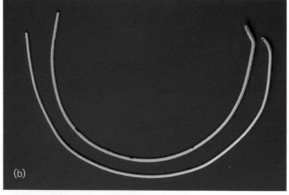

(b)

Figure 8.74 **(a)** The endotracheal tube introducer with coudé tip; **(b)** the Eschmann gum-elastic bougie and the blue single use Frova introducer from Cook®.

AIDS FOR INTUBATION/TUBE EXCHANGE

Bougies and stylets

Occasionally at direct laryngoscopy, the larynx may be only partially visualized or hidden behind the epiglottis and beyond reach with the normal curvature of an endotracheal tube. Intubation may then possibly be accomplished by either:

- altering the curvature of the endotracheal tube using a malleable plastic coated metal stylet; or
- initially inserting a long thin gum-elastic bougie (GEB) and using this as a guide over which the tube may be passed (rail-roaded) into the trachea (Fig. 8.74).

Credited to Dr P Venn, the GEB with a coudé tip was designed in the 1970s as the Eschmann Tracheal Tube Introducer (now available from Portex Ltd).[70,71] It has been hugely successful due to the angled tip and the memory of the material for holding a curve. Latto, in his surveys of UK anaesthetic practice, has found the preference for the GEB over other aids at difficult direct laryngoscopy to rise from 45% in 1984 to 100% in 1996.[72]

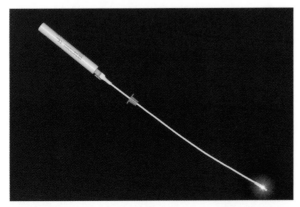

Figure 8.75 The lighted stylet.

Repeated autoclaving rapidly renders the material brittle. The new single use versions of the device in plastic do not generally have the same characteristics in use[73] and some are particularly unsatisfactory.

Cook have recently marketed the single use hollow Frova introducer (Fig. 8.74b) which has a comparable 'memory' to the GEB, and is supplied with a Rapifit adapter in Luer–Lok and ISO 15 mm fittings to allow gas sampling or oxygenation.

Light wand

A logical development from the stylet, is the lighted stylet, allowing transillumination of the neck tissues as a further aide to positioning of the tracheal tube (Fig. 8.75).

Trachlight

The Trachlight (Laerdal Medical) develops the concept one stage further by aiming to allow intubation using only transillumination of the neck (without laryngoscopy). As such, the stylet is more rigid than the aforementioned aids to permit some tissue retraction.

A re-usable handle houses the battery to which are attached particularly bright disposable lighted stylets of three different sizes. The tracheal tube is mounted on the stylet assembly and is held by the handle (Fig. 8.76). The stylet is bent into an L-shape before insertion into the mouth. The non-dominant hand grips and elevates the lower incisors and mandible and the Trachlight is rotated into place to transilluminate the thyroid cartilage in the midline. At this point the wire core of the stylet is held steady whilst the rest of the Trachlight and tracheal tube are advanced into the trachea. The device is then disconnected from the tracheal tube and removed.

Intubation in skilled hands appears simple and smooth enough for routine use, with some reporting only a 1% failure rate.[74,75] Sore throat and tracheal bleeding are

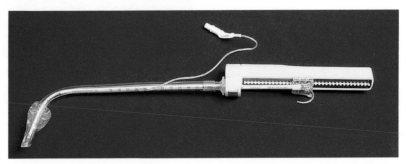

Figure 8.76 The Trachlight prepared for intubation.

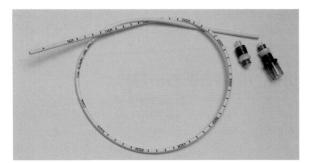

Figure 8.77 The Cook® Airway Exchange Catheter with Rapi-Fit® adaptors.

reported[75] and use in obese patients may not be straightforward.[76]

Airway Exchange Catheter

Endotracheal tubes can be more safely exchanged over a catheter or bougie that has been inserted through the tube into the trachea, the new tube then being simply railroaded into place over this. The Airway Exchange Catheter (AEC) by Cook® (Fig. 8.77), is long enough to allow comfortable removal of a nasal endotracheal tube without risk of losing hold of the catheter. Where there may be doubt as to the ability of a postoperative or sedated patient to maintain a patent airway following extubation, the AEC may be inserted first and extubation may be performed 'over' this. It may then be removed some hours later or used to guide re-intubation if needed. Because the plastic remoulds at body temperature and the AEC is smaller than the tracheal tube it replaces it is usually well tolerated[77] by patients. Oxygen insufflation or jetting is possible as with the Aintree Catheter (see above).

Retrograde intubation

The larynx may be intubated in the following manner. A cannula is introduced diagonally through the cricothyroid membrane with its tip pointing cephalad. A flexible 'J' tipped guide wire is then passed via the cannula and the tip grasped in the mouth or as it emerges from the nose. A plastic catheter is passed over the J tip and back along the guide wire to provide a stiffer guide over which the endotracheal tube may be railroaded. An epidural catheter and other disparate items may be used where dedicated kit (Fig. 8.78) is not available. This 'lo-tech' approach also has the advantage of being applicable where blood and secretions prevent use of the flexible fibrescope.

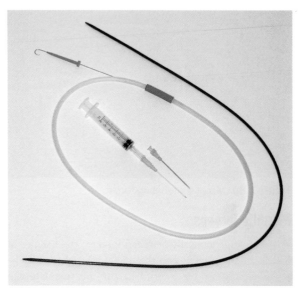

Figure 8.78 A retrograde intubation kit, the principle components of which are a stiff guide wire with a soft flexible J tip and an introducing cannula. A 70 cm 11 Fr Teflon catheter runs over the guide wire to give extra stiffness for railroading the endotracheal tube.

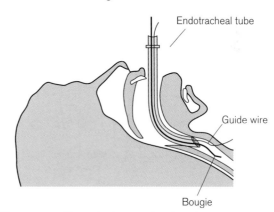

Figure 8.79 To assist in ensuring that the tracheal tube follows down the trachea after removal of the guide wire, a gum elastic bougie can be introduced through the tracheal tube first.

The very high entry point of the wire into the trachea means that only a short length of tracheal tube can be inserted before it abuts the anterior tracheal wall and the guide wire must be withdrawn (proximally). To insure being able to insert the tube further into the trachea before withdrawing the wire, a gum elastic bougie may be inserted through the endotracheal tube once it is within the trachea (Fig. 8.79), or the emerging guide wire from the larynx may be introduced up the operating channel of a flexible fibrescope with a preloaded tracheal tube.

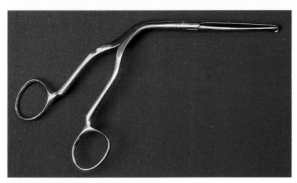

Figure 8.80 Magill's intubating forceps.

Magill's forceps

These are ergonomically designed forceps, the handles of which fit comfortably into the operator's right hand like a pair of scissors (Fig. 8.80). The tips are spatulate and ridged for gripping the tip of an endotracheal tube so that it can be lifted from the back of the pharynx and into the larynx.

DRUG DELIVERY SYSTEMS

Nebulizing sprays are used for the topical application of local anaesthetic solutions (e.g. 4% lignocaine to the larynx and trachea). The principles of the Forrester spray are shown in Figure 8.81. When the air reservoir bulb is compressed, a part of this is blown into the chamber containing the solution. This forces the latter up and along a narrow bore delivery tube to the tip of the apparatus. The rest of the air from the bulb is directed to the tip where it mixes with and nebulizes the solution. These sprays tend to block if they are not cleaned shortly after use, because the solution remaining at the nozzle dries

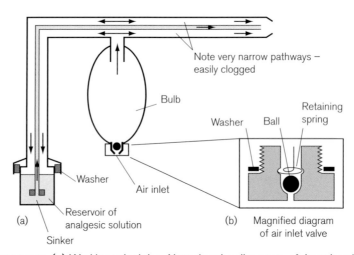

Figure 8.81 The Forrester spray. **(a)** Working principles. Note that the diameters of the tubes leading to the nozzles are very small and if analgesic solution is allowed to collect and crystallize out in this area the spray will be blocked. **(b)** The air inlet valve.

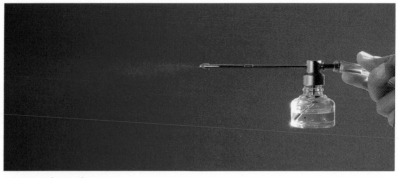

Figure 8.82 Oxygen powered atomizer.

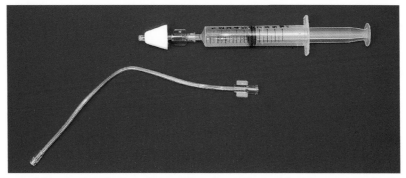

Figure 8.83 The Mucosal Atomization Device, above with syringe attached for intranasal application, and below for intraoral and laryngeal use.

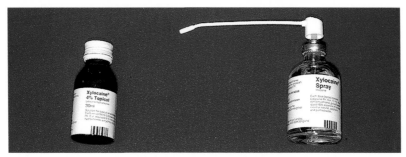

Figure 8.84 10% solution lignocaine in an oily base presented as a metered spray dispenser giving 10 mg lignocaine per spray (0.1 ml). The 4% solution is ideal for topical analgesia of the larynx and trachea.

out, leaving crystals that block the small orifice. This may be avoided by rinsing them out with distilled water or spirit, before cleaning and disinfecting for subsequent usage.

The same principles are used in atomizers using pressurized oxygen to drive the nebulization (Fig. 8.82).

For use through the fibrescope, single use dispensers are available with controlled dosing of drug from a small syringe using oxygen as the propellant.

The Mucosal Atomization Device (Wolfe Tory Medical; Salt Lake City, USA) (Fig. 8.83) simply relies on forcing solution through a very narrow orifice for atomization. Lignocaine is available for topical use as a 4% solution or as a 10% solution in a multi-dose metered dispenser (Fig. 8.84), in spite of the small volume delivered (0.1 ml), because of the concentration of drug care must be taken to avoid overdosage, particularly in children.

REFERENCES

1. Verghese C (1999). Airway Management. *Current Opinion in Anaesthesia.* **12**: 667–674.

2. Thomas DI (1999) Overcoming the beard. *Anaesthesia* **54**: 100.

3. Vincent C, Ames WA (1998) The bearded airway. *Anaesthesia* **53**: 1034–1035.

4. Brain AI (1983) The laryngeal mask – a new concept in airway management. *British Jounral of Anaesthesia* **55**: 801–805.

5. Ocker H, Wenzel V, Schmucker P *et al.* (2002) A comparison of the Laryngeal Tube with the Laryngeal Mask Airway during routine surgical procedures. *Anaesthesia and Analgesia* **95**: 1094–1097.

6. Asai T, Kawashima A, Hidaka I, Kawachi S (2002) The laryngeal tube compared with the larygeal mask: insertion, gas leak pressure and gastric insufflation. *British Journal of Anaesthesia* **89**: 729–732.

7. Brimacombe J (1996) Analysis of 1500 laryngeal mask uses by one anaesthetist in adults undergoing routine anaesthesia. *Anaesthesia* **51**: 76–80.

8. Nolan JD (2001) Prehospital and resuscitative airway care: should the gold standard be reassessed? *Current Opinion in Critical Care* **7**: 413–421.

9. Pandit JJ, MacLAchlan K, Dravid RM, Popat MT (2002) Comparison of times to achieve tracheal intubation with

three techniques using the laryngeal or intubating laryngeal mask airway. *Anaesthesia* **57:** 128–132

10. McNeillis NJ, Timberlake C, Avidan MS, *et al.* (2001) Fibreoptic views through the laryngeal mask and the intubating laryngeal mask. *European Journal of Anaesthesia* **18:** 471–475.

11. Keller C, Brimacombe J, Puhringer F (2000) A fibreoptic scoring system to assess the position of laryngeal mask airway devices. Interobserver variability and a comparison between the standard, flexible and intubating laryngeal mask airways. *Anaesth. Intensiv. Notfall. Schmerz.* **35:** 692–694.

12. Kihara S, Yaguchi Y, Brimacombe J, *et al.* (2001) Routine use of the intubating laryngeal mask airway results in increased upper airway morbidity. *Canadian Journal of Anaesthesia* **48:** 604–608

13. Keller C, Brimacombe J (2000) Mucosal pressure and oropharyngeal leak pressure with the ProSeal versus laryngeal mask airway in anaesthetized paralysed patients. *British Journal of Anaesthesia* **85:** 262–266.

14. Brimacombe J, Keller C (2000) The ProSeal Laryngeal Mask Airway: A Randomized, Crossover Study with the Standard Laryngeal Mask Airway in Paralyzed, Anesthetized Patients. *Anaesthesiology* **93:**104–109.

15. Miller DM, Light D (2003) Laboratory and clinical comparisons of the Streamlined Liner of the Pharynx Airway (SLIPA(tm)) with the laryngeal mask airway. *Anaesthesia* **58:** 136–142.

16. LippM, Thierbach A, Daubländer M, Dick W (1996) *Clinical evaluation of the Combitube.* 18th Annual Meeting of the European Academy of Anaesthesiology, August 1996: Copenhagen, Denmark. p. 43.

17. Vézina D, Lessard MR, Bussières J, *et al.* (1998) Complications assosciated with the Esophageal-Tracheal Combitube. *Canadian Journal of Anaesthesia* **45:** 76–80.

18. Klein, H, Williamson M, Sue-Ling HM *et al.* (1997)Esophageal rupture associated with the use of the Combitube(tm). *Anaesthesia and Analgesia* **85:** 937–939.

19. Asai T, Kawashima A, Hidaka I, Kawachi S (2002) The laryngeal tube compared with the laryngeal mask: insertion, gas leak pressure and gastric insufflation. *British Jounral of Anaesthesia* **89:** 729–732.

20. Cook TM, Gupta K, Gabbott DA, Nolan JP (2001) An evaluation of the Airway Management Device. *Anaesthesia* **56:** 660–664.

21. Sivasankar R, Bahlmann UB, Stacey MR, *et al.* (2003) An evaluation of the modified Airway Management Device. *Anaesthesia* **58:** 558–5561.

22. Ahmed SM, Maroof M, Khan RM, *et al.* (2003) A comparison of the laryngeal mask airway and PAXpress (tm) for short surgical procedures. *Anaesthesia* **58:** 42–44.

23. Cook TM, Rudd P, McCormick B, *et al.* (2003) An evaluation of the PAxpress Pharyngeal Airway. *Anaesthesia* **58:**191.

24. Gillespie NA (1941) *Endotracheal Anaesthesia.* USA: The University of Wisconsin Press. pp. 6–25.

25. Vesalius A (1542) *De Humanis Corporis Fabrica.* 1st edn. 658.

26. Trendelenburg F (1871) *Archiv f Klin Chirurg.* **12:** 121.

27. Waters RM, Rovenstine EA and Guedel AE (1933) Endotracheal anaesthesia and its historical development. *Anaesthesia and Analgesia* **12:** 196.

28. MacEwen W (1880) *British Medical Journal* 2: 122 and 163.

29. Meltzer SJ, Auer J (1909) *Journal of Exploratory Medicine* **11:** 622.

30. Koh KF, Hare JD, Calder I (1998) Small tubes revisited. *Anaesthesia* **53(1):** 46–50.

31. Stenqvist O, Sonander H, Nilson K (1979) Small endotracheal tubes. Ventilator and intratracheal pressures during controlled ventilation. *British Journal of Anaesthesia* **51(4):** 375–380.

32. Stout DM, Bishop MJ, Dwersteg JF, Cullen FC (1987) Correlation of endotracheal tube size with sore throat and hoarseness following general anaesthesia. *Anaesthesiology* **67:** 419–421.

33. Avrahami E, Frishman E, Spierer I, *et al.* (1995) CT of minor intubation trauma with clinical correlation. *European Journal of Radiology* **20:** 68–71.

34. Shapiro M, Wilson RK, Casar G *et al.* (1986) Work of breathing through different sized endotracheal tubes. *Critical Care Medicine* **14:** 1028–1031.

35. Nunn JF, Ezi-Ashi TI (1961)The respiratory effects of resistance to breathing in anaesthetised man. *Anaesthesiology* **22:** 174–185.

36. Thornton HL (1944) Vinyl-'Portex' Tubing. *British Medical Journal* **Jul 1:**14.

37. Mallick A, Smith SN, Bodenham AR (1996) Local anaesthesia to the airway reduces sedation requirements in patients undergoing artificial ventilation. *British Journal of Anaesthesia* **77 (6):** 731–734.

38. Andrzejowski J, Francis G (2002) The efficacy of lidocaine administered via the LITA(tm) tracheal tube in attenuating the extubation response in beta-blocked patients following craniotomy. *Anaesthesia* **57(4):** 399–401.

39. Diachun CA, Tuninck BP, Brock-Utne JG (2001) Suppression of cough during emergence from general

anaesthesia: laryngotracheal lidocaine through a modified endotracheal tube. *Jounral of Clinical Anaesthesia* **13(6)**: 447–451.

40. Ciaglia P, Firsching R, Syniec C (1985) Elective percutaneous dilatational tracheostomy: a new simple bedside procedure – preliminary report. *Chest* **87**: 715–719.

41. Cooper RM (1998) Use and safety of percutaneous tracheostomy in intensive care: Report of a postal survey of ICU practice. *Anaesthesia* **53(12)**: 1209–1212.

42. Susanto I (2002) Comparing Percutaneous tracheostomy with open surgical tracheostomy: both will coexist until robust evidence becomes available [editorial]. *British Medical Journal* **324(7328)**: 3–4.

43. Griggs WM, Worthley LIG, Gilligan JE, *et al.* (1990) A simple percutaneous tracheostomy technique. *Surgery* **170**: 543–545.

44. Fikkers BG, van Heerbeek N, Krabbe PF, *et al.* (2002) Percutaneous tracheostomy with the guide wire dilating forceps technique: presentation of 171 consecutive patients. *Head and Neck* **24(7)**: 625–631.

45. Fantoni A, Ripamonti D (1997) A non-derivative, non-surgical tracheostomy: the translaryngeal method. *Intensive Care Medicine* **23(4)**: 386–392.

46. Diba A (2002) Transtracheal Jet Ventilation. *Anaesthesia and Intensive Care Medicine* **3(6)**: 207–209.

47. Layman PR (1983) Transtracheal Ventilation in Oral Surgery. *Annual Review of College Surgeons of England* **65**: 318–320.

48. Benumof JL, Scheller MS (1989) The importance of transtracheal Jet Ventilation in the Management of the difficult airway. *Anaesthesiology* **71**: 769–778.

49. Patel C, Diba A (2004) Measuring tracheal airway pressures during transtracheal jet ventilation: an observational study. *Anaesthesia* **59(3)**: 248–251.

50. Dollner R, Verch M, Schweiger P, *et al.* (2002) Long-term outcome after Griggs tracheostomy. *Journal of Otolaryngology* **31(6)**: 386–389.

51. Skilton RWH, Parry D, Arthurs GJ, Hiles P (1996) A study of the brightness of laryngoscope light. *Anaesthesia* **51(7)**: 667–672.

52. Twigg SJ, McCormick B, Cook TM (2003) Randomized evaluation of the performance of single-use laryngoscopes in simulated easy and difficult intubation. *British Journal of Anaesthesia* **90(1)**: 8–13.

53. Evans A, Vaughan RS, Hall JE, *et al.* (2003) A comparison of the forces exerted during laryngoscopy using disposable and non-disposable laryngoscope blades. *Anaesthesia* **58(9)**: 869–873.

54. Levitan RM, Ochroch EA (1999) Explaining the variable effect on laryngeal view obtained with the McCoy laryngoscope. *Anaesthesia* **54(6)**: 599–601.

55. Chisholm DG, Calder I (1997) Experience with the McCoy laryngoscope in difficult laryngoscopy. *Anaesthesia* **52(9)**: 906–908.

56. Leon O, Benhamou D (1998) Improvement of glottis visualization with a McCoy blade. *Annales Francaises d Anesthesie et de Reanimation* **17(1)**:68–71.

57. Cook TM, Tuckey JP (1996) A comparison between the Macintosh and the McCoy laryngoscope blades. *Anaesthesia* **51(10)**: 977–980.

58. Foley LJ, Ochroch EA (2000) Bridges to establish an emergency airway and alternate intubating techniques. *Critical Care Clinics* **16(3)**: 429–444.

59. Pearce AC, Shaw S, Macklin S (1996) Evaluation of the Upsherscope. A new rigid fibrescope. *Anaesthesia* **51(6)**: 561–564.

60. Fridrich P, Frass M, Krenn CG, *et al.* (1997) The UpsherScope in routine and difficult airway management: a randomized, controlled clinical trial. *Anesthesia and Analgesia* **85(6)**: 1377–1381.

61. Halligan M, Charters P (2003) A clinical evaluation of the Bonfils Intubation Fibrescope. *Anaesthesia* **58(11)**: 1087–1091.

62. Wong P, Lawrence C, Pearce A (2003) Intubation times for using the Bonfils intubation fibrescope. *British Journal of Anaesthesia* **91(5)**: 757.

63. Liem EB, Bjoraker DG, Gravenstein D (2003) New options for airway management: intubating fibreoptic stylets. *British Journal of Anaesthesia* **91(3)**: 408–418.

64. Calder I, Pearce A, Towey R (1996) Classic paper: a fibreoptic endoscope used for tracheal intubation. *Anaesthesia* **51(6)**: 602.

65. Murphy P (1967) A fibreoptic endoscope used for tracheal intubation. *Anaesthesia* **22**: 489–491.

66. Popat M (2001) *Practical Fibreoptic Intubation*. Oxford: Butterworth-Heinemann. pp. 83–85.

67. Jones HE, Pearce AC, Moore P (1993) Fibreoptic intubation. Influence of tracheal tube tip design. *Anaesthesia* **48(8)**: 672–674.

68. Kristensen MS (2003) The Parker Flex-Tip Tube versus a Standard Tube for Fiberoptic Orotracheal Intubation: A Randomized Double-blind Study. *Anaesthesiology* **98(2)**: 354–358.

69. Atherton DPL, O'Sullivan E, Lowe D, Charters P (1996) A ventilation-exchange bougie for fibreoptic intubations with the laryngeal mask airway. *Anaesthesia* **51(2)**: 1123–1126.

70. Venn PH (1993) The gum elastic bougie. *Anaesthesia* **48**: 274–275.

71. Henderson JJ (2003) Development of the 'gum-elastic bougie'. *Anaesthesia* **58(1)**: 103–104.

72. Latto IP, Stacey M, Mecklenburgh J, Vaughan RS (2002) Survey of the use of the gum elastic bougie in clinical practice. *Anaesthesia* **57(4)**: 379–384.

73. Hodzovic I, Latto IP, Henderson JJ (2003) Bougie trauma - what trauma? *Anaesthesia* **58(2)**: 192–193.

74. Hung OR, Pytka MD, Morris I, *et al.* (1995) Clinical Trial of a New Lightwand Device (Trachlight) to Intubate the Trachea. *Anaesthesiology* **83(3)**: 509–514.

75. Tsutsui T, Setoyama K (1002) A clinical evaluation of blind orotracheal intubation using Trachlight in 511 patients. *Masui* **50(8)**: 854–858.

76. Nishiyama T, Matsukawa T, Hanaoka K (1999) Optimal length and angle of a new lightwand device (Trachlight). *Jounal of Clinical Anaesthesia* **11(4)**: 332–335.

77. Loudermilk EP, Hartmannsgruber M, Stoltzfus DP, Langevin PB (1997) A prospective study of the safety of tracheal extubation using a pediatric airway exchange catheter for patients with a known difficult airway. *Chest* **111(6)**: 1660–1665.

FURTHER READING

Cook TM (2003) Novel Airway Devices: Spoilt for Choice? [editorial] *Anaesthesia* **58**: 107–110.

Diba A (2002) Transtracheal JetVentilation. *Anaesthesia and Intensive Care Medicine* **3(6)**: 207–209.

Jaeger JM, Durbin CG (1999) Special Purpose Endotracheal Tubes. *Resp Care* **44**: 661–683.

Latto IP, Vaughn RS (eds) (1997) *Difficulties in Tracheal Intubation*. 2nd edn. London: W.B. Saunders.

Popat M (2001) *Practical Fibreoptic Intubation*. Oxford: Butterworth-Heinemann.

9

Equipment for the inhalation of oxygen and other gases

Daniel W Wheeler

The administration of supplemental oxygen is a fundamental part of the treatment of the acutely ill patient and those undergoing surgery. The equipment required has evolved to facilitate its use in a wide variety of circumstances.

The benefits of supplemental oxygen are:
- as a treatment for hypoxaemia due to hypoventilation, or due to gas transfer or ventilation/perfusion abnormalities (e.g. heart failure, anaesthesia);
- to improve oxygen supply to tissues, when a disease process causes oxygen demand to outstrip delivery (e.g. malignant hyperpyrexia);
- as a specific treatment for certain conditions, e.g. carbon monoxide poisoning, postoperative nausea and vomiting; and
- to allow humans to survive at very low atmospheric pressure, e.g. mountaineering and high altitude flying.

Oxygen is also administered in combination with other gases for therapeutic or other purposes. For example:
- *Entonox* A mixture of 50% O_2 and 50% nitrous oxide (N_2O) that is used in anaesthesia, as an analgesic both in labour and for short procedures such as reduction of fractures, removal of drains or dressing changes;
- *Heliox* A mixture of 21% O_2 and 79% helium that is used increasingly with additional oxygen entrainment as a temporizing measure in the treatment of acute exacerbation of obstructive pulmonary disorders;[1]

- *Diving gases* (e.g. *Trimix*) Mixtures of oxygen, helium and nitrogen at a variety of different ratios are used to allow deep sea diving.

The method of administration of supplemental oxygen will depend on the cause and severity of the conditions mentioned above. If supplemental oxygen at or just above atmospheric pressure is required to saturate the haemoglobin in the bloodstream, the treatment is normally referred to as *normobaric oxygen therapy*. If supplemental oxygen has to be delivered by dissolving it in plasma at pressures greater than atmospheric, it is classified *as hyperbaric oxygen therapy.*

NORMOBARIC OXYGEN THERAPY

There are almost as many devices that deliver oxygen as there are indications for its use. These devices may be classified by the extent that the patient relies upon the device to correct any deficiency in oxygen delivery (Table 9.1).

Low dependency systems

When supplemental oxygen alone is required, it may be delivered by a miscellany of devices. These can be divided into two groups by convention.

Table 9.1 A classification of oxygen delivery devices by degrees of dependency

	Definition	Respiratory pattern	Examples
Low dependency	When supplemental oxygen alone is sufficient to correct hypoxia	Spontaneous breathing	Nasal prongs, standard facemasks
Medium dependency	When supplemental oxygen and a degree of respiratory assistance is required	Spontaneous breathing but requires additional support, for example CPAP	CPAP mask and equipment
High dependency	When supplemental oxygen and full respiratory support is required	Unreliable or absent. Requires NIPPV or IPPV	Involves use of intensive care, operating theatre or non-invasive ventilators

CPAP = continuous positive airway pressure
NIPPV = non-invasive positive pressure ventilation
IPPV = intermittent positive pressure ventilation

Variable performance devices

With these devices, the oxygen concentration delivered to the upper airway varies with the phase and pattern of respiration (as well as the selected oxygen flow rate). As an example, consider a standard oxygen mask applied to the face (Fig. 9.1). Oxygen flows into the facemask from a continuous supply and quickly fills the relatively small volume of the mask (approximately 200 ml) when the patient is neither inhaling or exhaling. The oxygen then begins to escape through the mask's vents and where the seal against the face is imperfect.

When the subject breathes in, the oxygen-rich mask contents are inhaled first. If the tidal volume exceeds mask volume, air is then entrained from outside and mixes with the supplied oxygen before entering the subject's upper airway. The fraction of inspired oxygen (F_IO_2) is reduced during this phase as the air dilutes the oxygen, the extent of which depends on the ratio of the flow rate of supplied oxygen to the inspiratory flow rate of the patient. In physiological terms, this means that for a given oxygen flow rate, the F_IO_2 will be higher when the patient's respiratory rate, tidal volume, and peak inspiratory flow rate are low, and *vice versa*.

The concept of how the difference between peak inspiratory flow rate and oxygen delivery rate determines F_IO_2 is fundamental to the understanding of the performance of oxygen delivery devices and is a recurring theme throughout this chapter.

Mask construction and oxygen flow rate are also important in determining F_IO_2. If the mask volume

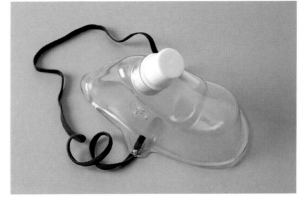

Figure 9.1 Standard adult facemask.

exceeds the patient's tidal volume, the F_IO_2 will be high as there is minimal air entrainment, although carbon dioxide accumulation and rebreathing will occur; especially at low oxygen flows. Masks with volumes substantially smaller than tidal volume tend to collapse during inhalation, making patients feel claustrophobic and thus likely to remove the mask. The ideal mask volume for an adult is approximately 200 ml with vents in the body through which air is entrained if peak inspiratory flow rate is high. Also, as the oxygen supply is increased, less air will be required for entrainment and the inhaled F_IO_2 will be higher.

The complex interplay between the factors that determine F_IO_2 (Table 9.2) means that most oxygen delivery devices deliver a variable F_IO_2. The extent of this

Table 9.2 The major determinants of F_IO_2 delivered by variable performance masks

Equipment factors	Oxygen flow rate Mask volume Quality of mask fit Area of holes in mask
Patient factors	Respiratory rate Tidal volume Peak inspiratory flow rate
Additional factors	Presence of other gases or vapours, e.g. humidifier

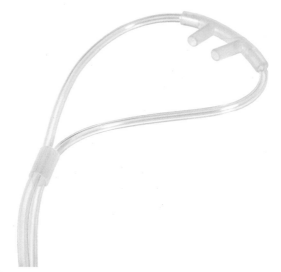

Figure 9.2 Nasal cannulae.

variability is difficult to quantify as normal methods of measuring breathing pattern are impractical in clinical practice. The latter require a mouthpiece that interferes with oxygen flow in the mask, and subjects are not able to breathe with a fixed respiratory pattern long enough for accurate measurements to be recorded. These difficulties explain why the factors most influential in determining F_IO_2 are still unclear.

As the volume of the mask as a reservoir plays an important role in its performance, low dependency oxygen delivery devices can be classified by their reservoir *capacity*.

No capacity oxygen delivery devices

Nasal cannulae (also known as nasal prongs or specs) deliver unhumidified oxygen to the nasopharynx (Fig. 9.2). They are more comfortable and less claustrophobic than facemasks, allowing talking, eating and drinking, making them the most suitable means of delivering long-term oxygen, especially at home. The main drawbacks are that F_IO_2 is unpredictable and oxygen flow greater than $2 \, l \, min^{-1}$ can cause discomfort and drying of the nasal mucosa. Clinical and laboratory studies have shown an enormous variability with respiratory pattern, with F_IO_2 ranging between 0.26 and 0.90.[2,3] An improved design is the nasal sponge (tipped) catheter, which is lodged in one nostril and effectively uses the nasopharynx as a small reservoir during the respiratory pause (Fig. 9.3).

Low capacity oxygen delivery devices (capacity <100 ml)

Facemasks for children, or tracheostomy masks (Fig. 9.4), have a volume of approximately 70–100 ml. Tracheostomy masks, especially, do not provide humidification without extra equipment, so are best suited for short-term use. In long-term use, oxygen may be humidified by

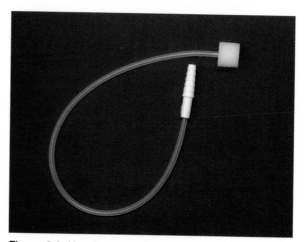

Figure 9.3 Nasal sponge tipped catheter.

using a 'Swedish nose' device (Fig. 9.5). This is essentially a small, light heat and moisture exchanger that connects to the tracheostomy tube by means of a 15 mm International Organization for Standardization (ISO) connector. Supplemental oxygen can be administered into this via a clip-on device. A Swedish nose may also provide 2.5–5 cmH$_2$O of positive end expiratory pressure (PEEP).

Medium capacity oxygen delivery devices (capacity 100–250 ml)

Standard adult facemasks are designed to cover the nose and mouth and have a capacity of approximately 175–200 ml (Fig. 9.1); there are a multitude of different designs. They are, almost without exception, made of transparent, soft plastic with an elastic strap to secure the

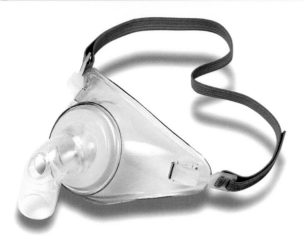

Figure 9.4 Tracheostomy mask.

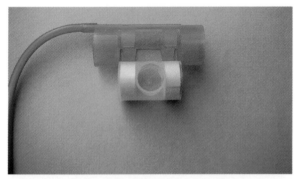

Figure 9.5 A 'Swedish nose' device for supplying supplemental oxygen on a long-term basis via a tracheostomy tube.

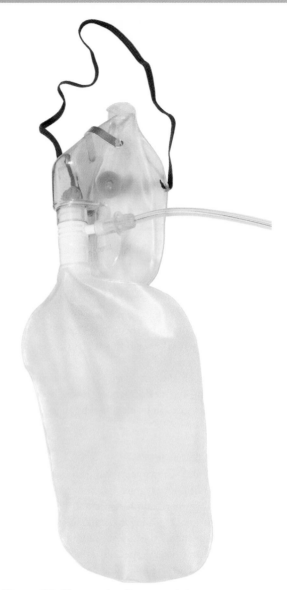

Figure 9.6 Facemask with reservoir bag.

mask in place. Some comprise a short deformable metal bar allowing the mask to be shaped around the nose to achieve a closer fit. Oxygen flow rates of $2-5\,l\,min^{-1}$ result in a highly variable and unpredictable F_IO_2. Rebreathing of CO_2 can occur with O_2 flow rates of less than $2\,l\,min^{-1}$ or if minute ventilation is very high.[4]

High capacity oxygen delivery devices (capacity 250–1500 ml)

Air is only entrained into a facemask when the patient's inspiratory flow rate exceeds the oxygen supply rate. To achieve a F_IO_2 near 1.0 (100% oxygen) by providing sufficient oxygen flow alone, rates in excess of $60\,l$ $O_2\,min^{-1}$ would be required, which is clearly impractical. Increasing mask size simply increases the risk of rebreathing CO_2. However, a great deal of oxygen delivered to the facemask is lost to the atmosphere whenever the patient's inspiratory flow rate is (a) *less* than the oxygen supply rate and (b) during exhalation. High capacity masks are designed to store some of this wasted oxygen in a 1100 ml reservoir bag attached to the facemask, thus providing a higher F_IO_2 (Fig. 9.6) With these devices, oxygen flows directly into the reservoir bag, which fills whenever the patient's inspiratory flow rate is less than the flow rate of delivered oxygen. The patient inhales oxygen preferentially from the reservoir bag and ambient air is not intentionally entrained. The incorporation of exterior flap valves on the vents in the body of the mask further reduces the possibility of air entrainment (some of which inevitably occurs between the mask edge

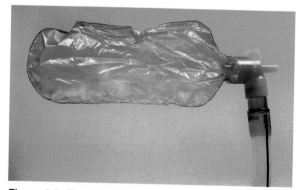

Figure 9.8 The T-Bag™ device for delivering supplemental oxygen via laryngeal mask airway or endotracheal tube.

Facemasks with reservoir bags probably deliver a F_IO_2 between 0.75 and 0.90 at oxygen flow rates of 12–$15\,l\,min^{-1}$. Some masks incorporate additional features, for example a small chimney containing a red polystyrene ball that moves up and down with respiration so that a patient's respiratory effort can be visualized and respiratory rate can easily be measured (Figure 9.7).[5]

A reservoir bag may also be attached to airway maintenance devices to improve the F_IO_2 delivered during emergence from anaesthesia. The T-Bag™ (Ultimate Medical Pty Ltd, Australia) (Fig. 9.8) consists of a reservoir bag with a capacity of 300 ml, attached via a 15 mm internal diameter ISO connector to a laryngeal mask airway (LMA) or endotracheal tube (ETT). There is a 3 mm connector to attach the oxygen tubing and a 10 mm port, which is open to the atmosphere. During inspiration, the reservoir bag, with its 15 mm aperture, provides a greater proportion of inspiratory gas. A smaller amount is entrained through the 10 mm port, which has a higher resistance to flow. During exhalation, this process is reversed until the reservoir bag is full. Subsequent exhalate leaves via the 10 mm port only. The T-Bag is light enough not to displace the LMA, provides visual confirmation of spontaneous ventilation and a F_IO_2 of up to 0.70 with an oxygen supply rate of $6\,l\,min^{-1}$. It is possible to ventilate patients briefly by occlusion of the 10 mm port, with additional volume being delivered by squeezing of the bag.

Very high capacity oxygen delivery devices (capacity > 1500ml)

Babies tolerate facemasks poorly and whilst small nasal cannulae are available, oxygen is frequently delivered in an incubator or via a head box or tent. Incubators make use of a metered oxygen source (see below) to allow F_IO_2 to be chosen with precision.

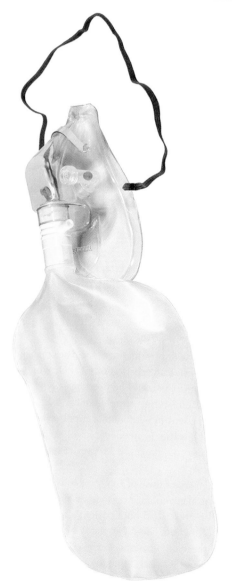

Figure 9.7 A Respi-Check facemask with device for detecting respiratory effort.

and the patient's face) but does not impede exhalation. Some manufacturers include a one-way valve between mask and reservoir bag, reducing rebreathing of CO_2. However, higher oxygen supply rates are required as exhaled dead space O_2 from the mask pharynx and upper trachea is prevented from entering the reservoir bag and is wasted. A valveless device is therefore most suitable when oxygen supplies are limited, but a valve is desirable if rebreathing of CO_2 would be detrimental, for example after head injury.

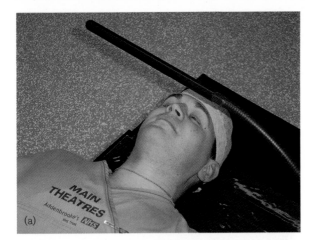

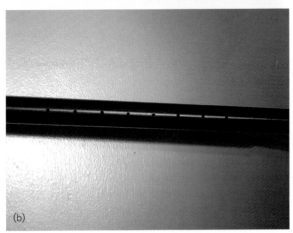

Figure 9.9 (a) Oxygen bar used for patients undergoing eye surgery under local anaesthesia. **(b)** Note the holes in the bar for the administration of oxygen.

During ophthalmic surgery under local anaesthesia, oxygen is sometimes administered under the drapes using an eye surgery bar (Figure 9.9a). The bar is hollow (Figure 9.9b). Oxygen is fed into the bar at one end and escapes through perforations in the bar where it is in close proximity to the patient. There are many different designs and some are 'home-made'. Oxygen flow under the drapes (which acts as a large reservoir) increases the F_IO_2, helps reduce rebreathing of CO_2, and provides a refreshing breeze on the patient's face, when otherwise they may begin to feel hot and claustrophobic.[6]

Fixed performance devices

When supplemental oxygen is delivered, the exact F_IO_2 is often irrelevant, as long as inhaled air is enriched with sufficient additional oxygen so that oxygen delivery to the tissues can meet their oxygen demand. However,

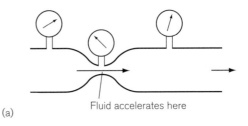

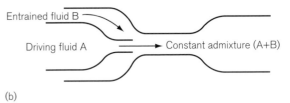

Figure 9.10 (a): Bernoulli Effect. **(b)** A Venturi.

there are circumstances when it is important to deliver a known F_IO_2 that does not vary with respiratory pattern. These are:

- When following guidelines for the management of patients with exacerbation of COPD, which state that an F_IO_2 of 0.28 should be used initially;[7,8]
- When administering supplemental oxygen to a critically ill patient in whom an accurate calculation of the P_aO_2/F_IO_2 ratio is needed to guide decisions about intubation or diagnose acute respiratory distress syndrome;[9]
- When an exact dose of oxygen needs to be prescribed, for clinical governance reasons. As oxygen is a drug that must be prescribed on a patient's chart, a dose rather than a flow rate should arguably be specified.

Under these circumstances, a fixed performance device will provide a F_IO_2 less dependent on respiratory pattern. These devices make use of a Venturi.

The Bernoulli Effect and the Venturi Principle

The Bernoulli effect (Fig. 9.10a) describes the change in pressure that occurs when a fluid flows through a constriction. The fluid accelerates, gaining kinetic energy at the expense of potential energy; hence pressure distal to the constriction is reduced. The Venturi principle describes how a second fluid can be entrained into the stream of the first, either through a side arm that opens into the area of low pressure or via a co-axial arrangement (Fig 9.10b).

Referring to Figure 9.10b, the degree of pressure drop is dependent on the flow rate of fluid A, the physical

Table 9.3 Fraction of inspired oxygen, oxygen flow rates and air entrainment of widely-used Venturi devices

F_IO_2 provided by Venturi valve		Oxygen flow rate to Venturi valve (l min^{-1})	Amount of air entrained (l min^{-1})	Total flow to patient (l min^{-1})
0.24		2	51	53
0.28		4	41	45
0.31		6	41	47
0.35		8	37	45
0.40		10	32	42
0.60		15	15	30

dimensions of the constriction and the density and viscosity of fluids A and B. Hence Venturis for oxygen delivery devices can be manufactured which entrain a known amount of air into a stream of oxygen of a specified flow rate, providing a fixed final F_IO_2 (Table 9.3).

The performance of Venturi devices is less dependent on respiratory pattern as they use relatively high oxygen flow rates to which is added the flow rate of entrained air. The total flow rate is close to or exceeds the patient's peak inspiratory flow rate, and is sufficient to flush away alveolar gas expired into the mask. The Venturi devices that entrain most air deliver a lower F_IO_2 and are thus most reliable, but those that deliver high F_IO_2, especially the 60% O_2 device, entrain less air and also have a lower total flow rate into the mask, which may be overcome by a patient breathing with a high peak inspiratory flow rate and may result in rebreathing. Hence the highest F_IO_2 Venturi devices may under-perform by 5–10%.[10]

Numerous manufacturers produce single-use clear plastic oxygen masks which come prepacked with a number of different Venturi devices (Fig. 9.11), typically giving overall flow rates of around 60 l min^{-1}, with each requiring a particular oxygen flow to give a fixed F_IO_2 (usually 24%, 28%, 31%, 35%, 40% and 60%).

A Venturi can also be attached to a 'T'-piece (Fig. 9.12) so that supplemental oxygen can be delivered to patients who are breathing spontaneously through an LMA or less commonly an ETT.[11] These devices are used on a short-term basis in recovery areas during emergence from anaesthesia. The segment of 22 mm diameter corrugated tubing has a volume of 56 ml, a compromise between oxygen enrichment and rebreathing. It provides a reservoir of oxygen-enriched air, which the patient inhales during the short period of the respiratory cycle in which peak inspiratory flow rate exceeds oxygen flow into the device. Pressure within the tubing is above atmospheric pressure as a result of the oxygen flow, creating a pressure gradient between the tubing and the room. Therefore the presence of the tubing also provides 1–2 cmH$_2$O of CPAP.

Medium dependency systems

Continuous Positive Airway Pressure (CPAP) may be applied:
- to improve oxygenation during respiratory emergencies that result in impaired gas exchange;
- on Intensive Care Units to aid weaning from ventilators;[12]
- as treatment for obstructive sleep apnoea.

The continuous pressure increases functional residual capacity of the lungs and reduces airway collapse.[13] CPAP may be applied to the face by means of a tightly-fitting mask, or directly to an endotracheal or tracheostomy tube. Under certain circumstances, such as acute pulmonary oedema, there is emerging evidence that bi-level positive airway pressure (BiPAP) improves ventilation and vital signs more rapidly than CPAP, but may cause haemodynamic instability.[14]

A CPAP or BiPAP facemask covers the mouth and nose. A variety of sizes are available as a good seal is essential; the mask is secured with a harness (Fig. 9.13). Because of the difficulty of achieving and maintaining a good seal, CPAP helmets have been developed to cover the entire head. Some designs of CPAP facemask have a single 22–mm female taper inlet similar to anaesthetic facemasks. In this case, a 'T'- or 'Y'-shaped connector on the mask allows oxygen delivery to one limb with the

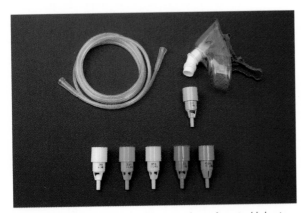

Figure 9.11 A facemask with a number of venturi injectors.

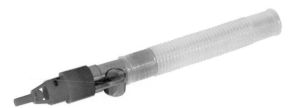

Figure 9.12 A 'T'-piece for delivering 40% oxygen to a patient breathing spontaneously through an airway device with a 15 mm ISO connector.

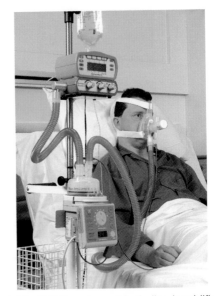

Figure 9.13 CPAP equipment including humidifier

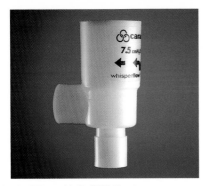

Figure 9.14 7.5 cm H_2O CPAP valve.

CPAP valve situated on the other. Other designs have two taper inlets, one for oxygen delivery and a second to accommodate the CPAP valve directly. For greater comfort and better tolerance, CPAP may be applied only to the nose, for example in neonatal respiratory distress syndrome (by means of nasal cannulae) and in the treatment of obstructive sleep apnoea. Under such circumstances pharyngeal valve mechanisms, including the soft palate, prevent loss of airway pressure through the mouth. Commercial CPAP valves can provide 2.5–20 cmH_2O of CPAP (Fig. 9.14).

The fresh gas flow in the CPAP circuit must exceed maximal inspiratory gas flow in order to maintain positive pressure throughout the respiratory cycle. Some systems incorporate a reservoir bag, otherwise a flow generator connected to the piped high pressure oxygen outlet (wall CPAP) is used (Fig. 9.15). The flow generator is a high-pressure oxygen driven Venturi injector and most devices of this nature tend to be quite noisy. To ensure that CPAP is maintained during all phases of respiration, it is important to check that the CPAP valve is being kept open by an adequate flow throughout the respiratory cycle. Humidification and oxygen monitoring units can be added to the system (Fig. 9.13).

Patients with a tracheostomy tube being weaned from a ventilator may receive oxygen and CPAP through a 'T'-piece with a CPAP valve connected to the distal end. This is most often a short-term arrangement due to the likelihood of disconnection. Most patients requiring long-term oxygen therapy by tracheostomy will receive it via a Swedish nose (see above).

High dependency systems

Positive pressure ventilation may be achieved by means of a nasal mask or facemask, avoiding the need for tracheal

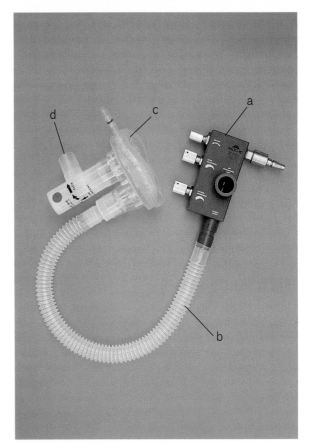

Figure 9.15 A CPAP device. The flow generator **(a)** plugs into a terminal outlet for oxygen. It has an ON switch, a flow adjustment and an oxygen concentration adjustment. A section of wide-bore tubing **(b)** connects it to a close-fitting facemask **(c)** that has two one-way valves in the body of the mask. One is an inlet valve and the other, fitted with a disposable CPAP valve **(d)**, is the outlet valve.

intubation with its associated complications. Non-invasive positive pressure ventilation (NIPPV or 'NIPPY') may be used electively to treat patients with central apnoea syndromes, neuromuscular or chest wall disease. It is increasingly used in acute respiratory failure and weaning.[15] The equipment used is the same as that required to provide CPAP, with the addition of a sophisticated Intensive Care ventilator capable of providing synchronized intermittent mandatory bi-level ventilation. For home use, highly sophisticated CPAP and BiPAP equipment is available, including some that use microprocessor control to adjust their own settings and can be controlled by telemetry.[16]

Metered sources of oxygen and air

The high flow rates required for CPAP, BiPAP and NIPPV require a metered source of fresh gas. The flow generator in the CPAP equipment (Fig. 9.15) plugs into a terminal outlet for oxygen via a Schrader device, typically the hospital piped oxygen supply or sometimes an oxygen cylinder. It has an 'on' switch and adjustments for F_IO_2 and flow rate. Air is entrained into the device through an adjustable Venturi orifice to determine F_IO_2 and flow rate is adjusted by means of a variable pressure regulator.

When providing NIPPV in hospital, a modern Intensive Care ventilator is normally used, which includes an electronically controlled oxygen blender allowing F_IO_2 to be manipulated precisely (see Chapter 12).

THE ADMINISTRATION OF OXYGEN IN A MIXTURE OF GASES

Entonox

The physical properties of this 50:50 mixture of oxygen and nitrous oxide (N_2O) are described in Chapter 2 and

the storage and supply in Chapter 3. This chapter will describe the equipment used for the self-administration of Entonox during labour and for short painful procedures such as fracture reduction, drain removal or dressing changes.

These devices are easy to use, allowing patients to breathe Entonox with minimal supervision and instruction from paramedics, midwives or nursing staff. However, staff must be aware that Entonox cylinders should not be stored in areas where temperature is liable to fall below 0°C. The pseudocritical temperature of Entonox is –6°C, at which N_2O separates out of the gaseous mixture and enters the liquid phase by lamination. The first breaths from such a cold cylinder are predominantly oxygen but as the cylinder empties a hypoxic mixture is delivered.

The BOC Entonox valve

This valve is no longer manufactured but many are still in use. It clamps directly to a pin-index Entonox cylinder. It consists of a first-stage pressure regulator and second-stage demand valve (Fig. 9.16). The demand valve consists of a sensitive rubber diaphragm that is deformed by negative pressure generated when a patient begins to

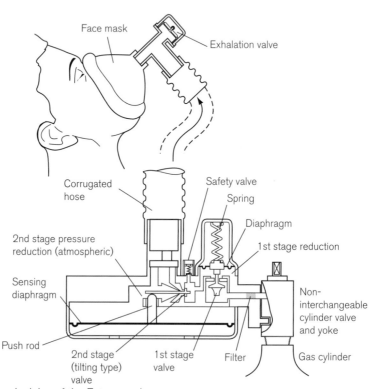

Figure 9.16 Working principles of the Entonox valve.

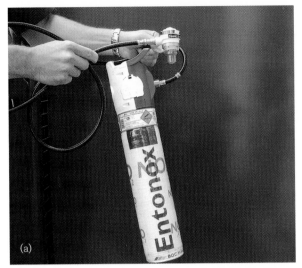 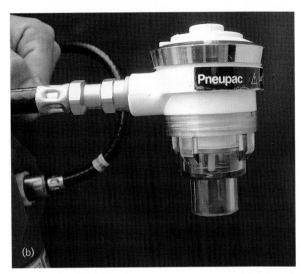

Figure 9.17 (a) Portable equipment for the administration of Entonox (here showing a composite cylinder with integral pressure reducing valve, see Chapter 3). **(b)** The demand valve showing the 22 mm connection for either a facemask or disposable mouthpiece.

inhale. The diaphragm operates a push rod that in turn tilts a lever to open the valve. A corrugated hose carries the Entonox to a facemask or mouthpiece, which contains an exhalation valve. An attendant can provide crude positive pressure ventilation in the event of respiratory arrest by depressing the sensing diaphragm manually.

The Pneupac Entonox valve

This equipment (Figure 9.17a,b) clamps directly to the Entonox cylinder and also consists of a first-stage pressure regulator connected by a sturdy narrow-bore delivery tube to the demand valve. The latter has a 22 mm male connector that may be attached to a mouth piece or facemask. The tubing may be several metres long so that the Entonox cylinder can be stored remotely from the demand valve. This allows the cylinder to be kept warm inside the ambulance when administering Entonox at the roadside in cold conditions. This model also incorporates a manual override button into the demand valve.

Heliox

Heliox is a commercially produced mixture of 21% oxygen and 79% helium. The low viscosity of helium makes it less likely to flow through an obstruction in a turbulent manner than air or oxygen alone, hence for a given pressure gradient (respiratory effort), higher gas flow rates are maintained (see Chapter 1, Types of Flow). Helium has been used in the specialist treatment of life-threatening upper airway obstruction such as acute epiglottitis and acute tracheal stenosis, where helium is enriched with additional oxygen in the breathing system of an anaesthetic machine under the supervision of an anaesthetist.[17]

In recent years there has been a great deal of interest in the use of Heliox as a temporizing treatment to improve gas exchange in acute exacerbations of asthma and COPD. Heliox may offer some benefit to patients with acute asthma within the first hour of use, but most conventionally treated patients improve to similar levels with or without it. It is still unclear whether Heliox can avert tracheal intubation, or reduce intensive care and hospital admission rates and duration, or even mortality.[1] Nonetheless, Heliox is now often administered routinely without the supervision of an anaesthetist or F_1O_2 monitoring. Supplemental oxygen and nebulized drugs can be added to the Heliox and delivered to variable performance facemasks by a number of different means (Fig. 9.18). However, it is impossible to determine F_1O_2 when patients may have profoundly abnormal breathing patterns. It should be remembered that the admixture of greater quantities of oxygen would increase the viscosity of the gas mixture and increase the work of breathing.

Heliox is sometimes administered to ventilated patients, especially children, via the air inlet of a ventilator. The altered viscosity of the fresh gas within the ventilator has a significant and unpredictable effect on delivered F_1O_2 and tidal volume.[18] Extra care should be

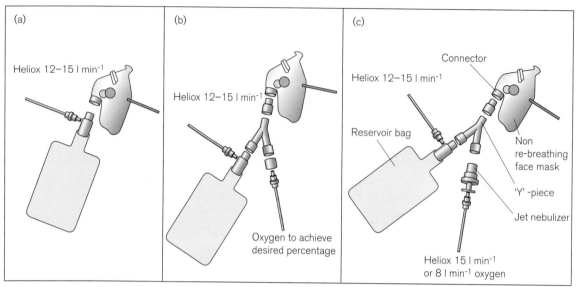

(a)

Heliox 12–15 l min^{-1}

(b)

Heliox 12–15 l min^{-1}

Oxygen to achieve desired percentage

(c)

Connector

Heliox 12–15 l min^{-1}

Reservoir bag

Non re-breathing face mask

'Y'-piece

Jet nebulizer

Heliox 15 l min^{-1} or 8 l min^{-1} oxygen

Figure 9.18 High capacity delivery device with a facility for the delivery of Heliox and nebulized drugs. **(a)** Using a 21% mix. **(b)** Oxygen admixture. **(c)** Drug nebulization.

taken in these circumstances to avoid volume trauma and detect over- or under-ventilation.

OXYGEN DELIVERY AT HIGH OR LOW ATMOSPHERIC PRESSURES

Hyperbaric medicine

Hyperbaric oxygen is most commonly used to treat decompression sickness and carbon monoxide poisoning.[19] Breathing oxygen at three times normal atmospheric pressure (absolute pressure) increases the amount of dissolved oxygen in plasma from a maximum of 2 ml 100 ml^{-1} to 6 ml 100 ml^{-1}, resulting in an extra 200 ml min^{-1} of oxygen delivery. As a result of this perceived physiological benefit, the US Food and Drug Administration (FDA) has approved 11 other application areas for hyperbaric oxygen, including the treatment of gas gangrene, necrotizing fasciitis, osteoradionecrosis, skin flaps and grafts, chronic refractory osteomyelitis, thermal burns and compartment syndrome.[20] However, the evidence for its efficacy in these latter conditions is unclear; most have not been investigated in clinical trials and many are based upon anecdotal case reports.

There are three types of hyperbaric chamber. Those in medical use tend to be divided into type A and type B on the basis of their size. The type A chamber (Fig. 9.19a,b) is large enough to accommodate one or more critically-ill ventilated patients, plus medical staff and equipment. The chamber shown is situated in the Hyperbaric Medicine Unit in the Royal Hospital, Haslar, UK. It can be adapted to accommodate ten or more sitting patients. Large chambers may have air conditioning and humidity control systems as the temperature of air rises as it is compressed. Hyperbaric chambers have multiple antistatic points to prevent build up of electrical charge, an essential safety feature as a spark in an enriched oxygen environment at 3 atm would result in a violent explosion. Compressing the chamber with air whilst the occupants breathe oxygen via a tightly fitting facemask (Fig. 9.19d) or head tent, further reduces risk of explosion.

Type B chambers are smaller and less suitable for ventilated patients. In the UK, hyperbaric chambers are often situated in deep sea diving centres although small, single patient portable chambers are also available (Fig. 9.19c). Lightweight and portable equipment has been developed to treat acute life threatening mountain sickness and decompression sickness on the scene, to transport patients suffering from decompression sickness and to pressurize patients during flight in non-pressurized aeroplanes.[21]

Diving

Divers face several problems when breathing underwater at increased atmospheric pressure.[22] Pressure increases by 1 atm for every 10 m of descent:

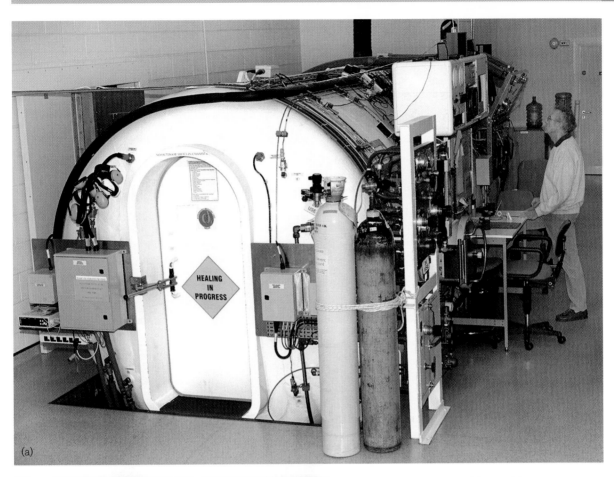

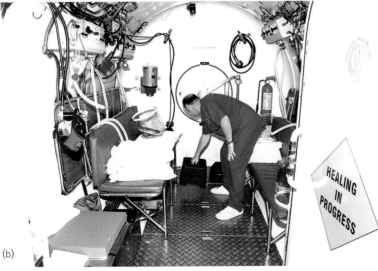

Figure 9.19 (a) and **(b)** The Type A hyperbaric chamber at Royal Hospital, Haslar (courtesy of Royal Navy and Qinetiq Ltd).

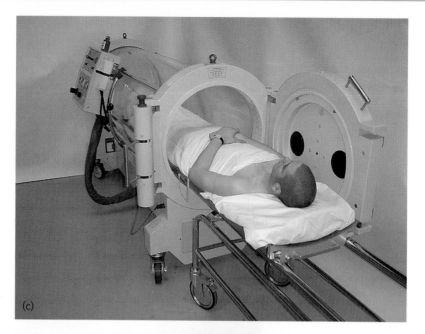

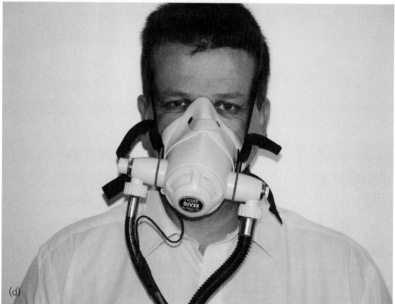

Figure 9.19, *cont'd* **(c)** Single patient portable hyperbaric chamber and **(d)** tightly fitting oxygen mask for use inside the chamber (courtesy of HYOX Ltd).

- *Nitrogen*: this poorly soluble gas is thought to be physiologically inert but at high pressure it is forced into solution in the tissues. If ascent is too rapid, bubbles of N_2 form, causing decompression sickness (the bends), which is potentially fatal. At depths of 50 m or more, N_2 causes narcosis by an unknown mechanism (rapture of the deep).
- *Oxygen*: high concentrations of oxygen cause lung injury and are toxic to the central nervous system. Convulsions can occur after breathing O_2 at 4 atm for 30 minutes.

To combat these problems, divers use a variety of gas mixtures to increase the amount of time that they may stay at depth without the need for decompression stops when ascending, to reduce the risk of decompression sickness by decreasing the amount of dissolved nitrogen in the body, and to avoid oxygen toxicity. Nitrogen may be partially or completely replaced by helium, which is not narcotic and reduces the work of breathing at very high pressures. For very deep dives, the oxygen content of the diving gas may be as low as 1%.[23]

Most divers use an open-circuit self-contained underwater breathing apparatus (Scuba).[23] The chosen gas is contained in steel, aluminium or titanium cylinders. Tank volume is normally about 10 litres but may be very small (bail out bottles) or up to 15 litres for deeper or longer exposures. A balanced first stage regulator situated on the tank reduces gas pressure to 10 atm. Gas then passes through an intermediate hose to a second regulator on the mouthpiece where it is balanced to the pressure of the surroundings and the lungs. When the diver exerts a slight negative pressure on the regulator at the start of inspiration, a non-return valve between the hose and mouthpiece opens and initiates fresh gas flow. Expiration and positive pressure closes the valve and expired gas is lost to the open water. Scuba equipment allows easy breathing with little resistance to inhalation and expiration independent of tank pressure. Safety is of paramount importance: tanks are visually inspected annually and subjected to a hydrostatic test procedure every 5 years and the resistance offered by each regulator, accuracy of instruments and integrity of hoses are checked regularly. An additional safety feature is a pinhole orifice in the proximal end of the high pressure hose, which prevents injury from a flailing hose should it rupture.

Military, cave and specialist divers may choose to use a closed circuit system in shallow dives when it is important not to produce bubbles.[23] The diver typically breathes 100% oxygen via a breathing bag, which is exhaled via a non-return valve into a canister containing a CO_2 absorber. The expired oxygen is recycled back into the breathing bag, which is supplemented by additional oxygen from the high-pressure supply. Use of mixed gases may allow deeper dives using a closed circuit system, with electronic monitoring of gas levels to ensure that their levels are maintained within safe ranges. A high degree of training and expertise is required to dive safely with such equipment. This system offers a higher resistance to breathing and CO_2 is liable to accumulate due to absorber inefficiency in moist, cold environments.

Mountaineering

Mountaineers require oxygen to facilitate climbing at very high altitude or to manage medical emergencies.[24] Closed circuit systems that use soda lime to absorb expired carbon dioxide have been used but are unreliable as internal valves tend to ice up before the soda lime begins to work. Constant flow systems have become most popular, mainly because of their simplicity. Weighing 3–7 kg in total, they comprise light titanium cylinders containing special no-water oxygen at 306 atm, pressure reducing valves and regulators. The regulator permits flow of 0.5–4 l min^{-1} into a rubber or plastic reservoir and facemask via light, non-kinking tubing. Finally, the mask is secured to the face in a helmet or with straps. All systems are checked and tested for several hours in a 'cold room' at –20°C before an expedition, paying particular attention to humidification, the collection of condensation and icing up of tubing.[25]

REFERENCES

1. Ho AM, Lee A, Karmakar MK, Dion PW, Chung DC, Contardi LH (2003) Heliox vs air-oxygen mixtures for the treatment of patients with acute asthma: a systematic overview. *Chest* **123(3):** 882–890.
2. Collis JM, Bethune DW (1967) Oxygen by face mask and nasal catheter. *Lancet* **1(7493):** 787–788.
3. Ooi R, Joshi P, Soni N (1992) An evaluation of oxygen delivery using nasal prongs. *Anaesthesia* **47(7):** 591–593.
4. Campkin NT, Ooi RG, Soni NC (1993) The rebreathing characteristics of the Hudson oxygen mask. *Anaesthesia* **48(3):** 239–242.
5. Breakell A, Townsend-Rose C (2001) The clinical evaluation of the Respi-check mask: a new oxygen mask incorporating a breathing indicator. *Emergency Medical Journal* **18(5):** 366–369.

6. Rayen AT (2000) A device for oxygen administration during ophthalmic surgery under local anaesthesia. *Anaesthesia* **55(5)**: 508–509.

7. Anon. (1997) BTS Guidelines for the Management of Chronic Obstructive Pulmonary Disease. *Thorax* **52**(Suppl 5): S1–S28.

8. Bach PB, Brown C, Gelfand SE, McCrory DC (2001) Management of acute exacerbations of chronic obstructive pulmonary disease: a summary and appraisal of published evidence. *Annuals of International Medicine* **134(7):** 600–620.

9. Bernard GR, Artigas A, Brigham KL, *et al.* (1994) The American-European Consensus Conference on ARDS. Definitions, mechanisms, relevant outcomes, and clinical trial coordination. *Americal Journal of Respiratory Critical Care Medicine* **149**(3 Pt 1): 818–824.

10. Jones HA, Turner SL, Hughes JM (1984) Performance of the large-reservoir oxygen mask (Ventimask). *Lancet* **1**(8392):1427–1431.

11. Campbell DJ, Fairfield MC (1996) The delivery of oxygen by a venturi T piece. *Anaesthesia* **51(6):** 558–560.

12. Duncan AW, Oh TE, Hillman DR (1986) PEEP and CPAP. *Anaesthesia and Intensive Care* **14(3):** 236–250.

13. Lindner KH, Lotz P, Ahnefeld FW (1987) Continuous positive airway pressure effect on functional residual capacity, vital capacity and its subdivisions. *Chest* **92(1):** 66–70.

14. Mehta S, Jay GD, Woolard RH *et al.* (1997) Randomized, prospective trial of bilevel versus continuous positive airway pressure in acute pulmonary edema. *Critical Care Medicine* **25(4):** 620–628.

15. Brochard L, Mancebo J, Elliott MW (2002) Noninvasive ventilation for acute respiratory failure. *European Respiratory Journal* **19(4):** 712–721.

16. Highcock MP, Morrish E, Jamieson S, Shneerson JM, Smith IE (2002) An overnight comparison of two ventilators used in the treatment of chronic respiratory failure. *European Respiratory Journal* **20(4):** 942–945.

17. Ho AMH, Dion PW, Karmakar MK, Chung DC, Tay BA (2002) Use of heliox in critical upper airway obstruction. Physical and physiologic considerations in choosing the optimal helium: oxygen mix. *Resuscitation* **52(3):** 297–300.

18. Berkenbosch JW, Grueber RE, Dabbagh O, McKibben AW (2003) Effect of helium-oxygen (heliox) gas mixtures on the function of four pediatric ventilators. *Critical Care Medicine* **31(7):** 2052–2058.

19. Tibbles PM, Edelsberg JS (1996) Medical progress – Hyperbaric-oxygen therapy. *New England Journal of Medicine* **334(25):**1642–1648.

20. Guo S, Counte MA, Romeis JC (2003) Hyperbaric oxygen technology: an overview of its applications, efficacy, and cost-effectiveness. *International Journal of Technological Assessments in Health Care* **19(2):** 339–346.

21. Dubois C, Herry JP, Kayser B (1994) Portable Hyperbaric Medicine, Some History. *Journal of Wilderness Medicine* **5(2):** 190–198.

22. Spira A (1999) Diving and marine medicine review part I: diving physics and physiology. *Journal of Travel Medicine* **6(1):** 32–44.

23. Egstrom GH (1997) Diving Equipment. In: Bove AA (ed.) *Bove and Davis' Diving Medicine*. 3rd edn. London: Saunders. pp. 26–38.

24. West JB (1982) Man at extreme altitude. *Journal of Applied Physiology* **52(6):** 1393–1399.

25. Hendricks DM, Pollock NW, Natoli MJ, Vann RD (2000) Mountaineering oxygen mask performance at 4572 m. *Aviation and Space Environmental Medicine* **71(11):**1142–1147.

10

Manual resuscitators

Andrew J Davey

Components	231
Other uses for manual resuscitators	239

There are occasions, both in and out of hospital, when a patient needs emergency ventilatory support that requires a device that is easily portable and that does not rely on a source of pressurized gas or electricity for its operation. A manual resuscitator fulfills these requirements. The number of different manufacturers marketing these devices bears testimony to their usefulness. Although there have been a plethora of designs from the first 'Ambu bag' in 1956, they all have three similar components:

1. a self-inflating bag;
2. a non-rebreathing valve; and
3. a facility for the admixture of oxygen.

COMPONENTS

The self-inflating bag

This bag may be made of silicone rubber or polyvinyl chloride (PVC), which is strengthened either by making its wall thicker, or incorporating circular 'ribs' of identical material during manufacture (Fig. 10.1), so that in the resting state it is expanded. Another design (Ambu mark III, Fig. 10.2) has an outer cover made from chloroprene or butyl rubber covering a thick foam lining, which also makes the bag expand in the resting state. All those produced now are latex-free. The PVC versions are designed to be for single use only and the others are made to be steam autoclaved.

The respirable gas inlet mechanism is housed at one end and the non-rebreathing valve at the other.

The respirable gas inlet

This inlet has a number of components (Fig. 10.3):

- *A one-way flap valve* (A). This is fitted to the inlet of the self-inflating bag. When the bag is squeezed, the gas pressure inside the bag rises and causes the flap valve to close. This prevents the escape of gas back through the inlet. When the bag is released, its self-inflating characteristic causes fresh gas from the respirable gas inlet to be indrawn. This may be either air, oxygen or a mixture of both.
- *A small bore nipple* (B). This is mounted on the inlet, to allow admixture of oxygen.
- *A wide bore inlet* (C). This supplies the bulk of the gas entering the bag and is usually air, unless oxygen is added, as above. In the latter situation, the final concentration of oxygen delivered is a function of the amount of added oxygen and its dilution with air in the self-inflating bag.
- *A reservoir system* (D). The inlet (C) may be fitted with a reservoir system. This feature is now widely used in almost all manual resuscitators. Its purpose is to store the oxygen fed into the system from the nipple (B). When the minute volume of oxygen supplied is greater than the volume given to the patient, the bag (D) will expand and will provide

231

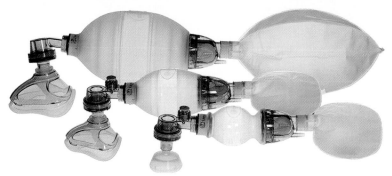

Figure 10.1 The Laerdal system in adult, child and infant sizes. The versions shown all have oxygen reservoir bags attached. The child and infant versions show overpressure safety valves fitted.

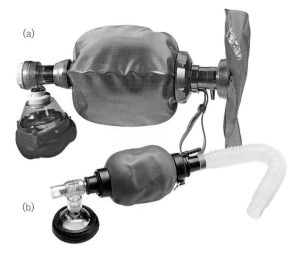

(a)

(b)

Figure 10.2 AMBU re-usable adult **(a)** and paediatric **(b)** resuscitators.

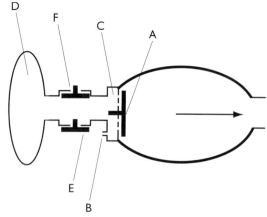

Figure 10.3 The respirable gas inlet of a self-inflating bag (see text). (A) One way flap valve; (B) 5 mm O$_2$ nipple; (C) wide bore inlet; (D) reservoir; (E) overpressure relief valve; (F) air entrainment valve.

all the gas for ventilation (i.e. 100% oxygen). The reservoir must be fitted with an overflow valve (E) to prevent overfilling from too high a flow of oxygen and an entrainment valve (F) to allow ingress of air for when oxygen is not available or when lower concentrations of oxygen are required. Tables 10.1 and 10.2 show typical oxygen concentrations that are delivered under a variety of conditions, with two popular makes of resuscitators. The differences reflect the size of the relevant reservoirs used.

The non-rebreathing valve

This valve is housed at the opposite end of the bag to the gas entrainment system described above. It has a number of components that ensure that during the inspiratory phase, gas flows out of the bag and only into the patient port. When the patient exhales, the valve also ensures that this exhaled gas escapes through the expiratory port without mixing with the fresh gas stored in the bag. Functionally, most non-rebreathing valves are similar, although there are some differences in their efficiency and their tendency to jam (see below).

Although primarily used in resuscitators, these valves may also be incorporated into anaesthetic breathing systems (see Chapter 29).

The Ruben valve (Fig. 10.4)

Now manufactured by Intersurgical in the UK, these valves may still be found in hospitals, particularly in developing countries. This valve has a spring-loaded bobbin within the valve housing and a one-way valve in the expiratory limb. In the resting position, the very weak spring holds the bobbin away from the expiratory port and against the inspiratory port, allowing relatively unhindered exhalation via the patient port. This prevents

Table 10.1 Oxygen concentrations (%) in a Laerdal resuscitator

Adult: Ventilation bag volume 1600 ml; reservoir bag volume 2600 ml

O₂ flow (l min⁻¹)	Tidal vol. (ml) × bag cycling rate per min					
	500 × 12	500 × 24	750 × 12	750 × 24	1000 × 12	1000 × 24
3	56 (37)*	39 (32)	47 (33)	34 (29)	41 (32)	30 (28)
5	81 (52)	52 (38)	62 (41)	42 (33)	52 (39)	38 (31)
10	100 (73)	84 (48)	100 (56)	65 (42)	84 (55)	53 (39)
12	100 (84)	97 (53)	100 (61)	74 (45)	94 (60)	59 (42)
15	100 (89)	100 (59)	100 (69)	86 (48)	100 (69)	66 (44)

*Data are O₂ concentrations using reservoir (without reservoir)

Child: Ventilation bag volume 500 ml; reservoir bag volume 2600 ml

O₂ flow (l min⁻¹)	Tidal vol. (ml) × bag cycling rate per min			
	250 × 20		100 × 30	
	w/reservoir	wo/reservoir	w/reservoir	wo/reservoir
10	100	75	100	90

Infant: Ventilation bag volume 240 ml; reservoir bag volume 600 ml

O₂ flow (l min⁻¹)	Tidal vol. (ml) × bag cycling rate per min			
	40 × 30		20 × 40	
	w/reservoir	wo/reservoir	w/reservoir	wo/reservoir
4	98	89	98	98

Table 10.2 Oxygen concentrations (%) in the Ambu system with reservoir

O₂ flow (l min⁻¹)	Ventilation volume (ml) × frequency			
	250 × 12	600 × 12	750 × 12	1000 × 12
2	74	43	38	34
5	100	76	65	54
10	100	100	100	87
15	100	100	100	100

any exhaled gases from mixing with inspiratory gas in the self-inflating bag. When the bag is squeezed, the bobbin is forced across the valve housing, so that the inspiratory port is joined to the patient port. This movement also occludes the expiratory port and allows inspiratory gas to enter the patient's lungs without leaking out through the expiratory pathway.

During spontaneous ventilation the spring-loaded one-way expiratory valve closes when the patient inhales. The resultant subatmospheric pressure in the main valve

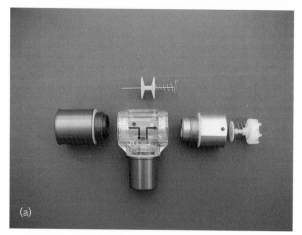

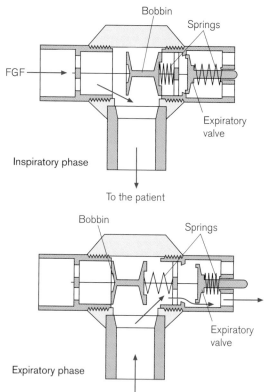

Figure 10.4 (a) The Ruben valve. **(b)** Working principles: (top) in the inspiratory phase the bobbin occludes the expiratory port; (bottom) during exhalation the spring causes the bobbin to occlude the inspiratory port.

moves the bobbin so that the inspiratory port opens to supply the patient with fresh gas. This valve has a tendency to jam in the inspiratory position if high upstream gas pressures are allowed to develop and can result in lung over-inflation. For example, if the valve is used to replace the APL valve in a Magill system during spontaneous ventilation, and the reservoir bag is allowed to over-distend, the valve will jam. In this situation, an APL valve upstream of the Ruben valve should always be fitted so as to provide a pressure relief facility if required. The valve may be disassembled for cleaning and autoclaving.

Ambu series of valves

The Ambu 'E' valve (Fig. 10.5)

This valve has been replaced by a newer design by the manufacturer but may still be encountered by anaesthetists visiting developing countries and so again is included. Although no longer marketed, the valve and spares are still advertized on the Internet. In this system, the unidirectional flow of gas is controlled by two labial flap valves:

- The upstream valve 'A', in the resting position, seals the inspiratory port but leaves the pathway into the expiratory port 'B' open, so that relatively unimpeded expiration can occur. During controlled ventilation, the valve 'A' is forced open and seals port 'B' so that inspiratory gas only enters the patient port.
- The labial valve 'D' is included to prevent the inhalation of downstream gas should the Ambu valve be used during spontaneous ventilation. This downstream gas may be air when the valve is used as a resuscitator but it could be exhaled gas if used in a circle breathing system.

When this Ambu valve is used for controlled ventilation, a high initial surge of gas is required to produce sufficient movement in valve 'A' to affect a complete expiratory seal. This model is relatively inefficient at lower inspiratory gas flow rates, and in this situation the seal may be incomplete, allowing some of the inspiratory gas to pass straight across the valve. This results in lower than expected tidal volumes. In fact, it is possible to occlude totally the patient port and gently squeeze the

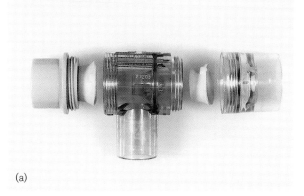

(a)

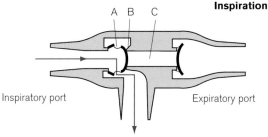

Inspiration

A B   C

Inspiratory port   Expiratory port

To the patient

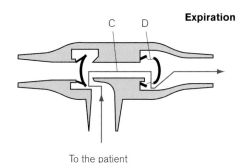

Expiration

C   D

To the patient

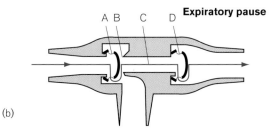

Expiratory pause

A B   C   D

(b)

Figure 10.5 (a) The Ambu E valve. **(b)** Working principles. (Top) During assisted inspiration. Note that the port B is closed by the pressure of the head of the 'mushroom' valve A. (Centre) During expiration. (Bottom) During the expiratory pause, excess gases may pass straight through the valve, so preventing excessive build-up of pressure. A, upstream (inspiratory) valve; B, expiratory port; C, expiratory pathway; D; downstream (expiratory) valve.

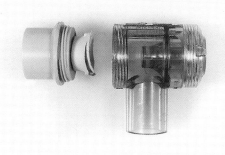

Figure 10.6 The Ambu E2 valve.

contents of the self-inflating bag out through the valve. This relative inefficiency greatly decreases the potential for valve jamming. For instance, if any high gas pressures were to begin to develop upstream, excess gas would be dumped across the valve. Because of this, the Ambu 'E' valve *should not be used* with automatic resuscitators that do not produce the initial high surge of gas required to produce an effective seal.

The Ambu E2 valve (Fig. 10.6)
This model contains only the main labial valve (A) seen in the E valve. Hence its function is similar to these valves when used with controlled ventilation, but behaves differently if used with spontaneous respiration. In this situation the absence of the downstream valve allows the patient to breathe ambient air via the expiratory port and not the gas mixture from the self-inflating bag.

Ambu Mark III valve (Fig. 10.7 a and b)   Again this valve has been superceded but is still in use in some countries and spare parts may still be purchased. This valve overcomes the potential problem of leakage across the E valve at low flow rates. The valve mechanism has three components: an inspiratory leaf valve, an expiratory leaf valve and a mushroom valve.

When this valve is used for controlled ventilation, a very small increase in pressure within the self-inflating bag, due to manual compression, expands the elastic mushroom valve, which then totally occludes the expiratory port, providing a complete seal. Further compression of the bag opens the inspiratory leaf valve, forcing gas from the bag into the inspiratory port, thus providing an inspiratory flow.

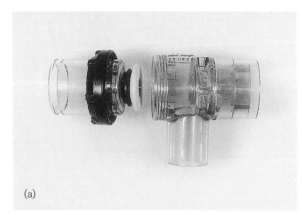

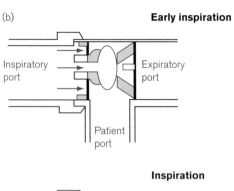

Early inspiration

Inspiratory port

Expiratory port

Patient port

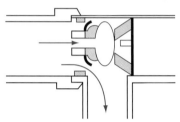

Inspiration

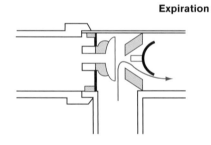

Expiration

Figure 10.7 (a) Ambu Mark III valve. **(b)** Working principles. (Top) Very early in inspiration, inspiratory gas causes the mushroom valve to balloon out and occlude the expiratory port. (Centre) Shortly afterwards, the inspiratory valve opens to allow inspiratory gas to enter the patient port. (Bottom) Expiratory phase, the mushroom valve retracts to its resting position and allows exhalation to occur.

At the beginning of the exhalation phase, the self-inflating bag starts to re-expand. The reduced pressure within causes the mushroom valve to collapse and the inspiratory leaf valve to close, sealing the bag off from the main valve. The exhaled patient gas then leaves the system through the expiratory port via the expiratory leaf valve.

If the valve is used on a spontaneously breathing patient, the negative pressure produced by the patient during inspiration causes the expiratory leaf valve to close, sealing the expiratory port. This ensures that the inspired gas is drawn from the bag contents and not from ambient air through the expiratory port.

This type of valve could jam in the inspiratory position if high upstream gas pressures were present at the end of an inspiratory phase. However, this is prevented by the self-inflating bag designed to be used with this valve. The gas-tight outer skin of this bag is made from thin,

distensible neoprene, which absorbs any build up of high pressure in the same way that an anaesthetic breathing bag does. As a further safety feature, the diameter of the inspiratory port of this valve (24 mm) prevents this valve being used with other breathing systems and prevents mis-assembly with other self-inflating bags.

Ambu Single Shutter valve (Fig. 10.8 a, b and c)

This valve is the version used in all current Ambu products. Compared to previous models, it has been simplified and now incorporates a single, multi-function shutter only. The valve shown here is re-usable and can be dismantled for cleaning and sterilizing. A disposable version is incorporated into the SPUR (Single Patient Use Resuscitator) system (Fig. 10.8b). The part of the valve body containing the expiratory pathway in both types may be unscrewed and a spring loaded PEEP valve substituted.

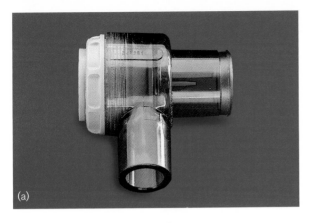

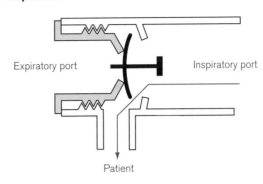

Inspiration

Expiratory port   Inspiratory port

Patient

Expiration

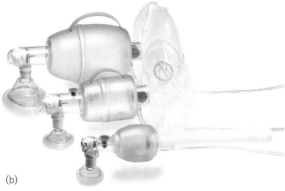

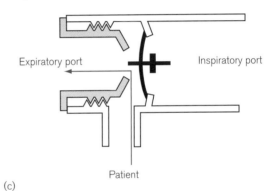

Expiratory port   Inspiratory port

Patient

(c)

Figure 10.8 **(a)** Ambu single-shutter valve. **(b)** A SPUR (Single Patient Use Resuscitator) system. **(c)** Working principles: upper part, the valve is pushed onto the expiratory port and occludes it so that gas can enter only the patient port; lower part, exhaled gas pushes the valve against the inspiratory port, occluding it so that the gas can escape only through the expiratory port.

When this valve is used for controlled ventilation, manual compression of the new self-inflating bag pushes gas against the concave aspect of the shutter causing it to move and occlude the expiratory port. The same movement opens the patient port to allow ingress of the gas.

At the beginning of the exhalation phase, exhaled gas impinges on the convex aspect of the shutter, causing it to move in the opposite direction, so that it opens the expiratory pathway as well as occluding the inspiratory port.

With spontaneous respiration, as inspiratory resistance ($0.7\,kPa$ at $10\,l\,min^{-1}$) through the valve is less than expiratory resistance ($0.8\,kPa$ at $10\,l\,min^{-1}$), gas will be drawn preferentially from the bag. Initial movement of gas will also cause the shutter valve to occlude the expiratory path so that the valve behaves in a similar manner to controlled ventilation.

The guide stem of the shutter is clearly visible through the transparent valve body and its 'to and fro' movement is an indicator of correct function.

The self-inflating bag supplied with this valve is made from silicone and the gas inlet is fitted with the two pressure relief valves described before.

Laerdal pattern valve

This high-efficiency non-rebreathing valve (Fig. 10.9) is made in three sizes (adult, child, infant). The valve itself has three components, a duck-billed inspiratory/expiratory valve, a valve body housing inspiratory and expiratory ports and a non-return flap valve sited in the expiratory port. Originally designed by Laerdal, it is now used by many manufacturers for their resuscitators. It may be made for single use only, in which case the valve

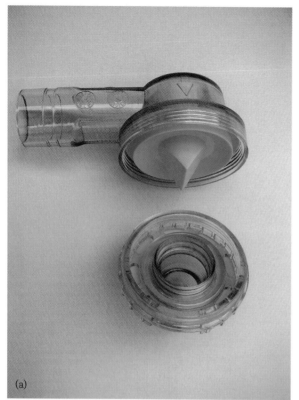

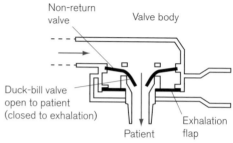

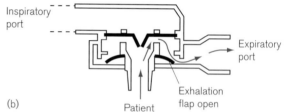

Figure 10.9 (a) The Laerdal valve; **(b)** working principles.

housing is sealed and cannot be opened. The reusable version made of autoclavable materials may be dismantled for cleaning and sterilizing. However, care must be taken to reassemble all the components correctly as there have been reports of misassembly:

- *Inspiratory Phase*. The central duck-billed portion of the main valve opens when the attached self-inflating bag is squeezed, or when a patient inhales through it. Almost simultaneously the outer disc-shaped portion of the valve is pushed against the apertures in the valve body, thus sealing the expiratory pathway.

- *Expiratory Phase*. Positive expiratory pressure from the elastic recoil of the patient's lungs causes the duck-billed section of the valve to close, thus preventing rebreathing it into the bag. It also lifts the outer disc-shaped portion off the expiratory apertures, allowing exhaled gas to escape. Escaping gas also lifts the flaps on a non-return valve in the expiratory port. This is a supplementary valve that prevents air from being aspirated into the expiratory port during spontaneous respiration.

- *Other Features*. All the sizes have a 23 mm external diameter expiratory port and a 22 mm external diameter/15 mm internal diameter inspiratory port so as to minimize the possibility of misconnection. The child and infant models have overpressure safety valves built into the inspiratory port of the valve and which are set to blow off at a pressure of 45 cmH$_2$O. If these pressures ever need to be exceeded, the safety valve can be overridden by finger pressure or a lock clip over the valve.

The self-inflating bag supplied with Laerdal resuscitators has thickened ribs of silicone rubber that provide the rigidity for the self-inflating action. These bags can be supplied with a supplementary reservoir bag (larger than that for the Ambu) for the supply of high oxygen concentrations to patients (Table 10.1). The entrainment port of the reservoir bags is fitted with a housing containing two valves. One is for air entrainment when little or no additional oxygen is used. The other is for the relief of any high-pressure build-up in the system from an excess of oxygen flow (see above).

OTHER USES FOR MANUAL RESUSCITATORS

Most of the devices described above can be used with draw-over anaesthetic equipment to provide controlled ventilation when required. An example of such a system is described more fully in Chapter 29.

FURTHER READING

Barnes TA, McGarry WP III (1990) Evaluation of ten disposable manual resuscitators. *Respiratory Care* **35**(10): 960–968.

Baskett P, Zorab J (2003) The resuscitation greats. Henning Ruben MD, FFARCS(I), FFARCS. The Ruben valve and the AMBU bag. *Resuscitation* **56**(2): 123–127.

Corley M, Ledwidge MK, Glass C, Grap MJ (1993) The myth of 100% oxygen delivery through manual resuscitation bags. *Journal of Emergency Nursing* **19**(1): 45–49.

Hermansen MC, Prior MM (1993) Oxygen concentrations from self-inflating resuscitation bags. *American Journal of Perinatology* **10**(1): 79–80.

Hess D, Simmons M (1992) An evaluation of the resistance to flow through the patient valves of twelve adult manual resuscitators *Respiratory Care* **37**(5): 432–438.

Hess D, Spahr C (1990) An evaluation of volumes delivered by selected adult disposable resuscitators: the effects of hand size, number of hands used, and use of disposable medical gloves. *Respiratory Care* **35**(8): 800–805.

Ho AM, Shragge BW, Tittley JG, Fedoryshyn JN, Puksa S (1996) Exhalation obstruction due to Laerdal valve mis-assembly. *Critical Care Medicine* **24**(2): 362–364.

Smith G (2002) Problems with mis-assembly of adult manual resuscitators. *Resuscitation* **53**(1): 109–111.

Smith G (2002) Problems with mis-assembly of adult manual resuscitators. *Resuscitation* **55**(3): 347–348.

Quintana S, Martinez Perez J, Alvarez M, Vila JS, Jara F, Nava JM (2004) Maximum FIO_2 in minimum time depending on the kind of resuscitation bag and oxygen flow. *Intensive Care Medicine* **30**(1): 155–158.

Automatic ventilators

Andrew J Davey

In order to inflate a patient's lungs adequately with a mechanical ventilator, sufficient pressure must be generated in the respirable gas within a ventilator or resuscitator (*positive pressure ventilation*) to overcome the elastic recoil of the lungs and chest wall (their *elastance*) and the resistance to flow within the airways. These may be normal in healthy patients, requiring the generation of only modest pressures for inflation, or may be grossly abnormal in disease, requiring the generation of much higher pressures in order to provide the same degree of ventilation. Furthermore, some surgical procedures may make it more difficult to inflate the lungs, for example, by restricting the movement of the diaphragm, due to posture or internal intervention. An additional factor during anaesthesia is the resistance of the artificial part of the airway, which may increase accidentally, for example, by mucus accumulation or kinking of the endotracheal tube.

A patient's lungs may also be inflated by using negative pressure. The patient's body (from the neck downwards) or thorax only, is encased in a gas tight container to which an intermittent sub-atmospheric pressure is applied. The thorax is 'sucked outwards' causing air/respirable gas to enter the lungs (*negative pressure ventilation*). Exhalation is achieved passively as a result of the elastance of the lungs and thoracic wall.

POSITIVE PRESSURE VENTILATORS

Methods of pressure generation

Respirable gas may develop sufficient pressure either:
- by being compressed in a ventilator bellows or bag. The bellows may be compressed *mechanically* by attaching it to a spring, weight, or piston. The piston may be driven by a compressed gas or via a cam, worm drive or gear chain connected to an electric motor. It may also be compressed *pneumatically* by placing the bellows in a gas-tight canister into which a separate pressurized gas source is fed;
- or by the adaptation of a suitable source of gas that is already pressurized (cylinder or pipeline supply). If the source is able to match the high flows required for ventilation, it may be fed directly into a ventilator to be divided up into suitable tidal volumes. If not, lower flows can be fed continuously into a reservoir that is pressurized by springs or weights to be used intermittently by the ventilator.

The pressure created within a bellows may be constant, as produced by a weight placed on top of it, or variable when produced by some of the other methods. Bellows attached to springs, produce pressures that steadily decline as the contents are released, whereas those attached to, say, an electric motor that progressively compresses the bellows, produce pressures that depend on the mechanical linkage and the regulation of the speed of the electric motor.

Ventilator designs fall into two categories: those developing modest pressures suitable only for relatively normal lungs (*low powered ventilators*) and those developing higher pressures that can cope with both normal and abnormal lungs (*high powered ventilators*).

Classification of ventilators according to their power

Low-powered ventilators (Fig. 11.1 a)

Low-powered ventilators generate only the modest gas pressures required to deliver reasonable tidal volumes to lungs with normal and near-normal compliances and resistances. These pressures are often insufficient to overcome the increase in airways resistance and/or the reduction in lung compliance that are seen in diseased lungs. As a result of this, the tidal volume delivered may well be less than the volume anticipated. Their use is therefore limited. When these ventilators are used, the need to monitor adequacy of lung ventilation must be emphasized. Either expired minute volume or capnography can be used to check that ventilation remains satisfactory throughout a procedure. However, these ventilators are simpler and more cheaply constructed and are also less likely to cause lung damage than those generating high pressures.

High-powered ventilators (Fig. 11.1 b and c)

In order to prevent a reduction in ventilator performance in the presence of deteriorating lung conditions, a ventilator needs to be powerful enough to develop a sufficiently high gas pressure so as to overcome the increases in airways resistance and reduction in compliance with little alteration in desired gas flow. These ventilators are more costly to produce and require also the addition of certain safety features to protect patients with both normal and abnormal lungs from excessive pressures. For example, a safety valve is always included in the gas pathway to the patient to release any build-up of potentially dangerous pressures that might damage the lungs. Figure 11.1b shows an example of a typical high-powered ventilator. The pressure-relief valve (S) can either be pre-set (usually at 4.4 kPa/ 45 cmH$_2$O) or, in more sophisticated machines can be adjustable (up to 7.8 kPa/ 80 cmH$_2$O) to cope with severe conditions such as

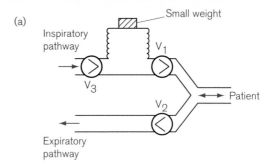

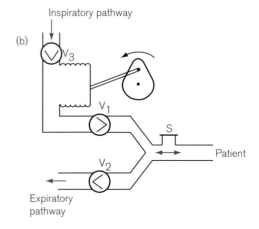

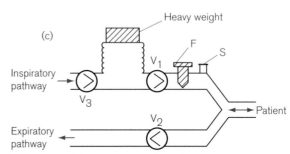

Figure 11.1 (a) Low-powered ventilator generating constant low pressure. **(b)** High-powered ventilator generating an increasing pressure. **(c)** High-powered ventilator generating a constant high pressure, V$_1$, inspiratory valve; V$_2$, expiratory valve; V$_3$, non-return valve; F, flow restrictor; S, overpressure relief valve.

asthma and the adult respiratory distress syndrome. The higher the pre-set safety limit, the narrower becomes the safety margin between safe ventilation and barotrauma.

Those high-powered ventilators that always generate high pressure of gas in the ventilator system prior to its delivery (by using powerful springs, heavy weights or a pipeline gas source (Fig. 11.1c)), require the presence of a further safety device, a flow restrictor, in the inspiratory pathway. This reduces the flow to the patient and prevents too rapid a build-up of pressure in the lung.

Alternative classifications

A popular classification with British anaesthetists has been described by Mushin.[1] Those ventilators that by their design produce a pressure sufficient only to ventilate normal or mildly abnormal lungs are classified as *pressure generators*, i.e. the tidal volume delivered to the patient is limited by the pressures generated. Those ventilators that develop pressures sufficiently high enough to deliver a desired flow even to grossly abnormal lungs are deemed *flow generators*. However, as most other electro-mechanical devices in common usage are described in terms of *power*, the author prefers the first classification.

Efficiency of ventilators

This may be defined as the ratio of the intended tidal volume (as determined by the settings on the ventilator) over the actual delivered tidal volume. For example, when a ventilator acts on a bellows containing patient gas at atmospheric pressure, the gas undergoes a degree of compression in order to raise the pressure sufficiently to provide an inspiratory flow. Part of the bellows travel is taken up in compressing the gas. If the bellows travel is calibrated for volume, it becomes apparent that the tidal volume actually delivered is less than that indicated on the bellows scale. The greater the pressure required to ventilate a patient's lungs, the greater will be the amount of gas lost in *compression*. This type of ventilator is regarded as relatively inefficient, as the discrepancy between anticipated and delivered tidal volumes may be as great as 25% in patients with significant pathological lung conditions.

Furthermore, the effective inspiratory time is shortened as initially, time is lost in compressing the gas to the required pressure. Inefficient ventilators (which include most anaesthetic ventilators that supply circle systems) may well require validation of the delivered tidal volume, using a spirometer or capnograph. With the advent of more sophisticated measurement of flow and electronic feedback to the ventilator, the compliance of this type of system, and therefore the compression volume, can now be calculated and automatic adjustment made for most of the apparent 'lost' volume.

More efficient ventilators store respiratory gas under a pressure greater than that required to ventilate a patient's lungs, so that the gas is already compressed prior to being released and, therefore, none is lost in a 'compression volume'. It is important to grasp this concept, as there may be a marked difference in the anticipated performance of ventilators.

Inspiratory characteristics of ventilators

Ventilators may produce a variety of pressure waveforms and inspiratory flow characteristics, depending on the method of generation of gas pressure and the resistance to flow that the gas meets during delivery of the intended tidal volume.

Low-powered ventilators

Low-powered ventilators (Fig. 11.2) normally generate their power from gas stored under modest pressure in a bellows or distensible bag. Those ventilators exerting a constant gas pressure (weighted bellows) on the patient airway, will have an inspiratory flow rate of gas that is greatest in early inspiration, when the pressure differential between the ventilator and the lung is wide, but that slows during expansion of the lung as the pressures approximate (Fig. 11.2a). Similar flow patterns will be seen with those ventilators exerting a gradually declining pressure (by storing gas in a distensible bag or bellows attached to a weak spring (Fig. 11.2b)).

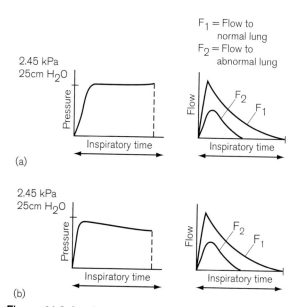

Figure 11.2 Inspiratory characteristics of low-powered ventilators. **(a)** Constant pressure (weighted bellows); **(b)** variable (declining) pressure (i.e. bellows attached to a weak spring).

High-powered ventilators

High-powered ventilators (Fig. 11.3) that function by creating a constant high pressure of gas (e.g. bellows compressed by a heavy weight, or by utilizing a high-pressure gas source), do not directly exert these pressures at the patient airway, as this would be potentially dangerous. The presence of an obligatory flow restrictor proximal to the patient (see above) determines both the pressure waveform, and the flow waveform of gas leaving the ventilator. A fixed performance flow restrictor produces a constant flow of gas through its orifice, resulting in a gradual pressure rise downstream of the device sufficient to deliver the pre-set tidal volume. As the lungs expand, the pressure rise that occurs within them is insufficient to alter the flow from the ventilator, which remains virtually constant (Fig. 11.3a).

Some high-powered ventilators generating a constant high pressure have flow restrictor apertures that can be varied electronically and so are able to respond to user-programmed inspiratory flow patterns (constant or decreasing flows (Fig. 11.3b)).

Ventilators may be designed to force their bellows to be compressed either mechanically, via a linkage from a suitable power source (Fig. 11.3c) or pneumatically, by

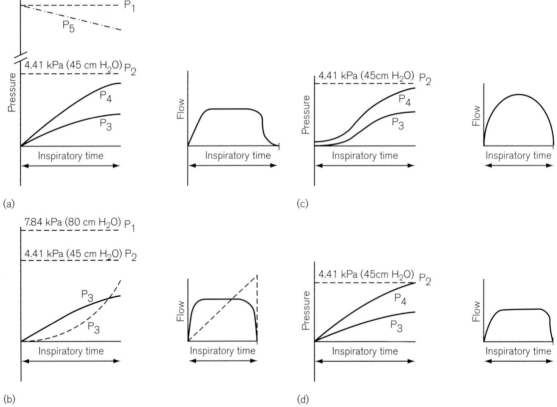

Figure 11.3 Inspiratory characteristics of high-powered ventilators. **(a)** Constant high-pressure generation (P_1) well in excess of that required to ventilate abnormal lungs (heavyweight pipeline gas supply) with fixed-performance flow restrictor. High-pressure generation produced by a bellows compressed by powerful springs provides a gradually declining pressure as the bellows empties (P_5 above). However, this is insufficient to affect the performance of the ventilator, which develops pressures and flows as if it were constant high-pressure generation. **(b)** Constant high-pressure generation using a varying orifice flow-restrictor (electronically controlled to provide different inspiratory flow patterns from the same ventilator). **(c)** Increasing high-pressure generation (no flow restrictor required) bellows compressed by a sinusoidally applied power source (i.e. electric motor driving a crank). **(d)** Increasing pressure generation (no flow restrictor required) bellows compressed by a linear power source (i.e. bag in bottle).

P_1, high constant pressure generated; P_2, safety valve release pressure; P_3, pressure rise downstream of restrictor as a result of flow to normal lungs; P_4 as above but to abnormal lungs; P_5, gradually declining high pressure.

placing the bellows in a gas-tight container into which a pressurized gas source is fed (bag-in-bottle arrangement (Fig. 11.3d)). The bellows in this type of ventilator normally fills with gas at near atmospheric pressures, so that when it is compressed, the pressure developed rises as it overcomes the resistive properties of the lungs. The resultant pressure waveforms can be sine wave (from a electric motor driving a cam) or ramp shaped (from any linear power source, e.g. gas piston). In either type the delivery of the intended tidal volume is assured owing to the power developed by the ventilator (unless the pressure relief valve opens). More sophisticated ventilators will provide an alarm signal if this occurs. The flow waveform produced depends in turn on the method of the pressure generation.

Great store has been placed on the ability of different flow waveforms to increase ventilatory efficiency in various clinical situations. However, in anaesthetic practice the claimed advantages are less demonstrable.

Classification of ventilators according to cycling

Intermittent automatic ventilation of the lungs consists of two phases: inspiratory and expiratory. A ventilator is said to *cycle* between the two phases.

Inspiratory cycling

During the inspiratory phase, the ventilator delivers a *volume* of gas into a patient's lungs. This takes place over a period of *time* producing an increasing airways *pressure*. There may also be a change in the pattern of *flow* (inspiratory waveform) at some stage in inspiration. However, the ventilator usually allows only one of these to terminate the inspiratory phase when its pre-determined value is reached. As all four variables are present in every inspiratory phase, it is sometimes difficult to decide which is the principle determinant of inspiratory cycling.

Volume cycling

A ventilator that uses this method of inspiratory cycling recognizes the point at which a predetermined volume of gas has left the ventilator and switches its internal mechanism to allow exhalation to occur. Many volume-cycled ventilators have a variable performance restrictor which slows down the inspiratory gas flow, introducing some element of timing during inspiration. However, volume remains the primary determinant of inspiratory cycling.

Time cycling

Ventilator cycling may be achieved using mechanical, pneumatic or electronic timers to operate the cycling mechanism which functions independently of the delivered tidal volume. This increases the sophistication of the ventilator. For example, it may allow the tidal volume to be delivered early in the inspiratory cycle, followed by a pause to allow better distribution of the gas prior to the start of the expiratory phase. Time cycling is now incorporated in most new ventilators.

Pressure cycling

Pressure-cycled ventilators sense a predetermined airway pressure in order to terminate the inspiratory phase. However, if the airway resistance increases and/or compliance of a patient deteriorates, a pressure-cycled ventilator will deliver a reduced tidal volume at the pre-set cycling pressure. The performance of these ventilators is thus very variable.

Flow cycling

Recognition of flow pattern changes has been used to cycle ventilators. However, this method is rarely employed nowadays.

Expiratory cycling

The expiratory phase may be similarly terminated by one of the above-mentioned variables. For example:

- *an expiratory volume-cycled* ventilator may have a mechanism for terminating the expiratory phase when the bellows has filled to the desired tidal volume required for the next inspiration;
- *an expiratory pressure-cycled* ventilator would be able to identify a selected airways pressure at the end of exhalation that would trigger the next inspiratory phase;
- *an expiratory flow cycled* ventilator would switch to the inspiratory phase when the desired flow rate at the end of exhalation was reached; or
- *an expiratory time cycled* ventilator is the most versatile as the phase may extend beyond the end of exhalation, unlike pressure and flow cycling. Nor is it limited by the fact that the inspiratory bellows is full, unlike a volume-cycled ventilator. It is therefore the most popular method of controlling the expiratory

phase and is achieved by using electronic or pneumatic timers within the ventilator to switch phases.

Further explanations are included in the individual ventilators mentioned below.

Ventilators may use one of the methods described above for inspiratory cycling and another for expiratory cycling, depending on the method of construction, and in some of them, limits may be set to one or more of the above functions.

Cycling mechanisms in ventilators

Gas flow to and from the patient from a ventilator (cycling) is usually controlled by a series of one-way valves that are operated and synchronized either:

- mechanically;
- electronically; or
- pneumatically.

Examples of these will be described where appropriate in the section on individual ventilators.

Ventilation modes

The terminology used to describe the way in which a ventilator combines its power capability and cycling to deliver a tidal volume has not been universally agreed upon. Originally it was termed *intermittent positive pressure ventilation* (IPPV). A desired tidal volume and rate delivered by a high-powered ventilator can be referred to by a number of terms, depending on the usage in a particular country or in the literature provided by a particular manufacturer. These include *Controlled Minute Ventilation* (CMV), *Volume Controlled Ventilation* or *Volume Ventilation*.

Low- or high-powered ventilators that have a pressure limit for the delivery of a tidal volume are said to deliver *Pressure Controlled Ventilation* (PCV), *Pressure Ventilation* or *Pressure Mode*.

Controlled ventilation, with the ability to synchronize delivered tidal volume with the patient's respiratory effort, may be termed *Synchronized Intermittent Mandatory Ventilation* (SIMV) or *Volume Mode plus trigger* (Vol Mode + Trigger) or *Synchronized Volume Ventilation* (Volume sync).

A sophisticated ventilator may have a facility that supports spontaneous respiration by sensing an inspiratory breath and assisting it by adding extra gas from the device. This may be termed *Assisted Spontaneous Breathing* (ASB) or *Pressure Support Ventilation* (PSV). This may also be used in conjunction with SIMV. There are a number of other similar terms used by manufacturers, which are for the most part self-explanatory.

Ventilator controls (general principles)

The three variables involved in setting the ventilatory parameters on a ventilator are traditionally arranged in the simple equation below:

Minute volume = tidal volume × rate (breaths per minute)

Armed with this equation, a user should be able to switch on and set up any ventilator in its basic mode for controlled ventilation. The equation can have only two pre-set variables, the third being dependant upon the other two. Hence a ventilator may only have two of the above variables assigned to knobs present on its control panel, i.e. it may have controls for tidal volume and rate (e.g. Blease 8500), minute volume and rate (e.g. Servo 900 series), or minute volume and tidal volume (e.g. Manley series).

The equation may be made slightly more complicated by the fact that *tidal volume* and *rate* are derived values (see below) and can be represented in a different form. For example, tidal volume is derived from the *inspiratory flow* delivered by the ventilator, and the *time* over which this is delivered. It may be expressed in the equation:

$$\text{Tidal volume} = \text{inspiratory flow rate} \times \text{inspiratory time}$$
$$\text{e.g.} = 0.5 \text{ litre per second} \times 2 \text{ seconds}$$
$$= 1 \text{ litre}$$

Hence a ventilator may have no tidal volume control, but will have a flow control and an inspiratory time control to perform the same function.

Rate is derived from the cycle time and expressed as the number of complete *cycles* per *minute*. It may be expressed in the equation:

$$\text{Rate} = \frac{\text{Time (1 minute)}}{\text{cycle time}}$$

For example, if the inspiratory time is 2 seconds and the expiratory time is 4 seconds then:

$$\text{Rate} = \frac{1 \text{ min or } (60 \text{ sec})}{(2\text{sec} + 4 \text{ sec})} = \frac{60}{6} = 10 \text{ cycles/min}$$

Hence a ventilator that has no rate control knob, will have an inspiratory and expiratory time control to perform the same function.

Classification of ventilators according to application

The miscellany of ventilator designs available and principles upon which they work is a result of (a) the wide spectrum of applications for which they are required and (b) efforts to harness the different power supplies that have been made available. However, there are four principle types of ventilator which are classified here according to their application in clinical practice:

1. 'mechanical thumbs';
2. minute volume dividers;
3. bag squeezers; and
4. intermittent blowers.

Mechanical thumbs

The most common source of pressurized gas is that found in cylinders and pipelines. This may be administered to a patient most easily as a continuous flow into the simplest of breathing systems, the T-piece (Fig. 11.4a). In Figure 11.4b, the anaesthetist has occluded the open end of the T-piece with his thumb. The force of the fresh gas flow (FGF) inflates the patient's lungs until the anaesthetist removes his thumb from the open end, which allows expiration to occur (Fig. 11.4c). By rhythmical application of the thumb to occlude the T-piece, intermittent positive pressure ventilation (IPPV) is achieved. The FGF has to be high enough to inflate the lungs during inspiration and, as it is not stored during exhalation, this method is wasteful of gas. Therefore, it is suitable only for use in neonatal anaesthesia. Furthermore, the advent of

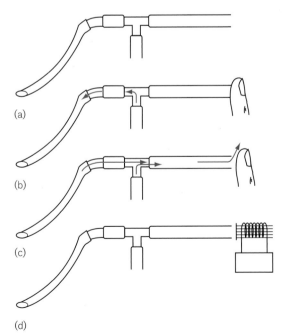

(a)

(b)

(c)

(d)

Figure 11.4 The T-piece principle and the 'mechanical thumb' (see text).

more efficient ventilators and gas monitoring has seen this usage of this type of ventilation decline.

However, in special care baby units the 'mechanical thumb' principle is still used in modern ventilators, albeit with greater sophistication.

In ventilators such as the Sechrist (Fig. 11.5d), the anaesthetist's thumb is replaced by a pneumatically-operated valve (Fig. 11.5e), the cycling of which is determined by the settings on the ventilator controls.

The exhalation valve may be electronically controlled (see Solenoids and Variable flow control valves, below) and by varying the degree of occlusion of the FGF is able to produce different types of inspiratory waveform (Bird VIP, Figs 11.5 a, b and c). Some designs use gas jets in the opposite direction to the fresh gas in place of the valve (SLE 2000).

Minute volume dividers

A more economical method of using a continuous source of pressurized gas is to feed it into a ventilator system (Fig. 11.6) to be collected by a reservoir R, which is continually pressurized by a spring, a weight or its own elastic recoil. Two valves, V_1 and V_2, are linked together and operated by a bi-stable mechanism. When V_1 opens, V_2 closes and causes the reservoir to discharge gas to the patient, i.e. this is the inspiratory phase. When V_1 closes, V_2 opens and expiration is permitted, allowing the reservoir bag to refill in preparation for the next breath.

All of the driving gas that is supplied is delivered to the patient. If, for example, the fresh gas flow delivered to the ventilator is 10 l min^{-1}, this is delivered to the patient as the minute volume. However, it is divided into a number of inspiratory volumes or 'breaths', depending on the settings of the volume and rate mechanisms of the ventilator, for example, 10 breaths of 1 litre, 20 of 0.5 or 25 of 0.4 and so on. These ventilators are referred to as *minute volume dividers* as they merely divide up the intended minute volume supplied by the driving gas. Ventilators based on this principle were the most common type used in the UK from the 1960s until the late 1990s. Setting an anticipated flow on the flowmeter bank and a vapour concentration on a vaporizer allowed a predictable flow of anaesthetic agent and gas mixture in the absence of gas and agent monitoring which was not readily available. The introduction of the latter into anaesthetic practice and the increase in cost of the more recently introduced volatile anaesthetics has resulted in a sharp decline in this type of ventilator. The most common type

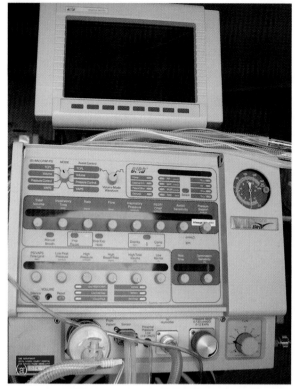

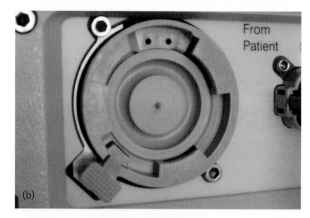

(b)

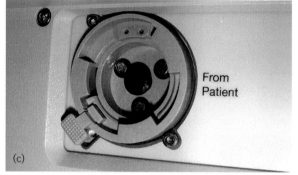

From
Patient

(c)

Figure 11.5 (a) Bird VIP neonatal ventilator; **(b)** Silicone diaphragm of Bird VIP acting as a variable flow valve; **(c)** Bird VIP Piston from flow valve that moves the diaphragm.

used is the series of ventilators designed by Dr Roger Manley.

The Manley MP3 (Fig. 11.7a)

This is the current and last version of a range of minute volume divider ventilators that have become the most popular of this type used in anaesthesia in the UK and in many other parts of the world as a result of its size, simplicity and reliability. These ventilators have ceased normal production but are still made to order.

Mode of operation

Inspiratory phase (Fig 11.7b) At the beginning of this phase, the main bellows (B_2) has filled to the pre-determined tidal volume. A lever (E) attached to the bellows slide (S) trips a bi-stable mechanical linkage (W), that operates the valves in the gas pathway so that:

- the valve V_1 closes and diverts the FGF to a storage bellows (B_1);
- the valve V_2 opens and allows the weight on top of

the bellows to expel the contents into the inspiratory pathway; and
- the valve V_3 closes in the expiratory pathway so that the inspiratory gas is directed to the patient through the inspiratory port I.

The inspiratory pressure is measured by the manometer, M.

Tidal volume: This is set by adjusting a sliding catch (E) over the calibrations on the lever D. Without the storage bellows B_1, the fresh gas would supplement that in the main bellows B_2, during inspiration, and so deliver an unknown tidal volume.

There is a weight (C) that slides along a rail (B) that is attached to the top of the bellows. By sliding the weight closer to, or further away from the pivot, the moment of force it exerts on the bellows causes the inspiratory pressure (within the bellows) to be altered.

During inspiration, the FGF is diverted into the spring-loaded storage bellows B_1, which expands, and when full trips the bi-stable mechanism via the lever (N). This in

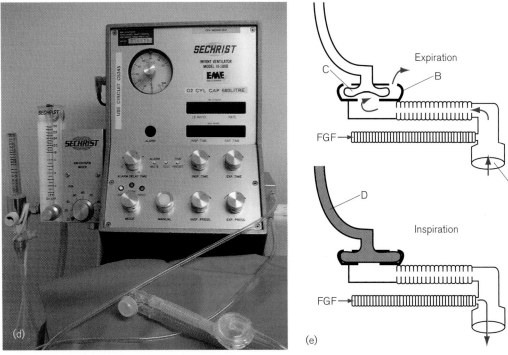

Figure 11.5, *cont'd* (d) Seechrist Infant ventilator; **(e)** Schematic diagram of the 'mechanical thumb'. A, patient connection; B, expiratory valve; C, deflated pneumatic valve; D, gas supply tube to pneumatic valve, which is now inflated.

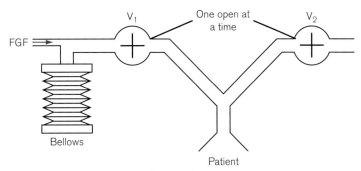

Figure 11.6 The principle of minute volume dividers (see text).

turn reverses all the valve positions and initiates the expiratory phase.

Expiratory phase
- V_3 closes, allowing the patient to exhale through the expiratory pathway K;
- V_2 closes preventing exhaled gas returning to the main bellows B_2; and
- V_1 opens allowing the contents of the storage bellows and the fresh gas flow to enter the main bellows.

Cycling controls
The *inspiratory phase* is determined by the *time* taken to fill the storage bellows B_1 to the predetermined volume required to trip the lever (N). The latter can be altered by adjusting the position of the trip mechanism with the 'inspiratory phase control' H. Also, a high FGF will fill the bellows more rapidly and so shorten the inspiratory time.

The *expiratory phase* is *volume cycled.* may be altered by adjusting the *tidal volume catch* that regulates

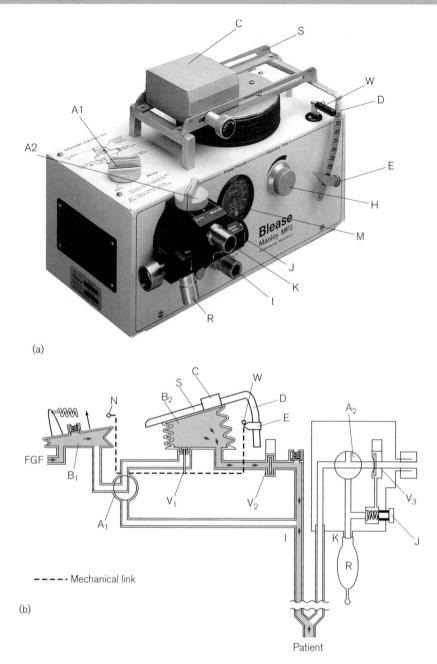

Figure 11.7 (a) Manley MP3 ventilator. **(b)** Working principles of the Manley MP3 ventilator in inspiration. A_1, auto/manual switch, for inspiratory limb; A_2, switch for expiratory limb to atmosphere/reservoir bag; B_1, reservoir bellows; B_2, main bellows; C, bellows weight; D, tidal volume selector; E, tidal volume catch for main bellows; FGF, fresh gas flow; H, inspiratory time control; I, inspiratory port; J, APL valve; K, expiratory port; M, airway pressure manometer; N, trip lever, for the reservoir bellows; R, reservoir bag; S, slide; V_1, V_2, V_3, valves; W, trip lever for main bellows.

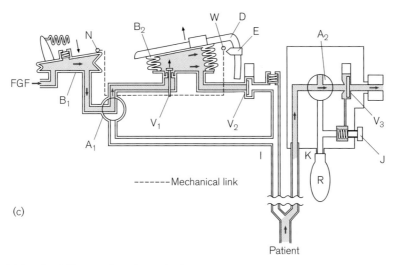

Figure 11.7, *cont'd* (c) Manley MP3 ventilator in expiration.

the degree to which B_2 is filled before the bi-stable mechanism is tripped to initiate inspiration.

Spontaneous respiration

When the ventilator is used in the mode for spontaneous breathing (by turning the tap T_1), fresh gases pass directly to the patient, and the expired gases pass through tap T_2, to the reservoir bag R and finally escape via the expiratory valve J. It therefore behaves as a Mapleson D system and will require the appropriately higher gas flows to avoid rebreathing.

Other features

The expiratory unit, complete with a condensation trap, may be detached very easily and autoclaved. This model also incorporates an airway manometer.

The ventilator produces a power output which depends on the position of the weight on the slider arm. Previous models (MN2 and MP2) used smaller weights and are classified as low-powered ventilators. However, the MP3 can develop pressures of 50 cmH$_2$O (5 kPa) and may be regarded as a high-powered ventilator.

Servo 900 Series ventilator

The Servo 900 Series ventilator is a sophisticated multi-mode ventilator (see Chapter 12, Figs. 12.19 a and b). Many of its functions are more relevant to an intensive care environment and are beyond the remit of this book. However, when used to ventilate anaesthetized patients it

is most frequently used as a pneumatically driven, electronically controlled minute volume divider.

Fresh gas from the anaesthetic machine is fed into the low-pressure entry port sited on the side of the ventilator and is stored in a spring loaded 2-litre bellows. The spring load can be varied with the front panel key to a maximum working pressure of 11.8 kPa/120 cmH$_2$O although a much lower pressure of 5.88 kPa/60 – 65 cmH$_2$O is normally used. If the bellows is overfilled, excess gas is vented through a pressure-relief valve linked to this bellows. This pressurized gas supplies the inspiratory flow to the patient; hence in this mode, the FGF from the anaesthetic machine should be set slightly (12–15%) in excess of ventilatory parameters set up on the ventilator so that the bellows remain optimally filled.

Alternatively, high-pressure gas (420 kPa in the UK) from a blender (nitrous oxide/oxygen) and a special high-pressure vaporizer may be fed into the bellows via the high-pressure inlet port, which is also sited on the side of the ventilator. Prior to entering the bellows, the gas passes through a demand valve that ensures that when any gas is removed from the reservoir bag it is immediately refilled from the blender and vaporizer. This extends the role of the ventilator from that of a simple minute volume divider to that of a machine that can respond to the extra gas demand caused by a patient breathing spontaneously, either with or between, controlled tidal volumes delivered by the ventilator (SIMV models 900C and E). It also allows a patient's respiratory efforts to be assisted by a variable amount when the 'pressure support' mode is selected (Servo 900C and D).

Bag squeezers

Most patients who require automatic ventilation during the course of an anaesthetic are connected to a circle or Mapleson D breathing system that employs a bag squeezer type of ventilator. It relieves the anaesthetist of having to squeeze the breathing bag and, apart from freeing him to do other things, offers the advantages of producing more regular ventilation, with controllable tidal volume and pressure.

The bellows (or bag) may be squeezed pneumatically by placing it in a gas-tight Perspex canister and feeding driving gas (under pressure) into the space between the bellows and canister (Figs. 11.8a and b). Figure 11.8a

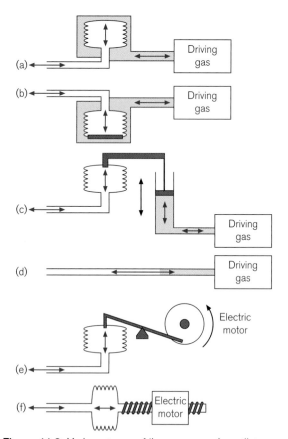

Figure 11.8 Various types of 'bag squeezer' ventilators: **(a)** rising bellows arrangement; **(b)** descending bellows arrangement. **(c)** pneumatic piston with mechanical linkage; **(d)** pneumatic piston; **(e)** cam driven linkage from an electric motor; and **(f)** screw threaded piston (worm drive) powered by electric motor.

shows a rising bellows arrangement. The bellows is filled by patient gas when in use and attached to a breathing system. For the rising bellows, the claimed advantage is that should it develop a leak, the bellows would collapse without any mixing of patient and drive gas. Its detractors claim that the pressure required to fill the bellows adds expiratory resistance and may prevent complete exhalation. Proponents claim that it provides a degree of positive end expiratory pressure (PEEP), which may be beneficial. However, this arrangement is very popular with many manufacturers (see below).

Figure 11.8b shows a descending bellows arrangement. The patient gas is sucked into the bellows by a weight placed in the base. The alleged advantage is the absence of expiratory resistance. This arrangement also allowed the drive unit to be placed above the bellows in the free-standing versions. It could be placed on the lower shelf of an anaesthetic machine with the controls easily to hand. However, a tear in the wall would not result in a bellows collapse and driving gas would be able to enter the bellows and dilute patient gas. Also, the bellows is normally full of air prior to connection to a breathing system and needs to be purged prior to use. This design is no longer popular. The Penlon Nuffield 400 series ventilator was the most common example used in the UK but is no longer produced.

The bellows may be both inflated and deflated by a gas-powered piston that is attached to the bellows by a lever (Fig. 11.8c). This removes the potential for drive and patient gas to mix. The piston may be driven by a smaller quantity of gas than in the methods described above. This could be important in situations where cylinders only are available. The expiratory phase is controlled by the travel of the piston. Here a second reservoir is required should exhalation be faster or slower than the ventilator so as to avoid respiratory embarrassment. This method is no longer popular with manufacturers. The most common models distributed in the UK were the Manley Servovent and the Oxford Mark 2 ventilators.

The bellows may also be squeezed mechanically, by means of a motor and suitable gears and levers (Figs 11.8e and f). Figure 11.8e shows a cam and piston arrangement. The movement of the cam produces a sinusoidal inspiratory pressure rise. In the expiratory phase the bellows may be re-expanded by the pull of the piston or if the piston rod is decoupled during this phase ('lost motion drive') by springs. This is no longer a common method.

Figure 11.8f shows a bellows whose travel is produced by the linear travel of a worm gear driven by an electric motor.

The speed of the motor can be altered both in inspiration and exhalation to produce a variety of flows. This is the method used in the Dräger E series of ventilators.

The bellows may be removed and a suitable length of wide-bore breathing hose substituted (Fig. 11.8d). In this arrangement, the ventilator may push the driving gas directly into the breathing system. This gas and patient gas are not physically separated but the length of hose ensures that the driving gas does not enter the patient part of the breathing system (see Chapter 9). The Penlon Nuffield 200 series has been the most popular ventilator in the UK that uses this method.

Advances in ventilator designs

Most of the recent advances in ventilator design have been seen in Intensive Care ventilators (intermittent blowers) and in anaesthetic ventilators for use with circle breathing systems (bag squeezers). Two key features need some preliminary explanation in order to understand how this new generation of ventilators function and perform. One of these is an electronic flow valve. This has become the major component in the driving gas pathway and has reduced greatly the number of working parts in the ventilator. The other, a programmable microprocessor controls the operation of this valve.

Electronic flow valves

There are three types of valve in common use.

Proportional (flow) valves (Fig.11.9a) When an electric current is fed around a wire coil (solenoid) E in the valve, the magnetic field produced displaces a ferromagnetic core D that acts as a piston and opens a small valve C normally held shut by a spring F. The aperture exposed can be varied depending on the size of the current used, hence the correct term 'proportional flow valve'. This type of valve is used in high-pressure gas pathways. The valve aperture is very small (1.5 mm^2) and the movement of the valve is also small so that: (a) the flow can be rapidly varied between 1–120 l min^{-1}: and (b) the size of the solenoid may be compact enough to fit into the equipment. The response time is usually less than 5 milliseconds.

Proportional valves may be used to control the whole of the inspiratory phase of a ventilator (including the size and duration of the tidal volume), the ventilation rate and the shape of the pressure waveform by varying the size of the valve aperture. Valves may also be used in parallel, each for an individual gas so that the unit behaves as a

(a)

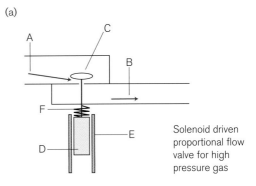

Solenoid driven proportional flow valve for high pressure gas

(b)

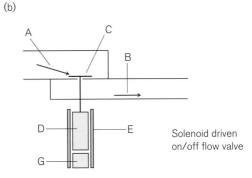

Solenoid driven on/off flow valve

(c)

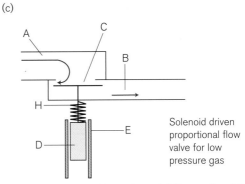

Solenoid driven proportional flow valve for low pressure gas

Figure 11.9 Electronic flow valves. **(a)** Proportional flow valve; A, gas input; B, gas output; C, valve; D, ferromagnetic core; E, solenoid coil. F, spring that holds the valve shut in the resting state. **(b)** Solenoid driven on /off valve instead of a spring magnet G attracts the core D and holds the valve shut. **(c)** A low-pressure proportional flow valve. The valve C and valve orifice is wide. A delicate spring H holds the valve open.

blender and can vary the gas concentrations in the mixture as well as the flow.

On/off valves (Fig 11.9b) These are constructed in a similar fashion to a proportional flow valve. However, they function only as on/off valves They may be used to switch a flow on or off. However, they can be pulsed on and off rapidly to produce a desired flow. Similarly, they may be used in parallel to blend gases to a desired concentration. The valve is held shut by a magnet that attracts the ferromagnetic core inside the solenoid. When a steady current is fed around the solenoid, the magnetic field induced in the core opposes the fixed magnet and the valve opens. When the current flow ceases the magnet attracts the core and the valve shuts usually with the help of the incoming gas flow.

Low-pressure proportional flow valves   This type of valve (Fig. 11.9c) is held open by a delicate spring H. The valve and valve aperture are large to allow a high gas flow at low pressure. When the solenoid is activated, the valve (C) may be partially or completely closed. These devices are used mainly in low-pressure gas pathways as expiratory and PEEP valves.

Microprocessors

These devices control the electrical signal to the proportional flow valve. They can be programmed to provide a wide variety of ventilatory parameters and modes and allow further enhancement of these to occur via reprogramming. Most ventilators now operate on the same principle. The differences seen are in the user display, quality of components and programming variables.

A few examples of 'bag squeezer' ventilators in common use in the UK are described below. The descriptions are not meant to be exhaustive but to point out the general working principles and some interesting features. User manuals for the individual ventilators will provide a greater depth of knowledge where required.

The Blease 8500/8700

This ventilator (Fig. 11.10) represents a type of pneumatically driven 'bag squeezer' with an ascending bellows arrangement. The driving gas is controlled by two proportional flow valves via a microprocessor to provide a wide range of ventilatory parameters (Fig. 11.10c).

Inspiratory phase   Driving gas from a pressurized source A (270–760 kPa (36–101 psi)) is passed through a filter B, a regulator D [set at 259 kPa (34.5 psi)] and fed through a pair of electronic proportional flow control valves E that are connected in parallel. The valves are held shut by the gas pressure upstream when not in use. The driving gas passes to a flow sensor G and to an airtight canister K that contains a rising bellows arrangement. As it enters the canister it compresses the bellows and forces the gas within

into a breathing system. The driving gas also supplies a small pneumatic valve L that closes the expiratory port N and prevents gas destined for inspiration from escaping.

The control of the driving gas through the proportional flow valves is via a microprocessor M. It receives information from three sources, the flow transducer G, the intended ventilation settings on the front panel of the ventilator and a second microprocessor S. The latter receives information from two other flow sensors (not shown in diagram). The first of these is fitted to the anaesthetic machine and measures the FGF. The second is fitted to the breathing system and measures the inspired flow to the patient. Changes in these flows (as a result of altering the FGF or a change in the lung elastance and airways resistance) will alter the delivered tidal volume. The second microprocessor recognizes these changes and applies a correction to the output of the main microprocessor M to restore the intended tidal volume.

Expiratory phase: At the end of the inspiratory phase, the microprocessor instructs the flow control valves E to close (if PEEP is required it remains partially open with a residual flow of 10 l min^{-1}) and a second valve J, to open. This opens the drive gas pathway to atmosphere and causes the pressure in the canister to fall. The reduced pressure of drive gas also allows a pneumatic expiratory valve H, in the ventilator gas pathway to open so that driving gas can escape from the canister as the bellows fills with exhaled gas. When the latter is full, it forces the pneumatic valve L open, so that any excess gas is vented to atmosphere through the expiratory pathway. Both phases are time-cycled by the microprocessor.

During this phase, the bellows behaves as a reservoir bag, allowing spontaneous respiration to take place if desired.

Ventilator controls: The front of the ventilator casing houses a flat panel TFT screen, similar to that found on a laptop computer (Fig. 11.10a). Also, there are two knobs, the bottom left switches the ventilator on in either the adult or paediatric mode. The right one is a rotary cursor (Trak^{TM}) wheel which, when rotated, highlights the adjustable parameters (contained in individual boxes) on the main screen in yellow. Pressing the wheel inwards changes the screen colour of the box to blue indicating that the parameter selected may now be adjusted. Rotation of the cursor wheel alters the parameter and when the value selected appears, it is activated by pressing the wheel inwards. The change is confirmed by the new colour of the box, which is white.

The screen is divided into three sections (Fig.11.10b). The top left has the facility for spirometry or pressure waveform display, mode of ventilation and adult/paediatric selection. The top right displays alarm limits. The bottom displays the adjustable parameters (tidal volume, rate, inspiratory/expiratory ratio, pressure limit, PEEP, trigger, pressure support) and those that are measured, such as peak/mean pressure, minute/tidal volume FGF from the anaesthetic machine and oxygen concentration if a sensor is used.

Above the cursor wheel there is a bank of six programming keys. Three of these control the alarm system, one is 'standby/on', another allows access to the main menu and the last configures the ventilator. The main menu performs the following functions:

- oxygen calibration;
- *features*: selects which parameters (in the white boxes) go into which space on the bottom of the main screen:
- *waveform select*: displays either pressure or pressure/flow/ or volume/flow loops and a pressure bar graph:
- *mode*: selects ventilatory modes such as (controlled minute ventilation (CMV), synchronized intermittent mandatory ventilation (SIMV), pressure-controlled ventilation (PCV), assisted spontaneous breathing

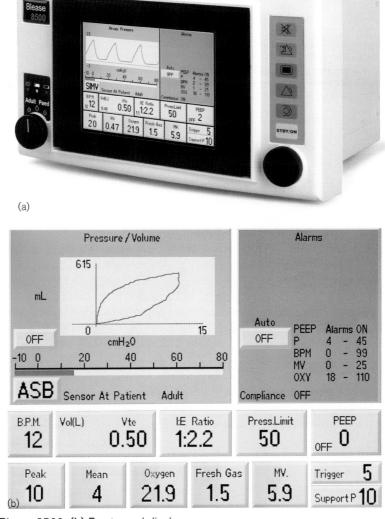

Figure 11.10 (a) Blease 8500. **(b)** Front panel display.

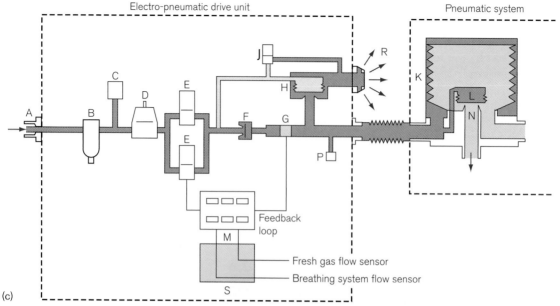

Electro-pneumatic drive unit

Pneumatic system

Feedback loop

Fresh gas flow sensor

Breathing system flow sensor

(c)

Figure 11.10, *cont'd.* (c) Working principles. A, drive gas input port (270–760 kPa (36–101 psi)); B, input gas filter (5 mm) and water trap; C, low supply pressure transducer (270 kPa); D, input pressure regulator; E, solenoid flow control valves; F, non-return valve; G, flow sensor; H, expiratory valve; J, solenoid dump valve; K, bellows assembly; L, pneumatic valve; M, microprocessor; N, patient gas expiratory port; R, driving gas exhaust; S, second microprocessor.

(ASB), end inspiratory pause (0–50%), sigh (tidal volume + 10% every 10 breaths) and inspiratory flow (adjustable from 2–99 l min^{-1}); and

- *configuration*: allows a different set of defaults settings to be used. There is an additional sub menu (also called 'configuration') that is password protected. This allows for language change, calibration of the ventilator and addition of a new set of defaults for individual users.

Adult ventilation   The ventilator is designed to operate with the manufacturer's absorber. When the ventilator is switched on in the adult mode, it asks the user to help perform a series of tests. These confirm that:

- the absorber is connected both electronically and pneumatically to the ventilator;
- that there is no leak in the absorber and breathing system; and
- the compliance of the absorber and breathing system is calculated (see below).

At the end of the sequence the ventilator is placed in the standby in the hospital default mode. When the on/off switch on the absorber is turned to the ON position, the ventilator starts to operate. The switch also automatically isolates the APL valve on the absorber.

Older systems did not have this facility and the APL valve had to be closed either manually or via a second isolating switch to stop patient gas from escaping during automatic ventilation. Ventilatory parameters may be changed 'on the fly' during ventilation.

Additional features   The ventilator has some interesting features worth mentioning.

Tidal volume: The ventilator receives information from flow transducers within the anaesthetic machine and the breathing system. This is passed on to the microprocessors in the ventilator. A calculation is made of the proportion the FGF makes to the intended tidal volume and the ventilator makes an adjustment to the bellows travel to deliver this. Therefore, the tidal volume set on the front panel is the actual volume delivered. In addition, the pre-use check calculates the compliance of the whole breathing system and factors this into the amount of gas required to maintain the set tidal volume. Furthermore, with each inspiratory cycle, using the peak inspiratory pressure, the set tidal volume and the system compliance, the ventilator calculates the compliance of the patient (which may change due to pharmacological or physiological reasons) and makes an adjustment with the next breath to restore the intended tidal volume.

Positive end expiratory pressure (PEEP): When PEEP is required, the main proportional flow valves allow a standing flow of $10 \, l \, min^{-1}$ to pass into the driving gas expiratory pathway. A low-pressure proportional valve J activates, partially occluding this flow to provide the desired level of PEEP. An electronic PEEP valve is available for certain countries that insist on this. To facilitate this, the expiratory one-way valve on the manufacturer's absorber is removed and replaced by one that is operated through the ventilator microprocessor (Fig. 7.18d).

Assisted spontaneous breathing: A flow transducer is usually fitted in the breathing system close to the patient to monitor inspiration and exhalation. This can be used to trigger the ventilator to assist a spontaneous breath and can be adjusted to recognize a flow of as little as $3 \, l \, min^{-1}$. The degree of assistance is determined by the amount of pressure support set on the ventilator. This can be a very useful tool in overcoming the higher inspiratory resistance of circle breathing systems when used for spontaneous respiration. In practice the system is more efficient when a degree of PEEP is also applied. This raises the functional residual capacity (usually low in an anaesthetized patient) and places the lungs on a better part of the compliance curve where a similar inspiratory effort produces a higher inspiratory gas flow of and therefore a quicker response time.

Paediatric ventilation The adult bellows and breathing hoses can be used for paediatric anesthesia. However, if the internal compliance is required to be small, the adult bellows may be easily removed and substituted by a smaller (300 ml) one. At the same time the hoses should be changed for narrower-bore ones (15 mm). The paediatric mode should then be selected from the front panel of the ventilator, as this alters the factory/hospital defaults. A new compliance calibration should be carried out as part of the start-up check. In PCV mode, the pressure limiter is adjusted to the peak inspiratory pressure required. The inspiratory flow will then reduce or cease in order to maintain the set pressure (even in the presence of a normal leak around the endotracheal tube), until the time cycled inspiratory phase has been completed.

The ventilator design can therefore be classified as a high-powered, time-cycled 'bag squeezer' ventilator.

The Ohmeda Aestiva 7100 and 7900

Both these ventilators work on similar principles. The 7900 is the more sophisticated and will be described here. Both are pneumatically-driven microprocessor controlled bag squeezers. Although the microprocessor handles the driving gas in a somewhat similar fashion to that described previously, the display and controls are somewhat different. The ventilator is powered up by turning on the master switch for the anaesthetic workstation. A light in the lower left of the control unit glows to indicate that the ventilator now has mains electric power available. The ventilator has two sections, the control unit and the rising bellows arrangement.

Control unit The control unit (Fig. 11.11a) houses a flat panel display surrounded by various keys and a single rotary control that the manufacturer calls a 'comm' wheel. The display (Fig. 11.11b) is divided into sections. The lower half of the screen has yellow boxes with displayed values for intended tidal volume, rate, inspiratory/expiratory ratio, maximum pressure limit and PEEP. Below each of these is a 'soft key' which when pressed, highlights that parameter. The latter may be adjusted to a new value by moving the comm wheel. The upper section of the display shows the measured ventilatory parameters (yellow numbering on a black background) and a graph of airways pressure. This information is retrieved from the twin flow transducers placed in the circle breathing system. Above the comm wheel is a menu key which when pressed produces a drop down menu showing ventilation mode, alarm settings, calibration screen, and audio setup and exit to normal screen. The comm wheel is rotated to select one of the options, for example 'ventilation' mode. Pushing the wheel inwards displays a sub-menu of the various modes available.

Above the menu key is another that turns the volume alarm on and off. On the lower left of the control unit is an 'end of case' key. When automatic ventilation is stopped, this may be pressed. This feature suspends the apnoea and low-volume alarm and restores the ventilation parameters, including PEEP, to either the hospital default or it keeps the current ventilator control settings (as requested in a pre-configured setup menu) The 7900 supports four modes of ventilation. These are volume-controlled ventilation, pressure controlled ventilation, synchronized intermittent mandatory ventilation and an assisted spontaneous breathing mode called *Pressure Support Ventilation Pro* (PSV Pro). The flow trigger for the latter may be adjusted for varying degrees of sensitivity (0.2–$10 \, l \, min^{-1}$).

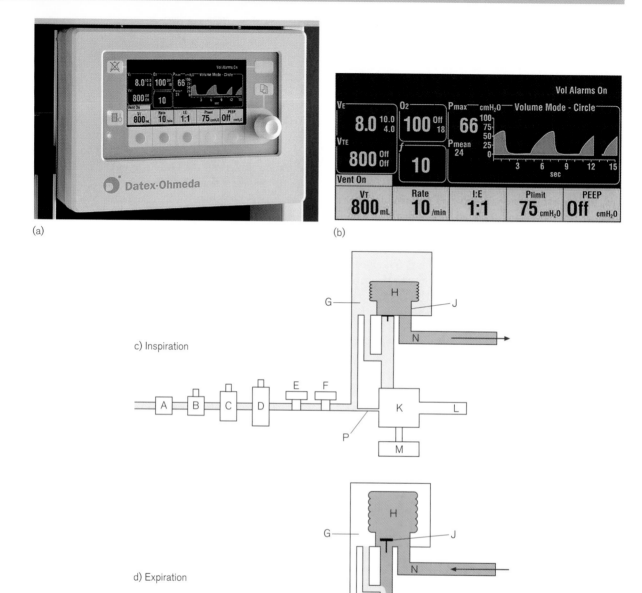

Figure 11.11 (a) Aestiva 7900 ventilator. **(b)** Front panel. **(c)** Working principles: A, 5 micron filter; B, electropneumatic switch; C, pressure regulator; D, flow control valve; E, electrically-operated overpressure relief valve; F, a mechanical dead weight valve for relief of overpressure; G, driving gas to bellows canister; H, bellows; J, exhalation dump valve; K, second exhalation valve for PEEP; L, expiratory pathway; M, exhalation safety valve (set at 30 cmH₂O); N, patient pathway; P, driving gas for PEEP valve (K).

The bellows unit This unit houses the manufacturer's circle absorber, a conventional rising bellows arrangement, inspiratory and expiratory flow transducers and an APL valve. The latter has a mandatory overpressure relief fitted for safety during spontaneous breathing.

Inspiratory phase (Fig 11.11c) Driving gas from a pressurized source, which may be air or oxygen at a pressure between 250–700 kPa (35 to 100 psi), is passed through a 5 micron filter (A) to an electrically operated pneumatic on/off valve which is turned on when the machine master switch is turned on. From here it passes through a regulator (C) that reduces the pressure down to 170 kPa (25 psi) and on to the flow control valve (D). The valve is closed when the ventilator is switched off but opens under the control of a microprocessor to deliver the appropriate flow for the intended title volume and cycling rate. The gas then passes across two safety valves (E) electrically operated and (F) a mechanical dead weight valve. It then enters the bellows canister where it puts pressure on the patient bellows, compressing it. A pilot line (not shown in diagram) goes to the exhalation dump valve (J) to close it. Gas from the bellows unit (H) is pushed into the wide bore hosing (N) which is attached to the circle breathing system.

Exhalation phase (Fig 11.11d) When the proportional flow valve is switched off, the gas pressure in the bellows canister decreases to zero. This allows the patient gas in the circle system to empty into the bellows. When this is full and pressure is raised above atmospheric, the dump valve (J) opens passively and the gas escapes through the exhalation valve (K) to atmosphere. At the same time the driving gas that was left in the bellows canister is also vented to atmosphere via the valve (K). If PEEP is required, a small bleed of driving gas (P) from the proportional flow valve pressurizes the exhalation valve (K) to provide the intended PEEP. The valve (K) is fitted with a pressure relief valve (M) which is set at 30 cm of water and which opens if the exhalation pathway is blocked.

Interesting features When used in volume controlled ventilation or SIMV mode, the inspiratory flow transducer in the breathing system measures delivered tidal volume. It passes this information back to the microprocessor, which updates the information every six breaths and adjusts the ventilation to ensure that the values set on the ventilator and the measured values match. This system compensates for changes in both lung compliance and

FGF from the anaesthetic machine. It even has a user selectable Heliox mode that compensates for the change in gas density and viscosity that would otherwise alter the information from the flow transducers.

Paediatric mode The ventilatory parameters available (tidal volume 20–1500 ml and rates of 4–100 breaths) and the compensation features mentioned above are sufficient to allow it to be used in infants and neonates. Most anaesthetists however use the ventilator in pressure control mode for such applications. Here, it may be beneficial to use narrow bore breathing hose (15 mm). The ventilator design can therefore be classified as a high-powered, time-cycled 'bag squeezer' ventilator.

Dräger anaesthetic ventilators (E Models)

The bag squeezer ventilators fitted currently to anaesthetic workstations marketed by Dräger (Primus, Fabius and Cicero) are electrically powered and controlled. These ventilators are made up from three modules, a control module, the ventilator module and the circle breathing system.

Control module (Fig. 11.12a) The ventilatory parameters available depend on the model used. The basic model, the Fabius CE allows volume-controlled ventilation only. The top of the range Primus has the facility for both volume and pressure controlled ventilation, either as stand-alone features or with the provision for spontaneous breathing with and without pressure support in these modes. It also allows a purely spontaneous respiration mode with triggered pressure support. The control unit shown is a mid-range model, the Fabius GS. Like the ventilator described above, it has a rotary control (bottom right) to alter selected variables. On the left of the unit are the keys that select the mode of ventilation. The middle of the unit has a thin film transistor (TFT) screen that displays all the relevant information. To the right of this are two banks of keys to select the alarms, menu set-up, home, alarm silence and standby. The home key restores the screen to the default after any sub menu called up is no longer required and the standby key stops the ventilator and keeps any ventilatory parameters selected for use again.

Ventilator module (Fig 11.12b) The ventilator has an electric motor (1) with a hollow spindle. The inside of the spindle has a screw thread. A rod (2) with a matching thread passes through the spindle. When the electric

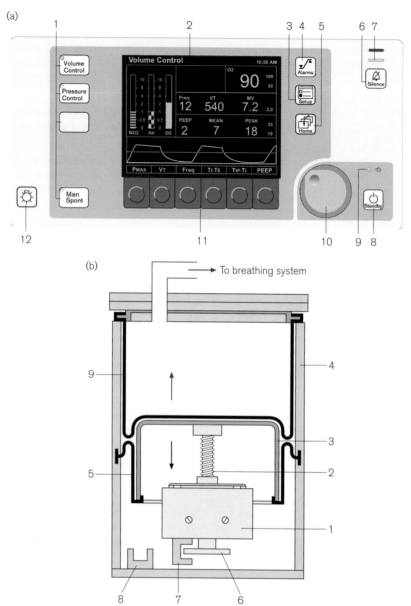

Figure 11.12 (a) Dräger E ventilator as fitted to the Fabius GS. 1, ventilation mode hard keys; 2, user interface display screen; 3, set up key; 4, alarm limits hard key; 5, home key; 6, alarm silence key; 7, alarm status indicators; 8, standby mode key; 9, power on indicator; 10, rotary knob; 11, soft keys (functions); 12, lamp switch. **(b)** Working principles. 1, electric motor; 2, rod with screw thread; 3, piston; 4, cylinder; 5, rolling rubber seal; 6, incremental encoder; 7, sensor; 8, light barrier; 9, ventilator bellows. (Figure 11.12a, reproduced with permission from Dräger Medical UK.)

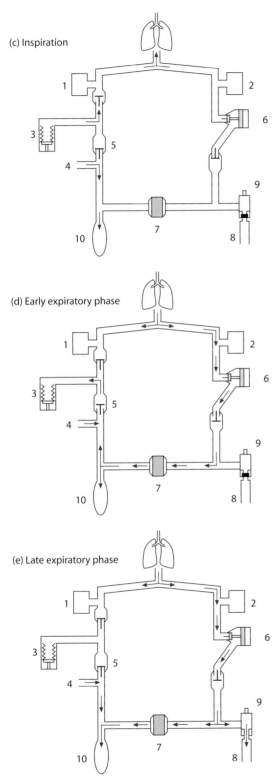

(c) Inspiration

(d) Early expiratory phase

(e) Late expiratory phase

Figure 11.12, *cont'd.* (c) Dräger circle system inspiratory phase: 1, inspiratory flow transducer; 2, expiratory flow transducer, 3, ventilator; 4, fresh gas; 5, fresh gas decoupling; 6, setting P_{max}/Peep; 7, absorber; 8, scavenging; 9, APL valve; 10, reservoir bag. **(d)** Dräger circle system early expiratory phase. **(e)** Dräger circle system late expiratory phase.

motor spins, the spindle rotates and the action of the two threads, which are interlocked, causes the rod to move through the spindle. This movement is referred to as either a recirculating ball screw or a worm drive. One end of the rod is connected to a piston (3) that moves backwards and forwards inside a cylinder (4), depending upon the direction and duration of current flow in the electric motor. The head of the piston is fitted with a rolling neoprene seal (5) so that on the downstroke is capable of producing a sub-atmospheric pressure to the bellows that sits above it. The position of the piston rod at any one time is sensed by a high-resolution incremental encoder (6) and allows precise volume (0.03 ml) delivery. The encoder consists of a metal disc that has 1024 perforations around the edge. When the electric motor is working, this disc spins between two arms of a sensor (7) that counts the passage of the perforations and then calculates the linear movement of the piston rod. At the bottom of the cylinder there is a light barrier to detect the lower stop position of the piston.

Interesting features

Inspiration (Fig.11.12c): During the inspiratory phase the ventilator delivers the intended amount of volume to the patient. It does this by diverting the FGF from the anaesthetic machine via a decoupling valve into the reservoir bag and not the patient. Furthermore, the delivered tidal volume from the ventilator enters the breathing system downstream of the absorber (which is isolated) and therefore minimizes the compression volume of the inspiratory pathway. The reservoir bag will be seen to expand with the addition of fresh gas, which may be a little unnerving for those not familiar with this system. There is a flow transducer in the inspiratory pathway that measures gas flow, which is then displayed on the control unit.

Exhalation (Fig. 11.12d): The expiratory travel of the piston is fixed by the I/E ratio of the ventilator. The sub-atmospheric pressure created by the downstroke of the ventilator sucks in gas from both the reservoir bag and the exhalation volume from the patient. Towards the end of the exhalation phase, the reservoir bag fills and surplus gas is dumped through the scavenging port. Again the reservoir bag will be seen to move. In the top of the range machine, information from the expiratory flow transducer is passed to the microprocessor, which in turn causes the movement of the piston backstroke in the ventilator to match the expiratory flow.

Paediatric mode: When these ventilators are switched on, the control unit software performs a leak and compliance test (except for the base model workstation). Compliance compensation, along with the low compliance of the bellows and breathing system, allows accurate delivery of small tidal volumes if required. More commonly, the ventilators may be used in the pressure support made that compensates for any small leak caused by an uncuffed endotracheal tube.

The ventilator design can therefore be classified as a high-powered, high-efficiency, time-cycled 'bag squeezer' ventilator.

Intermittent blowers

These ventilators are driven by a pressurized source of gases or air, at a pressure of 250– 400 kPa (37.5–60 psi). The driving gas pathway through it is very small with a low internal compliance that makes this type very efficient. The major component is an electronically timed and activated proportional flow valve or a pneumatically timed oscillator that divides the driving gas into tidal volumes the size and rate of which can be adjusted. Sophisticated ventilators such as those used in Intensive Care and anaesthetic workstations make use of a proportional flow valve (see above). Automatic resuscitators and more basic anaesthetic ventilators use the pneumatic oscillator principle (see below) as this is cheaper, does not require the same sophistication of operation and is powered by the driving gas requiring no electrical supply. Intensive Care ventilators are discussed in more detail in Chapter 12.

Pneumatic oscillator A typical example is seen in Figure 11.13. The diagram is a very simplified version and does not attempt to show the detailed pneumatics that are essential for its function. Driving gas enters at point (1). It divides into three pathways. The main one passes to a cylinder that contains a shuttle (2), which travels between the ends of the cylinder. In the inspiratory phase (Fig. 11.13a), the driving gas passes into the cylinder and through a hole in the shuttle into the gas pathway (3) to the patient. The other two pathways supply two

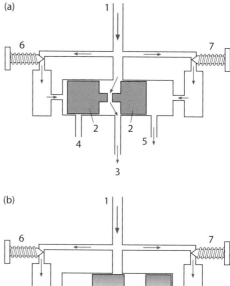

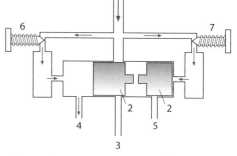

Figure 11.13 A pneumatic oscillator. **(a)** Inspiratory phase. **(b)** Expiratory phase. 1, Driving gas; 2, shuttle; 3, gas pathway to patient; 4, inspiratory timer vent; 5, expiratory timer vent; 6, inspiratory timer; 7, expiratory timer.

pneumatic timers (6) (inspiratory) and (7) (expiratory), each of which has a needle valve that regulates flow to the timer mechanism at the relevant end of the cylinder. When the flow causes sufficient build-up of pressure in the inspiratory timer, the shuttle is forced to the opposite end of the cylinder (Fig. 11.13b) and in doing so causes three events:

1. it blocks off the flow of driving gas through the cylinder terminating the inspiratory flow;
2. it opens a vent (4) to open on the inspiratory side of the cylinder that allows the pressure in the inspiratory timer to be released; and
3. it causes the shuttle to occlude the expiratory timer vent 5 so that a pressure can build up to reverse the direction of the shuttle and terminate the expiratory phase.

Working principles of pneumatically controlled intermittent blowers

A generic line diagram of a typical pneumatically powered and controlled 'intermittent blower' is show in Figure 11.14. High-pressure driving gas, (300–400 kPa) is

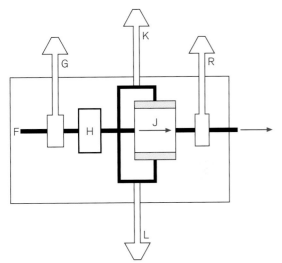

Figure 11.14 Schematic diagram of a pneumatically controlled intermittent blower (see text for details). F, high pressure driving gas input (300–600 kPa); G, pneumatic on/off switch; H, pressure regulator; J, oscillator; K, variable pneumatic inspiratory timer; L, variable pneumatic expiratory timer; R, inspiratory flow restricter.

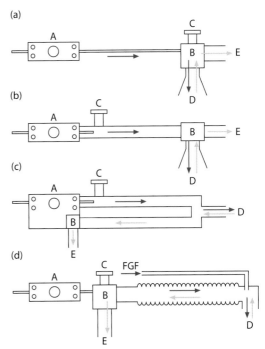

Figure 11.15 Classification of intermittent blowers: **(a)** Basic resuscitator. **(b)** Sophisticated resuscitator. **(c)** Ventilator for Intensive Care. **(d)** Anaesthetic ventilator for Mapleson D system. A, resuscitator/ventilator; B, patient valve; C, overpressure relief valve; D, patient pathway, E, expiratory pathway.

connected to the device at point (F). When the main pneumatics on/off switch (G) is turned on, gas flows through it to a regulator (H) that reduces the driving pressure to approximately 275 kPa. Gas flows on to the oscillator (J). The output from this passes through a variable flow restrictor and exits the device to be attached to a breathing system. The delivered tidal volume is a function of the inspiratory timer (K) which is calibrated in seconds and flow restrictor (R) which is calibrated in $l\,sec^{-1}$. The respiratory rate is determined by the *cycle time*: inspiratory time (adjusted at K) plus the expiratory time (adjusted at L).

Classification of intermittent blowers

Intermittent blowers are used in four different ways (Fig. 11.15) .

Basic resuscitators

The simplest design is used as a basic resuscitator (Fig. 11.15a). The working principles are shown in Figure 11.16a. It has no on/off switch and no flow restrictor and a fixed expiratory timer. It has a single control (K) for tidal volume, cycling rate and I/E ratio, which is actually the variable inspiratory timer. Since the flow rate is constant, when the inspiratory time is lengthened, the tidal volume is increased, the cycling rate

is reduced and the I/E ratio is prolonged and vice versa. The intended tidal volume travels along a narrow-bore tube as a small volume of high-pressure gas to a one-way spring-loaded patient valve (B) (Fig. 11.15a). The gas expands inside the body of the valve to provide a lower pressure and larger volume of gas to a patient. The valve body is provided with an overpressure relief valve (C). The advantage of this system is that the narrow-bore flexible pipeline can be many metres long which may be useful where there is limited access at the site of an accident.

An example of this type is the Pneupac adult/child resuscitator (Fig. 11.16b), which although a very old design, is still in production.

The working principles of the patient valve are explained in Figure 11.16c.

Sophisticated resuscitators

Figure 11.15b shows this more sophisticated version of the above. For reasons stated below, it is fitted with wide-bore hosing that supplies the patient valve.

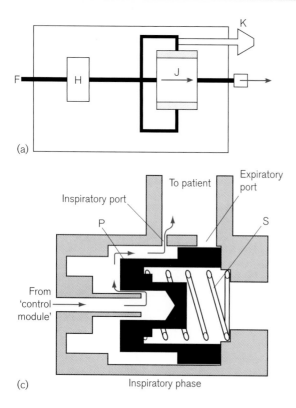

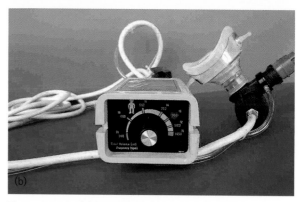

(a)

(b)

(c) Inspiratory phase

Figure 11.16 (a) Working principle of a basic resuscitator: F, driving gas; H, pressure regulator; J, oscillator; K, tidal volume and rate control. **(b)** A basic resuscitator: the Pneupac adult/child resuscitator. The overpressure relief valve with its red cap is seen connected to the patient valve. **(c)** Working principles of the Pneupac patient valve (inspiratory phase): P, piston; S, spring.

A typical example is the Pneupac Ventipac (Fig. 11.17a). The increased sophistication may be seen in the line diagram Figure 11.17b. The output from the oscillator (J) is passed via a variable flow restrictor (R) on to two coupled needle valves (P) and (Q), operated by a switch (O). If P (air mix mode) is selected, the driving gas is passed into a Venturi that entrains a fixed amount of ambient air from S (*this port has a non return valve*) and the total flow is fed into the patient breathing system. If Q (no air mix) is selected, both needle valves are activated. The bore of Q is such that its output matches the entrainment from S to supplement the flow from P so that no air is entrained and the delivered content is 100% driving gas (usually oxygen). The output of the ventilator is connected to the wide-bore hose of breathing system, the other end of which is attached to a lightweight low-resistance Laerdal pattern non-rebreathing valve. The device has separate controls for inspiratory time, expiratory time and inspiratory flow rate and so is able to provide greater ventilatory flexibility than the base model.

In addition, should the patient attempt to breathe, a demand detector (M) senses the pressure in the breathing system via a pilot line (W) and triggers the demand valve (N). This takes its gas supply from the high-pressure gas inlet upstream from the pneumatic switch (G) and allows the demand valve to function even if the ventilator is switched off. If the latter is switched on however, the demand valve operates in conjunction with the oscillator to integrate this signal and to extend the expiratory phase as a function of the spontaneous tidal volume up to a maximum time dictated by the frequency settings of the ventilator. Thus, if the patient demands a high flow for a short duration or low flow from a longer duration, (i.e. similar tidal volumes) an equal expiratory time will be allowed before the next breath. The cumulative effect of successive spontaneous breaths by the patient causes the ventilator to become inhibited although, in fact, this is only on a breath-by-breath basis. Inhibition starts at 150 ml and increases to a full inhibition of 450 ml. The level of spontaneous breathing required to fully inhibit the oscillator is fixed at that of the typical adult breathing spontaneously. This is taken as tidal volume of about 450 ml at 12 to 16 breaths per minute. Higher spontaneous ventilation rates can readily be taken and will result in complete inhibition of the ventilator. Lower rates will

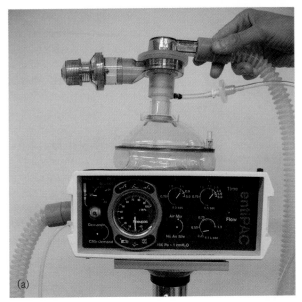

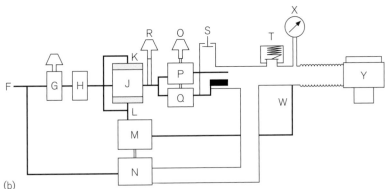

Figure 11.17 **(a)** A Pneupac Ventipac ventilator with the airways pressure line, Laerdal pattern non-rebreathing valve with a PEEP attachment. **(b)** Working principles: F, driving gas input; G, on/off valve; H, pressure regulator; J, oscillator; K, inspiratory timer; L, expiratory timer; M, demand detector; N, demand valve and demand gas pathway; O, air mix selector switch; P, needle valve for airmix; Q, needle valve to supplement flow from F for no airmix; R, variable flow restrictor; S, air entrainment port with non return valve; T, variable pressure relief valve; W, pilot line to demand detector; X, airways pressure display; Y, laerdal pattern non-rebreathing valve.

only give partial inhibition but providing the demand flow is above $15\,l\,min^{-1}$ the ventilator will still interact with the patient and synchronize its ventilation pattern with the spontaneous breathing.

The ventilator has a variable pressure relief valve (T). It also has battery operated multi-functional pressure alarm and pressure gauge.

Intensive care ventilators

Figure 11.15c shows a basic line diagram of an intermittent blower used as typical intensive care ventilator. These are discussed in more detail in Chapter 12.

Ventilators for anaesthetic breathing systems

Figure 11.15d illustrates the use of an intermittent blower with an anaesthetic breathing system. The patient valve may be placed adjacent to the ventilator and the output connected to a breathing system (Mapleson D or circle system) in place of the normal reservoir bag (see Chapter 7). It must be remembered that sufficient length of wide-bore hosing must be used between the ventilator and the breathing system to prevent any driving gas from diluting the anaesthetic intended for the patient. The ventilator that popularized this method in the UK is the Penlon Nuffield 200 series (Fig, 11.18).

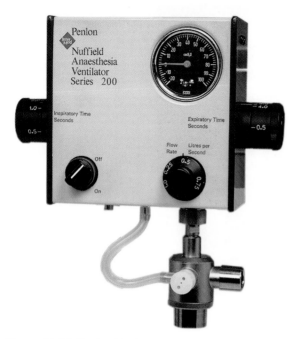

Figure 11.18 Penlon Nuffield Series 200.

Jet ventilation

Conventionally, the lungs of a patient are normally ventilated by providing a seal to the upper airway so that sufficient pressure may build up to provide movement of gas into the lungs. Alternatively, a high-pressure jet of gas may be directed into the airway without the need for a seal. The kinetic energy of the gas molecules is sufficient to overcome the elastic properties of the lungs and to cause them to expand. Furthermore, the speed of the molecules leaving the jet may act as a Venturi and entrain adjacent gas so as to increase the volume provided. The efficiency of the jet depends on a number of factors. The jet is at its most efficient in terms of gas delivery and ability to entrain when its path is in a straight line. Sharp bends dramatically decrease both of these. The amount of gas delivered is also increased as the driving pressure is raised.

Jet ventilation may be very useful in situations where the airway is so narrowed that only a small gas delivery device may be passed or in situations where conventional airway management devices would impede the view of a surgeon or the conduct of an operation.

There are two ways in which a high-pressure jet of gas may be used to ventilate a patient.

Manually controlled jetting

For short procedures such as rigid bronchoscopy, a patient may be paralyzed and then ventilated by applying an intermittent jet via the bronchoscope, using a manually-operated injector device such as the Manujet (see Airway management devices, Chapter 8)). The jet behaves as a Venturi causing air to be entrained by the driving gas. The latter is usually oxygen, at a pressure of up of 420 kPa (60 psi). Anaesthesia is normally maintained intravenously.

The tidal volumes, inspired oxygen concentrations and airway pressures are not easily measured. As the delivery system is placed in the supraglottis, barotrauma is very unlikely. If the jet is placed below the vocal cords, for example, by using a flexible catheter then caution must be exercised during the procedure. Any obstruction above the catheter will prevent exhalation and a dangerous build-up of pressure may result. If a manual method is used, a check should be made for a complete exhalation after each delivered tidal volume.

Automatically controlled jetting

Specially designed ventilators are available that can deliver a jet of gas automatically with the ability to monitor both the delivery pressure and the airways pressure with a safety cut-out should the latter exceed a set limit. The Acutronic jet ventilator (Fig. 11.19a) is a common example of this in Europe and the UK. There are two models. The 'Mistral' is a dry ventilator that jets dry gas only. It is suitable for surgical procedures. The 'Monsoon' has a built in humidifier system for use in longer procedures and the Intensive Care Unit. Both are based around a high-performance, electronically-controlled solenoid flow valve capable of frequencies up to 500 cycles per minute. The ventilator has three main controls. One alters the rate; another, the I/E ratio (by altering the percentage of the cycle that is inspiration); and the third operates a needle valve that controls the output pressure of the driving gas. The delivered tidal volume/minute volume depends on a combination of all three settings and all of these ventilatory parameters are displayed on a screen on the front panel of the device.

Normally double lumen catheters are used for ventilation and are placed subglottically. The jet is usually attached to the main lumen and the jetting pressure is adjusted until suitable chest movement is seen. The delivery pressure can be adjusted to a maximum pressure of 400 kPa, although 200 kPa is the norm. Higher

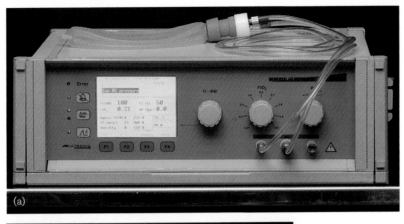

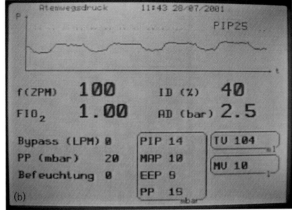

Figure 11.19 **(a)** Monsoon Universal Jet ventilator, Acutronic Medical Systems AG. **(b)** Ventilator display.

pressures may be required for supraglottic jets attached to an operating laryngoscope or bronchoscope. Here the jet is less efficient as it is attached to the side of the device, which reduces the efficiency of the Venturi.

The 'Monsoon' measures the airways pressures (from the second lumen of the catheter) throughout the respiratory cycle and displays them on the front panel of the device (Fig. 11.19b). These include peak inspiratory pressure (PIP), mean airway pressure (MAP), end expiratory pressure (EEP) and pause pressure (PP). The latter measures the decay in the pressure in the jet tube following an inspiratory phase. If this has not dropped sufficiently below a pre-set limit within 1 ms of the next jet, the ventilator stops. This is a safety feature designed to reduce the risk of barotrauma by preventing 'stacking of breaths' due to injected gas from consecutive jets being trapped in the lungs. The 'Mistral' has the latter feature only and none of the other displays.

Features of jet ventilation

Frequency

There are two modes of jet ventilation in use. Conventionally, jet ventilation may be carried out at rates up to 60 cycles per minute. Above 60 cycles per minute the technique is referred to as high-frequency jet ventilation. There are advantages and disadvantages to both methods.

Low-frequency jet ventilation Low-frequency jet ventilation at low rates (10–30 min), is simple and requires minimal equipment. A few key points are outlined below:
- normal tidal volumes are required for carbon dioxide elimination;
- the ventilation can be carried with a manual injector;
- there is sufficient time during exhalation for conventional methods to be used in the measurement of carbon dioxide elimination;

- larger movements of gas in and out of the laryngeal inlet may cause sufficient movement of the vocal cords to preclude any operative procedure; and
- inflation pressures may be high and may embarrass cardiac output.

High-frequency jet ventilation At rates above 60 and up to 300 cycles per minute, a number of advantages are claimed for jet ventilation. Some of these and other salient points are outlined below:

- more efficient alveolar ventilation with much lower tidal volumes;
- a substantial reduction in mean airway and alveolar pressures with a reduced potential for barotrauma;
- a minimal disturbance of cardiac output, and subsequent renal function;
- a reduction in leaks from broncho-pleural fistulae, often with an improvement in gas exchange;
- a more comfortable method of providing ventilatory support for patients in the intensive care unit;
- for surgical procedures the target site is more stable and only vibrates;
- expensive and unfamiliar equipment is needed; and
- altering ventilatory parameters causes less intuitive changes in physiological variables.

Inhalational anaesthesia

Current jet ventilation systems (the most popular method) do not readily lend themselves to providing inhalational anaesthesia. Although nitrous oxide and oxygen mixture can be used with the ventilators (via a high-pressure blender) there are no commercial high-pressure vaporizers available for the addition of inhalational agents. Furthermore, as the jet may sometimes act as a Venturi, entrained gas in any attached breathing system needs to be of the same composition as the driving gas in order to guarantee the desired final gas composition.

Humidification

Conventional hot-water or condenser humidifiers are impractical for use with high-frequency ventilation, as they have too high an internal volume. The small delivered tidal volumes with high-frequency ventilation get 'lost' in the humidifier and are not delivered to the patient. However, warmed distilled water or saline can be fed into the jet line by a peristaltic pump. As this emerges from the jet it is atomized to provide a degree of humidification which can be varied by adjusting the speed of the pump.

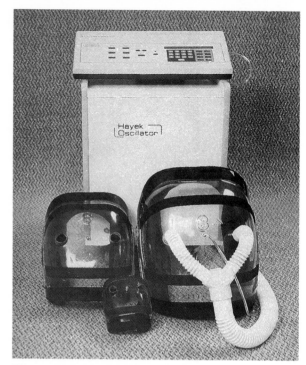

Figure 11.20 Hayek oscillator.

NEGATIVE PRESSURE VENTILATION

A patient's lungs may also be inflated by encasing the patient in a gas-tight container from the neck downwards (tank cuirass) or by a smaller device that surrounds the patient's thorax only (thoracic cuirass), and applying an intermittent sub-atmospheric pressure (*negative pressure ventilation*). The thorax is 'sucked outwards' during the inspiratory phase causing air/respirable gas to enter the lungs. Exhalation is achieved either by the elastic recoil of the thorax or by applying active compression to the cuirass.

This method has many attractions. It is non invasive. The patient does not require intubation either orally, nasally or through a tracheostomy, and unlike positive pressure ventilation, it does not reduce cardiac output. The smaller of the two types (thoracic ciurass) has been used in anaesthesia to ventilate patients requiring laryngoscopy and laser therapy without having to use conventional endotracheal intubation.

Hayek oscillator (Fig. 11.20)

This has three components:

1. The first is of a moulded lightweight shell made from clear plastic with soft foam edges that provide

a seal around the anterior chest wall and upper abdomen. It comes in three sizes, one for infants, one for larger children and one for adults. Each version has appropriately-sized wide-ore tubing that links it to the second component, the power unit.

2. The power unit houses a diaphragm pump that has a maximum stroke volume of 3.5 litres and which drives air backwards and forwards through the tubing to intermittently evacuate the shell when it is attached to a patient. A second pump can be used to vary the baseline pressure of the driving gas below atmospheric. This determines the negative end expiratory pressure within the shell and hence the functional residual capacity of the lungs.

3. The third component (the control unit) sets the frequency of oscillations (8–999 cycles/minute), the inspiratory pressure (–70 cm H_2O), the expiratory pressure (–70 to +70 cmH_2O and the inspiratory/ expiratory ratio (6:1 to 1:6). It receives information from a pressure transducer (that is connected to the shell) so that it can automatically compensate for any alteration in performance.

Although it can function at conventional rates and tidal volumes, it is designed to work in its higher-frequency range and with correspondingly smaller tidal volumes.

REFERENCES

1. Mushin WW, Rendell-Baker L, Thompson PW, Mapleson, WW (1980) *Automatic Ventilation of the Lungs*, 3rd end. Oxford: Blackwell Science.

FURTHER READING

Mushin WW, Rendell-Baker L, Thompson PW (1980) *Automatic Ventilation of the Lungs*, 3rd edn. Oxford: Blackwell Scientific.

Blease 8500 user and maintenance manual, October 2003.

Datex Ohmeda Aestiva 7900, 2nd.Line Biomedical Course Ohmeda Healthcare Academy.

Penlon Nuffield 200 Technical description (200 4tecNV200.ppt), 2004,

Glaister C (2003)Dräger Fabius GS Training notes. Dräger UK. February 2003.

Sims Pneupac Principles of operation of ventiPAC Pneupac Ltd.2002 Part No504-2101 Issue 1 07/2003.

Acutronic Technical: Service manual MONSOON II Software 4.0. 27 October 2003.

Ventilation in the intensive care unit

Martin Street

Originally Intensive Care Unit (ICU) ventilators were adapted from standard anaesthetic equipment, by the addition of a separate breathing system that allowed the patient to take a spontaneous minute volume over and above that delivered by the ventilator. With the widespread use of microprocessors and sophisticated pneumatic controls, modern ICU ventilators allow both mechanical ventilation and patient spontaneous breathing to take place through the same system.

IDEAL REQUIREMENTS

Despite the ideals that one machine should cope with all clinical situations, modern ICU ventilatory strategies require a range of ventilators with different operational modalities to accommodate the full range of requirements. Safe and easy-to-use machines are important for clinical practice with the ability to ventilate without restricting the patient's spontaneous breathing.

Of the numerous ventilators available for use in Intensive Care Units, each have dissimilar mechanical pneumatic and electrical components that influence their working and behaviour characteristics when used in the clinical situation. An ideal ICU ventilator should provide:

1. the ability to ventilate all sizes of patient from neonate to obese adult. However, specific machines have been designed to ventilate neonates and most ICU ventilators are manufactured to have the ability to only ventilate small infants to large adults.
2. operational versatility with the ability to provide different patterns of ventilation for varied clinical circumstances. The machines should offer the ability to alter such characteristics as inflation pressure, tidal volume, gas flow, respiratory rate and inspiratory to expiratory (I:E) ratio.
3. a facility for the patient to breathe spontaneously through the ventilator in spontaneously breathing mode without imposing an increased work of breathing;
4. the ability to augment patient efforts in spontaneously breathing modes to prevent respiratory muscle fatigue;
5. the ability to increase the pressure in the inspiratory limb of the breathing system for the application of Positive End Expiratory Pressure (PEEP) and Conti-

nuous Positive Airway Pressure (CPAP) in spontaneously breathing modes;

6. the ability to deliver its pre-set volume and flow pattern independent of changing patient lung resistance and compliance;

7. the ability to cope with large leaks from the breathing system without altering performance, thus allowing non-invasive ventilation;

8. the delivery of precise inspired oxygen concentrations varying from 21–100% in all ventilatory modes;

9. the ability to humidify inspired gases without changing ventilator characteristics;

10. the ability to add drugs and to nebulize bronchodilators into the inspiratory limb without altering the ventilator performance or inhaled oxygen concentration;

11. the ability to monitor accurately and reliably both patient and ventilator respiratory performance along with the capability to provide alarms, should these exceed predefined limits;

12. patient safety features such as high pressure relief valves and gas supply safety features in the event of either electrical or gas supply failure;

13. easy to use and intuitive operator controls;

14. the ability to ensure that patients are not exposed to cross-infection hazards with the use of disposable or simple-to-sterilize patient breathing systems and expiratory valves;

15. the ability to work independently of a fixed electrical or gas supply to facilitate patient transport; and

16. reliable component parts with infrequent routine maintenance schedules.

DIFFERENCES BETWEEN VENTILATORS FOR ANAESTHESIA AND INTENSIVE CARE

Ventilators used in anaesthesia are primarily designed to support the minute ventilation of a patient who is paralyzed or has a depressed respiratory drive as a result of anaesthetic agents and opiates.[1] In contrast, intensive care patients are normally encouraged to breathe alongside the mechanical ventilatory support, which is gradually reduced during a slow weaning phase, where as at the end of anaesthesia extubation is more precipitous with the rapid recovery of consciousness and return of spontaneous breathing. ICU ventilators, therefore, have to cope with the complexity of both machine and patient initiated respiration.

The pulmonary mechanics, in terms of airways resistance and total lung compliance in ICU patients, is rarely normal. ICU ventilators have been designed to support respiration using such techniques as inverse ratio ventilation and high levels of PEEP, which are rarely required during routine anaesthesia. Ventilation for prolonged periods of time may require humidification techniques other than the heat and moisture exchanger, which is common in the operative setting. These alternative techniques, such as hot water humidifiers, are associated with increased accumulation of fluid in the respiratory circuits, which may compromise ventilator function. Large air leaks from the lungs or around airway tubing are more common in the ICU setting, and monitoring facilities on ICU ventilators have to be adapted to function in these unusual circumstances to prevent the incidence of excessive false alarms.

DRIVING MECHANISMS

All ventilators require a driving force to deliver a gas flow into the patient. This force may come from a high-pressure source of gas that delivers the intended inspired volume directly to the patient or it may be indirectly responsible for gas delivery by compressing a bag or bellows containing the inspired gas mixture, which is then delivered to the patient. Driving mechanisms, which have been used in ICU ventilators, include:

1. Rotating electric motors – These may drive:
   a) *Pistons* that in turn deliver the inspiratory gas. The disadvantage of these systems is that they have difficulty in altering inspiratory flow characteristics, as the interconnecting cams produce sinusoidal shaft movement.
   b) *Low pressure blowers*. The advantage of this type of driving mechanism is that they can produce very high volumes of gas flow to cope with leaks from the patient circuit, in non-invasive ventilatory systems.
   c) *Gas compressors* producing high-pressure gas, which may in turn be manipulated by pneumatic controls:
2. *Linear electric motor* – These are devices that use the magnetic field generated by a solenoid to move a ferromagnetic core in and out of a wire coil. This can be used to drive either the pistons or diaphragms which are used in high-frequency oscillators.

3. *Tension springs* – These compress the gas in storage bellows prior to being delivered to the patient. The disadvantage of this mechanism is that the pressure in the bellows is not constant but varies with the tension in the springs.

4. *Weighted bellows* – The gravitational force on a mass will produce a constant driving pressure within the bellows; however, this mechanism is very susceptible to movement.

5. *Pneumatic* – these may be of two types:
   a) *Low-pressure systems* using gas supplied from electric blowers or venturi devices;
   b) *High-pressure systems* with the gas supplied from a compressor via a high-pressure gas pipeline or cylinder, which is connected to the ventilator.

MICROPROCESSOR ELECTRONIC CONTROL

The use of microprocessor control has become virtually ubiquitous in all modern ICU ventilators. At the heart of these ventilators is the control microprocessor whose function is to receive data from the analogue to digital converters that measure pressure and flow within the ventilator system. With this information and under soft-ware control, the microprocessor provides the commands for the circuit board to precisely control the inspiratory and expiratory flow valves and secondary functions (e.g. nebulizer control or to flush pressure measurement lines). Data is also received from the oxygen and carbon dioxide sensors, if fitted. Information may also be received from external sources and interface boards that allow ventilators to talk to each other for synchrony in ventilator modes, such as independent lung ventilation.

Some ICU ventilators use dual microprocessors to control the ventilator function. The advantage of using two processors in parallel is not only that such function as display and control of the valves can be separated, but each microprocessor can check the other to ensure maximum patient safety and ventilator reliability. One microprocessor can be tasked to constantly monitor the position of the user adjustable control settings, providing this information to the second control microprocessor (Fig. 12.1).

Information display

In the oldest ICU ventilators, the only information available to the operator was analogue measurements of pressure or volumes (Fig. 12.2). With the use of micro-processors, digital information monitoring both patient

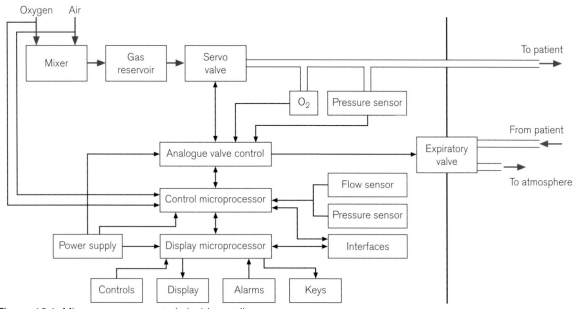

Figure 12.1 Microprocessor controls inside ventilator.

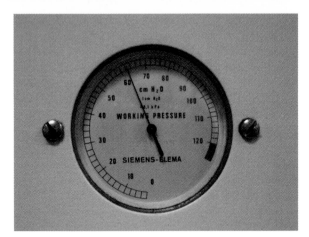

Figure 12.2 Analogue pressure display.

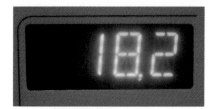

Figure 12.3 LED digital display.

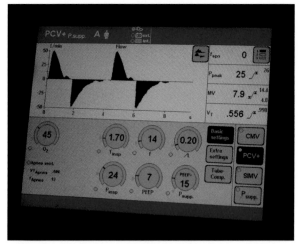

Figure 12.4 TFT panel display.

and ventilator variables is also provided. This information can be in two forms, either displaying a value or informing the user that an alarm condition has been triggered.

Digital information provided to the user was originally only in numeric format, such as pressure values (peak, plateau, PEEP, etc) calculations of tidal volume, machine or patient triggered breaths, differences between inspiratory and expiratory tidal volume and the quantity of gas leaking from the patient circuit[3] (Fig. 12.3). With the availability of LCD screens, more of this information, instead of being provided as single numerical displays, is demonstrated on a matrix screen which allows the user to view the numeric and graphical information such as flow, pressure and volume variation against time. Other graphical displays, often available, are pressure/volume or flow/volume loops. The increasing use of these graphical displays allows the user to more easily understand the effect of changes in ventilator controls on gas delivery to the patient. Although LCD screens have the advantage of lower power consumption, they are only readable over a narrow viewing angle and are now being replaced by TFT LCD screens that can provide similar information in colour. These are readable over a larger viewing angle and in lower lighting conditions.

INSPIRATORY FLOW VALVE

Inspiratory gas flow in most ICU ventilators is controlled by two types of solenoid valves. In one, the valve is designed to be either on or off. The other, when activated, opens in proportion to the electrical current supplied and is thus called a proportional flow valve.

High-speed proportional flow valves, that are servo-controlled, are used in several manufacturers' ventilators. They are capable of delivering flows from 20 to 3000 ml sec^{-1} and are adjusted by the ventilators' microprocessor control. A current flowing in the field coils of the solenoid generates the force to move the ferromagnetic core (piston) up and down. Connected to the piston is the valve orifice which opens to allow gas to flow. This type of valve has a quick response time of less that 5 msec and along with the small internal dead space of the ventilator, causes flow rates to change almost immediately in the patient system, allowing precise control of the desired flow pattern and tidal volume. The microprocessor monitors the position of the valve and the pressure drop across it to enable it to continually adjust the flow to the required setting, so that its performance characteristics are not affected by any back pressure in the circuit (Fig. 12.5).

Some manufacturers are now using high-pressure, high-speed on/off solenoids which control the flow of both oxygen and air. Under the microprocessor's control, these can be rapidly pulsed on and off to create the desired inspiratory flow pattern. Ventilators using these types

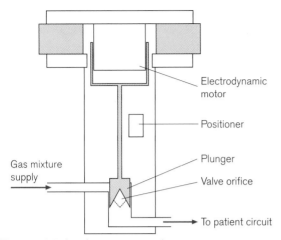

Figure 12.5 Inspiratory servo valve.

Labels: Electrodynamic motor; Positioner; Plunger; Valve orifice; Gas mixture supply; To patient circuit

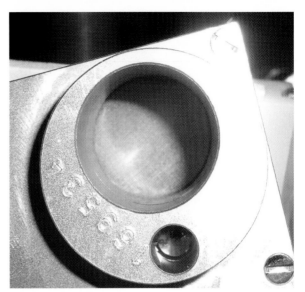

Figure 12.6 Wire mesh pneumotachograph.

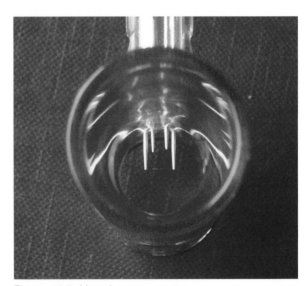

Figure 12.7 Hot wire anemometer.

of inspiratory solenoid no longer require a separate gas blender to create the oxygen air mixture, as this is produced directly by the solenoids from the high-pressure gas pipeline. Not having a separate gas blender and mixing chamber allows the ventilator to rapidly change oxygen concentration within the patient circuit in response to altered settings by the operator, facilitating 100% oxygen setting for use prior to tracheobronchial suctioning.

Flow sensors

Flows sensors are often placed in both the inspiratory and expiratory limbs of ventilators. These are used, not only by the ventilator control microprocessor to sense and adjust gas flow, but also provide the user with measurements of inspiratory and expiratory tidal volumes, whether ventilator delivered or patient initiated, together with information about leaks from within the patient circuit.

Manufacturers have used a variety of flow sensors. These can be a wire mesh pneumotachograph such as that incorporated into the Siemens 900C (Fig. 12.6), a hot wire anemometer which is used in the expiratory limb of the Dräger Evita ventilators (Fig. 12.7) or a bidirectional variable orifice device that is incorporated into the patient end of the ventilator breathing system in the Hamilton Galileo ventilators (Fig. 12.8). Flow sensors placed in the expiratory limb are susceptible to condensation and manufactures provide heating arrangement to ensure that these devices are kept free of water droplets. The physical principles behind these devices are further described in Chapter 4: Measurement of gas flow.

Patient triggering

To facilitate the patient's spontaneous ventilation alongside mechanically-driven breaths (in such modes as described under Intermittent Mandatory Ventilation and Pressure Support below), ICU ventilators have to be able to sense the start of the patient's own respiratory effort to then provide a suitable gas supply from which they can breathe. This can be achieved by sensing a change in either flow or pressure within the breathing system and

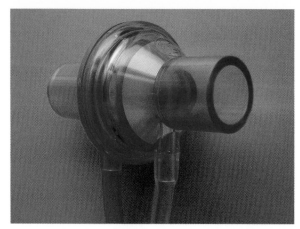

Figure 12.8 Bidirectional pneumotachograph.

triggering the ventilator to open the inspiratory valve. If the patient has to generate large changes of pressure within the system before obtaining any inspiratory gas supply, this will add significantly to their work of breathing. Together with the increased pressure changes, a time delay from the commencement of the patient's inspiratory effort to the start of gas flow will multiply the effect of any pressure drop, further increasing in the patient's work of breathing.[4]

Pressure triggering

Earlier ventilators, such as the Siemens Servo 900C, provided only pressure triggering, the pressure-sensing device being placed within the inspiratory pathway inside the ventilator. The trigger is activated by the pressure drop resulting from a patient's inspiratory effort. Its sensitivity is adjustable and is usually set at −1 to −2 cm of water. When this threshold is reached, an electronic control inside the ventilator opens the inspiratory valve allowing access to a gas flow from which the patient can breathe.[5] The disadvantage of this sensor position is that for the patient to activate the minimum threshold within the ventilator they may have had to generate a considerably greater effort at the patient end of the system. This is particularly apparent when a thin-walled highly compliant disposable plastic breathing hose is connected to the ventilator. Also, if a hot water humidifier is connected to the inspiratory limb, the added compliance and resistance further increases the pressure gradient and therefore the patient's work of breathing before obtaining any inspiratory gas supply.[6]

To overcome this problem, pressure sensing of the patient's inspiratory effort can be achieved more reliably

in the expiratory side of the ventilator, although this is still subject to the effects of condensation accumulating within the expiratory limb. Other manufacturers, such as the Hamilton series of ventilators, sense pressure directly at the patient end of the breathing system, thus avoiding these problems.

Flow triggering

To overcome the disadvantages of pressure triggering, most ICU ventilators now provide a form of flow triggering.[7] Flow triggering does not require change in the pressure within the inspiratory system to enable patient-initiated breath. The ventilator provides a continuous bias flow, frequently $10 \, l \, min^{-1}$, that is introduced into the inspiratory circuit through all phases of the machine's respiratory cycle. When the patient initiates a breath, the fall in bias flow in the expiratory limb is sensed and the ventilator opens the inspiratory valve to allow a patient-initiated breath. The change in flow required to trigger a patient breath can be adjusted by the operator and is often set between $1 \, l \, min^{-1}$ and half the bias flow.[8] The advantage of this mode is that it is not as affected by humidifiers placed in the inspiratory limb or a build-up of condensation in the tubing and so patient work of breathing is minimized.[6,9,10] Most ventilators allow the user to adjust the sensitivity of the flow triggering to achieve the minimum work of breathing without the delivery of falsely triggered breaths.[11]

EXPIRATORY PRESSURE GENERATION

The treatment of such conditions as Adult Respiratory Distress Syndrome (ARDS) requires the ventilators to be able to maintain a pressure in the patient circuit that is above atmospheric pressure during expiration, both for ventilator delivered breaths and for patient spontaneous respiration. PEEP/CPAP valves are incorporated into the expiratory limb and may be of two types; either fixed value or variable pressure:

- Fixed pressures can be generated by a spring-loaded valve, an underwater column or are a weighted valve leaflet. The function of the latter two types is severely impaired with movement and so these are no longer used.
- Variable pressure valves have the advantage that they can be controlled by the operator to produce the desired level of expiratory pressure and they can be closed completely by the ventilator and so may function as the expiratory valve as well.

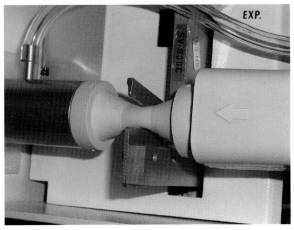

Figure 12.9 Scissor expiratory valve.

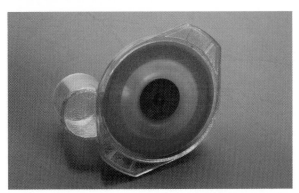

Figure 12.10 Expiratory valve diaphragm type.

Exhalation valves

Constriction type

PEEP/CPAP can be produced using a variable orifice device in which the pinching of the expiratory silicone rubber exit tube by an electromagnetic scissor valve can be used to control expiratory flow and pressure (Fig. 12.9). This also usually functions as the expiratory valve.

Diaphragm type – mechanically operated

Levels of PEEP/CPAP can be generated using a linear dynamic motor that operates a large-surface silicon membrane. Electrical current supplied to the dynamic motor during exhalation will produce a force on the diaphragm, which is proportional to the level of PEEP/CPAP required. During inspiration, the silicon diaphragm (Fig. 12.10) is forced hard onto the expiratory valve seat by the action of the actuator rod. In exhalation, the weight of the rod is balanced by an internal spring (Fig. 12.11) so the patient only has to overcome the weight of the membrane to exhale. The expiratory resistance in this type of valve is less than 2cm H_2O/l/sec.[12]

Diaphragm type – pressure operated

The force on the expiratory valve diaphragm can be generated pneumatically within the ventilator in a similar fashion to that of the inspiratory gas flow, although from a single gas source as it does not need to be a blend of air and oxygen. When this is applied to the downstream side of the expiratory valve diaphragm, it can be used to control the level of PEEP/CPAP delivered by the ventilator. The diaphragms used in these types of

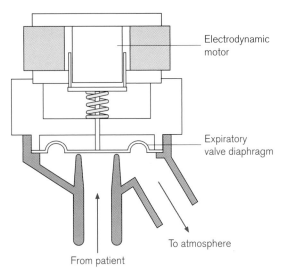

Figure 12.11 Expiratory valve.

expiratory valve have a larger central mass (Fig. 12.12), to provide the required damping to prevent inadvertent oscillations.

Nebulizer port

Ventilator manufacturers provide an additional gas supply (Fig. 12.13) with the same oxygen concentration as the patient's pre-set mixture, to drive a micro-nebulizer for the delivery of drugs into the breathing system. The advantage of these fixed outlets is that not only does the gas supply contain the same oxygen concentration, but that it can be made to be operational only during the inspiratory phase to maximize drug delivery. Unlike separate external gas flows, these will not interfere with the flow triggering sensitivity of the ventilators.

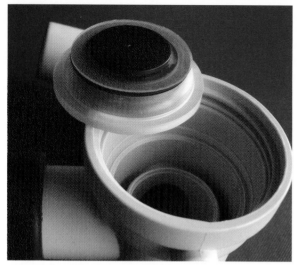

Figure 12.12 Expiratory valve Dräger Evita 4.

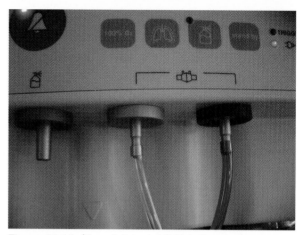

Figure 12.13 (From left to right) Nebulizer and pneumotachograph on Galileo ventilator (Hamilton Medical).

Overpressure valves

To ensure patients are protected from receiving gas supply above safe operating limits, ventilators have protection in the form of electronic control with a secondary mechanical device as backup. The electronically-controlled pressure limit can be set by the operator and this will prevent pressure rising within the circuit, even if the desired tidal volume is not delivered. Audible and visual alarms are triggered in any over-pressure condition.

Ambient air inlet

In addition, for patient safety, an atmospheric air inlet valve is incorporated into the inspiratory gas pathway. In the event of a gas supply failure or internal electronic dysfunction, these valves will open immediately, allowing the patient to spontaneously inhale from ambient air.

BATTERY BACKUP

Microprocessor ventilators go though a series of computer self-checks to ensure that the electronic and pneumatics are working correctly on initial power up; this checking process can take up to forty seconds in some ventilators. To prevent this occurring in the event of a temporary disconnection of power supply, manufactures provide a battery backup to allow the ventilator to continue functioning. To prevent these self-checks occurring in routine use, 'sleep' or 'suspend' buttons are provided which enable the ventilator to stop operating but then resume again with the same settings.

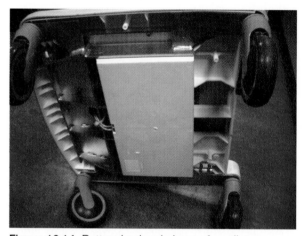

Figure 12.14 Battery backup in base of ventilator.

Additional batteries can be provided to allow for more prolonged periods of disconnection from mains electrical supply, to facilitate the movement of patients. These batteries are often stored in the base of the ventilator stand (Fig. 12.14). The addition of cylinder supplies of oxygen and air allow the ventilator to be easily transportable.

FLOW PATTERN GENERATION/ VENTILATION MODES

With the use of a sophisticated microprocessor and high-performance pneumatic controls, the gas flow characteristics of such ventilators is no longer primarily determined by the physical characteristics of the machines, as had been the case with anaesthesia ventilators in the past.

The characteristics of the inspiratory and expiratory cycle can be broken down into fundamental components and gas delivery characteristics can be pre-set by the manufacturer or adjusted by the clinician at the bedside. Further advances in microprocessor monitoring are employed in some ventilators in turn, allowing the patients own breathing characteristics to alter ventilator setting, whose control traditionally had only been accessible to the care provider. This ability allows ventilators to operate in a closed loop automatic fashion.

A classification for mechanical ventilators proposed three types of variables:[13]

1. *control variables*, which included pressure, volume, flow and rate;
2. *phase variables*, which defined how the change over points in the respiratory cycle occur, these being trigger, cycle and limit variables (Fig. 12.15): and
3. *conditional variables*, which define additional parameters, such as supplementary breaths.

Control of volume or pressure

In all ventilators, the primary control variable is either minute volume (usually set as tidal volume and rate) or airway pressure (settings usually include I:E ratio and respiratory rate). The ventilator delivers a pre-set tidal volume or inspiratory pressure, regardless of patient effort. Limits and alarms are then superimposed to ensure against unacceptable pressures or volumes being generated. If the patient is apnoeic or has limited respiratory effort, the controlled mandatory ventilation mode is the most reliable to ensure delivery of appropriate minute ventilation. As the patient's respiratory function

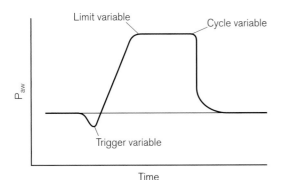

Figure 12.15 Inspiration showing position of phase variables.

improves, the control setting may be reduced to allow the patient to breathe alongside the minute ventilation delivered by ventilator. The control mode can be variably adjusted between full support and zero.

Volume pre-set control mode

In this mode, inhalation proceeds with a pre-set flow rate until the desired tidal volume is delivered. At the end of the predefined inspiratory time (the phase variable), either set directly or indirectly by the ventilator rate and inspiratory to expiratory ratio (I:E ratio), passive exhalation follows. Inspiratory gas follows a predefined flow pattern and the peak pressure measured in the airways is a result of airways resistance and the force required for lung distension. Since the volume delivered is constant, peak airway pressure will alter with changing pulmonary compliance and airways resistance; plateau pressure being a reflection of pulmonary compliance and the peak pressure being additionally influenced by airways resistance. To avoid excessive pressures resulting in pulmonary barotrauma in a volume pre-set mode, most machines have high airway pressure alarms to alert the user to the potentially dangerous situation. In addition, many machines have an over pressure release setting at which the ventilator will no longer deliver any additional tidal volume to the patient, but vent the excess to atmosphere. This results in only partial delivery of the pre-set tidal volume. Warning alarms are triggered to alert the user if this is happening.

When this mode of ventilation is used with hot water humidifiers in circuit, the rain out from these devices and subsequent pooling in the tubes may falsely trigger high-pressure alarms. A similar false alarm may occur if the patient coughs during the inspiratory cycle.

Pressure pre-set control mode

In this mode, often referred to as pressure controlled ventilation, a predefined peak inspiratory pressure is applied to the airways and the resulting pressure difference between the ventilator and the alveolus results in inflation until there is equilibrium between the two. After a pre-set inspiratory time, passive exhalation follows. In this mode the delivered volume, during respiration, is dependent on pulmonary and thoracic compliance. A potential disadvantage of this mode is that changes in pulmonary mechanics will result in varying tidal volumes and minute ventilation.[14] With accurate flow sensors within this circuit, close monitoring of tidal ventilation is employed and dramatic changes in tidal volume or minute ventilation can be signalled.

As this mode of ventilation pre-sets the pressures within the inspiratory system, flow pattern cannot be influenced by the user, and is usually of a falling flow pattern as the pressure gradient between the inspiratory circuit and the alveolus declines with lung inflation. This usually results in a more homogenous gas distribution throughout the lung and improved arterial blood oxygenation and may reduce the patient's work of breathing compared to volume pre-set modes.[15]

Ventilatory modes

Although some terminology referring to modes of ventilation has become standardized, manufacturers have tended to coin new terms for their own versions and variances. To fully understand what a ventilator will and will not allow a patient to do in each setting, there is the need to read the ventilator manual. For example, many modern ICU ventilators will allow spontaneous respiration, even during CMV mode (see below), and some will even apply pressure support to those breaths, whilst others will deliver a machine volume or pressure pre-set breath on detecting an inspiratory effort. The principles of the more common terminology are explained below:

Continuous Mandatory Ventilation (CMV). Breaths are delivered at pre-set time intervals, regardless of patient effort. This mode is similar to that of anaesthesia ventilators and is most often used for the paralyzed or apnoeic patient. Large increases in work of breathing for the patient are created if their respiratory efforts fail to coincide with the ventilators inspiratory cycle.

Intermittent Mandatory Ventilation (IMV). In this mode, breaths are delivered from the ventilator at pre-set intervals. However, a patient's spontaneous respiration is allowed between ventilator-administered breaths.[16] The IMV rate may be reduced, allowing increased time for the patient's spontaneous respiration during the weaning process.

Synchronous Intermittent Mandatory Ventilation (SIMV). In this mode, the ventilator tries to deliver its breaths in conjunction with the respiratory effort of the patient. Spontaneous breathing is also allowed between ventilator-administered breaths.

Synchronization of ventilator breaths is achieved by the ventilator attempting to detect the patient's inspiratory effort in a small time window prior to the initiation of its own inspiratory cycle. If patient inspiratory activity is detected, the ventilator synchronizes its mandatory breath in conjunction with the patient's own effort. This mode of ventilation improves the comfort of spontaneous respiratory efforts for the patient and reduces the incidences of patient ventilator disharmony where the patient appears to be 'fighting the ventilator'. Breath stacking may still occur where the patient wishes to exhale but is then subject to an additional mandatory ventilatory inspiratory tidal volume, potentially over-distending the lungs.

On its own, the SIMV mode has not been shown to improve patients' weaning from ventilatory support.[17] This may be the result of the increased work of breathing associated with spontaneous respiration through these mechanical circuits. The work is created by having to generate the pressures and flows within the ventilator tubing needed to trigger the ventilator into opening an inspiratory valve prior to gaining gas flow (see above, Patient triggering).

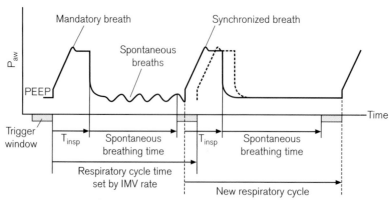

Figure 12.16 Synchronization of IMV breaths. The second tidal volume (synchronized breath) is delivered early because an inspiratory effort falls within the trigger window. The machine's next respiratory cycle timing is reset from this point.

Pressure support mode/assisted spontaneous ventilation

Pressure support ventilation has been shown to decrease the work of spontaneous breathing through ventilator circuits.[18,19] When triggered, the ventilator produces a pressure in the inspiratory pathway to support the patient's own inspiratory effort. This effort is detected either by flow or pressure triggering. With this mode of ventilation, a user pre-set pressure is generated in a circuit (not a fixed tidal volume) to assist every patient's spontaneous effort. This predefined airway pressure remains until the patient's own inspiratory flow falls below a predefined cut-off e.g. 25% of peak inspiratory flow[20] (Fig. 12.17). The disadvantage of this mode of ventilation is that if the patient fails to take any respiratory effort, no pressure-supported breaths will be initiated. To avoid the potentially disastrous consequences, most ventilators have a backup or 'apnoeic' SIMV rate should the patient's spontaneous respiration cease for a predetermined period.

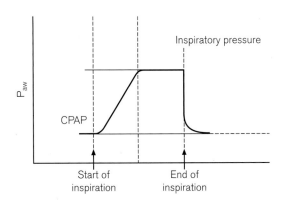

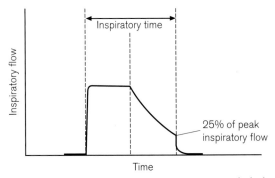

Figure 12.17 Expiration in pressure support mode being set at 25% of peak inspiratory flow.

For patients who have adequate respiratory drive and whose respiratory failure is not severe, pressure support ventilation may offer the patient considerable advantages, as all the breaths are patient-initiated; breath stacking and fighting the ventilator is almost abolished. Even patients who are initially tachypnoeic may be successfully managed in this mode, as the pressure support can be set sufficiently high to augment their own tidal volume and hence, reduce patient respiratory rate. As this is a pressure pre-set mode of ventilatory support, the risks of barotrauma associated with high airway pressures and fixed tidal volume ventilation are reduced.[21]

For patients who have severe respiratory failure, this mode of ventilation is commonly used in conjunction with volume pre-set or pressure pre-set SIMV modes.[22]

Closed loop controlled ventilatory modes

Historically, adjustments of ventilator settings were made by physicians, nurses or attending bedside staff, according to the patient's requirement. With the advent of microprocessor control, it is possible to design ventilators with closed loop control in which the setting is automatically adjusted using an algorithm and data obtained from patients.[3]

Early ventilators models adjusted either the tidal volume or inspiratory pressure to achieve a target end tidal carbon dioxide level. However, in intensive care, the end tidal carbon dioxide of a patient does not always correlate with arterial carbon dioxide tension and the target variable of minute ventilation is used instead. Most ventilator manufacturers provide a closed loop mode of control, implementing different versions of mandatory minute ventilation (MMV), in which the target minute ventilation is achieved by the ventilator adjusting inspiratory pressure support and mandatory breath frequency[23] (Table 12.1). More recent versions of MMV have incorporated algorithms that aim to reduce the patient's work of breathing while still achieving the desired minute ventilation, by encouraging the patient to breathe with larger tidal volumes and slower rates, this being more efficient than rapid shallow breathing[4] (Fig. 12.18). Ventilator manufactures have tried to produce other additional modes for spontaneously breathing patients, which attempt to reduce the work inherent with gas flows through the endotracheal tube, again this being achieved by adjusting inspiratory pressure according to inspiratory flow.

Table 12.1 Nomenclature and details of various closed loop ventilatory modes

Name of Mode	Ventilator	Operator preset variables	Ventilator controlled variables
MMV	Veolar (Hamilton)	MV	Pinsp
MMV	Evita 4 (Dräger)	MV, VT	F, Pinsp
Automode	Servo 300A (Siemens)	VT,F	Pinsp, Psupp, Mode
ASV	Gallileo (Hamilton)	%MV	Pinsp, Psupp, F, Ti

F: rate, VT: Tidal Volume, MV; Minute Volume, Pinsp :Inspiratory Pressure Level, Psupp: Pressure support level, MMV: Mandatory Minute Ventilation, ASV: Adaptive Support Ventilation

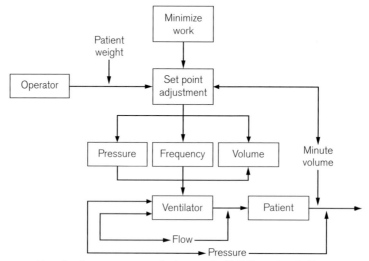

Figure 12.18 Algorithm used in adaptive support ventilation mode (ASB) on the Galileo ventilator.

Total closed loop ventilation has not found universal favour as ventilation is not solely about carbon dioxide elimination and oxygenation of blood, but involves complex interactions with the patient's musculature and cardiovascular system.

INDIVIDUAL VENTILATORS

900C

The Siemens 900C, which ceased production in April 2004, (Figs 12.19a and b) consists of two parts, the pneumatic and the electric section. The pneumatic section is mounted directly on top of the electronic section, which contains the ventilator controls and electronic displays. The two sections are connected by a cable and could be separated if desired. High-pressure gas

enters the pneumatic section from an external blender. A second gas inlet connection is provided that accepts low-pressure gas directly from an anaesthetic machine, if required. The gas then passes through the oxygen analyzer and main bacterial filter before entering a spring loaded bellows, which stores the gas prior to use.

From the bellows, gas passes through the inspiratory flow transducer and then through the inspiratory scissors valve, before leaving the unit to enter the inspiratory limb of the breathing hose. Exhaled gas, returning from the patient via the expiratory limb, re-enters the ventilator and passes through the expiratory flow transducer to an expiratory scissors valve, before exiting the unit via a one-way valve to the atmosphere. The inspiratory scissors valve consists of a flexible piece of silicone rubber tubing, which is compressed in the jaws of the scissors mechanism by the action of an electric stepper motor to control gas flow.

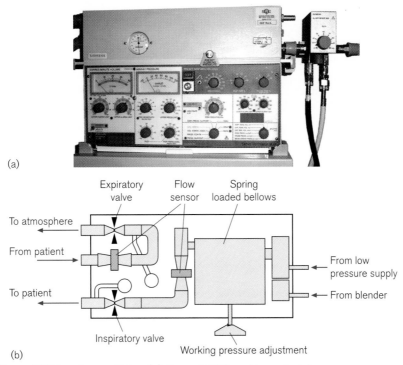

(a)

Expiratory valve   Flow sensor   Spring loaded bellows

To atmosphere

From patient

To patient

From low pressure supply

From blender

Inspiratory valve

Working pressure adjustment

(b)

Figure 12.19 **(a)** Servo 900C series ventilator. **(b)** Servo 900C working principles.

In contrast, the compression of the equivalent tube in the expiratory scissors valve is controlled by a pull of an electromagnet under the control of the ventilator's electronics. This force is adjusted to maintain the correct PEEP in the expiratory limb; during inspiration the valve remains shut.

During inspiration, the gas flow is measured at the inspiratory flow transducer and compared in the electronics section to that which is required to achieve the operator's pre-set volume. If the actual flow does not match the required value, the stepper motor either opens or closes the inspiratory scissors valve to adjust the flow delivery. The driving pressure for the gas flow is generated by the tension in the spring attached to the inspiratory bellows and this may be insufficient to achieve a desired high flow rate. Under such circumstances the working pressure is increased manually by turning the key (Fig. 12.20) on the front of the pneumatic section.

Servo 300

The Servo 300, which like the Servo 900C ceased production in April 2004 (Figs 12.21a and b), has two units, a patient pneumatic unit and a control unit which

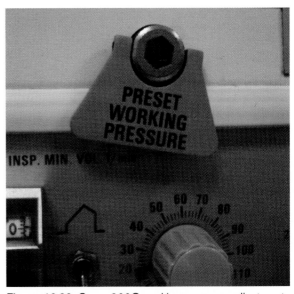

Figure 12.20 Servo 900C working pressure adjustment.

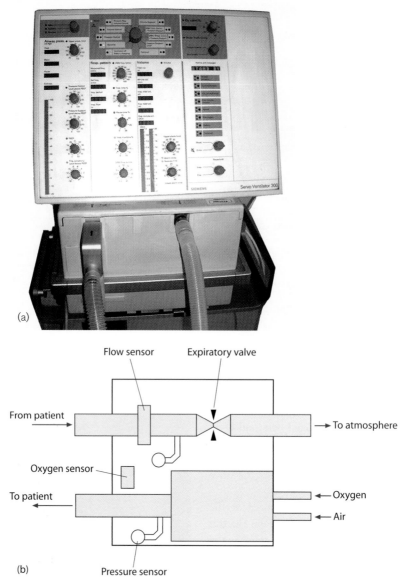

(a)

(b)

Figure 12.21 (a) Servo 300 series. **(b)** Servo 300 series ventilator working principles.

are connected by a cable. The electronic circuit of the control unit both controls and displays the ventilator settings used to operate the pneumatic unit. Oxygen and air are supplied by pipeline and are blended directly into the patient's circuit by high-speed gas solenoid valves. Unlike its predecessor, the Servo 900C has no bellows storage of inspiratory gas and no low-pressure port for anaesthetic gas.

The solenoid valves have a response time of 6 milliseconds; under microprocessor control they can be rapidly opened or closed to achieve the desired flow rate and pattern in the ventilator circuit. Exhaled gas from the patient returns to the unit and, as with the Servo 900C, passes through the expiratory flow transducer and expiratory scissors valve before exiting out a one-way valve to the atmosphere.

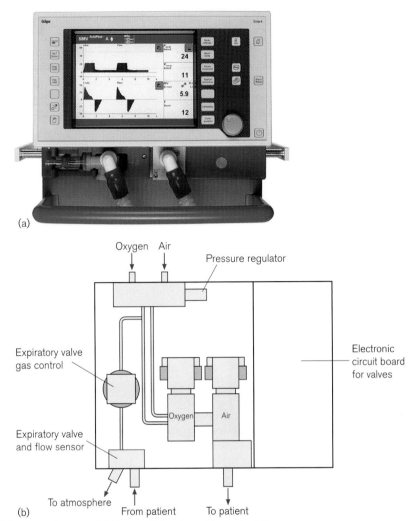

Figure 12.22 (a) Dräger Evita 4. **(b)** Dräger Evita 4 working principles.

Dräger Evita 4

The Dräger Evita 4 (Fig. 12.22a) ventilator has three sections; the electronic compartment, which sits directly on top of the pneumatic controls and a third detachable display unit, which houses the controls and touch sensitive screen. The screen displays both the ventilator information and the 'touch sensitive' virtual buttons and screen knobs.

Gas from the high-pressure pipe lines enters the ventilator via a filter and a non-return valve directly into two proportional flow valves which control the flow of oxygen and air to be blended directly into the patient circuit. Sensors measure the pressure of the oxygen and air supplied to the ventilator and with this information a central microprocessor is able to adjust the function of the valves to deliver the correct flow. The inspiratory gas enters the breathing system to produce an inspiratory breath. It returns to a diaphragmatically operated expiratory valve and then through the external hot wire flow sensor to atmosphere (Fig. 12.22).

The PEEP/CPAP pressure is controlled by a balancing pressure applied to the ventilator side of the expiratory diaphragm and is controlled by a valve connected to the oxygen supply. The gas flow of $9 \, l \, min^{-1}$ to drive the nebulizer is also obtained from this oxygen supply, with balance of the main two pneumatic valves adjusted to deliver the correct oxygen concentration.[25] During an oxygen pipeline failure, a switch-over valve is operated which allows the pneumatics to continue to function normally using the pressure from the air supply.

NON-INVASIVE VENTILATION

The application of mechanical ventilatory support, through a mask or helmet in place of endotracheal intubation, is becoming increasingly accepted and utilized in the Intensive Care Unit. This modality of ventilatory support can be used successfully for patients with mild to moderate respiratory failure, but the patient must be

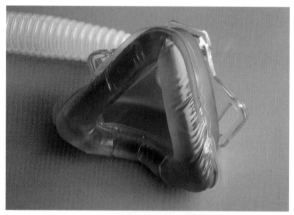

Figure 12.23 Nasal mask for non-invasive ventilation.

mentally alert enough to follow commands and without an endotracheal tube there is no mechanical method of preventing aspiration into the lungs. Clinical situations, in which it has proven useful, include acute exacerbation of chronic obstructive pulmonary disease (COPD) or asthma, and decompensated congestive heart failure (CHF) with mild to moderate pulmonary oedema. Conventional ICU ventilators, set in their PSV mode of ventilation with PEEP, are commonly used to support non-invasive ventilation through a mask[4] (Fig. 12.23) although special machines (see below) are now available for use in this technique in general acute wards. Conventional ICU ventilators have the advantage of precise control of the oxygen concentration and inspiratory flow pattern together with sophisticated monitoring, but are ill-adapted to cope with the large leaks of gas that may occur with poorly-fitting masks in awake patients.[26]

Specialist non-invasive machines (Figs 12.24, 12.25) use an electrically-driven blower to deliver the inspiratory gas supply and are capable of generating flows of 300 l min^{-1}.[27] The rotating speed of the electrical blower is adjusted by the ventilator's microprocessor to achieve the desired level of pressure for both inspiration and expiration. This bi-level pressure ventilatory mode is time cycled in a similar manner to the CMV mode on a conventional ICU ventilator. The only difference is that the patient is capable of breathing during the ventilator's inspiratory and expiratory cycle, as gas is supplied conti-

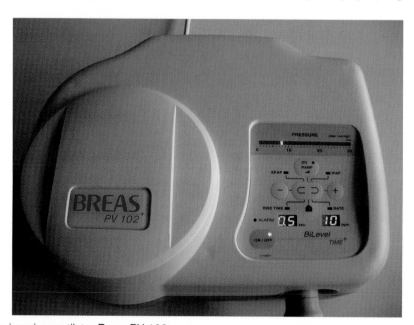

Figure 12.24 Non-invasive ventilator Breas PV 102.

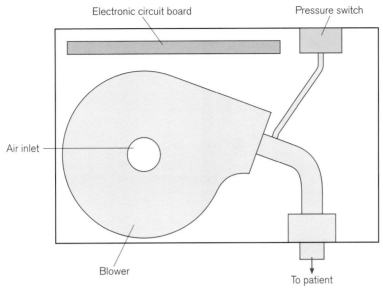

Figure 12.25 Working principles of a non-invasive ventilator.

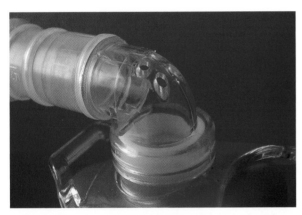

Figure 12.26 Expiratory holes on mask for non-invasive ventilation.

nuously during both phases of respiration. There is no expiratory valve in this type of ventilator, the gas exiting from the circuit through a series of holes or slits close to the patient mask (Fig. 12.26). Alterations in inspired oxygen concentration are achieved by entraining oxygen into the suction side of the blower or adding the oxygen flow directly into the patient circuit just before the mask. As a result, it is difficult to achieve high inspired concentrations, particularly when the ventilation is delivering its maximum flow rate.

With the addition of a pneumotachograph in the inspiratory limb, sensing changes of 40 ml sec^{-1} in the flow required to maintain the expiratory pressure, sophisticated non-invasive ventilators enable the patient to trigger the commencement of the inspiratory positive airway pressure. Large and variable leaks from the mask make the detection of patient expiration by flow sensing difficult and hence less comfortable for the patient than a time-cycled expiratory trigger.[28]

HIGH FREQUENCY OSCILLATORS

High frequency oscillators, such as the SensorMedics 3100B (Fig. 12.27), use a device similar to a loudspeaker as the driving mechanism; the diaphragm (Fig. 12.28) is made to operate at frequencies of 3–15 Hz or180–900 breaths per minute, although typical starting setting are in the range of 5–6 Hz for adults.

A fresh gas supply or bias flow is provided constantly down the inspiratory limb independent of the diaphragmatic oscillations and can be controlled by the operator in range up to 60 l min^{-1}. Altering the power setting (sometimes referred to as delta P) increases the amplitude of the diaphragmatic oscillations. Carbon dioxide elimination from the patient is achieved by a combination of altering the power setting or increasing the bias flow.[29] The inspiratory proportion of the total time can also be adjusted by the operator.

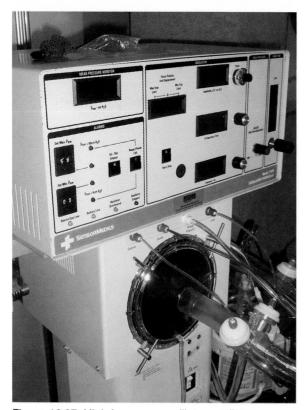

Figure 12.27 High-frequency oscillator ventilator.

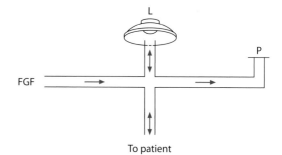

Figure 12.29 Schematic of high frequency oscillator ventilator. FGF, fresh gas flow; L, oscillator; P, PEEP valve.

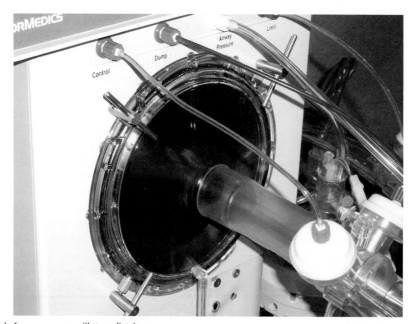

Figure 12.28 High-frequency oscillator diaphragm.

SUMMARY

Despite the ideals that one machine should cope with all clinical situations, modern ICU ventilatory strategies require a range of ventilators with different operational modalities to accommodate the full range of requirements. Safe and easy-to-use machines are important for clinical practice with the ability to ventilate without restricting the patient's spontaneous breathing.

REFERENCES

1. Del Valle RM, Hecker RB (1995) A review of ventilatory modalities used in the intensive care unit. *American Journal of Anesthesiology* **22**: 23–30.

2. Smallwood RW (1986) Ventilators – reported classifications and their usefulness. *Anaesthesia in Intensive Care* **14**: 251–257.

3. Chatburn RL (2004) Computer control of mechanical ventilation. *Respiratory Care* **49**: 507–517.

4. Nava S, Ambrosino N, Bruschi C, *et al.*(1997) Physiological effects of flow and pressure triggering during non-invasive mechanical ventilation in patients with chronic obstructive pulmonary disease. *Thorax* **52**: 249–254.

5. Sassoon CS, Gruer SE (1995) Characteristics of the ventilator pressure- and flow-trigger variables. *Intensive Care Medicine* **21**: 159–168.

6. Street MK, Hopkinson RB (1987) Evaluation of the comfort of spontaneous respiration through three ventilator systems. *Intensive Care Medicine* **13**: 405–410.

7. Prinianakis G, Kondili E, Georgopoulos D. (2003) Effects of the flow waveform method of triggering and cycling on patient-ventilator interaction during pressure support. *Intensive Care Medicine* **29**: 1950–1959.

8. Sassoon CS (1992) Mechanical ventilator design and function: the trigger variable. *Respiratory Care* **37**: 1056–1069.

9. Giuliani R, Mascia L, Recchia F, *et al.* (1995) Patient-ventilator interaction during synchronized intermittent mandatory ventilation. Effects of flow triggering. *American Journal of Respiratory Critical Care Medicine* **151**: 1–9.

10. Ranieri VM, Mascia L, Petruzzelli V, *et al.* (1995) Inspiratory effort and measurement of dynamic intrinsic PEEP in COPD patients: effects of ventilator triggering systems. *Intensive Care Medicine* **21**: 896–903.

11. Imanaka H, Nishimura M, Takeuchi M, *et al.* (2000) Autotriggering caused by cardiogenic oscillation during flow-triggered mechanical ventilation. *Critical Care Medicine* **28**: 402–407.

12. Techical Specification (1992) Veolar operators manual. Rhazuns: Hamilton Medical.

13. Chatburn RL. (1992) Classification of mechanical ventilators. *Respiratory Care* **37**: 1009–1025.

14. Kallet RH, Alonso JA, Diaz M, *et al.* (2002) The effects of tidal volume demand on work of breathing during simulated lung-protective ventilation. *Respiratory Care* **47**: 898–909.

15. Kallet RH, Campbell AR, Alonso JA, *et al.* (2000) The effects of pressure control versus volume control assisted ventilation on patient work of breathing in acute lung injury and acute respiratory distress syndrome. *Respiratory Care* **45**: 1085–1096.

16. Sassoon CS (1994) Intermittant mandatory ventilation. In: Tobin MJ (ed.). *Principles and practice of mechanical ventilation.* New York: McGraw-Hill. pp. 221–237.

17. Brochard L, Rauss A, Benito S, *et al.* (1994) Comparison of three methods of gradual withdrawal from ventilatory support during weaning from mechanical ventilation. *American Journal of Respiratory Critical Care Medicine* **150**: 896–903.

18. Brochard L, Harf A, Lorino H, *et al.* (1989) Inspiratory pressure support prevents diaphragmatic fatigue during weaning from mechanical ventilation. *American Review of Respiratory Disease* **139**: 513–521.

19. Esteban A, Frutos F, Tobin MJ, *et al.* (1995) A comparison of four methods of weaning patients from mechanical ventilation. Spanish Lung Failure Collaborative Group. *New England Journal of Medicine* **332**: 345–350.

20. Du HL, Amato MB, Yamada Y (2001) Automation of expiratory trigger sensitivity in pressure support ventilation. *Respiratory Care Clinics of North America* **7**: 503–517, x.

21. Moylan FM, Walker AM, Kramer SS, *et al.* (1978) The relationship of bronchopulmonary dysplasia to the occurrence of alveolar rupture during positive pressure ventilation. *Critical Care Medicine* **6**: 140–142.

22. Esteban A, Anzueto A, Alia I, *et al.* (2000) How is mechanical ventilation employed in the intensive care unit? An international utilization review. *American Journal of Respiratory Critical Care Medicine* **161**: 1450–1458.

23. Brunner JX (2001) Principles and history of closed-loop controlled ventilation. *Respiratory Care Clinics of North America* **7**: 341–362, vii.

24. Brunner JX, Iotti GA (2002) Adaptive Support Ventilation (ASV). *Minerva Anestesiology* **68**: 365–368.

25. Service manual Evita 4. 5th edn (2000) Lubeck: Drager Medizintechnik GmbH.

26. Mehta S, McCool FD, Hill NS (2001) Leak compensation in positive pressure ventilators: a lung model study. *European Respiratory Journal* **17**: 259–267.

27. BiPAP Vision (2003) *Respironics*.

28. Calderini E, Confalonieri M, Puccio PG, *et al.* (1999) Patient-ventilator asynchrony during noninvasive ventilation: the role of expiratory trigger. *Intensive Care Medicine* **25**: 662–667.

29. Fort P, Farmer C, Westerman J, *et al.* (1997) High-frequency oscillatory ventilation for adult respiratory distress syndrome – a pilot study. *Critical Care Medicine* **25**: 937–947.

13

Breathing filters, humidifiers and nebulizers

Antony R Wilkes

Most patients undergoing surgery and those in intensive care have an airway conduit device *in situ*. This allows the delivery of oxygen-enriched gases, sometimes with anaesthetic gases and vapours, and any necessary ventilatory assistance. In addition, a tracheostomy may be carried out on some patients to bypass the upper airways, either acutely or longer-term, whilst allowing the patient to speak, eat and drink. These devices bypass the normal physiological functions of the nasopharynx.

During normal breathing, the nasopharynx warms, humidifies and, particularly during nasal breathing, filters inspired gases. When the patient's nasopharynx is bypassed, these functions are lost. The trachea has a continuous stream of mucus, called the mucociliary elevator: this moves towards the pharynx, trapping and removing any particles that enter the trachea. The mucociliary elevator relies on optimum levels of temperature, and particularly humidification, to work effectively.

Gases supplied from cylinders or pipelines need to be very dry to reduce the risk of corrosion, condensation and frost forming in cylinders, pipes and valves. Gases delivered to the patient's trachea therefore need to be artificially warmed, humidified and filtered to prevent damage to the patient's airways,[1,2] to maintain the effectiveness of the mucociliary elevator[3] and to reduce the incidence of infection.[4] This chapter deals with devices that fulfill these functions.

BREATHING SYSTEM FILTERS

Filtration and mechanisms of filtration

Filtration is the removal of particles from either a gas or liquid suspension. Filters are used to remove particles from gases delivered to patients, to prevent microbes from patients cross-infecting other patients and staff, and to reduce the contamination of equipment. In addition, sputum expectorated by a patient, and condensation in breathing systems may harbour pathogens, and filters can also be used to reduce the risk of liquid-borne cross-infection.[5]

Mechanisms of filtration of gas-borne particles

Filter material generally consists of fibres formed into a non-woven wad or sheet. There are five main mechanisms by which the filter material removes particles from a flow of gas (Fig. 13.1):

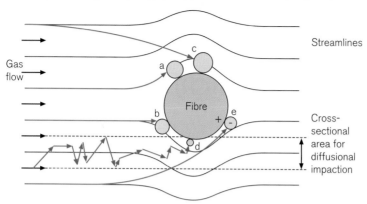

Figure 13.1 Mechanisms of filtration. **(a)** Interception; **(b)** inertial impaction; **(c)** gravitational settling; **(d)** diffusional impaction; **(e)** electrostatic attraction (see text for details). Adapted from Hinds WC (1999) Aerosol Technology. *Properties, behaviour, and measurement of airborne particles*, 2nd end. New York: John Wiley and Sons.

1. Interception

Particles will tend to follow streamlines in a flow of gas. However, if a particle in the gas stream comes within one particle radius of the surface of a fibre, the particle will adhere to the fibre.

2. Inertial impaction

Particles have mass, and are therefore not always able to follow a gas streamline around a fibre due to their inertia. The particles may therefore strike the fibre even though the gas streamline is more than one particle radius from the fibre.

3. Gravitational settling

Large particles in slow-moving air do not follow gas streamlines, but settle due to gravity, and can therefore fall onto, and adhere to, a fibre.

4. Diffusion

Small particles do not remain on particular streamlines in the gas but undergo Brownian motion due to interactions with gas molecules. This effectively increases their cross-sectional area and so increases the probability of them striking a fibre.

5. Electrostatic attraction

Some filter material (see below) is electrostatically-charged during manufacture to enhance the capture of particles. There are three mechanisms of capture: charged particles in the gas stream are attracted to oppositely charged fibres; neutral particles are attracted to a charged fibre as the electric field on the fibre induces a dipole in the particles (positive and negative charges on opposite sides of the particles); and charged particles are attracted to neutral fibres by inducing image forces on the fibres.

Most penetrating particle size

The relative efficiencies of the five mechanisms of filtration vary with the size of the particle (Fig. 13.2). In particular, particles of a certain size, typically in the range 0.05 to 0.5 μm, pass through the filter more easily than others. This size is known as the most penetrating particle size. Particles of this size are too small to be directly intercepted by fibres and too large to undergo substantial Brownian motion.

Types of filter

There are two main types of filter material used in breathing system filters:

Glass fibre filters

This filter material consists of a sheet of resin-bonded glass fibres. The fibres are packed densely (Fig. 13.3a) and hence the sheet has a high resistance to gas flow per unit area. A sheet with a large surface area is used to reduce the resistance to gas flow to an acceptable level. The sheet is then pleated to minimize the required volume, and hence dead space, for the housing. This type of filter material is hydrophobic and under normal clinical conditions, does not absorb water.

Electrostatic filters

There are two main types of electrostatic filter material. In both types, the fibre density is lower than in glass fibre filters and hence the resistance to gas flow is lower per unit area. The filtration performance is enhanced by using electrostatically-charged material, which attracts and binds with any particles passing through the filter material. Therefore, this type of filter material does not need to be pleated, and a flat layer is generally used in breathing system filters.

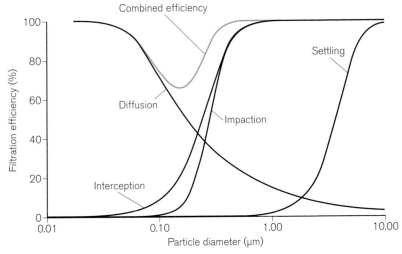

Figure 13.2 Filtration efficiency as a function of particle aerodynamic diameter due to the different filtration mechanisms. Note the minimum efficiency (maximum penetration) at a diameter of about 0.3 μm. Adapted from Hinds WC (1999) Aerosol Technology. *Properties, behaviour, and measurement of airborne particles,* 2nd end. New York: John Wiley and Sons.

1. Tribocharged filters

An electrostatic charge can be induced on two dissimilar fibres by rubbing them together during the manufacturing process, so that one type becomes positively charged and the other type negatively charged (*tribocharging*). One such filter material is made from fibres of polypropylene and modacrylic which can then be converted into a non-woven felt (Fig. 13.3b).

2. Fibrillated coronal-charged filters

An electrostatic charge can be applied to a sheet of polypropylene by using a point electrode emitting ions (*corona charging*). An opposite charge can be induced on the rear of the sheet. This type of material is often called an electret. If the sheet of polypropylene is now stretched, the strength of the molecular bonds is enhanced in the direction of the stretching, but reduced in a direction perpendicular to it. The sheet can then be split into fibres, a process called fibrillation, and made into a non-woven filter wad (Fig. 13.3c).

Measuring the performance of breathing system filters

The filtration efficiency of a filter is determined by measuring the number of particles passing through the filter as a percentage of the number of particles in an aerosol challenge to the filter. This percentage is the penetration value for the filter. Although challenges of microbes can be used,[6] the standard for breathing system filters specifies that the challenge should consist of a particular

quantity of an aerosol containing sodium chloride particles having diameters close to the most penetrating particle size.[7] The filter is challenged at a flow of 15 or 30 l min⁻¹ for filters intended for use with paediatric or adult patients, respectively. Typical penetration values for filters are shown in Figure 13.4.

HUMIDIFIERS

Humidity

Humidity is used to describe the amount of water vapour in air or gas. The mass of water vapour in the gas is the absolute humidity (g m⁻³). The maximum amount of humidity that gas can contain is limited by temperature (Fig. 13.5). At the maximum humidity for a particular temperature, the gas is said to be saturated with water vapour, and the level of humidity is the humidity at saturation. The relative humidity, RH (%) is the absolute humidity of the gas at a particular temperature as a percentage of the humidity at saturation at the same temperature.

Room air at 22°C typically has an absolute humidity level of about 10 g m⁻³. The humidity at saturation of air at 22°C is about 20 g m⁻³, so that the room air has a relative humidity of about 50% RH. If the air is cooled, a point is reached at about 11°C when the absolute humidity level equals the humidity at saturation, and hence the relative humidity is 100%. If the air cools to an even lower temperature, condensation will occur. If room air is inspired, the air is warmed to 37°C by the upper

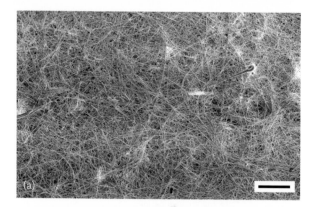

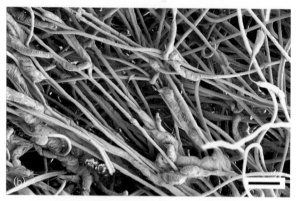

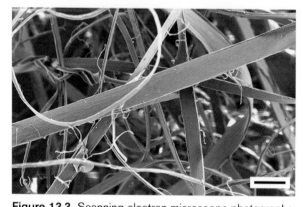

Figure 13.3 Scanning electron microscope photographs of the surface of different types of filter material.
(a) Glass fibre; **(b)** tribocharged electrostatic; **(c)** fibrillated electrostatic. Note the 100 μm scale marker in the bottom right corner of the photographs. Bacteria are about 1 μm in diameter.

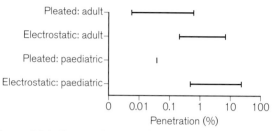

Figure 13.4 Range of penetration values for different filters when challenged with an aerosol of sodium chloride particles at the most penetrating particle size for the filters. Filters are tested at flows of 15 or 30 l min⁻¹ when intended for use with paediatric or adult patient, respectively. Note: only one pleated hydrophobic filter intended for use with paediatric patients was tested.

this deficit to 0 g m⁻³. If the room air is warmed from 22 to 37°C without any humidification, the relative humidity will fall to $100 \times (10 \div 44) = 23\%$. The massic enthalpy (latent heat) of evaporation of water is 2.4 kJ g⁻¹. To saturate inspired gases, which have a low level of humidity, a considerable proportion of the body's heat production must be used (up to a third for a neonate). This can then lead to a fall in the patient's core temperature of more than 1°C.

Humidification requirements

The level of humidity acceptable in gases delivered to patients, whose upper airways have been bypassed, depends on the length of time of the bypass. For short-term use, the level of humidity may only need to be 20 g m⁻³ (45% of BTPS conditions).[8] For longer use, for example, for patients in intensive care units, the level of humidity should be at least 33 g m⁻³ (75% of BTPS conditions)[9]. One group has proposed that the level of humidity should be close to BTPS conditions (44 g m⁻³).[3]

Humidification equipment

Gas can be humidified by using either passive or active systems. Passive systems, such as heat and moisture exchangers (HMEs), rely on the patient's ability to add moisture to the inspiratory gas. Active systems, such as heated humidifiers, add water vapour to a flow of gas independently of the patient. Combined passive and active devices are also now available.

Passive humidification systems

1. Heat and moisture exchangers (HMEs)
HMEs return a portion of the exhaled heat and moisture to the next inspiration. If the exhaled gas is at 34°C and

air passages by the time it reaches the lungs, and the humidity is increased from 10 to 44 g m⁻³ (BTPS conditions: body temperature and pressure, saturated). The difference between the two (−34 g m⁻³) is the humidity deficit: humidity must be added by the airways to reduce

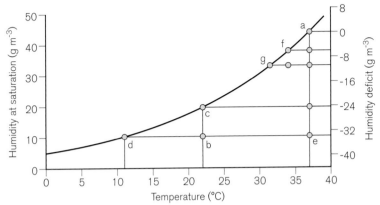

Figure 13.5 Humidity at saturation against temperature. Humidity deficit indicates the humidity that must be added by the airways to increase the humidity to **(a)** BTPS conditions (37°C, 44 g m^{-3}, 100% relative humidity). **(b)** Typical room air (22°C, 10 g m^{-3}, 50% RH); **(c)** room air saturated with water vapour (22°C, 20 g m^{-3}, 100% RH); **(d)** room air cooled so that condensation occurs (11°C, 10 g m^{-3}, 100% RH); **(e)** room air warmed to body temperature (37°C, 10 g m^{-3}, 23% RH); **(f)** expired gas (34°C, 38 g m^{-3}, 100% RH); **(g)** minimum moisture output for humidifiers intended for use with patients whose airways have been bypassed (33 g m^{-3}).

is saturated with water vapour (38 g m^{-3}) then, even if the HME is 80% efficient, only 30 g m^{-3} is returned to the patient.

These devices generally consist of a transparent plastic housing so that any obstructions and secretions in the device can be seen readily. The housing contains a layer of either foam or paper that is commonly coated with a hygroscopic salt such as calcium chloride. The expired gas cools as it passes through this layer and condensation occurs, releasing the massic enthalpy of vaporization, which is partly retained by the HME layer. The hygroscopic salt absorbs water vapour, hence reducing the relative humidity of the gas to below saturation level, although some moisture is always lost into the breathing system. During inspiration, the humidity level of the gas entering the HME is usually low, so that the condensate evaporates using the absorbed heat, which also warms the gas. The hygroscopic salt, to which the water molecules are loosely bound, releases the water molecules when the water vapour pressure is low. The inspired gas is therefore warmed and humidified to an extent that depends on the moisture content of the expired gas, and hence on the patient's core temperature.

A layer of filter material may also be added to the device (heat and moisture exchange filters, HMEFs). Devices are also available that consist only of a layer of filter material. An electrostatic filter layer used on its own has a very low moisture-conserving performance, but a pleated hydrophobic filter layer used on its own can return some moisture as a temperature gradient builds up

within the pleats, allowing condensation during expiration and evaporation during inspiration.

Classification of filters and heat and moisture exchangers There are, therefore, five broad types of filter and/or heat and moisture exchange devices (Fig. 13.6):
- a heat and moisture exchange-only device, without a filter layer;
- a filter-only device, without a heat and moisture exchange layer; which can be either:
  - electrostatic; or
  - pleated hydrophobic;
- combined devices with both a heat and moisture exchange layer and a filter layer (HMEF), which can be either:
  - electrostatic; or,
  - pleated hydrophobic.

The range of typical levels of moisture output available is shown in Figure 13.7. Devices available from some manufacturers are colour-coded to indicate particular types of device (Fig. 13.8).

Filters and HMEs are available with different connectors. These include angle-pieces, catheter mounts and gas sampling ports. The gas sampling port is a female Luer-lock connector. When the cap on the port is removed, it can be placed on a storage port (if one is available) or, on some devices, a tether prevents the cap from becoming mislaid. HMEs are also available that are intended to be connected to a tracheostomy tube (Fig. 13.9).

2. Circle breathing systems

In these breathing systems, a portion of the exhaled gas is usually returned to the inspiratory limb of the breathing system in order to recycle the anaesthetic agents. This gas is first passed through a container of soda lime that is used to remove the exhaled carbon dioxide. This reaction generates both heat and water (see Chapter 7).

The removal of one mole of carbon dioxide from exhaled gas generates one mole of water. If all this water vaporizes, and assuming ideal gas conditions exist, an identical volume of water vapour will replace the volume of carbon dioxide. If the exhaled gas contains 5% carbon dioxide, sufficient water vapour could be produced to saturate gas at 33°C, as saturated gas at 33°C contains 5% water vapour by volume (36 g m^{-3} water vapour). This is much more than the minimum of 20 g m^{-3} recommended

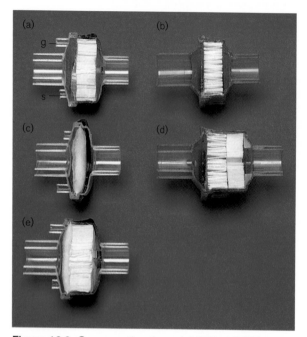

Figure 13.6 Cross-section through HMEs, HMEFs and filters. **(a)** HME only; **(b)** pleated hydrophobic filter only; **(c)** electrostatic filter only; **(d)** pleated hydrophobic filter and HME; **(e)** electrostatic filter and HME. Note the gas sampling port **(g)** and the storage port (s) for the cap from the port when the port is in use.

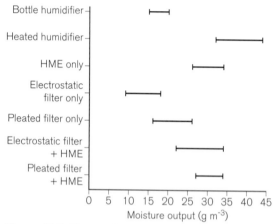

Figure 13.7 Range of humidification performance of different devices. The moisture output of bottle humidifiers depends on the ambient temperature and the degree of cooling. The moisture output of HMEs, HMEFs and filters varies for different devices and also depends on the tidal volume. In theory, a heated humidifier can be set to delivery any level of humidity if it has the appropriate controls. The values shown illustrate those that can be obtained when following the manufacturer's recommendations.

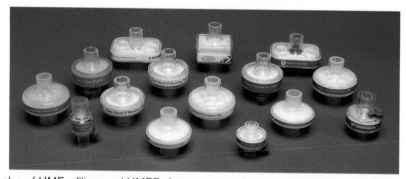

Figure 13.8 Examples of HMEs, filters and HMEFs from one manufacturer. Note the colour-coding: blue: HME-only; yellow: filter-only; green: HMEF. Other manufacturers use different colour-coding. The different sizes of devices are intended for use with paediatric and adult patients.

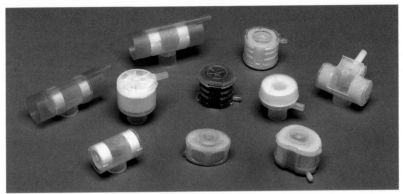

Figure 13.9 Heat and moisture exchangers intended to be attached to a tracheostomy tube. An oxygen tube can be connected to a port on some devices; some devices also have a port through which the patient's airways can be suctioned. One device has a valve which, when pressed closed, occludes allowing the patient to speak.

when the upper airways are bypassed during short-term procedures.[8] Hence, provided low fresh-gas flows are used with the circle breathing system (so that the humidity in the gas is not diluted excessively by the dry fresh-gas), adequate levels of humidity may be produced by the circle system alone (Fig. 13.10). During anaesthesia, the humidity of the gas in the circle system therefore increases, although it may take up to an hour or more to reach a maximum level. The humidity in the breathing system will augment the moisture content of the gas delivered to the patient from a filter or HME sited at the patient connection port.[10]

Active humidification systems

In these devices, water vapour is added to the inspired gases independently of the patient:

1. Bottle humidifier

The simplest type of active humidifier is the bottle humidifier (Fig. 13.11). In its simplest form, gas is directed over the surface of the water (Fig. 13.11a). The water evaporates and the water vapour mixes with the gas, increasing its humidity. The process is inefficient in that, unless the gas flow is very low, there is not sufficient time for the gas to become saturated with water vapour before it leaves the humidifier. The efficiency of humidification can be improved by increasing the surface area for evaporation. This can be achieved by bubbling the gas through the water, either through a tube (Fig. 13.11b) or through a sintered filter (Fig. 13.11c), or by placing a wick into the water: water is drawn up the wick again increasing the surface area for evaporation (Fig. 13.11d). Bubbling gas through the water increases the pressure drop across the

device, and the resistance to gas flow may therefore be unacceptably high for a spontaneously breathing patient who is required to draw gas through the humidifier.

However, in all these systems, the ambient temperature limits the maximum level of humidity that can be generated. For typical room air, the maximum level of humidity (humidity at saturation) that can be achieved is about 20 g m^{-3}. However, as the water will cool as evaporation occurs, the level is likely to be less than this. To achieve higher levels of humidity, either both the gas and water must be heated or a nebulizer must be used (see below).

2. Active heat and moisture exchanger

In this device, there is a heat and moisture exchange layer that retains and returns a portion of the exhaled heat and moisture as with passive versions. However, there is also a source of water that is heated within the device so that additional water vapour can be added to the inspiratory gases. One version of the device can be used with any HME or HMEF, and therefore, if a filter is used, the patient can be protected from inhaling any infective droplets (Fig. 13.12). This device adds about 5 g m^{-3} to the humidity provided by the HME or filter with which it is used.[11]

3. Heated humidifiers

Heated humidifiers typically consist of the following (Fig. 13.13). Water is heated in a chamber that includes a wick, which absorbs the water and increases the surface area for evaporation. The water vapour produced mixes with the supplied gas as it flows through the humidifier. The water lost by evaporation is either manually or

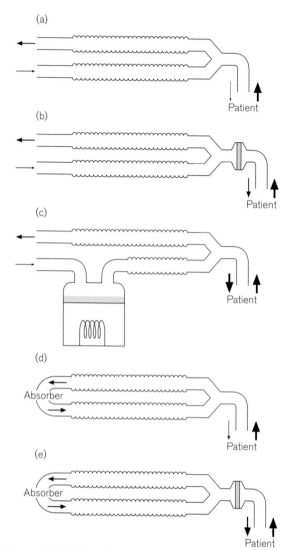

Figure 13.10 Breathing systems with different methods of humidification. **(a)** Open breathing system; **(b)** breathing system with HME; **(c)** breathing system with heated humidifier; **(d)** circle breathing system; **(e)** circle breathing system with HME. The width of the arrows indicates the level of humidity at various points in the breathing system. High levels of humidity can cause condensation if an appropriate temperature is not maintained.

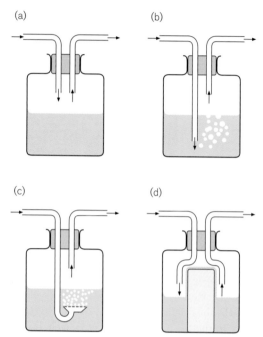

Figure 13.11 Ambient temperature or bottle humidifier. **(a)** Simple bottle humidifier; **(b)** bubble-through humidifier; **(c)** bubble-through humidifier with sintered filter to reduce the size of bubbles and hence increase surface area for evaporation; **(d)** wick humidifier.

automatically replenished from a reservoir. The humidified gas then flows to the patient through a delivery tube, which contains a sensor to monitor the temperature of the gas at the patient end. The temperature of the delivered humidified gas is set using a control knob. If this gas is allowed to cool as it flows through the delivery tube, condensation may occur. To reduce this cooling, a heater

wire in the delivery tube maintains the temperature of the gas. The temperature of the gas at the outlet of the humidification chamber is also monitored. The difference in temperature between the humidification chamber and the patient connection port is set on a second control knob. If the heater wire increases the temperature of the gas as it flows through the delivery tube, the risk of condensation forming is reduced, but the relative humidity of the gas also decreases. Alternatively, if the temperature of the gas falls, because of the settings on the two knobs, some condensation will occur, but the gas remains fully saturated with water vapour (Fig. 13.14).

Unless a second heater wire is used, condensation will also occur in the expiratory limb. Alternatively, a water trap can be fitted to collect any condensation that forms.

In one type of humidifier, the user has only to select whether the patient is intubated or receiving humidified gases via a facemask. The temperature and humidity of the gases are then controlled by the humidifier to provide the optimum level for the patient. The humidifier controls the humidity and temperature and also takes into account the flow of gas (Fig. 13.15).

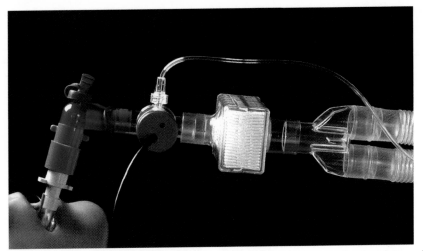

Figure 13.12 The Tomtec HME-Booster. Water is gravity-fed into a space between a heater plate and a Goretex membrane. The water is heated and evaporates: the water vapour then passes through the Goretex membrane.

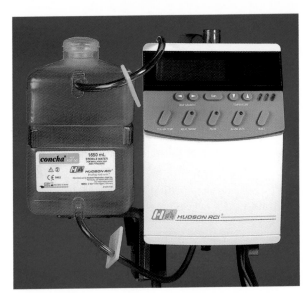

Figure 13.13 Hudson RCI Conchatherm IV heated humidifier. There are separate controls for 'TEMPERATURE' (temperature of the gas delivered to the patient) and 'TEMP GRADIENT' (difference between the temperature at the patient end of the delivery tube and the humidifier outlet).

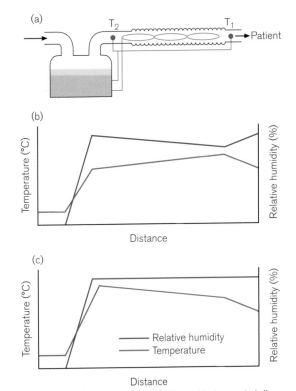

Figure 13.14 (a) Heated humidifier with heated delivery tube. **(b)** Humidifier set so that the temperature of the gas at the patient end of the delivery tube (T1) is higher than the humidification chamber outlet (T2). **(c)** Humidifier set so that the temperature of the gas at the patient end of the delivery tube (T1) is lower than the humidification chamber outlet (T2). In this case, condensation will occur in the delivery tube. The humidity of the gas delivered to the patient is the same in both cases.

Nebulizers

Nebulizers are used to humidify respirable gases by generating aerosols containing droplets of water from a reservoir of water (Fig. 13.16). The water may additionally contain medication. Some of these droplets evaporate as the gas flows to the patient so that the gas is likely to be fully saturated with water vapour when it reaches the patient's

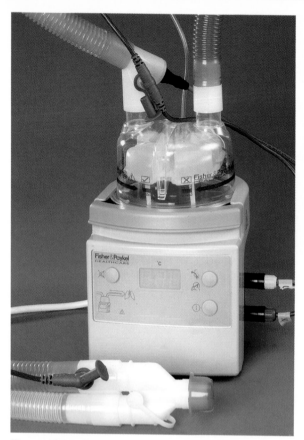

Figure 13.15 Fisher and Paykel MR850 heated humidifier. To use the humidifier, the user has merely to choose whether the patient is intubated or receiving humidified gas via a facemask. A heated wire in the delivery tube maintains the temperature of the delivered gas and reduces condensation.

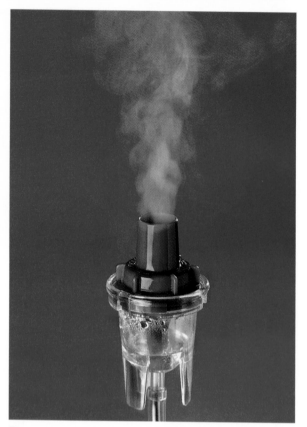

Figure 13.16 Aerosol generated by a nebulizer.

airways. However, as heat is required for evaporation, the temperature of the gas will fall. The temperature of the gas can be increased by warming the water in the reservoir.

There are two types of nebulizer: gas-driven or ultrasonic. Both types can generate large numbers of water droplets, equivalent to a moisture output of several hundred grams per cubic metre, compared to 44 g m^{-3} for humidity at saturation at 37°C.

1. Gas-driven nebulizers

When a flow of gas under pressure leaves a tube, the rapid expansion of the gas causes a fall in pressure (the Bernoulli effect, see Fig. 1.10). This effect is used in a gas-driven nebulizer to draw water up a second tube. The water is sucked into the gas stream and is broken up into droplets by the high flow of gas. An anvil, placed in the path of the

flow of gas, breaks up the larger droplets into smaller ones, suitable for delivery to the patient (Fig. 13.17a).

2. Ultrasonic nebulizer

In this device, a plate containing a piezo-electric crystal vibrates at an ultrasonic frequency, typically around 2 MHz. Water is either dropped onto the plate, or the plate is placed in water. The frequency of oscillations of the plate causes the water to break up into droplets. Gas flowing into the nebulizing chamber picks up the droplets to deliver them to the patient (Fig. 13.17b).

Deposition in the airways

Deposition of droplets in the airways depends on the same five mechanisms as deposition of particles in filters. Deposition therefore depends on the size of the droplets. Droplets with a diameter greater than 5 μm are deposited in the upper airways, droplets with a diameter in the range from 2 to 6 μm are deposited in the tracheo-bronchial airways, and droplets with a diameter in the range from 0.5 to 3 μm are deposited in the alveoli

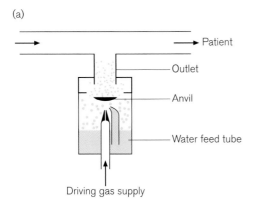

(a)

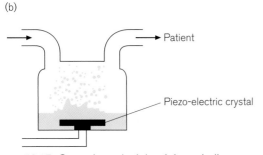

(b)

Figure 13.17 Operating principle of the nebulizer.
(a) Gas-powered; **(b)** ultrasonic. In **(a)** rapid expansion of
the gas at the end of the tube causes a reduction in
pressure, drawing liquid up the tube, which is then
broken up into droplets as it emerges. The droplets are
broken into smaller droplets when they strike an anvil. In
(b) a plate vibrates at an ultrasonic frequency (around
2 MHz) which breaks up liquid water into small droplets.

(Fig. 13.18).[12] As with particles and filters, deposition and
retention of droplets within the airways is a minimum for
droplets with an aerodynamic diameter of about 0.3 μm.
The mass of the droplets is also important. The mass of
the droplet is proportional to r^3, where r is radius. A
droplet with 10 times the radius will carry 1000 times the
mass, or 1000 times the medication. Deposition increases
for droplets with diameters less than 0.3 μm due to
Brownian motion. However, droplets of this size carry
only a very small mass of medication.

Deposition in the alveoli, particularly when breathing
nasally, is a small fraction of the overall deposition.
Deposition in the alveoli will be greater during oral
breathing and particularly when the upper airways are
bypassed.

PROBLEMS WITH FILTERS, HUMIDIFIERS AND NEBULIZERS

When added at the Y-piece of a breathing system, filters
and HMEs add dead space. A commonly-held view is that
the HME or filter should add no more than the equivalent
of one fifth of the tidal volume to the dead space, so that
for a tidal volume of 0.5 l, the maximum dead space of
the device should be 100 ml.

Filters and HMEs also increase the resistance to gas
flow in a breathing system. Also, if the dead space is
reduced, by using a smaller device, the resistance to gas

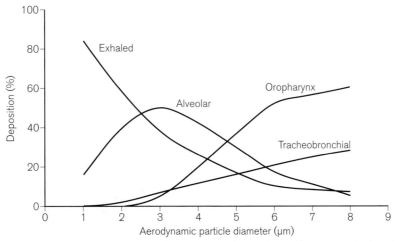

Figure 13.18 Deposition of particles in the airways. Note that maximum deposition occurs in the alveoli for particles
with an aerodynamic diameter of about 0.5 to 3 μm. Larger particles are predominantly deposited in the large airways.
In this size range, smaller particles are predominantly exhaled. Data from O'Callaghan C, Barry PW (1997) The
science of nebulised drug delivery. *Thorax* **52**: S25–S30.

flow increases, and the filtration efficiency and moisture output decreases. Filters can block if excessive water or sputum enter the housing, preventing adequate ventilation of the patient.[13,14]

In some early humidifiers, gas was bubbled through the water in the vaporization chamber. In addition to humidifying the inspired gas, this method produced droplets of water in the gas stream which occasionally contained microbes. This increased the risk of infection to a patient. The risk of infection from modern heated humidifiers is low, as the gas passes over, rather than through, the water.

Heated humidifiers rely on temperature sensors to ensure that the temperature of the delivered gas is that required by the user. The temperature of the gas in the delivery tube is generally warmer in the centre than towards the inner surface of the delivery tube. If the temperature sensors are not sited correctly in the middle of the gas flow, the temperature of the delivered gas may be much greater than that indicated on the humidifier and required by the user, and injury may result.

Condensation will occur in the expiratory limb of a humidification system. A heater wire can be used to reduce the condensation. However, this may cause excessive condensation to form within the expiratory valve of the ventilator, adversely affecting the performance of the expiratory flow sensor that may be sited there.

With nebulizers, it is relatively easy to add a large amount of moisture to the delivered gas, leading to excessive loading of the lungs with water and subsequent hypoxia due to blockage of the alveoli. In addition, the size of the droplets produced are very effective for the transmission of microbes, so care must be taken to ensure that the liquid water in the nebulizer is sterile. Some nebulized drugs can block some types of filter.[15] If the nebulizer is operating continuously, then a fraction of the medication will be lost into the expiratory limb of the breathing system during exhalation. This fraction depends on the inspiratory:expiratory ratio of the breathing pattern.

REFERENCES

1. Burton JDK (1962) Effects of dry anaesthetic gases on the respiratory mucous membrane. *Lancet* i: 235–239.
2. Chalon J, Loew DAY, Malebranche J (1972) Effects of dry anesthetic gases on tracheobronchial ciliated epithelium. *Anesthesiology* 37: 338–343.
3. Williams R, Rankin N, Smith T, Galler D, Seakins P (1996) Relationship between the humidity and temperature of inspired gas and the function of the airway mucosa. *Critical Care Medicine* 24: 1920–1929.
4. Rathgeber J, Keitzmann D, Mergeryant H, Hub R, Züchner K, Kettler D (1997) Prevention of patient bacterial contamination of anaesthesia-circle-systems. A clinical study of the contamination risk and performance of different heat and moisture exchangers with electret filter (HMEF). *European Journal of Anaesthesiology* 14: 368–373.
5. Wilkes AR (2002) The ability of breathing system filters to prevent liquid contamination of breathing systems: a laboratory study. *Anaesthesia* 57: 33–39.
6. Wilkes AR, Benbough JE, Speight SE, Harmer H (2000) The bacterial and viral filtration performance of breathing system filters. *Anaesthesia* 55: 458–465.
7. Wilkes AR (2002) Measuring the filtration performance of breathing system filters using sodium chloride particles. *Anaesthesia* 57: 162–168.
8. Kleemann PP (1994) Humidity of anaesthetic gases with respect to low flow anaesthesia. *Anaesthesia and Intensive Care* 22: 396–408.
9. British Standards Institution (1998) Humidifiers for medical use - general requirements for humidification systems (BS EN ISO 8185: 1998). London: British Standards Institution.
10. Henriksson B-Å, Sundling J, Hellman A (1997) The effect of a heat and moisture exchanger on humidity in a low-flow anaesthesia system. *Anaesthesia* 52: 144–149.
11. Medical Devices Agency (2001) 'Active' heat and moisture exchanger: Tomtec HME-Booster (Evaluation 01029). London: Medical Devices Agency.
12. British Standards Institution (2001) Respiratory Therapy Equipment - Part 1: Nebulizing systems and their components (BS EN 13544-1: 2001). London: British Standards Institution.
13. Williams DJ, Stacey MRW (2002) Rapid and complete occlusion of a heat and moisture exchange filter by pulmonary edema (Clinical report). *Canadian Journal of Anaesthesia* 49: 126–131.
14. Lawes EG (2003) Hidden hazards and dangers associated with the use of HME/filters in breathing circuits. Their effect on toxic metabolite production, pulse oximetry and airway resistance. *British Journal of Anaesthesia* 91: 249–264.
15. Stacey MRW, Asai T, Wilkes A, Hodzovic I (1996) Obstruction of a breathing system filter. *Canadian Journal of Anaesthesia* 43: 1276.

FURTHER READING

Branson RD, Campbell RS, Davis K, Porembka DT (1998) Anaesthesia circuits, humidity output, and mucociliary structure and function. *Anaesthesia and Intensive Care* **26:** 178–183.

Branson RD, Peterson BD, Carson KD (eds) (1998) Humidification: current therapy and controversy. *Respiratory Care Clinics of North America* **4:** 189–344.

Brown RC (1993) *Air filtration. An integrated approach to the theory and applications of fibrous filters.* Oxford: Pergamon Press.

Hinds WC (1999) *Aerosol Technology. Properties, behavior, and measurement of airborne particles,* 2nd edn. New York: John Wiley and Sons.

Muers MF (1997) Overview of nebuliser treatment. *Thorax* **52:** S25–S30.

O'Callaghan C, Barry PW (1997) The science of nebulised drug delivery. *Thorax* **52:** S31–S44.

Shelly MP (1993) Humidification. In: *Intensive Care Rounds.* Abingdon: The Medicine Group (Education) Ltd.

Wilkes AR (2001) Humidification: its importance and delivery. *British Journal of Anaesthesia CEPD Reviews* **1:** 40–43.

Wilkes AR (2002) Breathing system filters. *British Journal of Anaesthesia CEPD Reviews* **2:** 151–154.

Equipment for paediatric anaesthesia

Stephen Fenlon

Children neither look nor behave like small adults. Their requirements in the perioperative setting differ, including those of anaesthetic technique and equipment. In the UK, surgery for children constitutes less than 10% of the total surgery performed and for financial reasons, development of equipment centres on the market for adult patients. Despite this, there is a rich history of innovation in paediatric anaesthesia. Some of the items we take for granted appear too simple to have been the subject of invention, an example of this being the T-piece breathing system developed from Magill's system by Dr Phillip Ayre.[1] This system, modified by Dr Jackson Rees, has stood the test of time, remaining in use by paediatric anaesthetists the world over (Fig. 14.1).

The differences, both between adults and children, and within children of different ages, affect the design of equipment. This is particularly so for those items relating to control of the airway and breathing. Small pieces of equipment designed for use on small patients, must still be handled by large unwieldy adult hands, and be compatible with international standard fittings. Bulky equipment increases the chance of technical complications, particularly accidental extubation.

ANATOMICAL AND PHYSIOLOGICAL DIFFERENCES BETWEEN ADULTS AND CHILDREN

The magnitude of these differences relate to age. Neonates and infants present the largest variation, the older child increasingly approximates to adult parameters. For the purposes of this chapter, the most important variation is found in the anatomy and physiology of the respiratory system.

Anatomical differences in the airway between adults and children

Compared to the adult, in the child:
- the tongue is relatively large and the larynx in a higher position;
- the epiglottis is longer and U-shaped;
- in the younger child, the narrowest part of the upper airway is the cricoid ring. a tube passing easily through the laryngeal inlet may be too tight at the cricoid ring. Should insertion of a tracheal tube be necessary, its

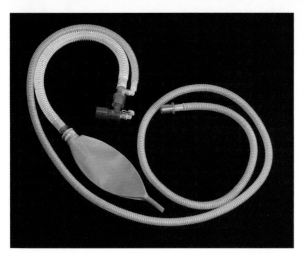

Figure 14.1 A modern T-piece system with rebreathing bag.

fit is critical. Too small a tube leads to an increase in resistance, large leak, and possible fluid ingress around the tube. Too tight a fit creates a risk of mucosal ischaemia and oedema, leading to stridor at extubation.

- the larynx is smaller, so the reduction in diameter imposed by a tracheal tube will have a significantly larger effect on airway resistance to flow (Poiseuille's Law, see Chapter 1). The significance of apparatus dead space in comparison to the child's total dead space becomes greater the smaller the child (Fig. 14.2). The two together may accommodate a high proportion of the tidal volume with a significant effect on carbon dioxide elimination.

Physiological differences in breathing between adults and children

- The chest wall of the child is more compliant, contributing little to ventilation. The diaphragm moves less efficiently and contains fewer fatigue-resistant muscle fibres. Alveolar ventilation is therefore dependant more on rate; hence respiratory rate in infants and younger children is higher than in adults. The high rate is achieved at the expense of the end expiratory pause. (The latter is important for the efficient action of anaesthetic partial rebreathing systems (see below).)

- The work of breathing is higher in children, consuming relatively more oxygen. Airway maintenance devices and breathing systems by presenting resistance to flow, contribute further to this. Though infants can cope with increased work of breathing in the short term, diaphragmatic fatigue will set in earlier than in adults.

- Closing capacity in small children may exceed and overlap functional residual capacity. This can be worsened by anaesthesia and the supine position, with resultant hypoxia. The ability to deliver positive end expiratory pressure or continuous positive airway pressure may help to overcome this.

- Compared to adults and older children, infants produce approximately twice as much carbon dioxide and consume twice the amount of oxygen relative to body weight.

EQUIPMENT

The anaesthetic machine

From its humble origins as a spartan trolley bearing just cylinders, vaporizers and the odd coffee stain, the anaesthetic machine has evolved into the anaesthesia workstation. The principles of the continuous flow machine remain the same, and this machine is most suited to paediatric practice. Draw-over apparatus presents too great a resistance to breathing to be used by children weighing under 20 kg and, if used, there must be some

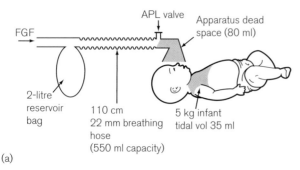

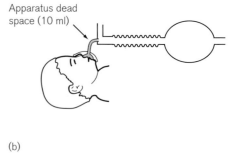

Figure 14.2 (a) A typical adult breathing system (Mapleson A system) with a typical dead space of 80 ml. **(b)** Apparatus dead space in a paediatric breathing system of less than 10 ml.

means of providing continuous flow, such as manual bellows.[2] Despite a long and largely safe record of use in anaesthesia, nitrous oxide may be superseded as carrier gas by air, only then will machines be ultimately incapable of delivering a hypoxic mixture. For certain congenital cardiac conditions, use of air without obligatory oxygen flow is needed to avoid the pulmonary vasodilatation seen with higher oxygen concentrations. This requires a specially adapted anaesthetic machine. Aside from this unusual application, any continuous flow machine will suffice.

Transmission of infection

In recent years, anaesthetic equipment has been changing to eliminate the risks of disease transmission between patients. The development of lightweight durable plastics has been particularly valuable for paediatric breathing systems, providing flexible low-resistance systems with a reduced tendency to 'drag' on other components. While items in intimate contact with the patient should be for single use, the need to discard whole breathing systems with each patient is less well proven. Unlike with adult anaesthesia, the use of breathing system filters to enable re-use of breathing systems is not encouraged in paediatric practice. Asides from the risk of transmitting infection, breathing systems may be manufactured to single-use standard, implying that repeated use leads to deterioration of components and a greater chance of failure (especially for tapered connectors). The situation is under continuous review and precautions evolve as understanding of disease transmission improves.[3]

Regulation of equipment manufacture

The development and testing of new apparatus, and its ease of use, have recently been reviewed.[4,5] Medical devices sold in the European Economic Area carry a CE mark (European mark of conformity assessment, Conformite Européene) placed by the manufacturer. To do this, the manufacturer must provide details of risk analyses, performance in standard tests and technical data relating to manufacture of an item of equipment. The Competent Authority, which in the UK is The Medicines and Healthcare Products Regulatory Agency, oversees this procedure (see Chapter 30). Medical devices are classified and tested according to risk of injury in the event of malfunction, e.g. a facemask is class 1 (low risk), a cardiac catheter class 3 (high risk).[6] It is important to be aware that the CE marking process does not always imply

specific clinical testing, therefore paediatric equipment may not be tested in the paediatric anaesthetic environment prior to release on the market.

Most pre-use testing is so-called bench testing, demonstrating equivalent or better function than existing similar equipment. Scaling down of adult equipment is acceptable on this basis, but may not produce the most effective devices in use. However, most manufacturers strive to thoroughly test their product and avoid, where possible, the incidence of post-marketing complications and inappropriate use. A good example of this is the laryngeal mask airway. Although directly scaled down from adult sizes, it was specifically tested to confirm it retained anatomical suitability for paediatric use.[7] CE marking is not always required before release of a product for use. Some novel devices need to undergo clinical trials before applying the mark and custom-made equipment is also exempt. Devices made within a hospital, for use within that same hospital, do not require a CE mark, but may be provided with an exemption certificate for specified use elsewhere.

Equipment for management of the airway

Apparatus for management of the paediatric airway, from facemasks through to tracheostomy tubes, is outwardly similar to the adult equivalent. Subtle changes are incorporated to try to achieve the ideals mentioned above. Management of the airway in both adult and paediatric practice has been revolutionized by the introduction of the laryngeal mask airway. Similar airway management devices introduced following the laryngeal mask have not so far enjoyed the same level of success.

Facemasks

These should be available in a range of appropriate sizes and form a good seal at the edges, with minimal dead space. Clear plastic masks are less frightening to awake children and can even be scented. They remain, however, unlikely to match the overpowering bouquet of volatile anaesthetic agents.

A variety of paediatric facemasks exist (Fig. 14.3). To reduce dead space, the Rendell–Baker-Soucek mask was designed anatomically, from casts of children's faces, in the same way as a dental plate is made.[8] This mask achieves a seal by virtue of its close approximation to the contours of the face. Other masks require some form of flexible lip or air filled cushion. The lipped round silicone mask is easy to apply, providing an excellent seal for infant use. Disposable masks generally employ a cushion seal,

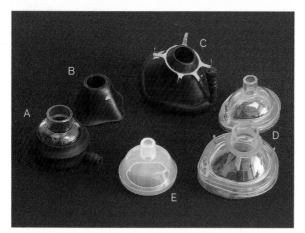

Figure 14.3 A gathering of facemasks. A, The Ambu facemask; B, The Rendell–Baker–Soucek facemask; C, The anatomical facemask; D, Disposable scented facemasks; E, The Laerdal silicone facemask

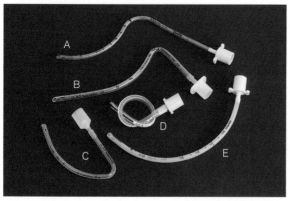

Figure 14.4 An assembly of tracheal tubes. A, Oral north facing tube; B, RAE tube; C, RAE south facing oral tube; D, reinforced tube; E, standard tracheal tube.

Table 14.1 Dimensions of some non-cuffed infant endotracheal tubes

Manufacturer	Int. diameter (mm)	Ext. diameter (mm)
Portex (silicone)	2.5	3.4
Sheridan (Ped-soft)	2.5	3.6
Portex (ivory)	2.5	3.6
Mallinkrodt (PVC)	2.5	3.6
Rusch (clearway)	2.5	4.0
Mallinkrodt (reinforced)	2.5	4.0
Portex (reinforced)	2.5	4.0
Rusch (rubber)	2.5	4.0
Portex (silicone)	2.5	4.2
Sheridan (Ped-soft)	3.0	4.2
Portex (ivory)	3.0	4.4
Mallinkrodt (PVC)	3.0	4.3
Rusch (clearway)	3.0	4.7
Mallinkrodt (reinforced)	3.0	4.7
Portex (reinforced)	3.0	4.7
Rusch (rubber)	3.0	4.7
Portex (silicone)	3.5	4.8
Sheridan (Ped-soft)	3.5	4.9
Portex (ivory)	3.5	5.0
Mallinkrodt (PVC)	3.5	4.9
Rusch (clearway)	3.5	5.3
Mallinkrodt (reinforced)	3.5	5.3
Portex (reinforced)	3.5	5.3
Rusch (rubber)	3.5	5.3

the rest of the mask being of rigid construction. Whichever is chosen, it must be easy to hold and seal on the face, and this may well be a matter of trial and error. Attempts to reduce facemask anatomical dead space may be less important than previously thought, the actual increase in physiological dead space with anaesthesia being less than predicted.[9]

Tracheal tubes

Tracheal tubes are available in sizes and shapes to suit different patients and surgical procedures (Fig. 14.4). Ideally the walls need to be as thin as possible, whilst remaining resistant to kinking. The tracheal tube is the site of greatest resistance in the paediatric airway. Different tubes of the same internal diameter have varying wall thickness, affecting the size of lumen available from a given tube fit (Table 14.1). Other factors affect tube resistance: connectors, tube length, shape of tube and tendency to collect secretions.

Therefore it is clear that the decision to intubate, and which tracheal tube to use, is of great significance. Previous attempts to circumvent the problem of tube resistance included the use of shouldered and tapered tubes (Fig. 14.5). However, the onset of turbulent flow at the narrowed part of the tube negates any benefit from

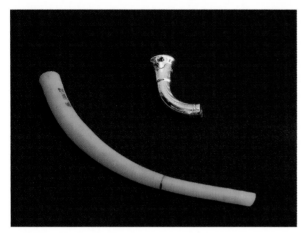

Figure 14.5 The Enderby tracheal tube, a tapered tube designed for use in cleft lip and palate surgery (no longer in use).

Table 14.3 A guide to tracheal tube dimensions

Age	Weight (kg)	Tube Diameter (mm)
Preterm	<2	2.5
Small Term	2–3	3.0
Term	3–3.5	3.5
3 months to 1 year	5–10	4.0
1 to 2 years	10–15	4.5
Over 2 years according to formula:		Age/4+4.5 mm
Tube Length (oral)	(Age/2)+12 mm	
Tube Length (nasal)	(Age/2)+15 mm	

Table 14.2 A comparison of cuffed and uncuffed tubes

	Uncuffed tracheal tube	**Cuffed tracheal tube**
Seal	Forms a seal in the cricoid ring, but seal may not be effective	Can completely seal the tracheal inlet
Effect on tracheal mucosa	May be less prone to causing damage	May cause damage
Available lumen	Maximizes available lumen	Cuff reduces the available lumen
Other		Generally only employed from 8–10 years of age

improved flow in the wider length.[10] Additionally, the wider section of these tubes can migrate into the cricoid ring, leading to oedema of the tracheal mucosa.[8] Reports of tracheal damage in children from tracheal intubation in the intensive care setting, gave rise to widespread use of uncuffed tubes around which an audible leak on lung inflation indicated correct fit. Uncuffed tubes also permit a wider lumen for a given internal diameter compared with cuffed tubes. Despite these perceived advantages, uncuffed tubes can permit aspiration of liquid around the tube and contribute to atmospheric pollution by leaking anaesthetic gases. A large leak is annoying as it will lead to inadequate ventilation and induce 'anaesthesia' in surgeons working around the upper airway.

Widespread use of uncuffed tubes has been questioned.[11] It may be that cuffed tubes, which give a better tracheal seal (Table 14.2), are safe to use in some children. Large studies of all age groups are needed to rule out low-incidence serious complications from applying this technique instead of the accepted practice. The development of novel non-compressive sealing for tubes may provide a solution.[12]

For the present, uncuffed, parallel-sided tubes are the norm, and a diameter should be chosen around which an audible leak of gas occurs at an inflation pressure under 25 cmH$_2$0. Although the presence of a tube leak is said to protect against mucosal damage, it may confer no benefit for the short periods of intubation needed for most operations.[13]

Whilst tube size selection is critical, formulae can only provide a rough guide to the correct tube size (Table 14.3). Coexisting medical conditions may influence tube size; children with Down syndrome often require a tube 1–2 mm smaller than expected for their age.[14] Likewise,

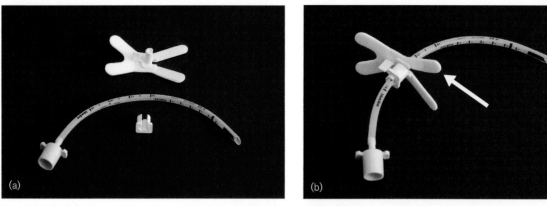

Figure 14.6 (a) A device for fixing tracheal tubes, The Portex RSP **(b)** The same device locked onto the tube, self adhesive strips (arrowed) are used to fix the device to the face.

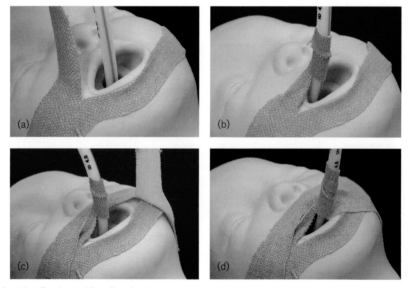

Figure 14.7 Simple tube fixation with adhesive tape.

the required length of tube can only be estimated. Some tubes incorporate marks intended to guide how far to advance the tube into the larynx under direct vision. Preformed tubes may have a mark indicating the position for fixation over the lip. The placing of such marks is inconsistent across tube sizes and manufacturers, and they should not be relied upon.

Fixation of the tube should aim to prevent displacement, maintain the tube position with head movement, and still be relatively easy to secure and adjust (Fig. 14.6). Simple tape fixation fulfills many of these criteria (Fig. 14.7). Nasal intubation in children is more secure and preferred in the intensive care setting, as the tube

tends to move less, reducing trauma to the tracheal mucosa.

Flow at the interface of breathing system and tube is disturbed by changes in diameter and direction. Connectors aim to minimize this by smooth internal surfaces, graduated reductions in diameter and gentle direction changes. The commonest tube connector is the ISO 15 mm, though another standard system is based on 8.5 mm connectors (Fig. 14.8). Connectors do not reduce the available lumen as they dilate the tube at the point of insertion. Problems can arise when assembling small thin-walled parts, with buckling of the walls and possible occlusion of the lumen.[15] Some older connectors remain

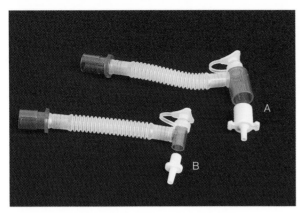

Figure 14.8 ISO fitting tracheal tube connectors and catheter mounts. A, 15 mm; B, 8.5 mm. Both are available for a range of paediatric tube sizes.

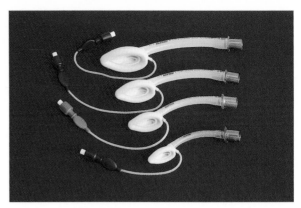

Figure 14.10 Paediatric sizes of laryngeal mask airway (sizes 1, 1.5, 2, and 2.5).

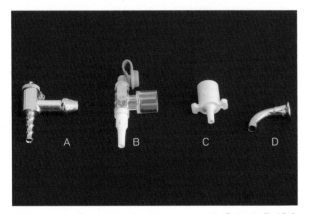

Figure 14.9 Tracheal tube connectors. A, Oxford; B, ISO 8.5 mm; C, ISO 15 mm; D, Magill oral.

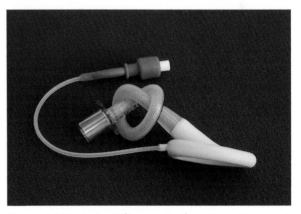

Figure 14.11 A size 2 (the smallest) reinforced laryngeal mask airway. The knot is for illustrative purposes only and is not recommended in use.

in use as they are compact and may offer less resistance to gas flow (Fig. 14.9). Endotracheal tubes allow suction to be applied to the lower airway. To select a suction catheter, doubling the tube diameter in mm, gives the appropriate French gauge catheter size.[16]

The laryngeal mask airway

Since its introduction, this piece of equipment has been credited with a revolution in anaesthetic technique. It is in wide use in paediatric practice with few problems,[17] and has been employed for both spontaneous and controlled ventilation.[18,19] The laryngeal mask has also proved valuable in managing the difficult airway, such as that encountered with Pierre Robin Sequence.[20] It can be used to guide fibreoptic intubation, or even blind passage of a tracheal tube,[21] though caution is advised with the

latter technique.[22] A range of sizes, from neonatal to older child, is available (Fig. 14.10), size selection being based on patient weight (Table 14.4). Where more flexibility of the tube is needed, a reinforced version is available down to size 2 (Fig. 14.11).

The laryngeal mask has lower resistance to gas flow compared with a tracheal tube, causes minimal stimulation of the airway and offers some protection against pulmonary aspiration of fluid from above. It does not protect against aspiration of regurgitated fluid. Though some authors suggest alternative methods, it is recommended the laryngeal mask be inserted in exactly the same way as for the adult patient.[7] Positioning and securing the laryngeal mask is generally easily accomplished in children, though some difficulties may be encountered with the smaller sizes, 1 and 1.5.[23] In any event, infants

Table 14.4 Recommended sizes and dimensions of laryngeal masks showing also the largest tracheal tube (TT) diameter that may be passed through each size

Mask Size	Patient Weight (kg)	ID/OD (mm)	Length (cm)	Max cuff volume (ml)	Largest TT ID (mm)
1	<5	5.25/8.25	8	4	3.5
1.5	5–10	6.1/9.6	10	7	4.0
2	10–20	7.0/11.0	11.5	10	4.5
2.5	20–30	8.4/13.0	12.5	14	5.0
3	>30	10.0/15.0	19	20	6.0 cuffed

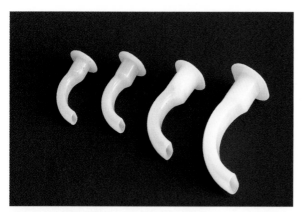

Figure 14.12 Various sizes of paediatric oropharyngeal airway, in order of increasing size: 000, 00, 0, 1.

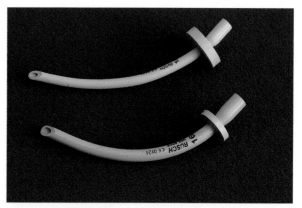

Figure 14.13 Paediatric adjustable flange nasopharyngeal airways.

usually need intubation and controlled ventilation for anaesthesia of longer duration.

When used for controlled ventilation, a small leak often occurs around the laryngeal mask and no attempt should be made to impede this by sealing the mouth, as gastric inflation may result. Loss of gas is minimal with normal inflation pressure; successful use with controlled ventilation and a circle absorber has been described.[24] Pressure controlled ventilation is advantageous, as it allows effective ventilation with lower airway pressures than volume controlled ventilation.[25] Oesophageal pH studies during controlled ventilation reveal no greater incidence of gastro-oesophageal reflux with the laryngeal mask compared to tracheal tube or facemask.[26]

Examination of the airway under anaesthesia and some surgery around the airway can be accomplished with a laryngeal mask in place.[27] This may allow better maintenance of anaesthesia and oxygenation during the procedure, compared with jet entrainment or apnoeic techniques. Care is needed with laryngeal mask cuff pressures, particularly if nitrous oxide is employed; high cuff pressures may result in nerve damage.[28] Despite this, there is a low rate of complications and the laryngeal mask has a place in anaesthesia for an increasingly wide range of paediatric patients.[29]

Airway adjuncts

Scaled versions of oral and nasal airway adjuncts exist for paediatric use (Figs 14.12 and 13) and are discussed in Chapter 8.

Tracheostomy tubes

A full range of uncuffed tracheostomy tubes exists for use in children (Fig. 14.14). To avoid endobrochial intubation, the intratracheal length is kept short; hence accidental decannulation is easily achieved.

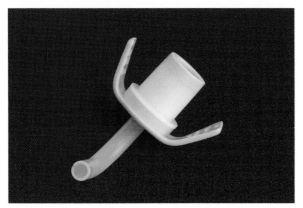

Figure 14.14 An uncuffed tracheostomy tube size 4 mm internal diameter.

Gaining access to the airway

Airway instrumentation and visualization differs in paediatric practice due to the anatomical differences previously mentioned. Difficulty visualizing the airway is unusual in paediatric practice overall. Management plans need to take account of the additional challenges posed by small and rightfully uncooperative patients.

The laryngoscope

The larynx is usually seen with the direct laryngoscope. A variety of laryngoscope blade profiles exist. The choice is usually dependant upon the age of the patient and the personal preference of the anaesthetist (Figs 14.15 and 16). Many practitioners use a straight blade for infant laryngoscopy: this blade picks up the relatively large epiglottis, affording a better view. For older children, a curved (small Macintosh pattern) blade will suffice. The little finger of the hand holding the laryngoscope may be used to apply external laryngeal pressure to improve the view. Flexible tracheal tube introducers can be used to railroad a tube into a larynx when a direct view cannot be obtained. These are available for use with tubes as small as 2.5 mm internal diameter.

A development of the bougie is the airway exchange catheter (AEC) (Fig. 14.17). A semi-rigid, hollow catheter with interchangeable 15 mm ISO male and Luer–Lok connectors, this is designed to allow tracheal tubes to be exchanged whilst retaining the ability to oxygenate the lungs. The AEC is inserted through the tube which is then exchanged over this. Once in place, the end connector can be fastened, gas sampled from the tip to detect carbon dioxide and correct position confirmed. Oxygen can then be insufflated through the catheter with

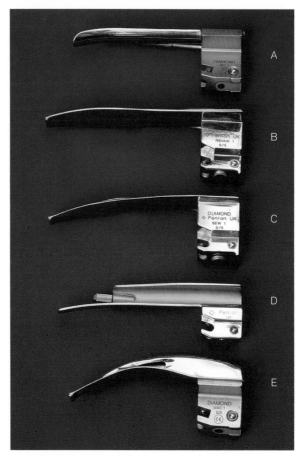

Figure 14.15 Paediatric laryngoscope blades in profile. A, Miller; B, Robertshaw; C, Seward; D, Wisconsin; E, Macintosh.

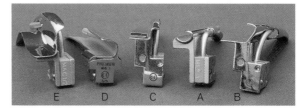

Figure 14.16 Paediatric laryngoscope blades, end-on view. A, Miller; B, Robertshaw; C, Seward; D, Wisconsin; E, Macintosh.

either a high-pressure injector or a standard anaesthetic breathing system. With the connector removed, a tracheal tube can be guided over the catheter and into the trachea.[30] The catheters are available to fit within tracheal tubes down to 3 mm internal diameter.

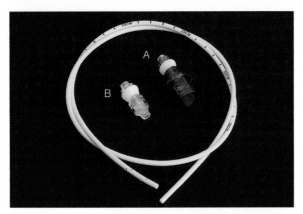

Figure 14.17 An airway exchange catheter suitable for paediatric use. The distal end with side holes is marked with an arrow. Also shown are the proximal Rapi-Fit® connectors, A, ISO 15 mm; B, Luer–Lok.

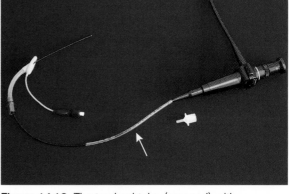

Figure 14.18 The tracheal tube (arrowed) with connector removed, is loaded onto the bronchoscope which is then advanced into the trachea using a laryngeal mask as guide.

The fibreoptic bronchoscope

Both the standard size and a smaller 2.2 mm fibreoptic bronchoscope can be used to aid intubation in children when the larynx is difficult to visualize. The standard bronchoscope incorporates a suction channel, ineffective for clearing secretions during intubation, but useful to thread a guide wire, which is then advanced into the trachea under direct vision. After removal of the bronchoscope, the wire remains in the trachea and is used to railroad a tracheal tube of the appropriate size.[31] Another technique with the standard bronchoscope is to guide a large tube over the bronchoscope until it abuts the laryngeal inlet. Holding the tube in position, the broncho-scope is withdrawn, a bougie passed down the tube into the trachea and the correct size tube passed over this.

Use of the 2.2 mm bronchoscope follows the adult pattern of fibreoptic intubation, whereby the tracheal tube (down to size 2.5 mm) is 'loaded' onto the broncho-scope prior to visualizing the laryngeal inlet. This technique is suited to difficult intubation in infants. A tracheal tube without its connector is passed along the bronchoscope (Fig. 14.18). Following induction of anaesthesia, the airway is maintained with a laryngeal mask. The right-angle connector in the breathing system incorporates a sealing port, through which the bronchoscope is advanced, passing through the bars of the laryngeal mask and into the trachea. The cuff of the laryngeal mask is deflated and it is then withdrawn back along the bronchoscope. The tube is advanced through the laryngeal mask, along the bronchoscope, and into the trachea (Fig. 14.19). The bronchoscope is withdrawn, the

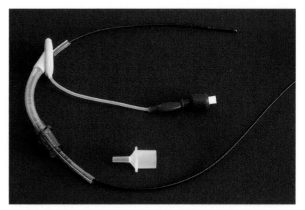

Figure 14.19 With the bronchoscope in the trachea, the laryngeal mask is withdrawn back onto the bronchoscope, the tube is threaded through it and on into the trachea.

tube connector replaced, and ventilation resumed when correct tube position is confirmed.[32] The tube may need changing over a suitable introducer, (see above) for one of better fit. If intubation is carried out with a long enough tube and the laryngeal mask does not impede the surgical view, the whole assembly can be left in position throughout surgery.

Instead of the laryngeal mask, a split oropharyngeal airway or modified tracheostomy tube can be used as a guide for the bronchoscope.[33] With all these techniques, components must be pre-assembled and compatibility confirmed, with particular attention to ensuring the components will fit through one another. When using fibreoptic intubation in children, oral intubation is usually

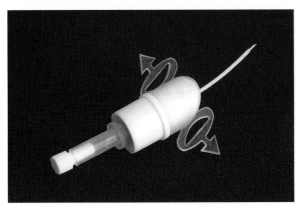

Figure 14.20 A paediatric cricothyroid cannulation needle.

preferable, as the nasal airway may be abnormal, and trauma to the nasal mucosa with subsequent bleeding can abolish the view completely.

A number of intubation aids are based on the rigid bronchoscope, with or without some curvature. These have been successfully employed to visualize and intubate the difficult airway.[34,35]

Trans-illumination techniques:

Passed blindly into the oropharynx, a light at the tip of a preformed curved stylet is visible through the skin of the neck. In darkened conditions the tip can be negotiated into the laryngeal inlet, and a tracheal tube mounted on the stylet advanced into the trachea. This equipment has the advantage of being cheaper, less prone to damage and requiring less maintenance than fibreoptic items. A single-use version is available to fit larger paediatric tracheal tubes.

Alternative approach to the difficult airway

Cricothyroid cannulation offers an alternative approach when difficulty maintaining and securing the airway is anticipated or experienced. Use of proprietary crico-thyroid cannulation kits (Fig. 14.20) has been described in children.[36] Unlike adult practice, these techniques are difficult to conduct on awake individuals. Certainly in small children, with a small trachea and large neck veins, this option presents a challenge and the safety of elective transtracheal ventilation has been questioned. For similar reasons, rapid formation of a tracheostomy may not be a straightforward option to fall back on.[37]

Anaesthetic breathing systems

The ability to continually and accurately measure inspired oxygen and end-tidal CO_2 has allowed attention to be re-focused on systems operating with low fresh gas flows and

reduced pollution. Early breathing system designs required clinical testing with invasive monitoring to generate safe operational limits for use in conjunction with the limited monitoring prevailing in clinical practice. Subsequently, patient monitoring has improved greatly. Pulse oximetry and end-tidal carbon dioxide monitoring, together with clinical observation, allow safer and more confident use of a variety of systems.[9]

Each breathing system has merits and limitations. Consideration of the major limitations helps to decide which is best in a particular situation. In no order of importance, these are apparatus dead space, rebreathing of exhaled gas, resistance and compression volume.

Apparatus dead space is difficult to determine with accuracy, though clearly should be minimized. Some items have recommendations for use based on their internal volume, e.g. breathing system filters. The contribution to dead space by a particular piece of equipment may differ from its measured volume, due to the effects of mixing by gas flows within the item. The term functional dead space incorporates this phenomenon.

Partial rebreathing of exhaled gas is a feature of some breathing systems, and is described in more detail in Chapter 7. The T-piece, classified as Mapleson E system, is an example of this. It is worth noting that it is similar in function to the D system.

Resistance is reflected in the pressure gradient required to drive gas through the breathing system to and from the patient. This translates to work done by the patient when breathing spontaneously. High resistance increases work and is tolerated particularly poorly by infants. Resistance arises from the components through which gas flows, including valves where fitted. As with apparatus dead space and rebreathing, resistance should be minimized where possible. This is best achieved by use of a valveless breathing system (such as a T-piece), avoiding acute angulation of connectors, and careful choice of tracheal tube (the source of greatest resistance). Where valved breathing systems are in use, the valves should be designed to be as light as possible.

Repeatedly reversing the direction of flow of relatively large volumes of gas provides additional inertial resistance in the system, reduced with the use of smaller-bore hoses. The latter may have a reinforcing coil placed around the outside (in place of the standard corrugated type) permitting a smooth internal surface, with lower resistance to gas flow. Although all tubing is designed to show marked resistance to deformation, this form may kink more easily on extreme flexion (Fig.14.21).

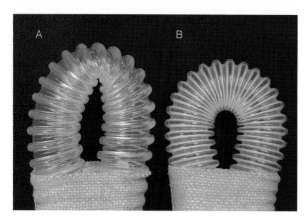

Figure 14.21 Deformation and reduction of tube lumen on extreme flexion. A, coil-over smooth bore tube; B, standard corrugated tube.

Table 14.5	Compression Volume
Definition	Volume lost during positive pressure ventilation due to compression of gas within the system
Features in	All breathing systems
Effects	More significant with large volume systems More significant with small tidal volumes Can be compensated for

Compression volume (Table 14.5) refers to a combination of system distension and internal compression of gas in a breathing system during positive pressure ventilation.

During inspiration, the pressure in the breathing system is raised above the expiratory pressure. This has two effects. Components such as the hoses of the breathing system tend to expand, but more importantly, according to Boyle's law, the gas within the system will reduce in volume. This is more noticeable, the greater the volume of the system. The overall result is that some of the gas intended for the patient remains in the breathing system and a smaller tidal volume is delivered at the patient end than that introduced into the system by the ventilator. The effects of compression volume are seen with all patients when the lungs are ventilated with positive pressure, but its significance is greater for children due to their smaller tidal volume in relation to total system volume.

As an example, consider a circle system of 5000 ml total internal volume. The ventilator adds 500 ml of gas to the system for inspiration, causing a pressure rise of 20 cmH$_2$O in the system. Taking atmospheric pressure to be 1000 cmH$_2$O, this pressure increase represents a fractional rise of 20/1000 cmH$_2$O or 2%. As pressure increases, volume decreases by the same proportion, here 2% of 5000 ml is 100 ml. Of the 500 ml added by the ventilator, 100 ml has been 'lost' to the compression volume, together with a further smaller loss to system compliance, leading to just under 400 ml reaching the patient. In this example, 20% of the inspiratory volume added by the ventilator is lost to compression. Consider a child with a tidal volume of 100 ml. Assuming the same pressure increase occurs on inspiration, the same volume is lost to compression and a total volume of 200 ml would need to be added to the system to achieve a tidal volume of 100 ml. Now, 50% of the inflation volume is lost to compression, thus for smaller patients a proportionately larger volume is added to the system in inspiration to maintain adequate tidal volumes.

Increased airway resistance or reduced lung compliance will increase system pressure in a patient ventilated with controlled volumes. At higher pressures, more volume is lost to compression, and the volume delivered to the patient falls, sometimes termed '*preferentially ventilating the compression volume*'.

A large compression volume results in high system compliance, reducing the 'feel' when hand ventilating. This may be why the 'educated hand' of the anaesthetist is a poor detector of changes in patient compliance and system occlusion.[9]

Systems such as the T-piece have a small internal volume, hence suffer less from the effects of compression volume. If the volume of the T-piece with bag is assumed to be 600 ml, with the same pressure change as above, the compression volume amounts to 2% of 600 ml or 12 ml. Thus, to achieve a patient tidal volume of 100 ml requires an inflation volume of just 112 ml, compared with 200 ml for the circle system previously described. Large volume systems may be used in paediatric practice with allowance for the effects of compression volume.

Ideal airway and breathing equipment for paediatric anaesthesia

For paediatric anaesthesia, equipment is modified to overcome the differences between children and adults. There may, of course, be conflicting demands: for example trying to reduce the internal volume of a breathing system may increase its resistance to gas flow. Equipment must be lightweight yet robust, with universal connectors, easily handled by adults.

Breathing systems for use with very small children should ideally:

- have minimal functional/apparatus dead space;
- be either valveless or fitted with very low resistance valves;
- have small internal gas volumes;
- be constructed in such a way as to minimize gas turbulence and subsequent flow resistance; and
- provide for heating and humidification together with filtration.

However, low flows of fresh gas, in combination with carbon dioxide absorption, will save on volatile agent consumption and pollution.

The materials used to manufacture this equipment should be compatible with human tissue, stable in use and may need to be sufficiently cheap and plentiful to allow single patient use. The considerable environmental impact from disposal of these non-biodegradable items is rarely considered.

Breathing systems in use

Breathing systems, their performance and classification are considered in detail in Chapter 7. For paediatric use, armed with knowledge of the features discussed earlier, it is possible to consider the reasons for and against use of any one breathing system in a particular context, such as varying age and size of child, altered lung compliance and need for spontaneous or controlled ventilation. There is no absolute as to when children become suitable for conventional adult systems. Some authors suggest that at 20–25 kg body weight, i.e. with a tidal volume of around 140 ml, some adult systems function satisfactorily.[38] If ventilation is controlled, adult systems can be used for smaller children than this.[39]

Mapleson A

This system is very efficient for spontaneous ventilation but much less so for controlled ventilation. The expiratory valve adds unwanted resistance to the system, and its position near the patient makes the apparatus dead space large, scavenging difficult and the assembly too cumbersome.

T-piece (Mapleson E and F)

The term 'T-piece' is commonly used to describe the Jackson Rees modification to the original Ayre's device. It is a valveless system with very low resistance, low apparatus dead space and is usually used with an open-ended bag (Jackson Rees' modification) on the expiratory limb (Fig. 14.1). A number of variants of the T-piece itself have been mostly superseded by the single-use disposable system in the form shown. It has a low compression volume and requires relatively high fresh gas flows (see Chapter 7) allowing rapid changes in composition of inspired gas. Classified as a Mapleson E without the bag and an F with it, this system functions in a similar way to the Mapleson D, though it lacks an expiratory valve. The T-piece is intrinsically very simple, lightweight and easy to use with few connections. It can be used for children of all ages for spontaneous ventilation, controlled ventilation and application of continuous positive airways pressure. If the bag is of the open-ended type, partial occlusion of the opening with the little finger against the palm of the hand allows the anaesthetist to carefully monitor and control ventilation with the body of the inflated bag manipulated between thumb and opposing finger(s).

Formulae exist for recommended fresh gas flows, but are for guidance only. For spontaneous ventilation, a fresh gas flow of up to three times predicted minute ventilation is required; for controlled ventilation this may be less, depending on the technique. If the fresh gas flow is used to drive inspiration by intermittent occlusion of the expiratory limb, higher flows are needed to provide adequate inspiratory flow. Manual ventilation with a reservoir bag or automatic ventilation with a ventilator, such as the Penlon Nuffield Series 200, enables use of a lower fresh gas flow. Ultimately, continuous monitoring of end tidal carbon dioxide is required for accurate use. The structure of the system makes it difficult to scavenge waste gas, though modifications exist to allow this.[40] To scavenge from the unmodified T-piece requires some form of collector but vigilance is needed to avoid occlusion of the outlet and subsequent high pressures in the system.

The T-piece is inefficient, requiring high fresh gas flows increasing with patient size. Scavenging is possible but detracts from the system's simplicity. These disadvantages, together with improvements in other systems and patient monitoring, have lead to reduced use of the T-piece in some centres. It remains very popular as a system to use during induction of anaesthesia, for short procedures and as a stand by if problems arise during anaesthesia. Its inherent simplicity and ability to provide both continuous positive airways pressure and 'feel' of airway dynamics are particularly valuable (Table 14.6). Most disposable T-piece systems are provided with a connector allowing them to draw fresh gas from wall or

Table 14.6 Advantages of the T-piece

Simple with few connections.

Low resistance, low dead space.

Rapid changes to inspired gas possible.

No 'wash in' of fresh gas required.

Cheap disposables.

No absorbant to become exhausted

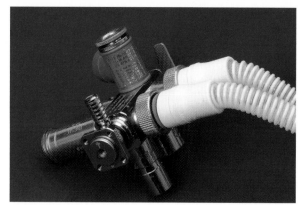

Figure 14.23 Valve block of the Humphrey ADE system.

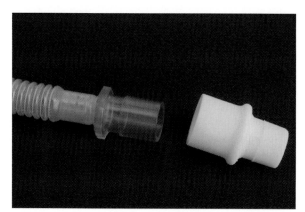

Figure 14.22 A connector (in yellow silastic) allowing the T-piece to be attached to the tapered oxygen fitting of flowmeters used on wall and cylinder supplies.

cylinder oxygen, again useful for emergencies or patient recovery (Fig.14.22).

Mapleson D

The Mapleson D system is similar in function to the T-piece, but possesses a valve at the end of the expiratory limb. This adds some resistance, but enables controlled ventilation and easier scavenging. The coaxial arrangement of the Bain system reduces the weight of tubing and allows better surgical access. Like the T-piece, the Mapleson D is inefficient for spontaneous respiration but more efficient for controlled ventilation.

Humphrey ADE

To maximize the advantages of different systems for different modes of ventilation, single systems have been designed which can perform essentially as a Mapleson A for spontaneous ventilation and a Mapleson D for controlled ventilation. This system was first described in 1983 (Fig. 14.23 and see Fig. 7.13). By employing parallel tubing and a low-resistance exhaust valve sited distant

from the patient, control and monitoring of ventilation, with scavenging, are easily accomplished. A lever at the machine end is used to switch from the spontaneous A mode to controlled ventilation in the D mode, achieved with a ventilator such as the Penlon Nuffield Series 200. For children weighing under 20 kg, breathing spontaneously in the A mode, a fresh gas flow of $3 \, l \, min^{-1}$ prevents rebreathing. In the controlled ventilation mode the system performs like a T-piece, a fresh gas flow of $3 \, l \, min^{-1}$ maintains normocapnia. If the fresh gas flow is adjusted for weight, a lower end tidal carbon dioxide can be achieved.[41] More recently, a carbon dioxide absorber has been incorporated, allowing even lower fresh gas flows.

Circle System

When the sweet smelling, explosive anaesthetic agent cyclopropane was in common use for anaesthesia, a circle system saved both money and lives. In current use, the perceived advantages of this system are a reduction in fresh gas flow, easy scavenging, reduced atmospheric pollution and addition and conservation of some heat and water vapour to inspired gas. Scaled-down circle systems or systems in which gas movement is assisted by some form of circulator are not usually necessary for paediatric use. When changes from adult to paediatric set-up are required, using the same system reduces the chances of assembly errors. However, it is worthwhile changing the breathing hoses from 22 mm to 15 mm diameter, and using smaller distal connectors with minimal dead space.

The circle system has been used successfully, even in infants, usually with assisted or controlled ventilation.[42] Reduction in fresh gas flow is less significant in small children, where all circuits employ a relatively low flow.

Table 14.7 Advantages of the Circle System
Very low fresh gas consumption
Reduces pollution
Warms and humidifies gases

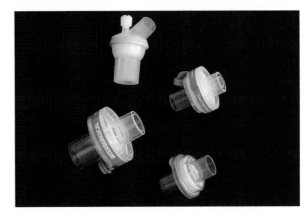

Figure 14.24 A selection of humidifiers and filter/humidifiers for paediatric use.

Additionally, leaks from the system around the tracheal tube or laryngeal mask will limit flow reduction, though in practice this rarely precludes efficient use of the circle system.[24] Gauging and rapidly changing the concentration of oxygen and volatile agent in the system is less easy than with the T-piece, and monitoring of these variables is mandatory. The large compression volume is reduced to some extent by the use of 15 mm tubing, but remains greater for this system.

The circle is a more complicated system than others used in paediatrics. However, used with appropriate monitoring and vigilance, it provides the added benefit of, amongst others (Table 14.7), significant reduction in wastage of anaesthetic agents.[43]

Breathing system humidification and filtration

Humidification of dry inspired gas by the patient is an important source of heat loss. Dry inspiratory gases may also increase tracheal mucosal damage and the incidence of tracheal tube blockage. A range of simple heat and moisture exchangers is now available and in common use by anaesthetists (see Chapter 13). The level of humidification and heat retention necessary to prevent the above problems is unknown. Furthermore, the performance of humidifiers varies significantly between manufacturers and during use.[44]

Anaesthesia circuits may become contaminated with microbes from the patient's respiratory tract; hepatitis C virus transmission has been reported between patients, linked to such contamination. This has lead to interest in the use of combined humidifiers and filters, aiming to prevent microbes entering the breathing system from the patient, whilst conserving heat and humidity (Fig. 14.24). Filters vary in their performance characteristics,[45] and they are not without problems. Even small filters contribute resistance and dead space to the breathing system, and may lead to more serious complications.[46] The dead space of breathing system filters is quoted by the manufacturer. At the time of writing, the smallest filter available has a volume of 10 ml, said to be suitable for tidal volumes as low as 20 ml. The actual contribution

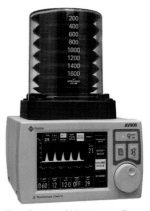

Figure 14.25 The Penlon AV900 ventilator (picture courtesy of Penlon Ltd).

to dead space may be more or less than this, though a worrying increase is seen in some situations.[47]

Ventilators for use during paediatric anaesthesia

Ventilators are described and classified in more detail in Chapter 11.

Ventilators designed specifically for paediatric use should ideally have a low internal volume and resistance, the ability to deliver small tidal volumes and high respiratory rates and a pressure control feature. However, increasing sophistication of control has allowed a number of ventilators with larger internal volumes, e.g. the Penlon AV900 (Fig. 14.25), to be suitable for both paediatric and adult patients and most modern anaesthesia workstation ventilators are currently suitable for use with small children.

This following classification is descriptive of the mode of action:

- Mechanical thumbs;
- Bag squeezers; and
- Hybrid systems (Newton valve)

Mechanical thumbs

Ventilators in this category are used with a T-piece (Mapleson E) system, the expiratory limb of which is intermittently occluded to allow lung inflation by continued fresh gas flow only. This is the mechanical equivalent of the anaesthetist using a thumb to intermittently occlude the expiratory limb. These ventilators are as simple and reliable as an anaesthetist, but only suitable for neonatal and infant use as they require a high fresh gas flow to ensure an adequate inspired volume. In fact, most of these are no longer produced specifically for paediatric anaesthesia. The Penlon Nuffield Series 200 ventilator with the Newton valve attachment is now probably the only type of device capable of this mode of ventilation in common use in the UK.

Bag squeezers

These ventilators incorporate a gas reservoir that takes the place of the bag on the breathing system.

They mimic the anaesthetist manually ventilating the patient via the reservoir bag, hence the name. Bag squeezers enable the use of automatic controlled ventilation with both the T-piece (Mapleson E), Mapleson D system and the circle system. They allow larger tidal volumes to be given whilst using a smaller fresh gas flow, as the latter is augmented with flow from the 'reservoir bag'.

There are two types of 'Bag squeezer'. In one, the reservoir bag of the partial rebreathing or more commonly circle system, is replaced by a 'bag in bottle' (bellows) arrangement that is also part of the ventilator system (see Fig. 11.8). The bellows may be either a standard 'adult' bellows (1500 ml) or it may be substituted for a smaller size (500 ml) so as to reduce the internal gas volume and therefore the compliance within the system. For a similar reason, the standard wide bore (22 mm) breathing hose may be replaced by a smaller bore (15 mm). Reducing the compliance was hitherto given greater priority as it reduced the 'compression volume' within the breathing system allowing more predictable tidal volumes to be delivered (see above and Chapter 11). However, modern ventilators incorporate microprocessor control and feedback monitoring, allowing the compliance to be calculated and adjustments made to restore the tidal volume to that desired.

In paediatric anaesthesia, there is additionally often a leak around the tracheal tube that prevents the accurate determination of tidal volume. Pressure controlled ventilation overcomes many of these problems (Table 14.8). The ventilator delivers gas into the system to rapidly reach the preset pressure and this is maintained until expiration occurs. This compensates for leaks around the tracheal tube, the effects of compression volume and changes in fresh gas flow. It also reduces the risk of barotrauma. Adequate ventilation is ensured by monitoring the end tidal CO_2 and adjusting the inspiratory pressure appropriately. However, pressure ventilation provides no compensation for reduced ventilation following changes in lung compliance or breathing system and airway resistance. Ventilation alarms, dependent on high system airway pressure, are obviously not activated when pressure control is employed, hence monitoring of expired gases at least for composition if not volume is important.

Many ventilators can deliver pressure control ventilation as a preset mode. Other ventilators delivering only volume control ventilation (Table 14.9) can be adapted to pressure control. This is usually achieved by setting a larger tidal volume and higher flow than is desired. The pressure limit control is then set at the desired inspiratory pressure so that flow ceases before the pre-set tidal volume is delivered.

Table 14.8 Advantages of pressure control

Reduced risk of barotrauma

Compensates for changes in fresh gas flow

Compensates for compression volume

Ventilate according to pressure rather than estimated tidal volume

Compensates for leaks

Table 14.9 Advantages of volume control

Set tidal volume delivered

Tidal volume maintained with changes in resistance or compliance

Pressure dependant alarms activated with above changes

In the second type of 'Bag squeezer', the reservoir bag is replaced by a suitable length of breathing hose one end of which is attached to the breathing system (see Fig. 11.8). The other end is connected to a valve that is fed by driving gas delivered from the ventilator. The gas is diverted into the breathing hose and acts as a gas piston mimicking the action of a manually squeezed reservoir bag. As the hosing also acts as the exit pathway for patient gas, its length must be sufficiently long to prevent driving gas entering the breathing system and diluting the anaesthetic gases (see below). The Penlon Nuffield Series 200 ventilator (see Chapter 11) popularized this method and there are now a number of similar ventilators that perform the same function.

Hybrid systems: the Newton valve

This ingenious device can function both as a sophisticated mechanical thumb or a bag squeezer and was designed for the Penlon Nuffield 200 ventilator (Fig. 14.26). The valve is attached to the expiratory limb of a T-piece system. The latter should have a minimum volume of 350 ml to prevent the driving gas from diluting the inspired gas.

In the inspiratory phase, gas from the ventilator enters the body of the valve according to the set parameters for flow and time. From here it can pass two ways, through the 3.5 mm diameter orifice to atmosphere, or into the patient limb of the valve. By altering the flow of gas from the ventilator, the pressure within the valve is controlled. The result of increasing the flow of driving gas is described below:

- At the recommended fresh gas flow rate for the T-piece and at a low inspiratory flow rate from the ventilator, the pressure developed inside the Newton valve is low as a result of the continuous leakage from the fixed orifice outlet. Therefore the valve only partially dams the outlet of the breathing system and so acts as a 'partial thumb occluder'. This transmits a small tidal volume to the patient at a rate depending on, but less than the fresh gas flow into the T-piece.
- As the flow of driving gas from the ventilator increases, at some stage, inflow to the valve will be equal to the leak through the orifice and at this time the valve behaves almost as a complete thumb occluder on the T-piece expiratory limb. The delivered tidal volume equals the fresh gas flow to the T-piece.
- Further increasing flow from the ventilator results in flow into the valve exceeding the leak, and some of the driving gas now passes back along the T-piece

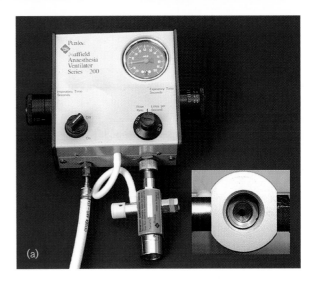

(a)

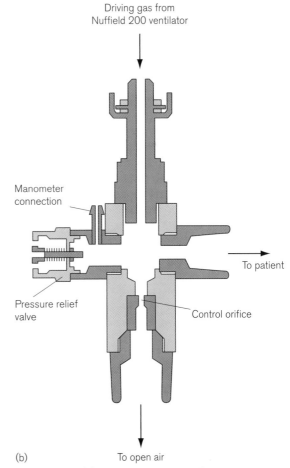

(b)

Figure 14.26 (a) The Penlon Nuffield Series 200 ventilator. Shown inset, the fixed expiratory orifice of the Newton valve. **(b)** Sectional view.

expiratory limb and can act as a gas piston. Tidal volumes will now exceed fresh gas flow and are altered by ventilator settings.

- During the expiratory phase, all gas passes out via the valve orifice, and for expiratory flows up to $15\,l\,min^{-1}$ pressure within the valve should not rise above $5\,cmH_2O$.

Modified with a Newton valve, the Nuffield 200 Series ventilator may be seen as the mechanical equivalent of the anaesthetist's hand in combination with the open-ended bag on a T-piece. The system is easy to understand, can switch rapidly from manual to automatic ventilation and permits scavenging of waste gas. It can deliver tidal volumes between 10 and 300 ml at frequencies from 10 to 85/min, making this a suitable ventilator for neonates and infants. The system requires high fresh gas flows and consumes large amounts of pressurized gas to drive the ventilator. The Newton valve is not suitable for patients over 20 kg.

Access to the circulatory system

Obtaining and maintaining secure venous access in small patients can be very challenging. As with adults, there are essentially two means to achieve this, the cannula over needle or wire through needle (Seldinger) techniques. Use of rigid indwelling needles alone is not recommended, as they tend to cut out of the vein resulting in extravasation. Much smaller cannulae are required for both peripheral and central access. Flow rates through narrow-bore cannulae are low (Table 14.10). In an emergency it may be impossible to cannulate a vein. Below the age of six year an intraosseous needle (Fig. 14.27) provides alternative access to the circulatory system for administration of drugs and fluid until venous cannulation is achieved. All contaminated sharps must be disposed of safely, and some cannulae incorporate a retraction device to ensure the needle end is covered after the vein is entered (Fig. 14.28). Cannulation of central veins, particularly the internal jugular vein, has traditionally been undertaken using surface landmarks as a guide. Ultrasound has been suggested to improve the success and safety compared to landmark techniques.[49] Two-dimensional ultrasound has not been adequately investigated in children, and the results with acoustic tipped needles in infants were inconclusive.[50] Where long-term venous access is required, peripherally inserted lines may be easier to site and can be threaded into central veins if necessary.

Positioning, environmental control and temperature monitoring

Great care is required with positioning during anaesthesia, including eye protection and protection of vulnerable peripheral nerves, etc. Padding under the shoulders of the supine infant prevents the large occiput from putting the head into flexion. Depending on the site of surgery, a bar or bridge placed over the patient prevents the surgeon from inadvertently leaning on the chest or face and allows

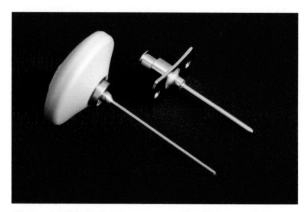

Figure 14.27 An intraosseus needle. On some designs the metal cannula has an outer screw thread for fixation into the cortical bone.

Table 14.10 Flow rates (ml min⁻¹) through intravenous cannulae			
Catheter Size (swg)	**Crystalloid (gravity)**	**Crystalloid (pressure)**	**Blood (pressure)**
24-gauge	14–15	42–47	20–30
22-gauge	24–26	65–77	44–50
20-gauge	38–42	103–126	69–81
18-gauge	55–62	164–214	150–164

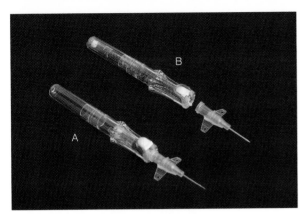

Figure 14.28 A sharp safe needle, The Insyte–N Autoguard. A, the cannula and needle prior to insertion; B, following successful venepuncture, the needle is retracted into the clear hub.

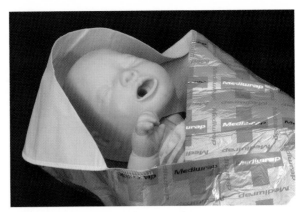

Figure 14.29 Foil wrap (Mediwrap).

improved access for the anaesthetist to monitor the patient, check line sites, etc. When a limb tourniquet is used, they must be of adequate width and exceed limb circumference by 7–15 cm. Padding is needed, particularly at the edges, and the tourniquet can be inflated to a lower pressure than that for adults. Skin preparing fluids must not soak under the tourniquet, as children's thinner skin is easily damaged.[51]

All patients can loose heat during anaesthesia, the thermoneutral temperature zone (about 28°C in an unclothed adult) being higher in neonates. Small children have limited thermogenesis, so heat loss may be difficult to recoup.[52] Depending on the operation and exposure, heat is lost through a combination of radiation, convection, conduction and evaporation of bodily fluids and can be prevented by a number of measures:

- Maintain the operating theatre at a higher temperature and humidity; this is rarely within the limits of staff comfort.
- Reduce evaporative loss by limiting exposure of wet areas at the operative site and humidifying inspired gas.
- Reduce radiation loss with foil blankets, correctly applied these reduce convective loss too (Fig. 14.29).
- Active warming, most commonly in the form of forced air warming, is a more effective way of maintaining temperature.[53] A warm air microclimate can be created around the child by use of forced warmed air, in combination with impervious clear plastic covers adapted for surgical access (Fig. 14.30).

Whatever methods are chosen, reliable monitoring is required as overheating of small children is easily

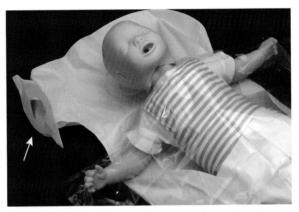

Figure 14.30 A child manikin lies still atop a forced air warming mattress (Bair Hugger). Clear plastic drapes help to create a warm microclimate. The hole at the top of the mattress (arrowed) connects to the warm air source.

achieved. Oesophageal, rectal, axillary and tympanic membrane temperatures all correlate well to central temperature.[19] For operations where a urinary catheter is needed, this can incorporate a temperature probe at the tip, providing an excellent means of monitoring.

Transfer of the critically ill child

An increasing trend for transferring critically ill children to centralized paediatric intensive care units requires safe and rapid transfer conditions, usually provided by a retrieval team from the accepting unit. Resuscitation is initiated at the referring unit, often under the guidance of the retrieval service. A challenge for practitioners with little exposure to sick children is to judge appropriate tube sizes, etc. This is made easier by some form of universal measuring device together with prepared packs of equipment[54] such as The Broselow Tape and The Broselow Paediatric ALS Organizer.

Transfer brings risks from moving a potentially unstable patient into an environment compromised by motion, cold, poor light, noise and limited electric power. Ideal equipment for this is lightweight, robust, compact and has a reliable power supply. All equipment can fail and manual backup, such as self-inflating bags, is vital. Transfer equipment is kept together in a series of clearly identified portable packs (Fig. 14.31), all batteries are continuously charged and packs are replenished and checked for immediate reuse after a transfer. Equipment requirements vary according to the size of child and the nature of the illness, but it is likely that ventilation and sedation will be needed together with inotrope infusions and intravenous fluids.

Portable ventilators (Fig. 14.32) need to be capable of delivering air/oxygen mixes, creating positive end expiratory pressure, displaying airway pressures, detecting and alarming for disconnections and must have adjustable tidal volumes for a range of patient sizes. They are usually driven from a high-pressure oxygen source and have high gas consumption (20 l min^{-1} for the example shown). Tubes and lines need to be secured sufficiently well to survive multiple transfers and movement. Temperature control can be difficult, rigorous use of foil helps, and highly insulating material such as 'bubble wrap' provides excellent thermal insulation. Single use heated mattresses are available for infants, heated by initiating a chemical reaction of the contents. Compact single module monitoring is available and even blood biochemistry and gases can be monitored with a portable machine (Fig. 14.33).

Monitoring

Adult monitoring equipment is usually simple to adapt for children. Old-style monitoring, such as the oesophageal stethoscope, is still valuable and almost free of technical complications. More ambitious surgery with large volume blood loss requires invasive monitoring of cardiovascular parameters. Arterial and central venous cannulation are useful, and means now exist for less invasive monitoring of cardiac output, e.g. by arterial waveform analysis following calibration by a dilution technique (see Chapter 18). In neonates, blood gases are monitored with transcutaneous sensors. This is less effective for older children, but fluorescent optical sensors sited on a catheter within a blood vessel can provide continuous readings of blood gases without the need for repeated sampling.[19] Mandatory modern monitoring has not been shown to improve the outcome from anaesthesia, but it does provide early warning of problems to the alert anaesthetist. Full monitoring of the awake child may be tricky, but once asleep it should be a formality.

FINALLY

In-depth knowledge of paediatric anaesthesia and the requisite equipment is fulfilling and vital. It will go unnoticed by your patients, whose admiration is saved for those *au fait* with the more complex fields of the latest children's toys, animals real, stuffed and extinct, and apparently banal television programmes.

ACKNOWLEDGEMENTS

The author would like to acknowledge the following people for their help: Mr Robin Baker BSc MIMI, Medical photographer, QVH; Mr John Cockerill, Chief Medical Technical officer, Paediatric Intensive Care Unit, Guys and St Thomas' NHS Trust; Mr Cedric A Russell FIM MRSC, Clinical Research Manager, Smiths Medical International Ltd, Hythe, Kent, UK.

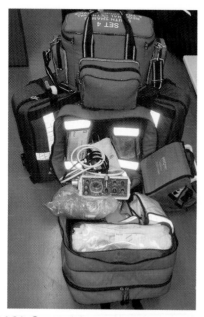

Figure 14.31 Some of the equipment needs for a paediatric transfer.

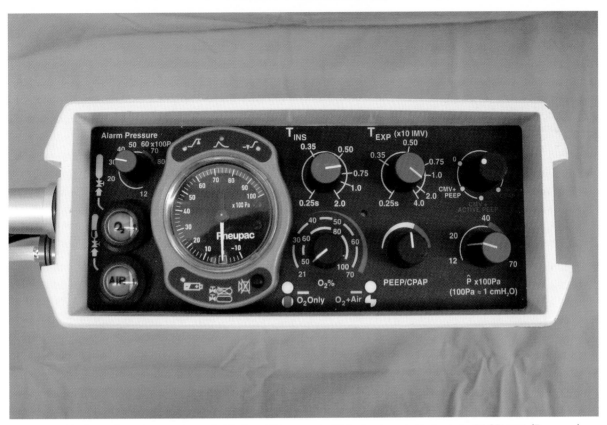

Figure 14.32 A ventilator for transfer, suitable for children up to 20 kg body weight: the babyPAC™ 100 (Pneupac).

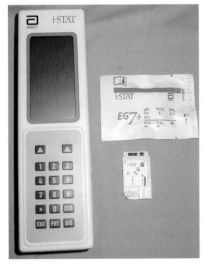

Figure 14.33 The iSTAT™, a portable blood analyser shown with single use cartridges.

REFERENCES

1. Ayre P (1937) Endotracheal anaesthesia for babies; with special reference to hare-lip and cleft palate operations. *Current Research in Anesthesiology* **16**: 330.

2. Hodges SC, Hodges AM (2000) A protocol for safe anaesthesia for cleft lip and palate surgery in developing countries. *Anaesthesia* **55**: 436–441.

3. Birks RJS (2001) Safety matters [editorial]. *Anaesthesia* **56**: 823–824.

4. Cook TM (2003) Novel Airway Devices: Spoilt for Choice? [editorial]. *Anaesthesia* **58**: 107–110.

5. Bridgland IA (2001) Monitoring Medical Devices: the need for new evaluation methodology [editorial]. *British Journal of Anaesthesia* **87(5)**: 678–680.

6. Grant LJ (1998) Regulations and safety in medical equipment design [editorial]. *Anaesthesia* **53(1)**: 1–3

7. Brain AI (1995) An evaluation of the laryngeal mask airway during routine paediatric anaesthesia [letter]. *Paediatric Anaesthesia* **5**: 75.

8. Rendell-Baker L, Soucek DH (1962) New pediatric facemasks and anesthetic equipment. *British Medical Journal* I: 1690.

9. Fisher DM (1989) 'Anesthesia Equipment for Pediatrics'. In: Gregory GA (ed.) *Pediatric Anesthesia*. New York: Churchill Livingstone. pp. 437–475.

10. Hatch DJ (1978) Tracheal tubes and connectors used in neonates-dimensions and resistance to breathing. *British Journal of Anaesthesia* **50**: 959–965.

11. James I (2001) Cuffed tubes in children. *Paediatrics in Anaesthesia* **11**: 259–263.

12. Reali-Forster C, Kolobow T, Giacomini M, *et al.* (1996) New ultrathin walled endotracheal tube with a novel laryngeal seal design. *Anesthesiology* **84**: 162–172.

13. Khalil SN, Mankarious R, Campos C, *et al.* (1998) Absence or presence of a leak around tracheal tube may not affect postoperative croup in children. *Paediatric Anaesthesia* **8(5)**: 393–396.

14. Allt JE, Howell CJ (2003) Down's Syndrome. *British Journal of Anaesthesia. CEPD Reviews* **3(3)**:83–86.

15. Gupta K, Harry R (1997) Cutting paediatric tubes – a potential cause of morbidity [letter]. *British Journal of Anaesthesia* **78(5)**: 627.

16. Mackway-Jones K, Molyneux E, Phillips B, Wieteska S (2001) *Advanced Paediatric Life Support*. 3rd edn. London: BMJ Books.

17. McGinn G, Haynes SR, Norton NS (1993) An evaluation of the laryngeal mask airway during routine paediatric anaesthesia. *Paediatric Anaesthesia* **3**:23–28.

18. Gursoy F, Algren JT, Skonsby BS (1996) Positive pressure ventilation with the laryngeal mask airway in children. *Anesthesia and Analgesia* **82(1)**: 33–38.

19. Booker PD (1999) Equipment and monitoring in paediatric anaesthesia. *British Journal of Anaesthesia* **82(0)**: 78–90.

20. Beveridge ME (1989) Laryngeal mask anaesthesia for repair of cleft palate. *Anaesthesia* **44**: 656–657.

21. Stocks RM, Egerman R, Thompson J, *et al.* (2002) Airway management of the severely retrognathic child: use of the laryngeal mask airway. *Ear Nose and Throat Journal* **81(4)**: 223–226.

22. Auden SM, Lerner GM (2000) Blind intubation via the laryngeal mask: a word of caution [letter]. *Paediatric Anaesthesia* **10(4)**: 452.

23. Bagshaw O (2002) The size 1.5 laryngeal mask airway (LMA) in paediatric anaesthetic practice. *Paediatric Anaesthesia* **12(5)**: 420–423.

24. Frohlich D, Schwall B, Funk W, *et al.* (1997) Laryngeal mask airway and uncuffed tracheal tubes are equally effective for low flow or closed system anaesthesia in children. *British Journal of Anaesthesia* **79**: 289–292.

25. Keidan I, Berkenstadt H, Segal E, *et al.* (2001) Pressure versus volume-controlled ventilation with the laryngeal mask airway in paediatric patients. *Paediatric Anaesthesia* **11(6)**: 691–694.

26. Ozlu O, Turker AK, Ozgun G, *et al.* (2001) Distal oesophageal pH measurement in children during general anaesthesia using the laryngeal mask airway, tracheal tube and face mask. *Paediatric Aneasthesia* **11(4)**: 425–430.

27. Baraka A, Choueiry P, Medawar A (1995) The laryngeal mask airway for fibreoptic bronchoscopy in children. *Paediatric Anaesthesia* **5(3)**: 197–198.

28. Sacks MD, Marsh D (2000) Bilateral recurrent laryngeal nerve neuropraxia following laryngeal mask insertion: a rare cause of serious upper airway morbidity. *Paediatric Anaesthesia* **10(4)**: 435–437.

29. Levy RJ, Helfaer MA (2000) Pediatric airway issues. *Critical Care Clinics* **16(3)**: 489–504.

30. Thomas PB, Parry MG (2001) The difficult paediatric airway: a new method of intubation using the laryngeal mask airway, Cook airway exchange catheter and tracheal intubation fibrescope. *Paediatric Anaesthesia* **11(5)**: 618–621.

31. Hasan MA, Black AE (1994) A new technique for fibreoptic intubation in children. *Anaesthesia* **49**: 1031–1033.

32. Ellis DS, Potluri PK, O'Flaherty JE, *et al.* (1999) Difficult airway management in the neonate: a simple method of intubating through a laryngeal mask airway. *Paediatric Anaesthesia* **9**: 460–462.

33. Wrigley SR, Black AE, Sidhu VS (1995) A fibreoptic laryngoscope for paediatric anaesthesia. *Anaesthesia* **50(8)**: 709–712.

34. Liem EB, Bjoraker DG, Gravenstein D (2003) New options for airway management: intubating fibreoptic stylets. *British Journal of Anaesthesia* **91(3)**: 408–418.

35. Ravishankar M, Kundra P, Agrawal K, *et al.* (2001)Rigid nasendoscope with video camera system for intubation in infants with Pierre Robin Sequence. British Journal of Anaesthesia **87(5)**: 728–731.

36. Depierraz B, Ravussin P, Brossard E, *et al.* (1994) Percutaneous transtracheal jet ventilation for paediatric endoscopic laser treatment of laryngeal and subglottic lesions. *Canadian Journal of Anaesthesia* **41(12)**: 1200–1207.

37. Seefelder C, Kenna MA (2000) Don't rely on the surgical airway: a case of impossible tracheostomy [letter]. *Paediatric Anaesthesia* **10(2)**: 224.

38. Hatch DJ (1985) Paediatric anaesthetic equipment. *British Journal of Anaesthesia* **57**: 672–684.

39. Brown TCK, Fisk GC (1992) *Anesthesia for children*. 2nd edn. Oxford: Blackwell Scientific Publications. pp. 53–76.

40. Dhara SS, Pua HL (2000) A non-occluding bag and closed scavenging system for the Jackson Rees modified T-piece breathing system. *Anaesthesia* **5(5)**: 450–454.

41. Orlikowski CE, Ewart MC, Bingham RM (1991) The Humphrey ADE system: evaluation in paediatric use. *British Journal of Anaesthesia* **66**: 253–257.

42. Rasch DK, Bunegin L, Ledbetter J, *et al.* (1988) Comparison of circle absorber and Jackson Rees systems for paediatric anaesthesia. *Canadian Journal of Anaesthesia* **35(1)**: 25–30.

43. Meakin GH (1999) Low-flow anaesthesia in infants and children. *British Journal of Anaesthesia* **83(1)**: 50–57.

44. Brock-Utne JG (2000) Humidification in paediatric anaesthesia [editorial]. *Paediatric Anaesthesia* **10(2)**: 117–119.

45. The Medicine and Healthcare Products Regulatory Agency. Breathing system filters: an assessment of 104 breathing system filters. *www.mhra.gov*. March 2004.

46. Lawes EG (2003) Hidden hazards and dangers associated with the use of HME/filters in breathing circuits. Their effect on toxic metabolite production, pulse oximetry and airway resistance. *British Journal of Anaesthesia* **91(2)**: 249–264.

47. Miller DM, Adams AP, Light D (2004) Dead space and paediatric anaesthetic equipment: a physical lung model study. *Anaesthesia* **59**: 600–606

48. Newton NI, Hillman KM, Varley JG (1981) Automatic ventilation with the Ayre's T-piece. *Anaesthesia* **36**: 22–36.

49. National Institute for Clinical Excellence (2002) *Guidance on the use of ultrasound locating devices for placing central venous catheters*. London: NICE.

50. Macintyre PA, Samra G, Hatch DJ (2000) Preliminary experience with the Doppler ultrasound guided vascular access needle in paediatric patients. *Paediatric Anaesthesia* **10(4)**: 361–365.

51. Kam PCA, Kavanaugh R, Yoong FFY (2002) The arterial tourniquet: pathophysiological consequences and anaesthetic implications (review article). *Anaesthesia* **56**: 534–545.

52. Crossley AWA, Holdcroft A (1999) 'Physiology of heat balance'. In: Jones RM (ed.) Royal College of Anaesthetists newsletter **47**: 155–158.

53. Giesbrecht GG, Ducharme MB, McGuire JP (1994) Comparison of forced-air patient warming systems for perioperative use. *Anesthesiology* **80(3)**: 671–678.

54. Cole R (1995) When every second counts. *Child Health* **3(2)**: 63–67.

FURTHER READING

Hatch D, Fletcher M (1992) Anaesthesia and the ventilatory system in infants and young children. *British Journal of Anaesthesia* **68**: 398–410.

Steven J M, Cohen D E, Sclabassi R J (1996) 'Anesthesia Equipment and Monitoring'. In: Motoyama EK, Davis PJ (eds) *Smith's Anesthesia for Infants and Children*, 6th edn. New York: Mosby. pp. 229–279

Walker I, Lockie J (1999) 'Basic techniques for anaesthesia'. In: Sumner E, Hatch DJ (eds). *Paediatric Anaesthesia* 2nd edn. London: Arnoldpp.165–210.

Equipment for local anaesthesia

Matthew R Checketts and J A W Wildsmith

Local anaesthetic drugs may be administered to a patient at any point along the pain pathway. However, the techniques and equipment required for placing the drugs to achieve the desired nerve blockade, depend on the anatomy of the area targeted. The latter can be used to classify the different types of block, namely:

- Neuraxial (spinal and epidural) Block;
- Major Nerve (brachial and lumbo-sacral and sciatic/femoral) Block;
- Minor Nerve (those of the head, neck, trunk and the limbs distal to the elbow and knee joints) Block;
- Field (circumferential infiltration of the surgical field) Block;
- Local Infiltration (direct injection into the tissues to be anaesthetized); and
- Topical (directly onto the skin or mucus membrane).

It is possible to perform many of these techniques, certainly the more peripheral, with hypodermic equipment, but there are good reasons for using specific needle and catheter systems whenever possible. Most equipment issues can be considered under the headings of neuraxial and major nerve block.

GENERAL CONSIDERATIONS

Needle design

Length

Most needles used in regional techniques are of a length suitable for their intended purpose, but longer devices may be required in the obese patient. For some blocks (e.g. caudal), it is traditional to use a needle with a bead on the shaft to prevent insertion to the hub because of the risk of breakage, although this is unlikely with modern equipment.

Diameter

Needle diameters are usually quoted in terms of standard wire gauge (swg), but Table 15.1 shows the metric equivalents of some of the commonly-used sizes. Standard notation is that the size is defined by the external diameter of the needle shaft, there being little or no standardization of internal diameters.

The diameter of needle required for a particular purpose will depend on two main factors:

Table 15.1 A comparison of standard wire gauge sizes with metric equivalent

27 G	26 G	25 G	23 G	22 G	21 G	19 G	18 G	16 G
0.36 mm	0.4 mm	0.45 mm	0.57 mm	0.64 mm	0.7 mm	0.9 mm	1.0 mm	1.3 mm

1. *The viscosity of fluid that is to be injected.* Local anaesthetics are usually prepared in aqueous solutions, which will pass through very small diameter needles, but needles which are too small may limit the speed at which other fluids (e.g. CSF or blood) can be aspirated. The latter may be required for confirmation of correct placement or for the early recognition of a potential complication. Oil-based agents (for neurolytic blocks) will only pass easily through the larger diameter needles (at least 18 swg).

2. *The rigidity required for its insertion.* The longer the needle the more flexible it becomes, making it more prone to deflection, bending, buckling or even breakage. Thus, epidural needles are usually of 16 swg or 18 swg size to minimize these risks. Spinal needles need to be even longer, but large diameter needles make post-dural puncture headache (PDPH) more likely and so finer needles are used and inserted through an introducer.

Bevel shape

Needles for neuraxial block require specialized bevels (Fig. 15.1a), but hypodermic needles, which have very long sharp bevels that cut tissue (Fig. 15.1b), are best avoided for peripheral nerve block. Because the latter advance easily through structures, subtle differences in the properties of tissues may not be appreciated. Therefore, in comparison to short bevelled needles, it becomes more difficult to identify tissue planes.

A shorter bevel is usually preferred, although there is some controversy surrounding the comparative risk of direct nerve damage with these two types of bevel. Theoretically, a short bevelled needle can touch a nerve eliciting parasthesia with less risk of nerve injury.[3] In general, it appears that long, flat bevels are more likely to cause nerve trauma,[1] but that the trauma will be more serious if a short bevel needle does make vigorous contact with a nerve.[2]

Hubs

All needles should have a standard Luer taper and lock to ensure that syringes and catheters fit tightly to prevent leakage during injection. Ideally, the hub should be made of clear plastic to aid identification of blood or CSF.

Catheters

Most catheters for continuous regional block are placed by insertion through a needle, but there are some catheter 'over' needle systems available. Whichever type is employed, the manufacturer's instructions must be followed to the letter to avoid shearing or breakage, which could result in a portion of catheter being left in the patient. It is wise to use only dedicated needle and catheter systems to avoid issues of incompatibility. The catheters must be made of inert material that will not produce any tissue reaction and have markings at intervals appropriate for the particular application, such that the length left within the patient can be readily identified. Most catheters have a single terminal opening, but other patterns are considered below under Epidural Block. The proximal end of the catheter should fit a Luer connector, ideally detachable, allowing the needle to be removed after the catheter has been inserted.

Filters

Filters should be used for continuous block techniques to exclude bacteria and other microscopic debris as small as 0.22 μm.

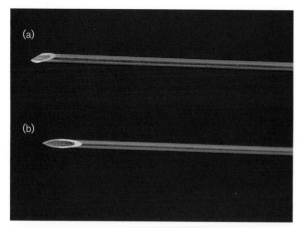

Figure 15.1 (a) Short bevelled needle for nerve block; **(b)** a typical hypodermic (cutting) needle.

Asepsis and disposability

Today, with the number of manufacturers providing high-quality single-use equipment for regional anaesthesia, there is little reason in modern economies for using anything but sterile, disposable products. If, for some reason, a re-usable needle is to be employed, it is essential that the interior is cleaned out thoroughly before sterilization, and that the needle and stilette are sterilized and disassembled.

Block packs

An aseptic technique is important in any regional anaesthetic procedure, but absolutely vital for neuraxial block and those involving the placement of an indwelling catheter. A number of items of equipment are required and matters are much facilitated by the use of purpose-made packs containing all the necessary items for that block, including perhaps, even the drugs. Such packs have economic advantages and involve less delay at the preparation stage compared to adding individually wrapped items to a sterile field. Such a pack should contain:

- a base of sufficient area to provide an aseptic field large enough for preparing the other items;
- sponges, swabs, disinfectant containers, etc for skin preparation and a drape to cover the area around the injection site with a central opening adequate for access to the patient;
- the hypodermic syringes and needles necessary for skin infiltration and preparation of the local anaes-thetic, including filter needles if glass ampoules are to be used; and

Some packs may contain the needle/catheter systems to be used for the block itself, but in many centres these are added to a basic preparation pack to minimize supply and storage problems. A number of manufacturers produce suitable packs, and many hospital sterile supply departments are happy to provide them. The choice is a matter for individual and departmental choice, with cost being an important factor.

Checking the equipment

It is essential to ensure that all the correct items are available before starting any procedure. Modern sterile disposable products are virtually 100% reliable; however, in an epidural kit for example, it may be prudent to check that:

- the syringe plunger moves freely in the barrel, and fits tightly the hubs of both needle and catheter;
- the tip of the stilette is flush with the bevel of the needle;

- the catheter passes easily through the needle; and
- the catheter and filter are patent. This is confirmed by injecting fluid through both.

EQUIPMENT FOR SPINAL ANAESTHESIA

The consequences of failure of aseptic technique are greater in spinal anaesthesia than any other block method and this should always be borne in mind.

Spinal needles

Diameter

The main consideration in the design of a spinal needle is the need to minimize the risk of post-dural puncture headache (PDPH), the incidence of which is lower with smaller diameter needles. Extremely fine 29 swg needles are produced but such needles are prone to bending on insertion, and identifying the back-flow of CSF can be extremely difficult. Such problems may be avoided by using needles of at least 22 swg diameter, but the inci-dence of headache with these is unacceptable, particularly in the obstetric population. Currently, most practitioners use a needle of around 24–25 swg as a reasonable compromise between these two extremes. The risk of bending can be minimized by using an introducer needle.

Bevel/tip shapes

The traditional lumbar puncture needle (e.g. Quincke) has a bevel with a sharp cutting edge (Fig. 15.2a), not unlike that of a hypodermic needle. Of more recent avail-ability are needles which end in a point that stretches and separates the tissues when it is advanced, so causing less trauma. Such needle tips are associated with a significantly lower incidence of PDPH than the older style. The two common versions of this tip are the pencil point (Whitacre; Fig. 15.2b) and the bullet shaped (Sprotte; Fig. 15.2c). In each case, the needle tip is solid with a side port cut into the lumen of the needle as close as possible to the tip.

Length

Most spinal needles are 10cm in length, but shorter (5cm for children) and longer (15cm for obese patients and for combined spinal/epidural anaesthesia, see below) are available.

Stilette

All needles for spinal anaesthesia must have a stilette, which should be in place whenever the needle is advanced. This is to prevent 'coring' of superficial tissues,

(a)

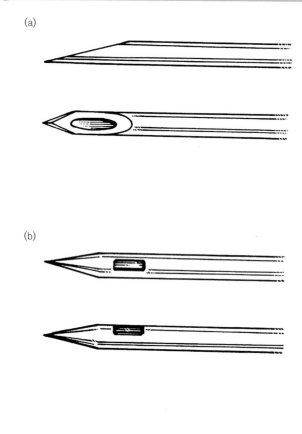

(b)

(c)

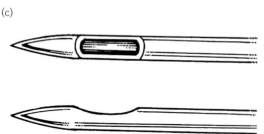

Figure 15.2 **(a)** Quinke tip spinal needle. Note the bevels giving it a sharp cutting tip. **(b)** Whitacre spinal needle. Note that the tip is shaped like a pencil point. **(c)** Sprotte spinal needle; the tip is bullet shaped and the side opening is larger than (b). (With permission from Wildsmith JAW, Armitage EN, McClure J (2002) *Principles and Practice of Regional Anaesthesia*, 3rd edn. Edinburgh: Churchill Livingstone

particularly skin, which could then be deposited in the CSF and develop into a cyst.

Practical problems

- The need for compromise in the diameter of a spinal needle was referred to above. Bending and breaking are ever present risks, even when an introducer needle is used, especially if there is contact with bone. The shape of modern needles may reduce the risk of PDPH, but the side port is a point of weakness, particularly the larger opening of the Sprotte pattern. Spinal needles should always be advanced with the minimum necessary force, and discarded if there is any suggestion of bending.

- Also the opening of a side port needle may straddle the dura mater such that CSF can be aspirated, but injected local anaesthetic may be deposited into the epidural, rather than sub-arachnoid space. Thus, it is particularly important to make sure that the opening is fully within the CSF. There is some concern however that this may increase the risk of traumatic contact with a nerve root because a greater length of needle must enter the sub-arachnoid space than with a Quincke needle.

Continuous spinal anaesthesia

It has always been possible to use the smaller catheter systems produced for epidural block for continuous spinal anaesthesia, but concerns about PDPH have limited use of the technique. In the 1980s, interest was rekindled by developments in plastics technology allowing the production of catheters in the range 28–32 swg, capable of being passed through a 22 swg spinal needle. Such a system allows both the extent and duration of a spinal anaesthetic to be titrated precisely, but the utility of such systems is limited by the difficulties in ensuring that such a fine catheter is correctly placed. In the past, a small number of patients have developed the cauda equina syndrome following continuous spinal anaesthesia. Although initially ascribed to the use of the indwelling microspinal catheters themselves, it now seems likely that the true cause was the repeated exposure of nerve roots to very high concentrations of local anaesthetic. Needle/catheter systems for continuous spinal anaesthesia are still available, but they are very much the preserve of the experienced practitioner. Most anaesthetists find that combined spinal/epidural techniques (see below) provide most of the benefits without the same concerns regarding catheter position.

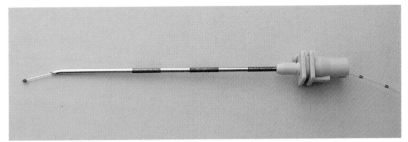

Figure 15.3 A Tuohy needle with a Huber tip and an epidural catheter emerging at an angle of 20 degrees to the shaft.

EQUIPMENT FOR EPIDURAL ANAESTHESIA

Epidural needles

Diameter

The external diameter of an epidural needle is a compromise between three factors. Firstly, the internal diameter should be sufficiently large, so as to allow a suitable size of catheter to be passed through it. Secondly, the external diameter should be as small as possible to provide ease of insertion, and thirdly, the thickness of its wall and the tensile strength of the material used should provide sufficient rigidity so as not to buckle or bend in use. Systems with 16–18swg needles are used in adults and there is a 19swg version available for children.

Bevel/tip shapes

The Tuohy needle is the one most commonly used. It has a Huber tip (Fig. 15.3 and see Fig. 15.6), causing the catheter to exit at an angle of about 20 degrees to the shaft, thus facilitating its entry into the epidural space. The Crawford needle has a short, conventional bevel and the catheter will emerge without any deflection in the axis of the needle and is likely to impinge directly on the dura, unless the epidural space has been reached more obliquely using the paramedian approach.

The tip of an epidural needle should be blunt, not sharp, to allow more ready identification of the changes in density as the needle passes through various inter-vertebral ligaments on its path to the epidural space. A blunt needle is also more likely to push away, rather than cut into, pliant tissue such as the dura mater.

Length

Standard epidural needles are approximately 10.5 cm in length (8 cm shaft and 2.5 cm hub), but shorter (5 cm for children) and longer (15 cm for obese patients) needles are available. The needle shaft should have 1 cm (0.5 cm in the paediatric version) markings on the shaft to help the anaesthetist gauge the depth of insertion.

Stilette

Epidural needles should be advanced through skin and subcutaneous tissue, with the close-fitting stilette in place, to prevent tissue blocking the lumen.

Loss of resistance devices

Historically, a number of devices for identifying the entry of the needle tip into the epidural space have been used. They have relied mostly on the (false) assumption that there is a negative pressure within the epidural space. It is now recognized that this negative pressure is in fact caused by 'tenting' of the dura by the tip of the needle. As a result, the *loss of resistance to injection* method of identifying entry into the epidural space is used almost universally. Once the needle tip is firmly embedded in the inter-vertebral ligaments, the stilette is withdrawn and a special low-resistance syringe (although some use an ordinary disposable one), filled with either air or saline, is attached to the hub. Further advancement of the needle is accompanied by constant pressure on the plunger so that, when the needle tip moves from the dense ligamentum flavum into the loose connective tissue of the epidural space, injection becomes significantly easier (the 'loss of resistance'). Detachable 'wings' may be used to advance the needle.

Catheters

Once the needle tip is in the epidural space, the catheter is fed through it, standardized (BS 6196) markings allowing precise identification of how much catheter lies within the space (Fig. 15.4). These markings are:

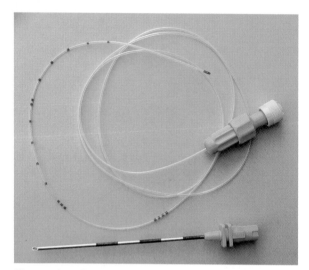

Figure 15.4 An epidural catheter. Note the markings as described in the text.

- a single marking at the tip;
- five single markings 1 cm apart from 5–9 cm;
- a double marking at 10 cm;
- four single markings from 11–14 cm;
- a triple marking at 15 cm; and
- a quadruple marking at 20 cm.

Two types of catheter tip are available. The standard catheter has a single end opening, but this may impinge on tissues and increase the resistance to injection. The alternative is to use a catheter with three 'side' holes situated in the first 2.5 cm of catheter. A minimum of 3 cm should be inserted to ensure that all the exit holes lie within the epidural space.

Displacement of a catheter is always a possibility, no matter how it is fixed to the patient's back. Some manufacturers supply special devices to aid fixation at the skin puncture point, these being shaped to reduce the risks of both displacement and kinking. It is standard practice in the UK to attach a bacterial filter at the hub end of the catheter.

COMBINED SPINAL/EPIDURAL TECHNIQUES

To obtain the benefit of the rapid onset of spinal anaesthesia, with the flexibility of a catheter technique, but without the technical problems associated with spinal catheters (see above), combined spinal/epidural techniques have become very popular, particularly in

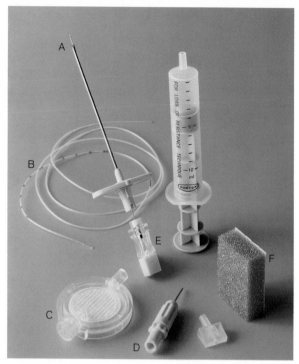

Figure 15.5 A combined Portex spinal/epidural kit. A, a 16 gauge 10.5 cm Tuohy needle with a Huber point, wings and 1 cm markings on the shaft. Inserted into the needle (for demonstration purposes) is a longer than usual 26 gauge spinal needle (11.7 cm); B, a 19 gauge epidural catheter with multiple side holes and markings; C, a bacterial/viral filter with luer locks at both ends; D, a connector that fits on one end of the catheter so that it can be connected to the filter; E, spinal needle; F, fixing (anti-kinking) sponge for the catheter.

obstetric anaesthesia. While separate punctures at separate inter-spaces may be used, the most commonly used technique involves insertion of a standard epidural needle, then the passage of a specially lengthened spinal needle (Fig. 15.5), followed by the insertion of the epidural catheter after the spinal anaesthetic has been injected. Tuohy needles should be used for this technique because the displacement of the catheter from its Huber tip will minimize the risk of the epidural catheter impinging on the puncture hole in the dura mater and entering the subarachnoid space.

EQUIPMENT FOR PERIPHERAL NERVE BLOCKS

These techniques are enjoying a renaissance in modern anaesthetic practice, partly because of the improvement in the quality of the equipment that is now commercially available. There has been a proliferation in the number of manufacturers producing needles and catheter systems for single shot and continuous peripheral major nerve block.

The equipment available for major nerve block can be broken down into:

- needles;
- catheter systems;
- nerve stimulators; and
- miscellaneous items, such as ultrasound machines.

Needles

A large number of peripheral block needles are currently available. There are a number of factors to consider when selecting a needle.

Bevel/tip design

The three major types of needle tip design are the faceted short bevelled type, the Tuohy with a Huber tip, and the Sprotte.

Faceted short bevelled needles

Traditionally, faceted short bevelled needles are used for reasons of increased safety. As discussed before, the short bevelled needle allows the user to 'feel' fascial planes more easily when performing a block. This is often important, for example, for ilioinguinal, cervical plexus or fascia iliaca blocks. A good example of a needle tip for these types of blocks can be seen in Figure 15.1a.

Tuohy with a Huber Tip

These needles mimic the design of a conventional epidural needle with a curved tip (Fig. 15.6). This design is useful when inserting peripheral nerve catheters through the needle, particularly when the nerve is approached at right-angles to its long axis, for example in posterior

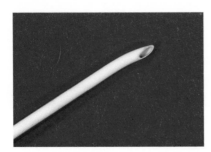

Figure 15.6 Tuohy type nerve block needle with Huber point. Note the white insulation material on the shaft.

approach lumbar plexus block. It may encourage the catheter to pass parallel to the nerve more easily.

Sprotte Tip

This pencil point tip was originally designed for spinal needles to reduce the incidence of PDPH because it is less traumatic to the dura than a cutting faceted tip. It has been developed for peripheral nerve block by Pajunk. The side hole orifice is about 1mm proximal to the tip of the pencil point and it is claimed that this aids passing a catheter parallel to the nerve. The potential problem with this design is that, because the orifice is some distance proximal to the needle tip, it may lie outside a fascial plane, resulting in block failure despite accurate nerve location either by nerve stimulation or paraesthesiae.

Needle length

Needles are available in lengths ranging from 30 mm to 150 mm. Some have centimetre markings on them which are helpful when placing catheters. The shorter needles (30–50 mm) are used for superficial nerve blocks, such as those involving the brachial plexus or femoral nerve and longer needles (100 mm) for deeper blocks, such as those targeting the posterior lumbar plexus or sciatic nerve. Very long needles (150 mm or longer) are awkward to use and are seldom required in clinical practice unless dealing with extremely large or obese patients, or when performing deep blocks such as the Labat approach to the sciatic nerve in the gluteal region. It is important to remember that very long needles can enter body cavities or penetrate organs, potentially resulting in major morbidity. They should be used with extreme care.

Insulation

A peripheral nerve stimulator (PNS) can be used to help locate major nerves. Use of a PNS in conjunction with good anatomical knowledge, significantly improves the success rate of regional anaesthesia.

When nerve stimulation was first used, the stimulator was simply connected to the uninsulated needle shaft by a crocodile clip. The problem with using needles in this way was that the current flow was spread over the whole needle surface and not concentrated at the tip of the needle near its orifice. Nerves could be stimulated by the shaft of the needle, but the block would fail when local anaesthetic was injected. Subsequently it was realized that some kind of insulation would need to be applied to the needle shaft, leaving only the very tip exposed to allow electrical stimulation only from this point. Modern stimulating peripheral nerve block needles are insulated with a Teflon® coating and have only a very small conductive area at the tip of the needle (Fig. 15.7).

Connections

Electrical: Stimulating needles should have an integrated electrical connection (Fig. 15.8a) that is compatible with the nerve stimulator. The connection should have no exposed conductive parts and must be long enough to take it out of the sterile field.

Injection Port: A side arm injection port (Fig. 15.8a) is desirable, because it helps the operator to keep the needle completely still while an assistant injects local anaesthetic incrementally. Very small movements of the needle at this crucial time can make the difference between block success and failure. One manufacturer has produced a side-arm injection port with a non-return diaphragm at its proximal end which allows a catheter to be passed through the needle without first removing the injection port (Fig. 15.8b). This helps to reduce needle movement.

Catheters

For many years, owing to the awkwardness of the equipment, peripheral nerve catheters were the preserve of the enthusiast. In the past five years, a variety of new kits for the placement of peripheral nerve catheters have been developed that are significantly more practicable. These kits include an insulated needle through which a catheter can be passed ('*catheter through needle'* technique) so as to lie alongside the nerve which has been located. The needle is then removed leaving the catheter in place. This catheter through needle technique is easier and more familiar to most anaesthetists than the '*catheter through cannula*' technique which was popular in the past (e.g. in B|Braun Contiplex D System).

Catheter design

The catheter should be a single end hole design (Fig. 15.9). Multiple side-hole catheters are unsuitable for continuous peripheral nerve block, because one or more of the holes may lie outside the fascial plane in which the nerve lies. Infusion of local anaesthetic will usually take the path of least resistance, which may be through an orifice that is either some distance from the nerve or outside a fascial plane. This leads to secondary block failure (the initial block which was administered through the needle works, but then wears off as the infusion fails to maintain anaesthesia).

Catheters normally have centimetre markings similar to those seen on epidural catheters (see above), to allow

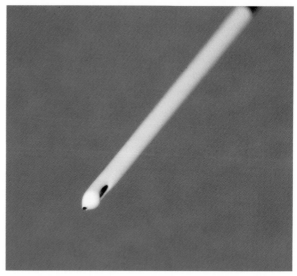

Figure 15.7 An insulated needle for peripheral nerve block. Note that the needle tip only is uninsulated.

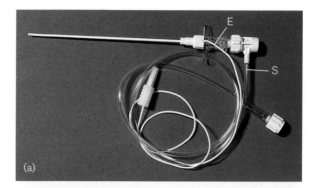

(a)

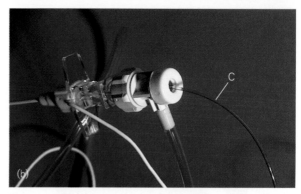

(b)

Figure 15.8 **(a)** An insulated Tuohy type needle with an integrated electrical connection (E) and a side arm injection port (S). **(b)** A catheter (C) can be seen entering the hub assembly ready to be passed through the needle.

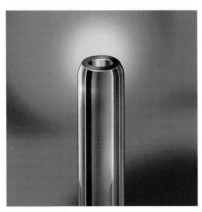

Figure 15.9 A catheter with a single hole at its tip for peripheral nerve block.

calculation of the length of catheter inserted distal to the needle. It is important to inspect the catheter carefully before starting the procedure. Particular attention should be paid to the distance marked on the catheter when the tip of it leaves the needle. Some catheters have a removable wire stiffener inside which makes passage between fascial planes easier. Unfortunately, this may also allow the catheter to pass *out* of the correct plane more readily, resulting in secondary failure of the block. Some catheters are radio-opaque (e.g. Arrow Stimucath) but if not, contrast may be injected to confirm accurate placement. A filter similar to that used with epidural catheters, should be included with the catheter system.

Stimulating catheters

There are catheters available that can be connected to a nerve stimulator in order to elicit nerve stimulation via the tip of the catheter itself. In theory this may allow even more reliable catheter placement and reduce the problem of secondary block failure. The catheter must have some kind of metallic element running through it to give it this capability. The Arrow Stimucath has a metallic spiral in its wall, while the Pandin catheter has an integrated fine conducting wire. (Fig. 15.10) However, the increased efficacy of stimulating catheters has yet to be proved and there is a significant price differential.

Nerve stimulators

A peripheral nerve stimulator (Fig. 15.11) allows localization of peripheral nerves electrically without the need to elicit paraesthesiae by direct contact between the needle and the target nerve. The technique was first described in 1912 and is now in common use.

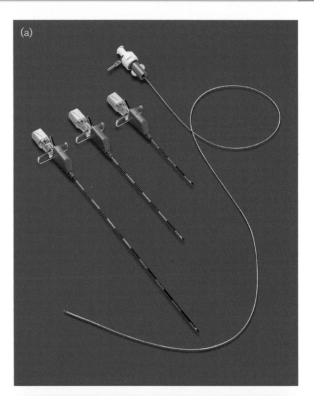

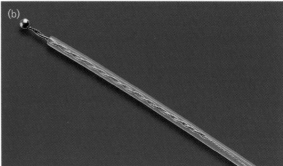

Figure 15.10 (a) A Pandin stimulating catheter and selection of Huber tipped insertion needles.
(b) Magnified view of the catheter tip to show conducting parts. Photos courtesy of HDC Corporation, USA.

Desirable characteristics of a nerve stimulator for localization of peripheral nerves include;[4]

1. adjustable constant current output from 0–5 mA. It should be easy for the operator or an assistant to adjust the delivered current.

2. a short stimulation pulse. The shorter the stimulation pulse, the greater the ratio of the current required to stimulate when the needle tip is 1 cm away from the nerve compared to when the needle

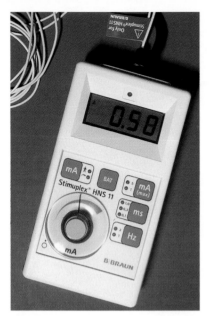

Figure 15.11 A Braun Stimulplex peripheral nerve stimulator.

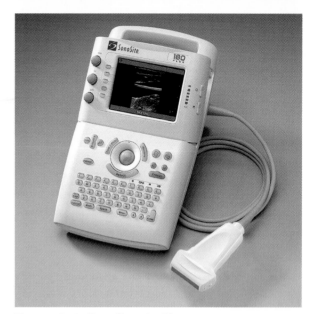

Figure 15.12 SonoSite 180 Plus.

is immediately adjacent to the nerve. Most commercially available nerve stimulators produce monophasic square wave impulses of between 0.1 and 1.0 ms.

3. clearly marked polarity. The needle should be connected to the cathode (−) and the anode (+) to the surface of the patient's skin.
4. display showing the current being delivered, and
5. audible alarm if a break in the circuit is occurs.

The reader is also referred to Chapter 19, Nerve Stimulators.

Ultrasound

Ultrasound guided peripheral nerve blocks are now possible, following the development of high-resolution portable ultrasound machines such as the SonoSite 180 Plus, which are portable and affordable enough to be used in the operating theatre (Fig. 15.12). When used with a 5–10 Mhz broadband probe, it can give good-quality images which allow the anaesthetist both to visualize the nerves (such as those of the brachial plexus) and the spread of the local anaesthetic during injection. A high-frequency probe such as this gives optimal resolution for locating superficial nerves to a depth of 4–5 cm. There have been a number of publications describing this technique to be very effective[5] with higher and more

consistent success rates than with the use of a nerve stimulator.[6] Lower-frequency ultrasound has greater tissue penetration, allowing visualization of deeper structures, but gives poorer image resolution.

Visualization of the block needle may be difficult, as most of the ultrasound beam is scattered by the smooth needle shaft. The needle is either perceived as a hyperechoic line or an echoic shadow in the deeper tissues. Needle movement may also often be implied by the displacement of tissues. There are also specific needles for ultrasound use with specially treated surfaces to make them 'visible', but they have been developed for interventional radiological techniques and are so far not suitable for regional anaesthesia.

It is likely that the use of ultrasound guided regional nerve block will become more popular in the future, although the learning curve appears to be longer compared with location by the use of anatomical landmarks and nerve stimulation.

REFERENCES

1. Selander D, Dhuner KG, Lundborg G (1997) Peripheral nerve injury due to injection needles used for regional anesthesia. *Acta Anesthesiology of Scandinavia* **21**: 182.

2. Rice ASM, McMahon SB (1992) Peripheral nerve injury caused by injection needles used in regional anaesthesia: Influence of bevel configuration, studied in a rat model. *British Journal of Anaesthesia* **69**: 433.

3. Selander D, Dhuner KG, Lundborg G (1977) Peripheral nerve injury due to injection needles used for regional anesthesia. *Acta Anaesethesiology of Scandinavia* **21**: 182.

4. Kaiser H, Niesel HC, Hans V (1990) Fundamentals and requirements of peripheral electric nerve stimulation. A contribution to the improvement of safety standards in regional anesthesia. *Regional Anesthesia* **13**: 143–147.

5. Sandhu N.S., Capan LM (2002) Ultrasound guided infraclavicular brachial plexus block. *British Journal of Anaethesia* **(2)**: 254–259.

6. Marhofer P, Schrögendorfer K, Koinig H, *et al*. (1997) Ultrasonographic guidance improves sensory block and onset time of three-in-one blocks. *Anaesthesia and Analgesia* **85**: 854–857.

Physiological monitoring: principles and non-invasive monitoring

Patrick T Magee

Monitoring the state of both the patient's physiology and the function of the anaesthesia delivery system is now an integral part of anaesthetic practice in the developed world. In some countries standards of monitoring are not enforced by law, yet it is difficult to prove that the absence of such monitoring is responsible for significant morbidity, since the trials required to prove this would be unethical. However, numerous studies have shown that anaesthesia has become safer in many countries over the last few decades. The cost of purchasing and maintaining such monitoring means it is unavailable to anaesthetists in many countries throughout the world and so the clinical monitoring skills of the anaesthetist remain crucial. Nonetheless, even in the developed world, all such standards emphasize the need for the continual presence of trained anaesthetic personnel.

The purpose of the monitoring is to advise the clinician of deviations from the normal and to warn of any unexpected, physiologically threatening events. In a study of closed claims in relation to deaths and cerebral damage under anaesthesia, two-thirds were found to be due mostly to human error; of these, two-thirds were deemed to be due to problems with securing the airway, endotracheal intubation, ventilation and hypoxia. A recent series of studies concluded that of the errors reported, 80% could be avoided by routine use of the pulse oximeter which, if used in conjunction with a capnometer, would lead to avoidance of 93% of such errors.[1] Figure 16.1 shows a graphical representation of the development of a critical incident and avoidance of the harmful results which might follow.[2] Arguably, it is the function of monitors to help the anaesthetist detect a critical incident early and avoid development of injury to the patient.

There are a number of guidelines, published by various authorities, such as the Association of Anaesthetists of Great Britain and Ireland (AAGBI), on minimum monitoring standards. These help the clinical anaesthetist select monitoring appropriate to the circumstances. It is notable how much the AAGBI guidelines defer to the anaesthetists' own clinical judgement in this respect, since the ultimate 'monitors' are the anaesthetists themselves.

CLASSIFICATION OF MONITORING EQUIPMENT

There are numerous ways of classifying monitoring equipment relevant to the anaesthetist. One way might specify the physiological system that it monitors: respiratory (including gas concentration, volume, flowrate and pressure); cardiovascular (e.g. ECG, arterial and venous pressures, cardiac output); nervous (e.g. EEG, neuro-

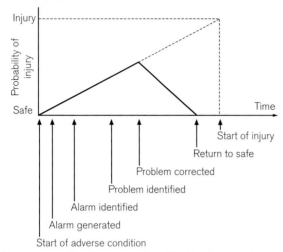

Figure 16.1 Development of a critical incident and its detection by a monitor. From Magee P, Tooley M (2005) The physics, clinical measurement and equipment of anaesthetic practice. By permission of Oxford University Press.

muscular junction); or metabolic (e.g. temperature or blood sugar). Another might include the degree of invasiveness of the monitoring: non-invasive monitoring, such as blood pressure and electrocardiogram (ECG); partially invasive, such as naso-pharyngeal temperature; or invasive, such as central venous pressure and arterial pressure. A third method might include classification according to whether the electrical signal being monitored is naturally generated by the body (e.g. a biological electrical potential such as the ECG), transduced from another signal modality (e.g. invasive arterial blood pressure to waveform), or a manifestation of some form of energy input to the body (e.g. pulse oximetry, ultrasound or magnetic resonance imaging) (Fig. 16.2).

Important components of a monitoring system, such as an automatic non-invasive blood pressure monitor, may therefore include some or all of the following (Fig. 16.3):

- an energy input source to the body (e.g. mechanical electrical, electromagnetic, infrared, ultrasound);
- a transducer to convert the signal from a measured physiological variable, usually to an electrical signal which can be processed; transducers need to be zeroed and calibrated. Calibration nowadays is often done at the factory of origin and the clinician merely has to zero the transducer;
- signal processing hardware and software, which amplifies the input signal, ensures the patient is safe from electrical hazards (see Chapter 25), is robust

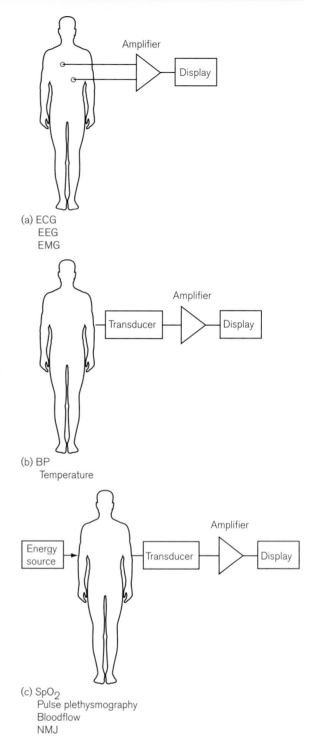

Figure 16.2 Basic classification of monitoring systems and some examples. **(a)** Monitoring electrical signals generated by the patient. **(b)** Conversion of measured variable to an electrical signal with a transducer. **(c)** Passing energy through a patient and measuring the effect the patient has on it.

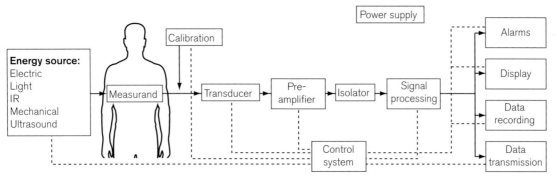

Figure 16.3 Generalized monitoring system showing the major components.

enough not to be damaged by other equipment such as diathermy apparatus or devices containing electromagnetic fields, and provides a good-quality output, free from electrical interference;

- a display for easy reading and interpretation by the clinician, who should not be obliged to become preoccupied with the monitor;
- an alarm system, with visual display and annunciation which is helpful rather than distracting, and with reasonable default limits and the ability to change those limits;[3]
- modern monitoring systems also have data storage ability for subsequent data analysis, and a means of data transmission to allow the data to be used by other parts of an integrated system such as an automated record keeping system; and
- a monitoring system must be intuitive and easy to use, ergonomically designed, and reliable when used under the conditions for which it is intended.

Almost all monitoring equipment is now controlled by microprocessors, making it possible to design equipment that needs minimal user calibration, offers self-diagnostics for fault conditions and also almost endless variability in user configuration of parameters. Single modality monitoring is becoming increasingly rare as a result of the flexibility and miniaturization possible with microprocessor control. Even greater user variability is offered in integrated monitors (one display for several variables) by the use of a modular system, in which the module for each monitored modality may be replaced by the user in the event of a fault or exchanged to perform a different function.

The remainder of this chapter will cover non-invasive monitoring, whatever the physiological system being monitored or the source of the electrical signal being

Table 16.1 The range of amplitudes and frequencies generated by biological potentials from different sources

Source of biological electrical potential	Amplitudes	Bandwidth (Hz)
ECG	0.5–4.0 mV	0.01–250
EEG	5–300 µV	DC-150
EMG	0.1–5.0 mV	DC-10000

processed. Chapter 17 covers gas monitoring and Chapters 18 and 19 cover other aspects of cardiovascular, neurophysiological and other monitoring.

MONITORING BIOLOGICAL ELECTRICAL POTENTIALS

All living cells have a potential difference between the outside and the inside of the cell membrane, which generates small electric currents within and between cells. Such a potential difference, when associated with excitable cells acting in unison, such as muscle or nerve, generates a current sufficient to be detected by a measurement system. Depending on the origin of the biological potential, there is a wide range of amplitudes and frequencies to be measured, processed and displayed, as shown in Table 16.1.

The quality of the electronics within these monitors must therefore be of a high order to measure accurately the currents produced by such small electrical potentials within a wide range of frequencies. Amplifiers used to process biological electrical potentials should have the following properties:[4]

- The *signal to noise ratio* of the amplifiers should be high. This is the ability of an amplifier to ensure preferential amplification of the signal being measured in comparison to any electrical noise interfering with this process;

- The *common mode rejection ratio* should be high; this is achieved by having two input ports, one of which inverts the input signal, so that any random noise signals, such as inductively or capacitatively coupled signals, which are common to both ports, cancel each other out before entering the amplifier, while signal inputs, which are not common to both inputs to the same extent (such as the biological potential itself), are allowed to enter the amplifier. The difference between the two inputs is then subjected to electronic amplification. Figure 16.4 shows single and double input amplifiers:

  - Where there are several amplifiers in a system, the *input impedance* of any single amplifier should be as high as possible so that the amplifier itself does not draw too much current from that being measured, thereby reducing its value.

  - The *output impedance* of an amplifier should be low so that the partially-processed signal can be passed to the next stage with minimum attenuation.

- In order to process preferentially that component of the signal within the appropriate range of frequencies without attenuation or distortion and to eliminate inappropriate frequencies, the amplifier should have appropriate filtering in its circuitry to give adequate *bandwidth*.

Even surface electrodes must be carefully designed in order to minimize degradation of the small surface electrical potentials. A further requirement of the monitors is high-quality *electrical isolation* between any parts touching the patient, such as the electrodes, and any other electrical components within the device, which might lead to an electrical hazard to the patient. This is particularly important, since it is the only situation where there is a deliberate electrical connection made between the patient and a device, which might be connected to a high voltage mains frequency source. If it is even remotely possible for a fault to develop in the ECG monitor or other electrical equipment simultaneously attached to the patient, an unwanted earth pathway can occur, which might lead to electrocution or diathermy burns. This is discussed in detail in Chapter 25.

This section covers the electrocardiogram and monitoring of the neuromuscular junction, while other chapters cover the electroencephalogram and its derivatives.

The electrocardiograph (ECG)

The electrical depolarization and repolarization of the myocardium is manifest on the surface of the skin, by the electrocardiogram in the form of the familiar PQRST complex. This can be detected by the use of electrodes connected to limbs and chest, which look at the electrical vector of the ECG from slightly different points of view. The relationship between the electrical axis of the heart and its detection by different limb leads was described by Einthoven in 1901. The signal from the electrodes is then fed into an amplifier, which meets the requirements discussed above.

As indicated in Table 16.1, the electrical potential from a surface ECG is in the range 0.5 to 4 mV, lying in the frequency range (bandwidth) of 0.01 to 250 Hz. The ECG is a complex waveform, which consists of a series of sinusoidal waves with different amplitudes, frequencies and phase relationships to each other. The ability of the ECG monitor to process the ECG waveform depends on its ability to respond to the range of different frequencies of these sinusoidal components, with faithful, unattenuated and undistorted reproduction of the signal, and with the desired amplification or gain. This is a measure of

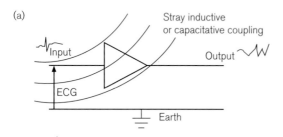

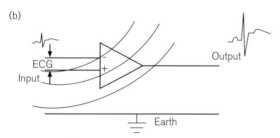

Figure 16.4 (a) The output of a single input amplifier is adversely affected by stray signal coupling. **(b)** The output of a differential input amplifier is relatively unaffected by stray signal coupling.

the bandwidth of the monitor and the ECG monitor should ideally have a bandwidth of 0.01 to 250 Hz. This is not practicable without also allowing amplification of noise within that bandwidth, thereby interfering with the ECG signal. Noise can originate from the amplifier circuit itself, from chest muscle electrical activity, from electromagnetic interference (inductive coupling), or from capacitative coupling to neighbouring electrical equipment such as diathermy apparatus (see Chapter 27). It is therefore more common to reduce the bandwidth to 0.05–100 Hz in a monitor with which the clinician wishes to make a range of diagnoses and to an even narrower bandwidth of 0.5–40 Hz in a monitor used in the operating room. The effect of this narrower bandwidth is to exclude high and low frequency components of electrical signal, which interfere with the ECG, without adversely affecting its quality or the clinician's ability to diagnose ischaemia and arrhythmias.

Figure 16.5 shows graphically the effect of electronic filtering, which is achieved by the addition of appropriate electronic components to an amplifier circuit. A low pass filter allows low frequency components to pass through the amplifier, blocking high frequency components. A high pass filter does the converse, allowing through high frequency components. A band pass filter allows through a range of frequencies, blocking signals of frequencies above and below this bandwidth. There is a significant DC voltage of up to 25 mV at the skin-electrode interface, partly due to the resistance in the layers of the skin and partly due to the electrolytic reaction between the Ag/AgCl gel and metal component of the electrode assembly. An ECG amplifier has to eliminate this DC voltage as well as the high frequency noise and therefore a band pass filter is appropriate.

Figure 16.6 shows a block diagram of the components of a modern ECG monitor. As discussed above, the

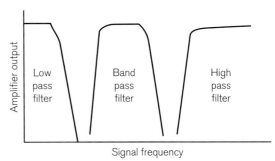

Figure 16.5 The effect of different electronic filters in allowing signals of different frequencies to pass through the amplifier.

characteristic features include a differential input to ensure common mode rejection. Electrical isolation of the amplifier is also important for reasons discussed earlier, using either an isolation transformer with good insulation between primary and secondary windings, or an optical isolator, in which the output signal from the amplifier is converted by a light emitting diode into a light signal and converted back into an electrical signal by a photodetector, with good insulation between the two.

Even these design features may allow the ECG signal to be overwhelmed by high power radio frequency diathermy signals. To deal with this, an additional technique is *adaptive noise filtering*. This is a digital electronic technique in which the noise signal is separately detected and digitally subtracted from the output signal, theoretically leaving a clean ECG signal. As Figure 16.6 shows, analogue to digital conversion of the signal occurs to allow microprocessing of the signal. One of the many things a microprocessor provides is the storage, in digital form in the random access memory (RAM), of enough signal information to reproduce a screen width's worth of

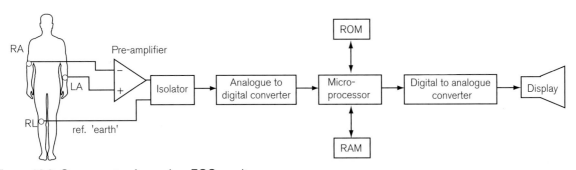

Figure 16.6 Components of a modern ECG monitor.

signal. This produces a more persistent and more easily readable screen than the previous phosphor dot screen. The RAM allows continual updating of the stored information so that the most recent 5 or 10 seconds of data is available. At the same time, the complete RAM storage is rapidly read through the microprocessor and a digital to analogue converter to a display. Thus, a rolling display of the most recent information is available and can be frozen on the screen for closer examination. Modern ECGs have adjustable rate alarms.

The causes of erroneous traces on an ECG include inappropriately positioned electrodes, left to right misconnections, poor electrode contact, capacitative and inductive interference, and voluntary and involuntary movement, such as shivering and excessive muscle tone.

Neuromuscular junction monitoring

The neuromuscular junction is monitored in order to determine onset and recovery from pharmacological neuro-muscular blockade. A supra-maximal electrical stimulus of between 10 and 50 mA is applied near an accessible peripheral motor nerve (for example, the ulnar or facial nerve) and the response of the appropriate muscle group is assessed, either clinically, mechanically or electromyographically. The stimulus has a square waveform of width 0.2 ms, to avoid the nerve firing repeatedly. The electrical stimulus applied in a clinical situation is either a single twitch or, more commonly, a *train of four* twitches (TOF), delivered at 2 Hz, or as a tetanic stimulus of duration not more than 5 s, delivered at 50 Hz. *Double burst stimulation*: two 40 ms tetanic bursts 750 ms apart, should also be available.

In non-depolarizing neuromuscular blockade, there is a characteristic fade on the muscle response to a TOF, and a characteristic temporary augmentation of the muscle response to further twitches delivered 3 s after a tetanic stimulus. The responses are distinguishable from no neuromuscular blockade or a depolarizing block. Application of the stimulus is painful and should not be carried out on an awake patient.

The nerve stimulator should have a constant current output.[5] This is desirable to ensure a constant current between the electrodes of the stimulator, whatever the changes in electrical impedance of the tissues to which they are applied. Many devices deliver constant current up to a tissue impedance of 2.5 kΩ. However, in some patients, the tissue resistance may be higher, causing a drop in current output, delivering a stimulus which is no longer supramaximal.

The electrodes may be of the type incorporating Ag/AgCl gel, used for ECG recording. Since a supramaximal response is required, an adequate current density is necessary at the electrodes, the surface area of which should not be too large.

The most common way of assessing the muscular response to a supramaximal nerve stimulus is to make a visual clinical assessment of the responding muscle (e.g. levator palpebrae superioris in the case of the facial nerve or adductor pollicis longus in the case of the ulnar nerve), which is usually adequate. If a mechanical assessment is made, it is usually done on the adductor pollicis longus muscle in response to ulnar nerve stimulation. The arm is rigidly clamped and a force transducer is placed in contact with the thumb, correctly orientated, with a preload of 100–300 g applied to ensure isometric thumb contraction. The transducer converts the force of contraction of the thumb into an electrical signal, which can be processed and displayed.

Electromyographic (EMG) assessment in response to nerve stimulation is now more commonly used than previously because of advanced signal processing and computer data handling techniques.[6] The EMG represents a collection of muscle action potentials, which diminishes in number in response to a neuromuscular blocking drug. Recording electrodes are placed over the muscle (usually a forearm muscle on the ulnar side of the arm if the ulnar nerve is stimulated), with an indifferent electrode on the second finger. The evoked EMG signal, in response to nerve stimulation, is a high-speed event, with very high frequency components as Table 16.1 indicates, and requires considerable processing before any display can record it. The modern EMG monitor can analyze, process and digitize the signal, displaying the result of the evoked EMG response digitally as a TOF ratio or as a percentage. See also Chapter 19.

BLOOD PRESSURE MONITORING

Monitoring blood pressure (BP) in the perioperative period has been routine since 1903 and is part of contemporary minimum monitoring standards. It is usually done non-invasively, except where there is a clinical need dictating 'beat to beat' invasive monitoring. Arguably, cardiac output would be a more useful measure of cardiovascular well being, but has always been more complex to carry out than blood pressure measurement. Non-invasive blood pressure measurement became relatively easy to do early on in the history of clinical monitoring, but the earliest blood pressure measurements were invasive, using a manometer (see below). The manometer is still used in many settings, as a mercury manometer attached to a non-invasive sphygmomanometer cuff (see below) or as a water manometer attached to a central venous catheter to measure pressure directly. The manometer is a column of fluid, at the bottom of which the pressure is equal to the weight of fluid above it, divided by the cross-sectional area of the tube. Hence the pressure P is given by:

$$P = \frac{\text{weight of fluid}}{\text{cross-sectional area of tube, A}} = \frac{\rho\, g\, h\, A}{A} = \rho\, g\, h$$

where ρ is fluid density, g is acceleration due to gravity, h is the height of fluid in the manometer column and A is the cross-sectional area of the tube. Hence the colloquial use of a column height (e.g. mmHg, cmH$_2$O) to describe pressure has evolved. The hydraulic pressure being measured is applied to the bottom of the manometer column or to one side of the 'U-tube' form of the manometer, shown in Figure 16.7.

The venous circulation is a low-pressure system, and in the upright or partially upright patient, the venous pressure at the head will be significantly less than at the feet; this should be remembered in deciding where to site the pressure transducer, when measuring central venous pressure. This difference in arterial pressure from top to bottom may not be so apparent, because the arterial circulation is a high-pressure system, with regionally adjustable resistance to flow.

Non-invasive arterial blood pressure measurement techniques include auscultation using a sphygmo-manometer, the oscillotonometer, the oscillometer and the volume clamp method (Peñaz technique). Invasive methods of measurement are discussed in Chapter 18.

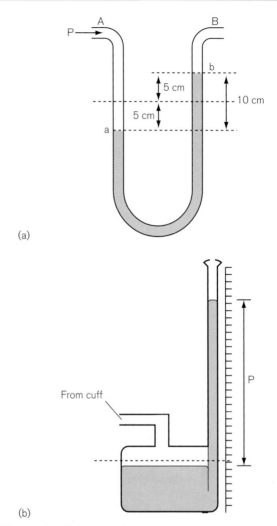

(a)

(b)

Figure 16.7 Two sorts of manometers to measure pressure, **(a)** a U-tube differential manometer; **(b)** a single tube manometer, of the type used in a sphygmomanometer.

Non-invasive arterial blood pressure (NIBP) measurement

NIBP methods all function by inflating an occlusive cuff around a limb to a pressure above the expected arterial pressure and, on subsequent, gradual, stepwise or continuous deflation, detecting the return of the pulse downstream of the cuff. Detection methods are described below in more detail. Most non-invasive methods are necessarily intermittent, although the volume clamp method (Finapres; see later) is continuous. In all non-invasive methods using a cuff, the cuff size is important for accuracy; the width of the inflatable bladder of the cuff should be 40% of the mid-circumference of the limb concerned and its length should be twice this width. A cuff, which is too narrow, overestimates the blood pressure, while a cuff which is too wide or too loosely wrapped around the limb, underestimates it.

The sphygmomanometer

The sphygmomanometer is a device that uses a combination of a pneumatic cuff to wrap around the limb in which the arterial pressure is to be measured, an inflating bulb, release valve, and a mercury manometer of the type shown in Figure 16.7b. The classical method of pulse detection is *auscultation*. If the cuff is used on the upper arm, the sounds of the pulse returning are heard over the brachial artery. These sounds are known as

Korotkoff sounds and their onset corresponds to the occurrence of turbulent flow in the artery as the cuff pressure falls below systolic blood pressure; the muffling or disappearance of these sounds corresponds to diastolic pressure.

The reason that Korotkoff sounds correspond to these pressures is unclear, but it is therefore not altogether surprising that it correlates poorly with invasive BP measurement. It has been shown that this method overestimates at low pressure and underestimates at high pressure, and has large inter-observer variation.[7] On the other hand, the method is simple using low level technology, and has a long history of use. Other methods of pulse detection with the sphygmomanometer include palpation and ultrasound. Palpation is more prone to error in the presence of bradycardia or too rapid cuff deflation and it has been shown that this method underestimates systolic pressure by 25%.[8]

The oscillotonometer

Figure 16.8 shows the double cuff system used in oscillotonometry. The upper cuff performs the same function as that in the sphygmomanometer, namely limb occlusion. The lower cuff is wider and acts as the pulse detection system. Both cuffs are connected via an inflating bulb and air release valve to an airtight box containing two aneroid barometers. One aneroid (B_1) is relatively rigid and its inside is connected to atmosphere to measure the absolute pressure. The other aneroid (B_2) is relatively sensitive and its inside is connected to the distal cuff.

Both aneroids are connected together by a lever, which is also toggled to the dial pointer. When the system is pressurized by manual inflation (using the bulb), both cuffs, the airtight box and the aneroid B_2 are filled to the same pressure This causes the aneroid B_1 to be compressed and via its mechanical linkage moves a pointer to display the pressure in the system.

By switching on the release valve, a narrow diameter tube connecting the inside of aneroid B_2 to the atmosphere is opened and air is allowed to leak gradually out of the system. This allows deflation of the lower cuff to be marginally delayed behind the upper cuff. As the upper cuff pressure falls below systolic pressure, arterial pulsations impinge on the lower cuff and these are transmitted to aneroid B_2; with the release valve switch in this position, aneroid B_2 is also connected to the pointer and the pulsations, which are shown on the dial, increase significantly as systolic BP is reached. On releasing the valve switch, the pointer is reconnected to aneroid B_1 and the actual BP is indicated at this point. With the valve reswitched to air leak mode, the pulsation fluctuations gradually disappear as diastolic pressure is approached, and the actual pressure at which this occurs is once again read by reconnecting the pointer to aneroid B_1. Its accuracy is better at systolic pressure than diastolic.

Oscillometry

This method uses a single cuff that both compresses the limb and detects pulsations and uses hydraulics linked to modern electronics to obtain BP measurements. Some

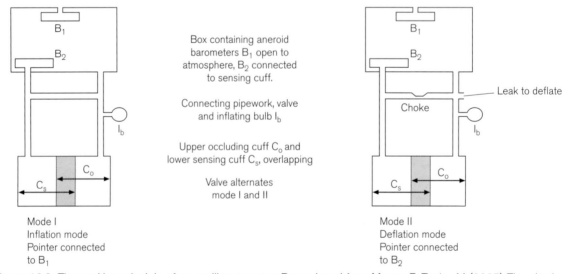

Mode I
Inflation mode
Pointer connected
to B_1

Box containing aneroid
barometers B_1 open to
atmosphere, B_2 connected
to sensing cuff.

Connecting pipework, valve
and inflating bulb I_b

Upper occluding cuff C_o and
lower sensing cuff C_s, overlapping

Valve alternates
mode I and II

Mode II
Deflation mode
Pointer connected
to B_2

Figure 16.8 The working principle of an oscillotonometer. Reproduced from Magee P, Tooley M (2005) The physics, clinical measurement and equipment of anaesthetic practice. By permission of Oxford University Press.

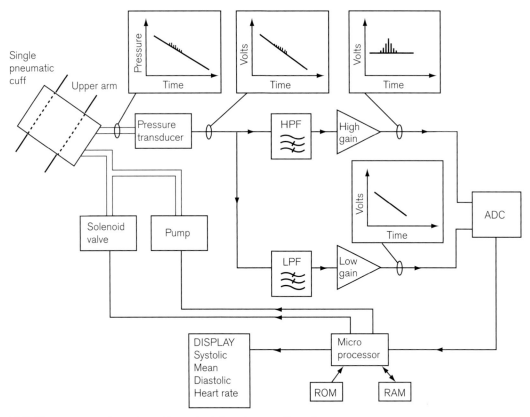

Figure 16.9 The components and working principles of an oscillometer.

systems use a single tube for both inflation and detection, and others use two. Figure 16.9 shows the components of the system. The hydraulic system consists of a pump to pressurize the system and a solenoid valve through which to depressurize the system, either in discrete steps or continuously, connected to a microprocessor. The detection system consists of a pressure transducer, whose output signal is fed through filters to amplifiers. On deflation, one part of the transducer signal goes through a high pass filter to pass only the high frequency pulsation components to a high gain amplifier that amplifies the pulsations due to the oscillations of the arterial wall.

The onset of the rapid increase of pulsations corresponds to systolic pressure, maximum pulsations to mean pressure, and the rapid offset of pulsations to diastolic pressure. The other part of the transducer signal goes through a low pass filter and a low gain amplifier to produce a signal proportional to the cuff pressure. The outputs from both amplifiers are passed through an analogue to digital converter to the microprocessor, which calculates systolic, mean and diastolic pressures. Depend-

ing on the exact algorithm being used, the microprocessor may also compare the measured systolic and diastolic values to the values calculated from the mean value, at which the device has the greatest accuracy, as the oscillations are maximum at mean pressure. The microprocessor also controls the pump and solenoid valve and connects to a display.

The Finapres

This is the manufacturer's name given to the device, which uses the *Peñaz volume clamp technique*. It depends on the hypothesis that if the transmural pressure of an artery (the difference between the externally and internally applied pressure across the arterial wall) is kept constant, then the diameter of the artery also remains constant, as will the volume of blood within it and the absorption of infrared light across its lumen. The device consists of a low compliance finger cuff and tubing connected to a rapidly responding solenoid valve and air pump. It also has a light emitting diode as an infrared light source, which transmits light through the finger; the transmitted light is detected on the opposite side by a photodetector. The pump, the solenoid valve and the microprocessor function together to keep the light transmission through the finger constant, by maintaining the transmural pressure. The device does this by altering the compression in the finger cuff throughout the cardiac cycle. At any instant the cuff pressure is the same as arterial pressure, and the low compliance of the system ensures rapid response. The output on the display therefore resembles an arterial trace. The Finapres is shown schematically in Figure 16.10. There have been reports of varying accuracy[9] and it is no longer in extensive clinical use.

PULSE OXIMETRY

Principles Table 16.2 shows that it is surprisingly difficult even for trained anaesthetists to ascertain accurately the patient's state of oxygenation, particularly where the oxygen saturations have fallen below optimal levels. Arguably pulse oximetry, first introduced in the early 1980s, has revolutionized clinical monitoring in this respect. It should not be thought of as a replacement for other oxygen monitors, such as those on anaesthetic workstations, but it does provide the best non-invasive monitor of patient oxygenation. The pulse oximeter uses two technologies; one is pulse plethysmography to detect a pulse waveform; the other is infrared spectroscopy to detect the absorption by the tissue under the probe of light at two wavelengths in the red and infrared wavebands.

Pulse plethysmography detects the cyclical change in volume of the artery as change in light absorption across it, an increase in one being an increase in the other. Red or infrared light is used for the same reasons as in clinical spectroscopy, namely that there are absorption spectra in this waveband across an artery. The absorption signal is then electronically processed, including amplification and display. In a modern pulse oximeter, this signal processing and display scaling occurs automatically, so the size of the plethysmographic signal cannot be taken as a quantitative indicator of pulse volume; a pulse volume below a certain threshold may not be amplified at all.

Table 16.2 The ability of experienced anaesthetists to detect hypoxaemia

SpO$_2$ reading	Percentage of anaesthetists detecting cyanosis
96–100	1.1
91–95	12.3
86–90	22.5
81–85	29.2
76–80	12.3
<75	22.5

Reproduced from Magee P, Tooley M (2005) The physics, clinical measurement and equipment of anaesthetic practice. By permission of Oxford University Press.

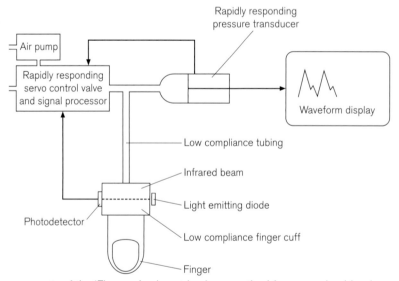

Figure 16.10 The components of the 'Finapres' volumetric clamp method for measuring blood pressure.

Apart from the objective indication of SpO_2, pulse oximetry may be described as tending to 'fail-safe', in that the technique fails and therefore alarms if the pulsatility of the pulse waveform decreases to below a critical level. Further information may be gained by the display of a plethysmograph trace, which enables the differentiation between the pulse waveform and artefacts. No pulse oximeter reading should be accepted, unless the plethysmograph trace can confirm lack of artefact (see below, under Limitations).

The spectroscopic aspect of the technology is based on the absorption of light by a 'dye' in tissues, in which absorption is proportional to concentration of the dye and the path length through the tissue, and which also depends on the wavelength of light used; these factors are embedded in the *Beer–Lambert laws* (see Chapter 17). Figure 16.11 shows the absorption spectra in the red and infrared wavebands of a number of haemoglobin species, including oxygenated and reduced haemoglobin, as well as the less common species, which can nevertheless contribute to a pulse oximetric signal.

The pulse oximeter has light emitting diodes (LEDs), which transmit light alternately at two wavelengths, 660 nm (red) and 940 nm (infrared). It can be seen that at 660 nm, the absorption of reduced haemoglobin exceeds that of oxygenated haemoglobin and at 940 nm, the converse is true. The absorption scale in Figure 16.11 is logarithmic, so the differences in absorption are large. The device uses two wavelengths, because it needs to distinguish between absorption of light in pulsatile and non-pulsatile tissues under the probe. Ideally the two wavelengths used should correspond to those at which absorptions of both haemoglobin species (reduced and oxygenated) are equal (the *isobestic point*) and at which they are furthest apart. LEDs of 660 and 940 nm are used because of their ease of production, constant outputs and narrow bandwidths.

The probe is put on a digit, an earlobe, the bridge of the nose or the forehead and the more peripherally placed it is, the longer the delay in the device detecting an event causing oxygenation change.[10] Probes should be appropriately designed for paediatric use because of the *penumbra effect* where, because of the small size of the digit to which the probe is attached, the path length of the light at the two wavelengths differ significantly.[11] The LEDs rate of alternating on and off is 400 Hz, with a measurable 'off' phase, so the photodetector allows for ambient lighting. The photodetector measures the light transmission (1 – absorption) of both pulsatile (AC) and non-pulsatile (DC) components at both wavelengths. The pulsatile components are assumed to come mainly from the arterial blood and non-pulsatile components from all other tissues including venous blood. The AC component of absorption represents 1 to 2% of the total, which puts significant demand on the accuracy of the device. Figure 16.12a shows the raw signal, with different transmissions of each component at each wavelength. The first stage of signal processing is to change the amplitude of the signal at one of the wavelengths in order to equalize the DC components. The AC components, which are the signals of interest in this context, are now measureable against comparable denominators. The microprocessor in the device calculates the ratio of absorption of the AC component at 660 nm to the absorption of the AC component at 940 nm.

The microprocessor has stored in its memory a number of discrete values of oxygen saturation of arterial blood samples from healthy subjects, measured by a multi-wavelength co-oximeter. Figure 16.12b shows this ratio plotted against the oxygen saturation and represents the calibration curve for the pulse oximeter. The term S_pO_2 is used to describe the oxygen saturation derived from this curve. Note that an absorption ratio of 1.0 corresponds to a S_pO_2 of 85%. The S_pO_2 displayed is a value averaged over a number of beats, so a change in saturation may not immediately be displayed.

Limitations

Clearly most values on the calibration curve shown in Figure 16.12b are either interpolated or extrapolated. Since it would be unethical to collect blood from subjects who had been exposed to life threatening hypoxia, it is

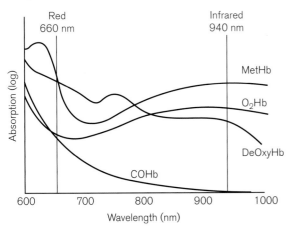

Figure 16.11 The absorption spectra in the red and infrared region for different species of haemoglobin.

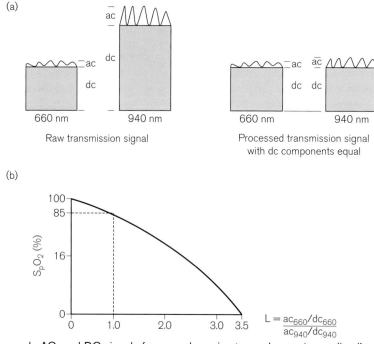

Figure 16.12 (a) The crude AC. and DC signals from a pulse oximeter probe are 'normalized' to make the DC components equal. **(b)** The curve of absorption ratio to S_pO_2. Reproduced from Magee P, Tooley M (2005) The physics, clinical measurement and equipment of anaesthetic practice. By permission of Oxford University Press.

to be expected that S_pO_2 values below about 80% will be less accurate. In normal clinical circumstances, this is tolerable because values below 90% would be acted upon.

Pulse oximeters are designed to take account of two haemoglobin species, oxygenated and deoxygenated haemoglobin, to calculate *functional* saturation. As Figure 16.11 shows, the presence of other haemoglobin species, such as methaemoglobin or carboxyhaemoglobin will affect the measured absorbances at the two wavelengths used. In particular, it can be seen that carboxyhaemoglobin resembles oxyhaemoglobin at 660 nm. This means that the pulse oximeter may give a falsely high S_pO_2 in smokers, in whom COHb levels can reach 20%. Clearly a pulse oximeter should not be used to assess the oxygenation of a patient who has suffered from carbon monoxide poisoning. Similarly, methaemoglobin, caused by a number of drugs including local anaesthetics and nitrates, resembles deoxygenated haemoglobin at 660 nm. Only a co-oximeter with a minimum of four wavelengths can distinguish these four species, to calculate *fractional* saturation.

Other factors which limit the accuracy of the pulse oximeter include:

- movement and vibration[12] artefact to which these devices are particularly susceptible; electromagnetic interference from diathermy or from mobile telephones;[1]
- hypertension and vasoconstriction;[13]
- hypotension and hypovolaemia, e.g. in sepsis;[14]
- hyperdynamic venous circulation, e.g. in tricuspid regurgitation;[15]
- ambient light; and
- IV dyes, e.g. methylene blue, indocyanine green.

Foetal haemoglobin has the same properties of light absorption as adult haemoglobin within the wavebands being discussed, so the pulse oximeter should be as accurate in neonates as adults. Bilirubin does not absorb light significantly in the waveband of interest, therefore jaundice does not affect the accuracy of the pulse oximeter. Both foetal haemoglobin and bilirubin, however, affect the accuracy of a multi-wavelength co-oximeter. Skin pigmentation does not usually affect accuracy, but some dark nail polish does. It is inappropriate to compare S_pO_2 measured by a pulse oximeter with the value of oxygen saturation derived from the oxygen dissociation curve following measurement of pO_2, pCO_2 and pH.

BODY TEMPERATURE MONITORING

At both physiological and biochemical levels, the human body functions optimally at 37°C. Anaesthesia and surgery both militate against this by tending to allow body temperature to fall and recovery to be delayed after prolonged surgery. On the other hand, malignant hyperthermia is a potentially fatal condition caused by some anaesthetic drugs in patients pharmacogenetically predisposed to it. It is therefore essential for the anaesthetist to monitor body temperature by several devices.

A traditional way of measuring the temperature of a patient is to use a glass thermometer. This consists of a glass fluid filled bulb attached to a calibrated glass tube. The glass bulb is placed against the tissue where temperature needs be measured, causing the fluid contained therein to heat up to the same temperature as the tissue. The resultant expansion of the fluid causes it to move into the calibrated glass tube as a column. The temperature can be read off the tube at the point where the head of the fluid column stops. A constriction is placed at the base of the tube so that when the bulb temperature drops and the bulb fluid contracts, the fluid column breaks allowing the final reading of the thermometer to be maintained.

Mercury is frequently the fluid used as its expansion characteristics allow it to cover a wide range of temperatures. Alcohol is also used, covering a narrower measurement range.

A *thermistor* is a semiconductor device, whose electrical resistance changes with temperature in an almost linear fashion. It is the basis of both the nasopharyngeal temperature probe and the tympanic membrane thermometer.[16]

A *thermocouple* consists of two dissimilar metals, connected together at both ends; one end is kept at a known reference temperature, the other at the temperature to be measured. A potential difference is generated between the two junctions, proportional to the difference in temperature between them, although the relationship is a non-linear one. This is the *Seebeck effect*, and is the basis of thermocouple function.

Liquid Crystal Displays are made of materials which change colour with temperature change. They have been shown to demonstrate hysteresis and are sensitive to draughts.[17]

The infrared tympanic thermometer (Fig. 16.13) is a recently-developed device which consists of a series of thermocouples (*thermopile*), which detect the infrared

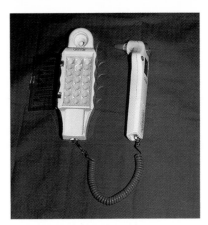

Figure 16.13 A tympanic thermometer.

radiation from the tympanic membrane. The thermopile generates a potential difference proportional to tympanic membrane temperature.

REFERENCES

1. Runciman WB, Barker L, *et al* (1993) The pulse oximeter: applications and limitations. The first 2000 AIMS reports. *Anaesthesia in Intensive Care* **21**: 543–550.
2. Schreiber P, Schreiber J (1987) *Anesthesia Systems Risk Analysis and Risk Reduction*. Telford PA: Dräger.
3. ISO standard 9703-3 (1998) *Anaesthesia and Respiratory Care Alarm Signals part 3 – Guidance on Application of Alarms*. Geneva: ISO.
4. Smith RJ (1971) 'Circuits, Devices and Systems: A First Course in Electrical Engineering', 2nd edn. ch.11 *Electronic Amplifiers*. New York: Wiley; pp 343–390.
5. Ford DJ, Pither CE, Raj PP (1984) Electrical characteristics of peripheral nerve stimulators. Implications for nerve localization. *Regional Anaesthesia* **9**, 73–77.
6. Epstein RM, Epstein RA (1975) 'Electromyography in evaluation of the response to muscle relaxants'. In: Katz RL (ed.), *Muscle Relaxants*. Amsterdam: Excerpta Medica. pp.299.
7. Pereira E, Prys-Roberts C, Dagnino J, Anger C, Cooper GM, Hutton P (1985) Auscultatory measurement of arterial blood pressure during anaesthesia: a reassessment of the Korotkoff sounds. *European Journal of Anaesethia* **2**: 11–20.
8. Van Bergen FH, *et al.* (1954) Comparison of indirect and direct methods of measuring arterial blood pressure. *Circulation* **10**: 481–490.

9. Farquhar IK (1991) Continuous direct and indirect blood pressure measurement (Finapres) in the critically ill. *Anaesthesia* **46:** 1050–1053.

10. Ralston AC, Webb RK, Runciman WB (1991) Potential errors in pulse oximetry III. The effects of interference, dyes, dyshaemoglobins and other pigments. *Anaesthesia* **46:** 291–295. SJ

11. Howell SJ, Blogg CE, Ashby MW (1993) Modified sensor for pulse oximetry in children. *Anaesthesia* **48:** 1083–1095.

12. Langton JA, Hanning CD (1990) Effect of motion artefact on pulse oximeters: evaluation of four instruments and finger probes. *British. Journal of Anaesthesia* **65:** 564–570.

13. Langton JA, Lassey D, Hanning CD (1990) Comparison of four pulse oximeters: effects of venous occlusion and cold induced vasoconstriction. *British Journal of Anaesthesia* **65:** 245–247.

14. Secker C, Spiers R (1997) Accuracy of the pulse oximeter in patients with low systemic vascular resistance. *Anaesthesia* **52:** 127–130.

15. Stewart KG, Rowbottom SJ (1991) Inaccuracy of pulse oximeters in patients with severe tricuspid regurgitation. *Anaesthesia* **46:** 668–670.

16. Edge G, Morgan M (1993) The Genius infrared tympanic thermometer. *Anaesthesia* **48:** 604–607.

17. MacKenzie R, Asbury AJ (1994) Clinical evaluation of liquid crystal skin thermometers. *British Journal of Anaesthesia* **72:** 246–249.

Physiological monitoring: gases

Patrick T Magee

Gas analysis during anaesthesia requires continuous monitoring of respired gases and at times, intermittent sampling of blood gases. The different techniques described in this chapter utilize different physical or chemical properties of the gas molecules, both to detect and quantify the gas. As with all clinical measurement techniques, it is important to understand the principles on which the gas analyzers are based, so that their applications and limitations are recognized.

RESPIRATORY GAS SAMPLING

A number of factors may affect or complicate gas sampling. Common to all methods is the delay in the sample reaching the analyzer and the response time of the analyzer itself. Not all analyzers return the sample to the breathing system. This is advantageous when the gas analyzer alters the integrity of the gas molecule. However, if low fresh gas flows are being used in a circle breathing system, the non-return of gas samples being removed at 100 ml min^{-1} significantly reduces the circulating fresh gas flow.

Following a step change in the gas concentration, delay in response time of the analyzer is due to two factors. The first is the *delay time* or *transit time*: the time it takes for the sample to get from the patient's airway to the gas analyzer. The second is the *response time* or *rise time* of the analyzer. The response time is usually considered to be the time taken for the analyzer to respond to within 90–95% of an actual step change in gas concentration. A step change can be produced in one of three ways: by moving a gas sampling tube rapidly into and out of a gas stream; by bursting a small balloon within a sampling volume containing a gas sample; or by switching a shutter to a gas sample volume using a solenoid valve. Figure 17.1 shows how these are related.

Most modern analyzers use side stream sampling, where the sampling tube takes the gas sample to the analyzer. It is important that only the recommended sample tubing be used for the analyzer concerned, because various types of tubing may absorb some of the gas mixture as well as water vapour to different extents; calibration of the analyzer will have allowed for this only with the recommended tubing. Gas analyzers sample gas at a rate of between 50 and 200 ml min^{-1}. If the sampling rate is higher than this, or if the tubing is too long or too wide, the sampling waveform will be distorted, thereby reducing accuracy. The delay time depends to great extent on the sampling rate and on the length of the sampling tube, which should be as short as possible.

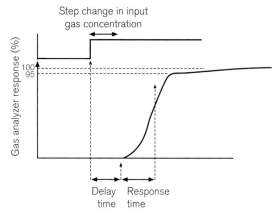

Figure 17.1 The response of gas analyzers to a step change in gas concentration.

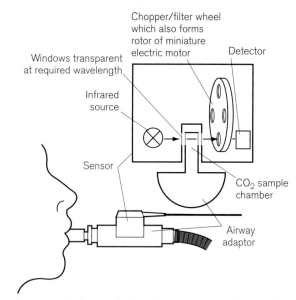

Figure 17.2 The Hewlett Packard IR gas analyzer, using mainstream sampling.

In trying to sample gases at the end of expiration, it is important to sample as close to the patient's trachea as possible, particularly where the tidal volume is small and the respiratory rate is large, as when anaesthetizing infants. Some systems have a sampling catheter that extends down the endotracheal tube, but this adds to airway resistance where that tube is of small diameter. Most systems, however, have a sampling port attached to the catheter mount adjacent to the artificial airway. It is important that the software within the analyzer can detect minima and maxima in the respiratory waveform, and associate with these, inspiratory and expiratory gas concentration values appropriately. It is still possible, however, for a gas sample, taken from the patient end of a coaxial Mapleson D breathing system, to give erroneously low end tidal readings, due to confusion between inspiratory and expiratory gas flows.

Some analyzers have used mainstream sampling instead, where the analyzer itself sits astride the artificial airway. This is a bulky addition to the airway but it eliminates transit time. There is also less of a problem dealing with water vapour in the sample. The sample is not degraded by the analyzer. An example, the Hewlett Packard infrared CO_2 analyzer, is shown in Figure 17.2. The sensor fits onto a sampling chamber inserted into the breathing circuit. The miniaturized unit contains a motor with filter wheel, an infrared (IR) source and detector, and IR transparent glass for the optical pathways. A second isolated optical window on the airway adapter provides a reference for calibration.

GAS CONCENTRATION MONITORING

Refractometry

Refractometry is a technique that detects the difference in refractive indices between two media, one of which contains the gas sample of interest (air and anaesthetic vapour), the other which is otherwise of identical constitution (air only). The refractive index of a medium is a measure of the ratio of velocity of light in a vacuum to the velocity of light in that medium. The molecules of the medium delay the path of the light wave through it; the delay depends on the number of molecules and hence on the density of the medium; thus refractive index for a gas medium depends on its concentration, pressure and temperature. When a light beam passes through a slit whose diameter is of the same order of magnitude as the wavelength of the light, interference patterns are produced by light waves arriving in phase (bright fringe) and 180° out of phase (dark fringe) with each other. When two such sets of fringes are formed from light passing through gas samples with differential velocities, they are displaced relative to each other and the displacement between them can be measured as refractive index difference.

The refractometer is included, not because it is frequently used as a clinical gas analyzer, but because it is a standard of gas analysis against which others are compared. All gases and volatile agents can be quantified using this method, since all possess the physical property of refractive index. Laboratory refractometers are used by vaporizer manufacturers to calibrate vaporizers. However, a diagram of the portable version of the refractometer (the Riken refractometer) is shown in Figure 17.3. Light from a small light source is collimated into a beam, which is split into two parallel beams by prisms. One beam is passed through the reference chamber containing, say air, and the other is passed through the measuring chamber containing air and another gas/vapour species, say isoflurane, whose concentration is to be measured. The beams are reflected back through the chambers to enhance the effect. Each beam is passed through a slit, producing interference fringes. As discussed above, the effective path lengths of the two beams differ and two sets of fringes are produced. These can be realigned by a knob controlling a vernier scale and the amount of realignment is taken as a measure of refractive index change from the reference sample, and thus of concentration of the gas under test.

Infrared absorption spectroscopy

The interatomic bond between dissimilar atoms of a molecule absorbs radiation in the infrared (IR) range. Thus, molecules such as nitrous oxide, carbon dioxide, water vapour and the volatile agents absorb infrared light, but oxygen, nitrogen and helium do not. Polyatomic molecules of different species absorb IR radiation across a range of IR wavelengths and there is frequently overlap between species. However, different polyatomic species absorb maximally at characteristic wavelengths within the IR bandwidth, which means that it is possible to identify the gas molecule as well as quantify the gas concentration. The amount of absorption (A) of any radiation by any

substance is governed by the *Beer–Lambert* law, which links A to the intensity of the incident radiation I_i, the non-absorbed, transmitted radiation I_t, the extinction coefficient ε, the path length L and the concentration C of the absorbing substance, where:

$$A = \log_{10} \frac{I_i}{I_t} = \varepsilon L.C$$

Since CO_2 analysis is important in anaesthesia, such devices are available in most anaesthetic locations in modern operating rooms. Figure 17.4 shows the principle of the *Luft* or non-dispersive type of IR gas analyzer, which uses a differential technique to minimize error. An IR light source emits radiation at between 1 and 15 μm. A 'chopper' wheel, with small windows at the rim, rotates in front of the light source at 25 to 100 Hz to prevent the gas sample from overheating; additionally the windows allow through IR light of a narrower bandwidth than the source itself, to match the wavelength of maximum absorption of the gas under study. This window might contain a 4.26 μm filter for CO_2, a 3.3 μm filter for halothane, isoflurane and enflurane, and a 4.5 μm filter for N_2O. The light passes through this to two chambers, a reference chamber and a sample chamber; the sample chamber contains the same background gas as the reference chamber, but additionally contains the gas under analysis. The light, which is not absorbed (the transmitted light) in each sample cell, is passed to a pair of air filled detector chambers, separated by a diaphragm. Because different amounts of IR light are absorbed in the reference and sample chambers, different amounts of light are therefore transmitted to the detector chambers, heating the air in them differentially. Because the chopper wheel produces an oscillating IR source, the changing air pressure in the two detector chambers causes the diaphragm separating them to oscillate. The diaphragm usually forms half of a capacitor and is, therefore, a component of electrical circuitry, which amplifies and processes the signal, to produce an output signal, which is proportional to the gas concentration.

There are a number of sources of error in IR spectroscopy. Although CO_2, N_2O and CO absorb IR light maximally at 4.3, 4.5 and 4.7 μm respectively, there is considerable overlap in the absorption spectra of these gases, particularly in the 3 to 5 μm range. There is also the phenomenon of *collision broadening*, where the presence of one gas may broaden the IR absorption spectrum of another. This effect is not only caused by IR absorbing agents themselves (such as CO_2 and N_2O) on the

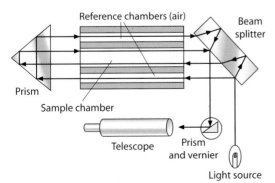

Figure 17.3 The principles of the portable refractometer.

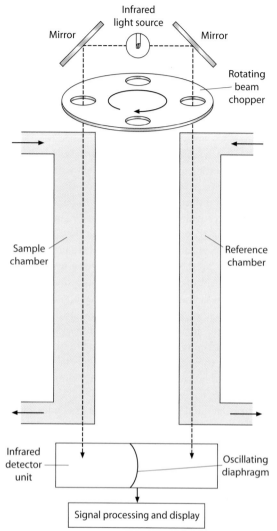

Figure 17.4 The principles of the infrared spectrophotometer.

absorption spectra of other IR absorbing agents, but by other non-IR absorbing carrier gases, such as helium, argon or hydrogen. It has been reported, for example, that in a gas mixture containing 79% helium in oxygen, an IR analyzer under-reads CO_2 values.[1] Desflurane,[2] cyclopropane,[3] acetone and alcohol[4] all produce errors in IR spectroscopy. There are electronic correction factors in the analyzers to allow for the presence of N_2O in the gas mix containing CO_2. Since water is a strong absorber of IR across the bandwidths of interest, it must be eliminated in the sampling process, in order to avoid some inaccuracy. If one wavelength is used for all volatile agent detection, then that agent must be selected manually, or the device

will be inaccurate, if either the wrong agent is selected or if there is a mixture of agents present. Some analyzers use the 10 to 13 μm bandwidth to detect volatile agents, where there is less chance for interference between absorption spectra.

Infrared spectroscopy detects numbers of molecules in a gas sample and thus constitutes a partial pressure analyzer. Therefore, error can be introduced if the pressure of the gas sample changes or if there is ambient pressure change, against which the device is calibrated. If the gas sample pressure changes due to back pressure from a ventilator, or if there is significantly low pressure in a sampling tube, the partial pressure of the gas being analyzed will change, without there being a real change in the fractional concentration of the gas. Similarly, if the device is calibrated at sea level and subsequently used at altitude, there will be an error in calculating gas concentration. Therefore, calibration should be carried out frequently and under the conditions of intended use, or the device should be calibrated to measure partial pressure rather than concentration.

The 90–95% response time of IR analyzers to a step change, including transit time and rise time, should be under 150 ms. Water vapour blocking the sampling tube sometimes causes the response time to increase. To deal with water vapour, most devices have either a water trap or use sample tubing, which absorbs water vapour. IR capnographs are accurate to about 0.1% in a range of CO_2 up to 10%.

A variant of the IR analyzer described above utilizes a combination of IR and photo-acoustic spectroscopy. In such a device, the chopper wheel contains three concentric rings of windows instead of one, that results in three different chopping or sampling rates for three different gas species CO_2, N_2O and volatile agent. This provides one means of allowing the software to differentiate the species. Each component of the chopped beam is then delivered through a separate narrow band optical filter, which allows through light of wavelength corresponding to the maximum absorption of the gas concerned. The components of the light beam then enter the sample chamber and the components of the IR light, now differentiated both by sampling frequency and wavelength, are absorbed by the gas molecules, which are caused to vibrate at different frequencies, leading to a set of audible, fluctuating pressure waves. The families of audible pressure waves are detectable by microphone. Figure 17.5 shows the Bruel and Kjaer model of the photo-acoustic IR spectroscope. Note that, since oxygen does not absorb

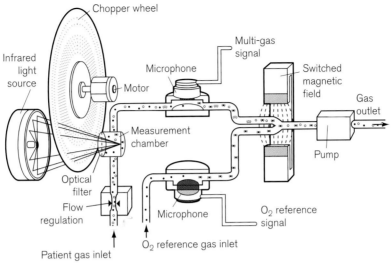

Figure 17.5 The components of the Bruel and Kjaer photo-acoustic and magneto-acoustic spectrophotometer.

IR light, this device uses magneto-acoustic spectroscopy for oxygen (see the section on Paramagnetic Oxygen Analyzers).

The signal from all gaseous components is taken from the microphone and filtered electronically into the four components of O_2, CO_2, N_2O and volatile agent. Separation and therefore gas identification occurs by audio frequency identification and quantification of the gas occurs by audio-amplitude. Note that the device does not distinguish between different volatile agents. The advantages of photo-acoustic IR spectroscopy over conventional IR spectroscopy include stability, zero drift, reduced need for calibration over prolonged periods and fast response time.

Mass spectrometry

Mass spectrometry identifies gas molecules by bombarding them with electrons (which converts them into charged particles) and separates them in a magnetic field according to the ratio of their mass and charge. The method can, therefore, identify and quantify all molecular species, providing there are no unexpected components in a gas mixture, such as the propellant in a bronchodilator or acetone in the expired breath of a diabetic. It is still considered to be the standard against which other gas monitoring techniques are compared, and is more frequently used as a laboratory technique than a clinical one. However, it was available for use as a time-shared, multi-site sampling device before the advent of cheaper IR spectroscopy. One example of a mass spectrometer is shown in Figure 17.6a. Essentially it has three stages: the first stage is where the sampled gas is drawn into a low-pressure chamber. In the second stage, which is the main part of the device, the sample is drawn into an ionization chamber by an even lower pressure (about 1 mmHg), where the gas molecules are bombarded with electrons. Finally they are drawn into a dispersion chamber, where they are influenced by a magnetic field. This third stage is where the deflected and separated beams of charged molecules are detected and the signal is processed and displayed.

In the vacuum chamber of the second stage of the device, the bombardment of the molecules, by a transverse beam of electrons, results in ionization of the molecule, usually to a single positive charge. The ions of the different molecular species then accelerate towards an electrically negatively-charged plate, the acceleration plate, and out through a small hole, *the molecular leak*, into the dispersion chamber. From here the path of the ions is influenced by a magnetic field. The ions are deflected according to mass, the lightest being deflected the most. The different species of gas are thus separated according to their mass:charge ratio. In the third stage, the ions reach the photo-voltaic detectors, where the rate of arrival of the ions is proportional to the partial pressure of the gas. The signal is processed, amplified and displayed.

Two different types of mass spectrometer exist, depending on the way in which the magnetic field is produced in the second stage and the mechanism of ion detection in the third stage.

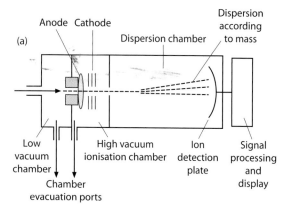

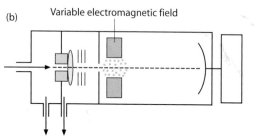

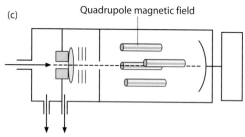

Figure 17.6 (a) Principles of a mass spectrometer. **(b)** Components of a magnetic sector mass spectrometer. **(c)** Components of the quadrupole mass spectrometer.

In the *magnetic sector mass spectrometer* (Fig. 17.6b), the magnetic field lies at right angles to the path of ions and is produced by a combination of electrical and fixed magnetic fields. By varying the voltage on the acceleration plate, the velocity of the ions entering the magnetic field can be changed. This allows the deflected ion beam to be directed across a single detector plate and different components to be detected in turn. It is, therefore, possible to separate components of the gas sample according to their mass:charge ratio.

More commonly seen these days, is the *quadrupole mass spectrometer*. This device is more compact and allows better discrimination between the ionic components from a gas mixture. The magnetic field is produced by a combination of DC electrical and AC radio frequency fields. As shown in Figure 17.6c, the quadrupoles consist of four rods with opposite pairs electrically connected. By careful tuning of the radio frequency component of the magnetic field, only ions of a given mass:charge ratio proceed through the quadrupole to the detector, all other ions oscillating and colliding with the device. By a combination of changing the voltage on the acceleration plate and of judiciously tuning the magnetic field, a spectrum of mass:charge components can be detected and quantified. By scanning at 50 Hz, it is possible to produce a continuous record of gas concentrations.

The respiratory mass spectrometer is accurate, giving good gas identification and quantification, requiring only 20 ml min^{-1} gas sampling rate, with a 100 ms response time. However, it does have some disadvantages. The second stage of the device operates under almost vacuum conditions; this requires a high-quality, continuously running pump. If the device itself is at some distance from the sampling site, as it used to be in the days of time-sharing of a single device, significant delay time may be added to the response time. Water condensation can be avoided by heating the sampling tube, but the response time for water vapour may still be longer than for other components.

Some molecule types may lose two electrons rather than one in the ionization process, and therefore become doubly charged ions rather than single. They then behave within the magnetic field like an ion with half the mass, which leads to confusion in interpretation. Furthermore, the ionization process can lead to fragmentation of a molecule, so that a mass spectrum appears at the output rather than a peak. However, this anomaly is useful to distinguish the gas components with the same molecular mass, which would otherwise be difficult to distinguish. These include N_2O and CO_2 (44 Da), or N_2 and CO (28 Da). N_2O is fragmented into NO, O_2, N_2, N and O, while CO_2 is fragmented into O_2, C_2, C and O. Rather than try to detect and distinguish both gases at 44 Da, N_2O can be detected at a subordinate peak of 30 Da and CO_2 at 12 Da. Because the fragmentation is predictable, the amplitude of the subsidiary peak can be used as a measure of the parent peak and, therefore, of gas concentration. Using appropriate low pass and high pass filters, obfuscating peaks in the spectra can be removed.

Raman spectroscopy

Rayleigh scattering refers to the scattering of light by particles of size up to one-tenth the wavelength of the

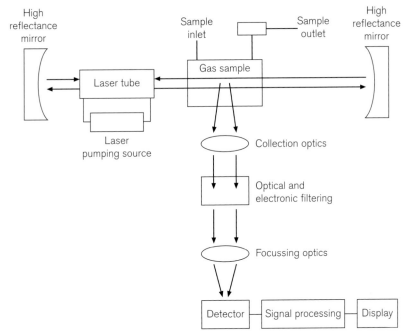

Figure 17.7 The components of the Raman spectroscope.

light and occurs without any loss of energy or change of wavelength. Being wavelength-dependent, this phenomenon gives us the blue sky because of the increased scattering of blue light. A small fraction of the incident light, about 10^{-6}, is scattered with a loss of energy and a change of wavelength characteristic of the molecule off which the light is being reflected; this is *Raman scattering*. Raman spectroscopy has been used in industry for years as a means of identifying solids, liquids and gases, but has had to await the advent of powerful laser light sources and sensitive photocell detectors to be useful in a clinical setting for breath-by-breath analysis.

Figure 17.7 shows a diagram of a Raman spectroscope, incorporating an Argon laser source of wavelength 485 nm, high reflectance mirrors to concentrate the laser beam, a gas sampling chamber, appropriate optics, a detection system, and microprocessor and display system. Table 17.1 shows characteristic wavelength or frequency changes, which identify different gases. If plotted graphically, the amplitudes of the frequency shifted peaks are proportional to the gas concentrations.

In Raman spectroscopy, each gas is independently analyzed, including CO_2, N_2O, volatile agents, O_2, N_2 and water vapour. This is done by first filtering out the Argon laser light at 485 nm, then passing the light through a system of optics to collect and focus the scattered low

Table 17.1 Frequency shifts in different gases detectable by Raman spectroscopy (N_2O and CO_2 give two characteristic frequency shifts).

Gas	Frequency shift Wave number (cm^{-1})
Isoflurane	995
Halothane	717
Enflurane	817
Nitrous oxide	1285, 2224
Carbon dioxide	1285, 1388
Oxygen	1555
Nitrogen	2331
Water	3650

level light, and through an electronic filtering system. The very low levels of light are then detected by a photomultiplier tube. The response time is 100 ms and the device is therefore capable of breath-by-breath analysis. The sample is not altered by the process and can therefore be returned to the breathing system, which is a significant advantage in low flow anaesthesia,[5] although there is some overlap between gas species.[6] However, the devices require a great deal of electrical power and are noisy.

The piezoelectric (Engstrom Emma) gas analyzer

A pair of piezoelectric crystals connected to an electrical power source is made to resonate, with a characteristic frequency difference. The frequency difference occurs because one of the crystals is coated in silicone oil, which absorbs a volatile anaesthetic agent to which it is exposed. This changes the natural frequency of the crystal, and the frequency difference between the crystals changes by an amount dependent on the amount of volatile agent absorbed. Manual identification of the agent is required, but the device is remarkably accurate and stable.[7]

The paramagnetic gas analyzer

Most gas molecules are repelled by a magnetic field and are, therefore, termed diamagnetic. Two gases, oxygen and nitric oxide, are attracted into the field and are termed paramagnetic. This property enables oxygen concentrations to be analyzed and is due to the presence of unpaired electrons in the outer shell of an oxygen molecule, which is able to generate force in a magnetic field. A paramagnetic oxygen analyzer of the original type is shown in Figure 17.8a. Two glass spheres, suspended between the poles of a magnetic field, are filled with nitrogen, a weakly diamagnetic gas. The glass spheres are arranged in a dumb-bell shape, suspended by a thread, tensioned to keep the dumb-bell in the plane of the magnetic field. Zeroing should be carried out in the carrier gas destined to have oxygen added to it at a later stage. When a gas mixture containing oxygen is drawn through the analyzer, oxygen is attracted into the magnetic field, displacing the nitrogen filled spheres away from it. The detection system can either be a deflection measurement (Fig. 17.8a) or a null deflection type (Fig. 17.8b), which measures the current required in the circuitry to restore the pointer to its null point. These devices are accurate to within 0.1% O_2, but are adversely affected by pressurization, vibration, water vapour and high flow rates; there is also a slow response time of up to one minute.

An analyzer has been developed to overcome these disadvantages (Fig. 17.9). A sample of gas to be measured is drawn continuously through one of two capillary tubes at the same rate as a reference gas sample (usually air) is drawn through the other. A powerful electromagnet, which produces a pulsed (on/off) magnetic field is placed

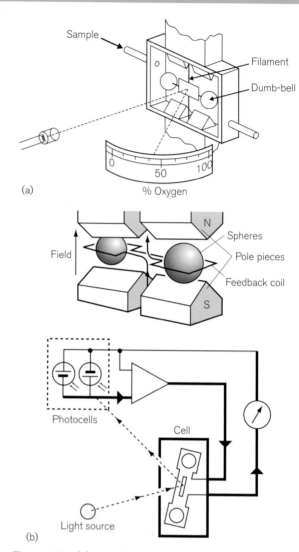

(a)

(b)

Figure 17.8 (a) A simple paramagnetic oxygen analyzer. **(b)** A null deflection paramagnetic oxygen analyzer (with permission from Kenny GNC, DavisPDD (2003) *Basic Physics and Measurement in Anaesthesia*, 5th edn. London: Butterworth Heinemann).

over the junction of the two tubes. The magnetic field, when switched on, attracts the oxygen from both tubes in proportion to their concentrations. This causes an intermittent differential reduction in pressure upstream in the tubes that is detected and measured by a pressure transducer, and can be calibrated so it displays oxygen concentration. This is the basis of the Datex paramagnetic oxygen analyzer.

The pulsed magnetic field may be replaced by an alternating one that has a frequency of 110 Hz. This produces

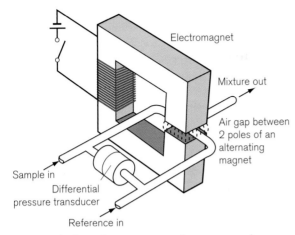

Figure 17.9 A modern paramagnetic oxygen analyzer.

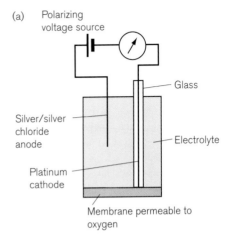

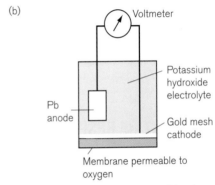

Figure 17.10 (a) The Clarke polarographic electrode. **(b)** The Galvanic fuel cell.

differential oscillating pressures of 20–50 μbar in the capillary tubes. The oscillations are transduced into a sound signal, the amplitude of which is directly proportional to the O_2 concentration in the sample. This is magneto-acoustic spectroscopy and forms the oxygen analyzing device in the Bruel and Kjaer gas analyzer.

It has been reported that a gas mixture containing Desflurane interferes with the accuracy of a paramagnetic oxygen analyzer.[8]

Fuel cells and polarographic cells

These techniques are used for analyzing oxygen and are included together, since they are similar electrochemical techniques.

The Clarke polarographic electrode is shown in Figure 17.10a. It consists of a cellophane covered platinum cathode and Ag/AgCl anode in a phosphate and KCl electrolyte, between which a potential difference of –0.6 V is applied by the battery as shown. At the cathode the following reaction takes place:

$$O_2 + 2H_2O + 4e^- \rightarrow 4OH^-$$

Electrons are provided by the cathode, to be consumed by the O_2 in the gas or blood sample. At the anode the following reactions take place:

$$4Ag \rightarrow 4Ag^+ + 4e^-$$
$$4Ag^+ + 4Cl^- \rightarrow 4AgCl$$

The rate of diffusion of oxygen into the electrolyte solution is a rate limited process, generating a current proportional to the pO_2 of the gas sample.

The problem with the polarographic electrode is the dependence on a battery and the reduction of any N_2O present at the cathode when it is contaminated by Ag^+ ions. A fuel cell is a similar device, which consists of a gold cathode and a lead anode (Fig. 17.10b). The same reaction occurs at the cathode as in the polarographic electrode. No polarizing voltage is required in this circuit. The fuel cell's response time is slow, making them acceptable but less suitable for breath by breath analysis than other methods.[9]

Nitric oxide measurement

Nitric Oxide (NO) is a pulmonary vasodilator and as such, has found its place in an intensive care environment. Since NO causes methaemoglobinaemia, it is important to be able to measure its concentration. Since nitrogen dioxide (NO_2) is a degradation product of NO and causes pulmonary oedema, it too must be detectable.

All industrial analyzers developed for NO analysis are designed for use in environmental control and, therefore, for gas mixtures containing 21% or less of oxygen. Medical gas mixtures frequently contain more oxygen than this and the accuracy of devices available is not guaranteed. The two methods available are the *chemoluminescent* and the *electrochemical* methods.[10]

The chemoluminescence analyzer is based on the reaction of NO with ozone (O_3) in a chamber to produce energized NO_2 molecules, which emit photons of light in the range 590–2600 nm. The amount of light emitted is proportional to the original concentration of NO. In a parallel system there is a catalytic converter before the reaction chamber to reduce NO_2 in the sample to NO. The total oxides of nitrogen are then measured as NO and the difference in the two readings is the NO_2 concentration.

The electrochemical analyzer generates a potential difference proportional to the NO_2 concentration. This is due to the migration of ions generated from the reaction between NO or NO_2 and the electrolyte. A separate cell is used for NO and NO_2.

MEASUREMENT OF RESPIRATORY VOLUMES

Measurement of respiratory volumes is carried out by one of a number of techniques, most of which involve integration of flow measurement. These include hot wire anemometry, ultrasonic detection of flow vortices, and venturi flow measurement. Devices for volume measurement, which can be considered not to be flow integration techniques, include a turbine respirometer (Wright's) and the positive displacement volume meter (Dräger). The principles of these techniques are discussed in Chapter 4.

BLOOD GAS ANALYSIS

Although it is now possible to continuously measure oxygen saturation with pulse oximetry, mixed venous oxygen saturation, and even pO_2, pCO_2 and pH with intravascular electrodes, it is still much more common to measure these variables by *in vitro* blood gas analysis.

The blood gas analyzer needs a very small, heparinized blood sample, 100–300 μl, and the blood is passed through four electrodes simultaneously in a temperature stabilized cuvette, shown in Figure 17.11. The electrodes measure the partial pressure of dissolved oxygen using a Clarke electrode, carbon dioxide using a Severinghaus electrode and pH with a conventional glass electrode; the fourth electrode is a reference electrode. Such a blood gas analyzer frequently measures Hb and some biochemistry as well.[10] Derived values from such a device include O_2 saturation, O_2 content, bicarbonate, base excess and total CO_2.

The Clarke polarographic electrode for measuring pO_2 has been described in the section above on gas analyzers and is suitable for both respiratory and blood O_2 analysis. The membrane is designed to allow only oxygen to cross it, rather than blood.

pH electrode

A *pH unit*, which is the measure of hydrogen ion activity in a liquid, is defined in as:

$$pH = \log_{10} \frac{1}{[H^+]}$$

In words, this can be described as 'the negative logarithm, to base ten, of the hydrogen ion concentration'.

The physical principle, on which the pH electrode is based, depends on the fact that when a membrane separates two solutions of different $[H^+]$, a potential difference exists across the membrane. In a pH electrode, the membrane is made of glass and the development of a potential difference between the two solutions is thought to be due to the migration of H^+ into the glass matrix. If one solution consists of a standard $[H^+]$, the pH of the other solution can be estimated by measurement of the potential difference between them. The glass membrane used is selectively permeable to H^+. No current flows in this device, which therefore does not wear out, in contrast to the Clarke electrode, in which current does flow and which does need periodic replacement.

The pH measurement system is shown diagrammatically in Figure 17.12, and consists of two half electrochemical cells. It has, in one half, an Ag/AgCl electrode and in the other, a Hg/HgCl$_2$ (calomel) electrode. Each electrode maintains a fixed electrical potential. The Ag/AgCl electrode is surrounded by a buffer solution of known pH, surrounded by the pH sensitive glass. Outside the glass membrane is the test solution, usually blood, whose pH is to be measured. It is the potential difference across the glass, between these two solutions, which is variable. The blood or other solution is separated from the calomel electrode by a porous plug and a potassium chloride salt bridge to minimize KCl diffusion. The

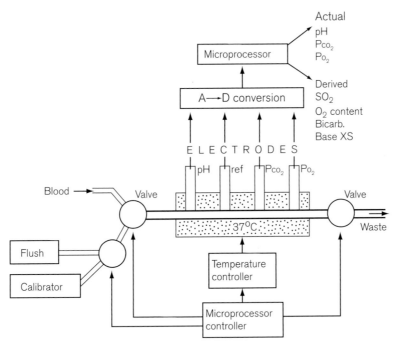

Figure 17.11 The components of a blood gas analyzer.

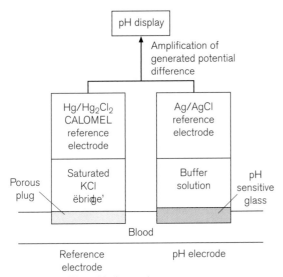

Figure 17.12 The pH electrode.

potential difference across the system is about 60 mV per unit of pH change at 37°C. The internal electrical resistance is high and in order to maximize the device's accuracy, a voltmeter (or other measuring device) of very high internal resistance must be used to minimize current drawn from the system.

The pH electrode actually responds to hydrogen ion activity rather than hydrogen ion concentration. These two variables coincide at infinite dilution of solution, but might otherwise differ, because of molecular interaction between ionic species. The electrode is therefore calibrated against standard buffer solutions of pH 6.841 and 7.383.

The glass of which the pH sensitive electrode is made consists of 72% SiO_2, 22% Na_2O and 6% CaO.

The Severinghaus pCO₂ electrode

There is a dynamic equilibrium between H^+ and CO_2. The *Henderson–Hasselbalch* equation describes this relationship:

$$pH = pK_a + \log_{10} \frac{[HCO_3^-]}{[H_2CO_3]}$$

$$= pK_a + \frac{\log_{10}[HCO_3^-]}{\alpha\, pCO_2}$$

where α is the Ostwald solubility coefficient, 0.003 mmol L^{-1} mmHg^{-1} at 37°C. pK_a, the association constant of the chemical reaction concerned is 6.1. Both α and pK_a vary with pH and thus lend the calculation some inaccuracy. It was Astrup who noticed that there was a linear relationship between pH and pCO_2.

The pCO_2 electrode is essentially a pH electrode with a difference. The sensitive glass membrane is covered with another membrane, which is selectively permeable to CO_2. In the original design, a layer of water was trapped between the two membranes, allowing the reaction described above to occur. A later modification had salt and bicarbonate solution in this space (Fig. 17.13). A pCO_2 electrode, therefore, allows a pCO_2 change to generate a pH change, which is measured by the electrode.

Derived variables from a blood gas machine

Buffer base is the sum of all bases in the blood capable of buffering pH changes. These include HCO_3^-, Hb, PO_4^{3-} and the anionic parts of protein. A respiratory driven change in status, marked by, for example, the addition of CO_2, results in the formation of carbonic acid, which produces H^+ and HCO_3^-. The hydrogen ions are buffered by the total buffer base, namely (HCO_3^- + Hb^- + PO_4^{3-} + $Protein^-$).

The buffer base can be considered to be a limitless source of buffering capacity, unless the haemoglobin component is significantly reduced. The base excess, an indication of metabolic rather than respiratory acid-base disturbance, is defined as the amount of titratable acid required to correct a blood sample to a pH of 7.40 at a pCO_2 of 5.3 kPa and at 37°C.

Standard bicarbonate is the bicarbonate in a fully oxygenated blood sample at a pCO_2 of 5.3 kPa and at 37°C.

Errors in blood gas measurement include:
- air bubbles in the sample;
- excess heparin;
- gas storage in container plastic walls;
- failure to store samples at low temperature;

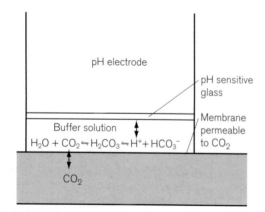

Figure 17.13 A pCO_2 electrode.

- metabolism in the sample
- signal processing errors
- at the O_2 electrode:
  - O_2 consumption in a Clark electrode
  - material used in electrode membrane
  - polarizing voltage
- at the pH electrode:
  - protein deposition on the electrode

Temperature and blood gas analysis

Blood gas analyzers measure blood gas variables at 37°C. A fall in body temperature means that CO_2 is more soluble in blood and that CO_2 production slows, leading to a fall in pCO_2. This shifts the O_2 dissociation curve to the left, increasing the O_2 content. However, O_2 solubility also rises, decreasing pO_2 and O_2 content. pH increases with a fall in temperature. Hypothermia itself does not alter the blood gas values at 37°C and arterial blood taken at lower temperatures should be corrected to 37°C before clinical decisions are made on the results.[12]

Other ion selective electrodes

By carefully selecting the proportions of constituents in the glass, glass ion-selective electrodes can be constructed for detection of other ions. For example, a glass electrode for measuring Na^+ concentrations consists of 71% SiO_2, 18% Al_2O_3 and 11% Na_2O. The K^+ sensitive glass electrode consists of 69% SiO_2, 4% Al_2O_3 and 27% Na_2O.

Transcutaneous blood gas analyzers

pO_2 can be measured transcutaneously by applying a Clarke polarographic electrode to the skin. If the skin is 'arterialized' by heating it, a reasonable value for pO_2 can be obtained. A modified pCO_2 electrode is used to measure transcutaneous pCO_2. A common O_2/CO_2 permeable membrane and electrolyte solution is used, ensuring a common pH for both measurements. Actual measured values do not correlate well with arterial values, but trends are clinically useful and these devices are used particularly in neonatology and when patients are ventilated outside the intensive care setting where arterial blood gas sampling is problematic. Care must be taken to avoid burns due to the heated electrodes.

Intravascular blood gas analyzers

These are microminiaturized versions of the devices described above.

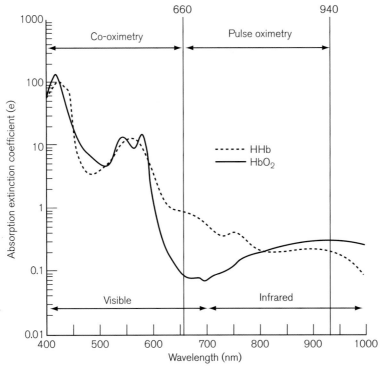

Figure 17.14 Absorption spectra for reduced and oxygenated haemoglobin showing the range of operation of a co-oximeter and of a pulse oximeter.

The co-oximeter

The co-oximeter is usually considered alongside the blood gas analyzer. The co-oximeter measures the fractional oxygen saturation of haemoglobin, taking account of the numerous different species of haemoglobin present in the blood, such as reduced Hb (HHb), oxygenated Hb (HbO), methaemaoglobin (MetHb), sulphaemoglobin and caorboxyhaemoglobin (COHb). The co-oximeter is a spectroscope, which therefore needs four or five different wavelengths to distinguish these different species. The Beer–Lambert law relating to light absorption is more closely adhered to than the pulse oximeter, which measures functional oxygen saturation, using only two wavelengths of light, and assumes the sample only contains reduced and oxygenated haemoglobin.

A small sample, 200–400 µl, of heparinized blood is injected into a cuvette of known path length. The red blood cells are disrupted by ultrasound or a soap solution, releasing free haemoglobin. Conventional spectroscopy then takes place on the sample at up to 17 wavelengths, which are produced either by a filter wheel with multiple narrow band filters, or by scanning with a diffraction grating or a prism. Figure 17.14 shows the spectrum covered by a co-oximeter as well as that covered by a pulse oximeter. The result is usually available within 30 seconds and includes SO_2 %, total haemoglobin (Hb) concentration, oxygen content, methaemoglobin (MetHb) %, sulphaemoglobin %, carboxyhaemoglobin (COHb) %. Some devices are capable of distinguishing foetal haemoglobin (HbF). As Figure 17.14 shows, the pulse oximeter and the co-oximeter operate in different spectra and therefore, strictly speaking, SO_2 and SpO_2 should not be compared.

REFERENCES

1. Ball JAS, Grounds RM (2003) Calibration of three capnographs for use with helium and oxygen mixtures. *Anaesthesia* **58**: 156–160.
2. Scheeren TWC, *et al.* (1998) Error in measurement of oxygen and carbon dioxide concentrations by the Deltatec II metabolic monitor in the presence of desflurane. *British Journal of Anaesthesia* **80**: 521–524.
3. Mason DG, Lloyd-Thomas AR(1991) Cyclopropane and the Datex Capnomac. *Anaesthesia* **46**: 398–399.
4. Foley MA, *et al.* (1990) The effect of exhaled alcohol on

the performance of the Datex Capnomac. *Anaesthesia* 45: 232–234.

5. Lockwood GG, London MJ, Chakrabarti MK, Whitwam JG (1994) The Ohmeda Rascal II. A new gas analyser for anaesthetic use. *Anaesthesia* **49**: 44–53.

6. Lawson D, Samanta S, Magee PT, Gregonis DE (1993) Gas monitoring in the OR: stability and long term durability of Raman spectroscopy. *Journal of Clinical Monitoring* 9: 241–251.

7. Humphrey SJE, Luff NP, White DC (1991) Evaluation of the Lamtec anaesthetic agent monitor. *Anaesthesia* 46: 478–481.

8. Scheeren TWC, *et al.* (1998) Error in measurement of oxygen and carbon dioxide concentrations by the Deltatec II metabolic monitor in the presence of desflurane. *British Journal of Anaesthesia* 80: 521–524.

9. Roe PG, Tyler CKG, Tennant R, Barnes PK (1987) Oxygen analysers. Evaluation of five models. *Anaesthesia* 42: 175–181.

10. Etches PC, Harris ML, McLinley R, Finer NM (1995) Clinical Monitoring of inhaled nitric oxide: comparison chemoluminescent and electrochemical sensors. *Biomedical Instrumentation and Technology* **29**: 131–140.

11. King R, Campbell A (2000) Performance of the Radiometer OSM 3 and ABL 505 blood gas analysers for the determination of Na, K, and Hb concentrations. *Anaesthesia* **55**: 65–69.

12. Rupp SM, Severinghaus J (1986) 'Hypothermia', In: Mipler R *Anesthesia*, 2nd edn, Ch. 57. New York: Churchill Livingstone. p. 2000.

FURTHER READING

Sykes MK (1982) 'The determination of pH'. In: Scurr C, Feldman S. *Scientific Foundations, Anaesthesia*, 3rd edn, Ch. 9. London: Heinemann. pp. 108–114.

Hutton P, Hahn C, Clutton-Brock TH (1994). Gas and Vapour Analysis. In: Hutton P, Prys-Roberts C. *Monitoring in Anaesthesia and Intensive Care*, Ch. 13. London: WB Saunders Co. Ltd, pp. 194–203.

18

Monitoring of cardiovascular and coagulation systems

Robert Sekun Kong and Nilesh Nanavati

Many anaesthetic drugs adversely affect the cardiovascular system to some degree. This response is often exacerbated by pre-existing medical or surgical conditions. Failure to take account of all of these may lead to irreversible organ dysfunction in the perioperative period. Monitoring the efficiency of the cardiovascular system and taking therapeutic steps to improve its function has become an essential part of high-quality anaesthesia. In the past, non-invasive measurements of parameters such as blood pressure and pulse gave some indirect information as to cardiovascular status. However, it is now recognized that inferences of cardiac output made from these measurements can be wildly inaccurate. Newer methods of assessing and optimizing cardiovascular function have been developed that allow vastly improved therapeutic intervention by anaesthetists in the perioperative period. Some of these are discussed below.

Blood loss at operation may also affect cardiac output and, particularly in combination with any resultant severe anaemia, may also lead to irreversible organ dysfunction. Early detection of coagulation abnormalities with 'bedside apparatus' may prevent this.

PULMONARY ARTERY CATHETER

Introduced over 30 years ago, the pulmonary artery flotation catheter (PAC) has been the most commonly used technique for cardiac output (CO) measurement at the bedside. The standard PAC is a balloon-tipped multi-lumen catheter, 110 cm in length and 7 or 7.5 French in external diameter, depending on the model. The distal lumen is used to monitor pulmonary artery pressure. More proximal lumens are used for central venous pressure measurement and administration of fluids and drugs. A rapid-response thermistor located near the tip of the PAC allows temperature measurement.

The catheter is inserted via an 8.5 French introducer sheath into the internal jugular, subclavian or femoral vein. After inflating the balloon with air (1.5 ml), the PAC is advanced with continuous monitoring of pressures transduced from the distal lumen (Fig. 18.1a). The location of the PAC tip, as it traverses the right atrium, right ventricle and pulmonary artery, is indicated by the typical pressures in these structures (Fig. 18.1b). The catheter is advanced beyond the main pulmonary artery until it is wedged in one of the medium-sized branches to measure the pulmonary artery wedge pressure (PAWP), which under normal circumstances is an estimate of left ventricular end diastolic pressure and reflects left ventricular end diastolic volume. The balloon must be deflated as soon as the PAWP measurement is completed, to minimize the risk of causing pulmonary ischemia. Successful passage of the catheter into the pulmonary artery is usually dependent on an adequate blood flow (i.e. cardiac output).

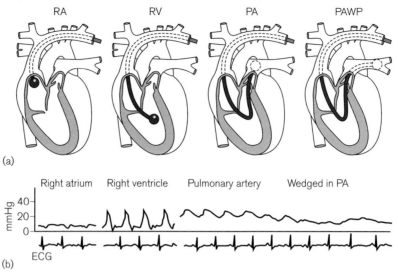

Figure 18.1 **(a)** Catheter advancing through right heart chambers and **(b)** corresponding pressures in right atrium (RA), right ventricle (RV), pulmonary artery (PA) and wedged (PAWP).

Cardiac output and other measurements

The original method of measuring cardiac output was proposed by Fick in 1870. His principle states that in a steady state, the amount of substance taken up by an organ (e.g. the lungs) in unit time is equal to its arterial concentration (i.e. amount going to the lungs) minus its venous concentration (i.e. amount leaving the lungs) multiplied by the blood flow. If the amount of substance is known and the two concentrations can be measured, then the unknown variable, the blood flow, can be calculated. The principle is also valid in non-steady states but the calculations are complex and require a computer. A non-steady state may be created, for example, by injecting a known volume of cold saline into the bloodstream and measuring its cooling effect (thermodilution) on the blood at a point downstream.

Cardiac output measurement by the PAC is based on the principle of thermodilution. A known quantity of cold saline or 5% dextrose solution is injected into the proximal port of the catheter. The temperature change in blood caused by the cold injectate flowing past the thermistor is measured and plotted against time. The shape of the curve produced is determined by the cardiac output. Low output states have a larger temperature change, with a longer delay from the time of injection. The thermistor is connected directly to a cardiac output computer (or CO module of a patient monitor), which displays the calculated cardiac output, together with the average of several readings and allows rejection of outlying values.

Variations of the standard catheter, with revised analysis software, have resulted in catheters with enhanced monitoring capabilities. Oximetric catheters contain a fibreoptic cable and permit continuous measurement of mixed venous oxygen saturation (SvO_2). Catheters that incorporate a microfilament heating element use a modified thermodilution principle to measure CO continuously, though not 'beat to beat' as the value is averaged over the previous 3–5 minute interval. Nevertheless, this makes the technique more convenient and less prone to operator-dependent errors when compared to intermittent measurement. Data from the continuous CO catheter can be synchronized with the electrocardiogram to obtain right ventricular stroke volume, right ventricular end-diastolic volume, and calculate right ventricular ejection fraction.

Limitations

Despite these advances, the PAC has several fundamental limitations, some of which are:

1. invasive procedure with risks of arterial puncture and haemorrhage;
2. the indwelling introducer sheath and PAC are potential causes of sepsis and thrombus formation;
3. the catheter may cause arrhythmias;
4. cardiac output measurement may be inaccurate in

the presence of intracardiac shunts or tricuspid insufficiency; and

5. PAWP may be an unreliable indicator of left ventricular preload.

Other cardiac output measurement techniques

In recent years, doubts have been raised over the true clinical benefits of PAC monitoring perioperatively and in the intensive care unit. Reduction in mortality cannot be demonstrated in patients managed with the PAC. This has contributed to the growing interest in less invasive techniques of CO measurement, such as oesophageal Doppler and arterial pulse contour analysis. These devices demonstrate an acceptable level of agreement for CO measurement compared to the PAC.

OESOPHAGEAL DOPPLER METHOD FOR MEASUREMENT OF CARDIAC OUTPUT

The oesophageal Doppler monitor measures blood flow velocity in the descending thoracic aorta. A flexible probe, with an ultrasound transducer mounted at the distal tip, is inserted into the oesophagus via the mouth or nose. Three oesophageal Doppler devices that utilize similar principles are commercially available: CardioQ (Deltex Medical, UK), Hemosonic (Arrow International, USA) and TECO (Medicina, UK). The description below is based on the CardioQ and key differences from the other devices are mentioned.

Doppler effect

Detection of blood flow in the descending aorta is based on the Doppler effect. That is, the frequency of sound waves reflected from or emitted by a moving object is altered proportionately to the relative velocity between the object and the observer. When the observer and object are moving towards each other, the perceived frequency is higher than the emitted frequency, but lower if they are moving apart.

In the oesophageal Doppler devices, ultrasound of a known frequency (Fe) transmitted by the monitoring probe is backscattered by red cells travelling in the descending aorta and returns to the transducer at a slightly different, lower, frequency. The difference – the Doppler shift or frequency (F) – is proportional to the velocity of blood flow (V) and other factors as seen in the equation:

$$V = \frac{CF}{2FeCos\phi}$$

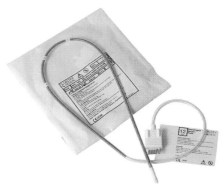

Figure 18.2 Doppler Probe (CardioQ). Note the flexible probe shaft, three depth markers and patient interface connector.

Where:

V	Velocity of red blood cells (blood flow)
C	Speed of ultrasound travelling through biological tissues
F	Doppler frequency shift
Fe	Emitted frequency from ultrasound device
Cosϕ	cosine of angle (ϕ) between the sound beam axis and the direction of blood flow (angle of insonation)

Doppler probe

The oesophageal Doppler probe of the CardioQ (Fig. 18.2) consists of a 55 cm length of steel spring and a piezo-electric crystal assembly (4 MHz continuous wave) mounted at the distal end. This whole is encased in silicone rubber, giving an outer tip diameter of 6.3 mm (19 French). The 45° bevel of the distal tip defines the angle of insonation (relative to the axis of blood flow in the aorta) in most patients. The probe ends proximally in an asymmetric connector that contains a memory device and connects to the monitor via an electrically isolated 'Patient Interface Cable'. The design of the Doppler probe allows it to be longitudinally flexible yet torsionally rigid, which permits rotation of the transducer at the distal tip by manipulating the probe from the proximal end. Markers on the probe indicating 35, 40 and 45 cm from the distal end are used to guide the initial depth of probe insertion via the mouth (35–40cm) or nose (40–45 cm).

There are several variants of Doppler probe for use with the CardioQ. The essential difference between the single-use, adult probes is the 6, 12 or 240 hours monitoring time limit allowed by the memory device. The 6- and 12-hour probes are aimed primarily for use in the operating room, while the 240-hour probe is for monitoring in critical care units. The Awake Doppler Probe, with a more flexible design, is for nasal insertion in the awake patient. The Paediatric Doppler Probe is currently suitable for use in paediatric patients above 15 kg in weight.

Probe insertion

The lubricated probe is inserted into the oesophagus using the depth markers as an initial guide. After connection to the monitor and input of patient data, the aortic signal is found by a combination of rotation and slight advancement or withdrawal of the probe. The optimal signal is obtained by attention to both the visual and audio characteristics of the spectral display.

The TECO probe and larger Hemosonic probes are not single-use and therefore must be covered with a disposable sterile jacket filled with acoustic gel. The Hemosonic device uses pulsed wave Doppler and M mode ultrasound, the latter to locate and measure the diameter of the descending aorta.

Signal acquisition and monitor

Flow signals acquired by the probe are processed by Fast Fourier Transform (FFT) and represented on the monitor as a spectral display of the distribution of red blood cell flow velocities (vertical axis) against time (horizontal axis). Descending aortic blood flow is shown as a positive deflection and is approximately triangular in shape. Correct identification of the descending aortic waveform is a prerequisite for oesophageal Doppler monitoring. Note that blood flow in the descending aorta occurs predominantly during systole; there is minimal forward flow in diastole. Ideally, the aortic waveform should appear as a triangular waveform with the 'brightness' confined to the peripheral edge and an absence of signal in the central region of the triangle (Fig. 18.3). This type of waveform is characteristic of a plug flow profile (present in the descending aorta) with a narrow spread of red cell velocities. Turbulent flow or unsatisfactory orientation of the transducer towards the descending aorta would show evidence of spectral dispersion (Fig. 18.4).

Signals from other vessels (e.g. pulmonary artery, celiac artery, azygous vein) may be encountered, although these are significantly different in appearance from the descending aortic waveform.

Speakers transmit the associated Doppler frequency, which is in the audible range. The two rotary controls on the CardioQ (Fig. 18.5) adjust the volume of the audio

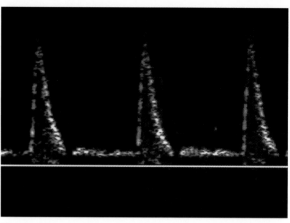

Figure 18.3 Ideal aortic waveform. The brightness of the signal is on the periphery of the waveform.

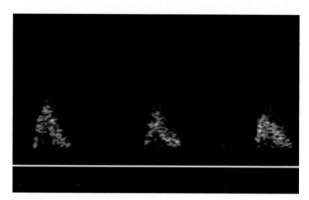

Figure 18.4 Unsatisfactory aortic waveform. This waveform shows spectral dispersion (see text).

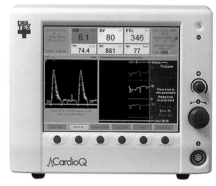

Figure 18.5 The CardioQ monitor.

Table 18.1 Adult and paediatric nomogram limits in the CardioQ

	Adult	**Paediatric**
Age (years)	16–99	0–15
Weight (kg)	30–150	15–60
Height (cm)	149–212	50–170

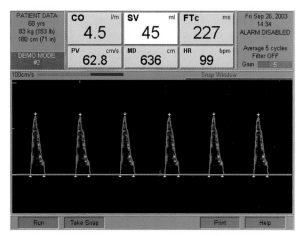

Figure 18.6 Characteristic waveform obtained from a hypovolemic patient: shortened flow time and low stroke volume.

output and amplify the signal (gain) or navigate through the menu options.

Cardiac output measurement by oesophageal Doppler

The patient's age, weight and height are entered in the monitor and stored in the memory of each new probe. This nomogram produces a calibration constant used to convert flow velocity measurement to a volumetric total CO estimation, inferences being made for blood flow to the upper limbs and head and neck. Note that the cross sectional area of the descending aorta necessary to convert flow velocity to volume is derived from a nomogram or 'look-up table' based on the patient's age, weight and height. The algorithm has been validated in adult and paediatric populations and thus allows CO measurements to be made in a wide age range. Analysis of other parameters of the waveform, such as 'corrected Flow Time' (FTc), 'Peak Velocity' (PV), and 'Mean Acceleration' (MA) are useful indicators of left ventricular preload, afterload and contractility. CardioQ adult and paediatric nomogram limits are given in Table 18.1.

The TECO measures CO using a similar algorithm in adults. The Hemosonic differs significantly in that the algorithm relies on measurement of aortic diameter by M mode ultrasound.

Oesophageal Doppler parameters

In addition to Cardiac Output (CO) and Stroke Volume (SV), the CardioQ can display these values indexed to body surface area (Cardiac Index and Stroke Volume Index). Other key parameters are detailed below.

Corrected Flow Time (FTc)

Flow time (FT) is the duration of blood flow in the descending aorta resulting from each cardiac ejection. It is indicated by two white triangles at the base of each waveform (Fig. 18.6). Flow occurs in systole, which occupies approximately one-third of the cardiac cycle. Corrected flow time is inversely related to heart rate and also affected by left ventricular (LV) preload and afterload. Corrected flow time (FTc) indexes the measured FT to a heart rate of 60 bpm and thereby permits interpretation of the influence of loading conditions on FT independent of heart rates. At a heart rate of 60 bpm, the cycle time is 1 second and the corresponding FT is therefore approximately one-third of 1 second. In similar manner to adjusting the time interval between ECG waves according to the prevailing heart rate (e.g. "corrected QT" instead of the QT interval), Bazett's formula is use to calculate FTc from FT. Thus FTc is obtained from FT divided by the square root of the cycle time (RR interval). The normal FTc is taken as 330–360 msec.

$$FTc = \frac{FT}{\sqrt{Cycle - time}}$$

A low FTc (<330 msec) is seen in hypovolaemia, decreased LV preload states due to major circulatory 'obstruction' (e.g. pulmonary embolus or isolated right ventricular failure). A low FTc may also reflect an elevated LV afterload, as may occur with significant peripheral vasoconstriction (Fig. 18.6). A prolonged FTc (>360 msec) is seen with decreased LV afterload, such as in a vasodilated circulation (e.g. sepsis, epidural anaesthesia) (Fig. 18.7).

Peak Velocity (PV)

The Peak Velocity is the highest velocity of descending aortic flow, indicated by the white arrow at the top of the waveform (see Figs. 18.6 and 18.7). Peak velocity

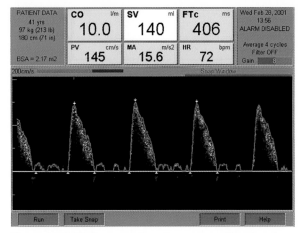

Figure 18.7 Typical waveform from a vasodilated patient: increased stroke volume and flow time longer than 360 ms.

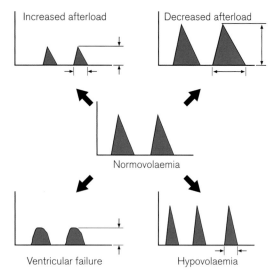

Figure 18.8 Predominant changes observed in the aortic waveform due to alterations in preload, afterload and contractility.

Table 18.2 Peak velocity decreases with age	
Age (years)	**Peak Velocity (cm/s)**
20	90–120
50	70–100
70	50–80

decreases linearly with age, as it is affected by LV contractility, which also declines with age. Peak Velocity is affected by LV preload (low preload = low PV) and afterload (high afterload = low PV). The normal ranges for peak velocity are shown in Table 18.2. An erroneous, low peak velocity may be recorded if the angle of insonation is significantly greater than 45°. This may occur in the presence of an abnormal anatomical relationship between the axes of the oesophagus and thoracic aorta.

Mean Acceleration (MA)

The Mean Acceleration is the average rate of change of velocity of blood flow from the start until the time at peak velocity. Mean Acceleration reflects LV contractility, but is also affected by changes in afterload and, to a lesser extent, preload.

Changes in contractility and loading tend to produce a predominant change in peak velocity or flow time. These are indicated in Figure 18.8.

Limitations

Readjustment of probe position, to ensure optimal aortic

waveform, is usually required before each measurement. The presence of air or other devices (e.g. nasogastric tube) in the oesophagus may interfere with signal acquisition. Cardiac output monitoring is unreliable or impossible in some conditions: aortic dissection (turbulent flow and interference due to the intimal flap), coarctation, during cross clamping of descending aorta, or concurrent intra-aortic balloon pump. Pharyngo-oesophageal pathology is a relative contraindication for the use of oesophageal Doppler monitoring.

PULSE CONTOUR ANALYSIS

Left ventricular ejection leads to an increase in aortic pressure during systole. As the magnitude of the increase is determined by stroke volume and aortic compliance, relative changes in cardiac output (CO) can be monitored by analysis of the arterial pressure waveform – the pulse contour. To obtain an accurate CO, this method has to be calibrated with reference to CO measured by a validated technique.

The PiCCO (Pulsion Medical Systems, Germany) and LiDCO™ Plus (LiDCO Ltd, UK), are both CO monitors based on pulse contour analysis, but differ in the mathematical modelling for stroke volume calculation and the reference technique used for CO calibration. Neither requires the insertion of a pulmonary artery catheter.

PiCCO

The PiCCO uses a 5 French, 20 cm proprietary cannula to monitor arterial pressure and temperature in the femoral, brachial or axillary artery. For calibration purposes, CO is measured by intermittent transpulmonary thermodilution. Cold saline or 5% dextrose solution is injected as a bolus via a central venous catheter. Cardiac output is calculated from the thermodilution curve obtained by measurement of temperature change at the arterial cannula. The reference CO is used to calibrate the pulse contour data and obtain the pulse contour-derived cardiac output (PCCO), as shown (Fig. 18.9). The displayed PCCO is the mean value of the previous 12 seconds. The manufacturer recommends that a CO calibration is performed every 8 hours.

LiDCO™

In the LiDCO™ device, the pulse contour analysis is calibrated with CO obtained by lithium dilution. A 2 ml bolus of lithium chloride (0.15%) is injected into a peripheral or central vein. Blood is then drawn from a peripheral artery at a constant rate by a battery-operated peristaltic pump. Lithium concentration is measured by allowing the sample past an ion selective (here lithium-sensitive) electrode. The voltage response of the electrode is related to the change in lithium concentration and from this a lithium concentration-time curve can be plotted. Cardiac output is calculated, as with any indicator dilution method, from the initial dose of lithium and the area under the lithium concentration-time curve.

The LiDCO™ Plus haemodynamic monitor is connected to the bedside monitor via a standard analogue output. Thus, the arterial waveform is slaved from the existing arterial transducer system. The LiDCO™ can, therefore, be used with any arterial cannula and a peripheral or central venous catheter.

The lithium selective sensor is primed with saline and connected via a three-way tap to the arterial line. The internal wick, now soaked in saline, makes the electrical connection between the blood in the cell and the remote reference external electrode. The electrode flow past assembly is connected to a blood collection bag, and this tubing, also primed with saline, is placed in a peristaltic pump, which controls the flow of arterial blood past the sensor (Fig. 18.10). A cable connects the sensor via an interface to the LiDCO™ monitor using a USB port.

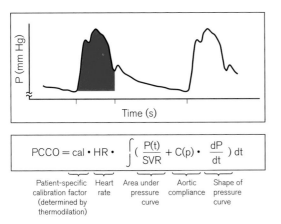

$$PCCO = cal \cdot HR \cdot \int (\frac{P(t)}{SVR} + C(p) \cdot \frac{dP}{dt}) \, dt$$

Patient-specific calibration factor (determined by thermodilation) · Heart rate · Area under pressure curve · Aortic compliance · Shape of pressure curve

Figure 18.9 Cardiac output calculation in the PiCCO. PCCO = pulse contour cardiac output, SVR = systemic vascular resistance.

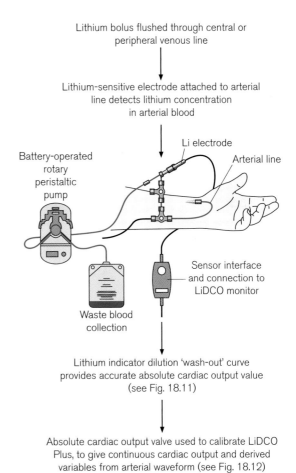

Lithium bolus flushed through central or peripheral venous line

Lithium-sensitive electrode attached to arterial line detects lithium concentration in arterial blood

Li electrode

Battery-operated rotary peristaltic pump

Arterial line

Waste blood collection

Sensor interface and connection to LiDCO monitor

Lithium indicator dilution 'wash-out' curve provides accurate absolute cardiac output value (see Fig. 18.11)

Absolute cardiac output valve used to calibrate LiDCO Plus, to give continuous cardiac output and derived variables from arterial waveform (see Fig. 18.12)

Figure 18.10 The set up for the LiDCO™ Plus Haemodynamic Monitor (see also Figs 18.11 and 18.12).

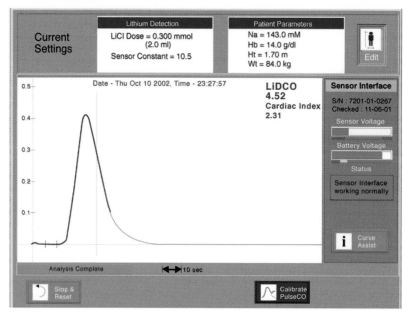

Figure 18.11 LiDCO™ Plus Haemodynamic Monitor display of the CO value, which is used to calibrate the waveform analysis.

A 4.5 ml volume length of tubing (the 'Park and Ride') is primed with saline and connected to the venous side. A 2 ml bolus of lithium chloride (0.15%) is 'parked' (injected into the Park and Ride) and a 15 ml flush attached. This ensures that all of the lithium is delivered to the patient promptly on injection of the flush. Blood is then drawn from a peripheral artery by pushing the red tension levers together on the pump. Once blood is seen at the internal part of the electrode, the levers are released and the pump switched on. Once the baseline voltage of the sensor stabilizes, which generally takes about 5–15 seconds, the lithium is flushed into the patient. A CO value is then displayed, which is used to calibrate the waveform analysis (PulseCO) (Fig. 18.11). The PulseCO software in the monitor uses power analysis of the arterial waveform to observe changes in cardiac output. Calibrated real time values of CO (averaged over a chosen number of cardiac cycles) and derived values, are shown in a number of displays that are designed to indicate the hemodynamic status of the patient (Fig. 18.12).

Preload responsiveness is assessed using stroke volume variation in the arterial waveform display. Response to fluid administration can be seen by observing changes in the stroke volume display.

The principal limitations of both pulse contour analysis devices are the requirement for and potential problems associated with arterial and venous cannulation. Signifi-cant distortion of the arterial waveform due to kinking or occlusion of the cannula will affect the accuracy of CO measurement. Intermittent recalibration with the reference CO method is necessary. The LiDCO device cannot be used in patients on lithium therapy or immediately following the administration of non-depolarizing muscle relaxants the metabolites of which interfere with the lithium estimation. Long-acting agents have an affect for 20 minutes – short-acting agents for up to 2 hours. The way around the problem is to paralyze the patient after calibration.

Intracardiac shunts will also introduce errors in any CO measurement that relies on an indicator dilution principle.

THROMBOELASTOGRAPHY

Thromboelastography evaluates the hemostatic capacity of blood by measuring the mechanical strength of the clot during clot formation. In contrast to traditional tests of blood coagulation (e.g. prothrombin or activated partial thromboplastin times, fibrinogen concentration and platelet count), which assess discreet components of the coagulation system, thromboelastography takes into account the dynamic interaction of plasma (clotting factors) and cellular (platelets) elements that occurs during *in vivo* clotting.

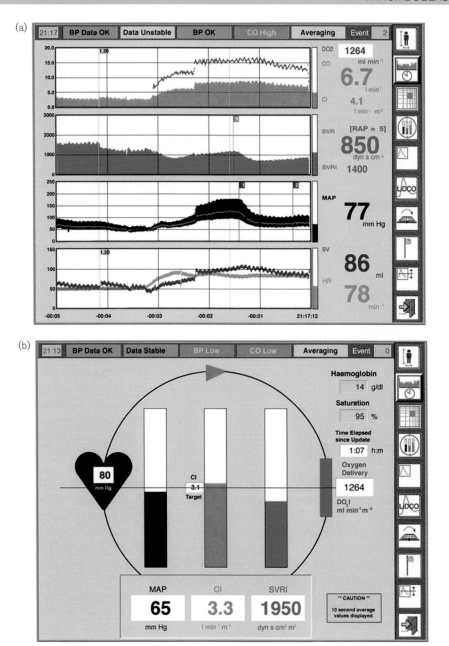

Figure 18.12 Two PulseCO display screen shots from the LiDCO Plus Haemodynamic Monitor.

Extensive development of the apparatus, since the original description of the technique by Hartert in 1948, has resulted in semi-automated and computer-driven devices. These are easy to use, portable, and robust enough to be sited in proximity to patient care areas (operating rooms and intensive care units). Test results are stored on the computer's hard disc and can be retrieved or exported in both graphic and database formats. A major practical benefit of using thromboelastography follows from the use of the devices as 'point-of-care' analyzers, which avoids some of the logistic problems inherent in laboratory-based testing. Apart from demonstrating abnormal patterns of coagulation, test protocols can use reagents that selectively inhibit

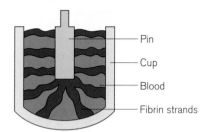

Figure 18.13 Fibrin strands, at the start of clot formation, link the cup and pin.

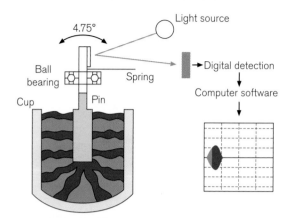

Figure 18.15 The detection principle in the ROTEM. The cup is stationary and the pin rotates.

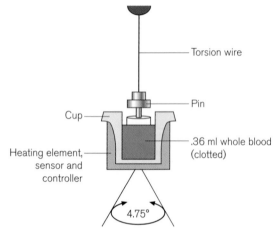

Figure 18.14 Schematic of the cup and pin in the TEG Analyzer. Note that it is the cup that oscillates in this device.

heparin, platelets, or fibrinolysis to determine the cause of the coagulopathy.

Thromboelastography has found application in two areas in particular, liver transplantation and cardiac surgery. Its use is increasing in intensive care, and in the evaluation of bleeding in obstetric and major trauma cases.

Measurement technique

A precise sample of blood is pipetted into a small 'cup'. A 'pin' is then suspended vertically in the blood sample within the cup. As the clot forms and fibrin strands attach the inner surface of the cup to the pin (Fig. 18.13), any movement of the cup or pin relative to each other will be impeded.

In the Thromboelastograph Coagulation Analyzer (Haemoscope Corp, USA), the cup oscillates periodically at 6 cycles/min through an arc of 4.75°. As the blood clots inside the cup, an increasing torque is transmitted to the pin, reflecting the strength of the fibrin-platelet bonds linking the cup to the pin. A torsion wire attached to the stationary pin forms part of an electromechanical system that monitors the torque and the output of this signal is directly related to the clot strength (Fig. 18.14). To ensure proper alignment of the pin and cup, this instrument has to be placed horizontally, a position that can be checked by a spirit level incorporated into the device. The current version of this device, Haemoscope 5000, contains two channels that can be used independently.

The ROTEM (Pentapharm, Germany), named from 'rotational thromboelastometry', is a modification of the classical thromboelastography. Unlike the Thromboelastograph Coagulation Analyzer, the cup in the ROTEM is stationary and coupled to a pin that rotates 4.75° in the longitudinal axis (10 seconds in each direction). The low shear force applied by the pin in the ROTEM is, therefore, similar to that applied by the oscillating cup in the first device. As the blood clot forms, rotation of the pin is restricted and this is transduced by an optical system linked to a charge-coupled device (Fig. 18.15). The ROTEM has four channels and uses a different nomenclature for the measured variables.

Thromboelastograph

The strength of the blood clot, specifically its shear elastic modulus, is represented in a real-time graph. The classical nomenclature, used in the Thromboelastograph Coagulation Analyzer, for the most frequently measured parameters, has been updated in the ROTEM and is indicated below.

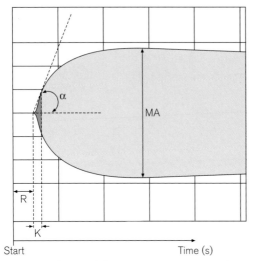

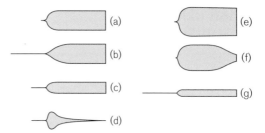

Figure 18.17 Characteristic thromboelastograph traces **(a)** Normal **(b)** Anticoagulants or factor deficiency **(c)** Thrombocytopenia or platelet dysfunction **(d)** Fibrinolysis **(e)** Hypercoagulability **(f)** Disseminated intravascular coagulation (DIC), early stage **(g)** DIC later stage.

Figure 18.16 Some of the parameters measured on a thromboelastograph (ROTEM nomenclature and units of measurement): R (Clotting Time, sec), K (Clot Formation Time, sec), MA (Maximum Clot Firmness, mm), α α-angle, deg).

From the start of the test, the initial trace (Fig. 18.16) is a horizontal line, which then branches symmetrically as soon as fibrin is formed. The time taken to reach this point is denoted R (from Reaction) or Clotting Time (ROTEM). The tracing then branches in the shape of a tuning fork. The alpha angle, α, is a measure of the rate of clot formation and has a lower value when the process is prolonged. The duration K (from Kontrol) or Clot Formation Time (ROTEM) is the time taken for the tracing to reach a 20 mm amplitude. The two branches reach their widest separation point when the clot has reached its greatest strength. This is given by the MA (Maximum Amplitude) or Maximum Clot Firmness (ROTEM). Subsequent clot retraction leads to a narrowing of the two branches. Hyperfibrinolyis is indicated by a short duration at the MA followed by a rapid diminution of this value. Comparison of these parameters in the test sample with normal ranges permits quantitative analysis of coagulation. Interpretation of the parameters is fairly straightforward. A prolonged R time is due to the presence of heparin or a clotting factor deficiency. Fibrinogen deficiency is indicated by a prolonged K duration, decreased α and, to a lesser extent, decreased MA. The strength of the clot, indicated by the MA, is decreased in the presence of reduced platelet number or significant dysfunction. Common causes of coagulopathy are associated with characteristic thromboelastograph patterns (Fig. 18.17).

FURTHER READING (CARDIAC OUTPUT)

Dark PM, Singer M (2004) The validity of trans-esophageal Doppler ultrasonography as a measure of cardiac output in critically ill adults. *Intensive Care Medicine* 30(11):2060–2066.

Gan T (2000) The esophageal Doppler as an alternative to the pulmonary artery catheter. *Current Opinion in Critical Care* **6(3):** 214–221.

Godje O, Hoke K, Goetz AE, *et al* (2002) Reliability of a new algorithm for continuous cardiac output determination by pulse-contour analysis during hemodynamic instability. *Critical Care Medicine* 30(1): 52–58.

Jonas MM and Tanser SJ (2002) Lithium dilution measurement of cardiac output and arterial pulse waveform analysis: an indicator dilution calibrated beat-by-beat system for continuous estimation of cardiac output. *Current Opinion in Critical Care* 8(3): 257–261.

Marik PE (1999) Pulmonary artery catheterization and esophageal doppler monitoring in the ICU. *Chest* **116(4):** 1085–1091.

Sandham JD, Hull RD, Brant RF, *et al* (2003) A randomized, controlled trial of the use of pulmonary artery catheters in high-risk surgical patients. *The New England Journal of Medicine* **348(1):** 5–14

Singer M (1993) Esophageal Doppler monitoring of aortic blood flow: beat-by-beat cardiac output monitoring. *International Anesthesiology Clinics* 31(3): 99–125.

Valtier B, Cholley BP, Belot JP, et al (1998) Noninvasive monitoring of cardiac output in critically ill patients using transesophageal Doppler. *American Journal of Respiratory and Critical Care Medicine* 158(1): 77–83.

FURTHER READING (THROMBOELASTOGRAPHY)

Harding SA, Mallett SV, Peachey TD, *et al* (1997) Use of heparinase modified thromboelastography in liver transplantation. *British Journal of Anaesthesia* **78(2):** 175–179.

Shore-Lesserson L, Manspeizer HE, DePerio M, *et al* (1999) Thromboelastography-guided transfusion algorithm reduces transfusions in complex cardiac surgery. *Anesthesia and Analgesia* **88(2):** 312–319.

Whitten CW and Greillich PE (2000) Thromboelastography: Past, Present and Future. *Anesthesiology* **92(5):** 1223–1225.

19

Depth of anaesthesia and neurophysiological monitoring

Andrew Morley

Neurological function may be monitored for a variety of purposes in anaesthesia and intensive care. For example, electrical stimulation of peripheral nerves can assist in the assessment of pharmacological neuromuscular blockade, anatomical localization during peripheral nerve blockade and confirmation of the integrity of neural pathways during spinal surgery.

Also, in the central nervous system, analysis of electrical activity in the cerebral cortex is the principle underlying most devices which purport to reflect anaesthetic depth. Cerebral activity is dependent on an adequate supply of oxygenated blood. In situations where this supply is potentially compromised (e.g. carotid endarterectomy or neurosurgery), monitors are available which may reduce the risk of cerebral ischaemia and consequent neurological deficit.

NERVE STIMULATORS

Nerve stimulators are designed to administer electrical stimuli to peripheral nerves. The responses may be assessed in different ways. The strength of an electrical stimulus applied to a nerve is defined by its charge (coulombs, Q). This is equivalent to the product of the current passed (amperes, A) and the duration (seconds, s) of that pulse of current.

Most nerve stimulators employ constant current circuitry, in which the difference between the current set by the user and the actual current delivered is detected. Voltage output from the device is automatically adjusted to minimize any disparity. A high impedance, which may occur with a dried-out skin electrode for example, causes low initial current flow. As a result, the nerve stimulator generates a compensatory increase in voltage output to restore the desired current.

Assessment of neuromuscular blockade

During assessment of neuromuscular blockade a *supramaximal stimulus* (i.e. one in which all axons in the nerve are made to discharge) is administered to a motor nerve through a pair of ordinary adhesive silver/silver chloride electrodes, applied to the overlying skin. Typically, the stimulus pulse duration might be 0.2 ms, the current 60 mA and the resulting charge, 12 μC. With pulses shorter than 0.2 ms, the amplitude required to generate a supramaximal stimulus may be beyond the capacity of the stimulator. Pulses longer than 0.3 ms run the risk of repetitive nerve or muscle stimulation. The charge required to deliver a supramaximal stimulus is significantly less when the negative electrode is placed distally.[1]

The motor response evoked by peripheral nerve stimulation may be measured in different ways. In clinical situations, subjective visual evaluation of the motor response to peripheral nerve stimulation is widely practised (usually contraction of adductor pollicis is observed following ulnar nerve stimulation at the wrist). Facial nerve stimulation on the cheek is also used but the resulting contraction may be due partly to direct electrical stimulation of facial muscles.

Basic hand-held devices provide a stimulus with a fixed current and pulse width and permit a limited range of stimulation patterns (Fig. 19.1). Other models have liquid crystal screens and user-variable current, enabling both neuromuscular monitoring and nerve localization. More advanced devices attempt to quantify the muscular contraction elicited by peripheral nerve stimulation. Methods for objective assessment of the motor response are:

- Electromyography;
- Mechanomyography;
- Accelerometry; and
- Piezoelectric methods.

Electromyography

The Datex Relaxograph is probably the best-known commercial electromyographic monitor used in anaesthesia. It records the muscle action potential in response to a supramaximal stimulation of the appropriate nerve. Datex stopped production of the Relaxograph in 1996, but continued to support the product until 2003.

Mechanomyography

In mechanomyography (MMG), the monitored muscle is fixed, to ensure a constant preload, and the force of muscular contraction is measured following supramaximal nerve stimulation. The Organon Myograph 2000 and the Relaxometer, developed by the University of Groningen, are monitors that work on this principle. Production of both has recently been discontinued. Anaesthetists conducting research involving MMG, often use non-specific commercial force-transducers.

Accelerometry/acceleromyography

Force is the product of mass and acceleration. During assessment of neuromuscular blockade, mass is relatively unchanged so acceleration is proportional to force. An accelerometric monitor is shown in Figure 19.2. An accelerometer comprises a small mass suspended on a

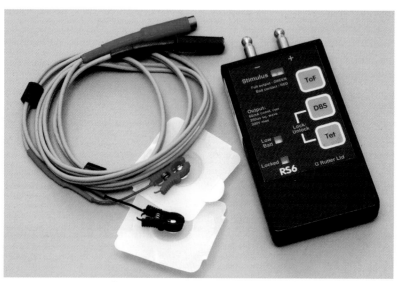

Figure 19.1 RS6 neuromuscular monitor (G. Rutter Ltd). Current (60 mA) and pulse width (0.25 ms) are fixed. A train-of-four, double-burst or tetanic stimulus may be selected. The leads may be removed to reveal probes for direct application to moistened skin.

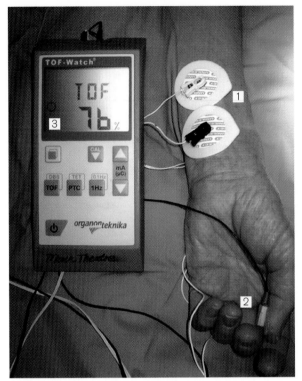

Figure 19.2 The TOF-Watch monitor (Organon Teknika). Stimulating current from 0–60 mA is set by the user. Accelerometric assessment of neuromuscular blockade or nerve localization may be performed. For the former, the device is calibrated after induction and before administration of muscle relaxant. (1) Stimulating electrodes applied over ulnar nerve; (2) accelerometric transducer taped to thumb; (3) display screen indicating train-of-four ratio: when less than four responses are detected, the number is indicated instead.

strain gauge within a 'box' attached to the accelerating object to be studied, the acceleration then being derived from the force exerted on the strain gauge.

Piezoelectric methods

Datex–Ohmeda have recently incorporated piezoelectric technology in a plug-in neuromuscular transmission module, for their S/5 anaesthesia monitor. Piezoelectric materials produce a charge when compressed or distorted. They are usually crystals or specially designed plastic films. The size of the charge is proportional to the degree of alteration in shape. In the M-NMT module, a piezo-electric sensor is incorporated into a clip placed on the patient's thumb and index finger. Thumb movement evoked by ulnar nerve stimulation is converted to an electrical signal (Fig. 19.3). Monitoring should be started after induction of anaesthesia but before neuromuscular blockade. On starting, the module automatically determines the current required for a supramaximal stimulus and sets a reference response level. The module also allows electromyographic recording and, with appropriate settings, can be used for nerve localization as well.

Comparative studies suggest that the methods above are not reliably interchangeable in assessing the response to a train-of-four stimulus. Most currently available monitors use accelerometric or piezoelectric technology.

Nerve stimulators for regional anaesthesia

Some peripheral nerve stimulators are designed specifically for nerve localization during regional anaesthesia (see Chapter 15, Fig. 15.10). A positive surface electrode is applied to the skin and the negative electrode cable is plugged into a unipolar stimulating needle.

User-adjustable constant current is necessary and the ability to adjust stimulus frequency and duration is desirable. The stimulus delivered is generally a monomorphic square pulse, though this becomes distorted as resistance increases. Usually an initial current of 1–2 mA with a frequency of 2 Hz is appropriate as the needle is advanced toward the nerve. Lower frequencies increase the risk of going past the nerve but may be desirable to reduce discomfort secondary to movement in traumatized patients.

Once contractions of the relevant muscle are seen, the current can be reduced. The stimulator-delivered charge required to generate a nerve impulse is proportional to the square of the distance from needle tip to nerve (by Coulomb's law). Local anaesthetic injected at the point where the threshold current for contractions is 0.3 mA or less, is likely to be effective.[2] Because chronaxie (the minimum stimulus duration required to elicit a response) is longer in sensory than in motor nerves, pulses longer than 0.15 ms are selected when attempting to locate a purely sensory nerve by inducing paraesthesia.

The accuracy with which peripheral nerve stimulators deliver the selected current tends to deteriorate as the current decreases. Manufacturers often quote accuracy (typically 1–5%) for a current setting of 1 mA. This is of limited relevance, as amplitudes used for peripheral nerve localization are less than 0.5 mA, where variability may be more than 80%.[3] A stimulator which delivers less than the set current may increase the risk of nerve damage during peripheral nerve block – with one that delivers more, a failed block may be more likely.

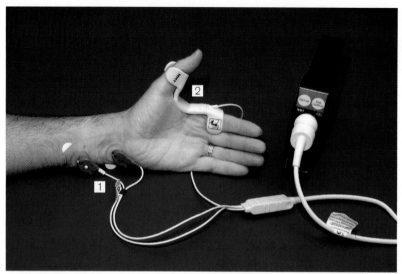

Figure 19.3 The mechanosensor for the Datex–Ohmeda M-NMT neuromuscular transmission module. (1) Stimulating electrodes applied over ulnar nerve; (2) piezoelectric mechanosensor.

Assessment of neural integrity

The incidence of neurological damage, secondary to traction and ischaemia of the spinal cord during scoliosis correction, is approximately 0.5%. This may be reduced by monitoring somatosensory evoked potentials (SSEP).[4] The monitors are complex and require an experienced operator. Typically a pair of stimulating electrodes is placed over each posterior tibial nerve at the ankles for lumbar surgery, or over the median nerves for cervical surgery. Stimuli are administered at about 30 mA and 5 Hz. Recording electrodes may be applied at various points adjacent to the ascending tracts, proximal to the site of surgery. The epidural space provides particularly robust potentials but application here is invasive. More usually, two or more scalp electrodes are used – e.g. one frontal and one cervical – together with a reference and a ground electrode. The recorded responses are passed through a digital signal converter and a band-pass filter (20–1000 Hz). An average response is calculated from as many as 200 individual ones and the result displayed on the monitor screen.

The period of interest is the first 100 ms after the stimulus, during which a characteristic W-shaped potential is seen in recordings from cortical electrodes (Fig. 19.4). The latency of each wave depends on the distance between the point of stimulation and the recording electrode. For example, long latencies will be seen in a tall patient, where the posterior tibial nerves are stimulated and the cortical response recorded. Shorter latencies will be seen in a short patient with median nerve stimulation and cervical recording electrodes.

The operator will usually record a baseline SSEP before induction of anaesthesia. This can be stored for the purposes of comparison. If intraoperative spinal manipulation completely prevents conduction of the ascending impulse, the SSEP disappears altogether. When conduction is merely impaired, an increase in SSEP latency and a decrease in amplitude are observed. A 50% increase in latency compared to baseline would be regarded as a critical change and the operator would inform the surgeon accordingly. Surgical disruption apart, a number of factors affect SSEPs, including volatile anaesthetic agents, nitrous oxide, hypothermia, hypoxia and hypotension.

By definition, SSEPs provide information only about the integrity of sensory tracts. In some circumstances, motor nerve function is of particular interest. During neck dissection or cerebropontine angle tumour resection, the surgeon may electrically stimulate the facial nerve, its integrity being confirmed by a motor response. Motor evoked responses have also been employed in a similar fashion to SSEPs with needle stimulating electrodes placed in the interspinous ligaments proximal to the surgical site and recording needle electrodes adjacent to distal motor nerves.[5] Some have advocated the use of electromyography during pedicle fixation to detect mechanical irritation of nerve roots.[6]

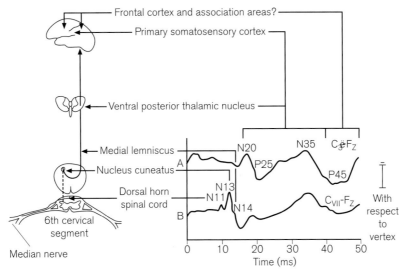

Figure 19.4 Somatosensory evoked response. The stimulating electrode is over the median nerve. Recording electrodes are over **(a)** the somatosensory cortex and **(b)** the seventh vertebra. The sequential peaks and troughs in the evoked response are named according to their latency (ms) and direction. Particular periods of the response correspond to specific neuro-anatomical regions as shown. (Thornton C, Sharpe RM (1998) Evoked responses in anaesthesia. *British Journal of Anaesthesia* **81**: 771–781. © The Board of Management and Trustees of the *British Journal of Anaesthesia*. Reproduced by permission of Oxford University Press/British Journal of Anaesthesia.)

MONITORING 'DEPTH OF ANAESTHESIA'

For decades, anaesthetists have sought a monitor which might reflect the conscious level of patients undergoing general anaesthesia. A number of different variables, which may relate to consciousness, can be derived from the electrical activity of the cerebral cortex. Ideally, in variables of this sort, the range of values seen in the conscious state should not overlap with that seen in the unconscious state (i.e. a cut-off value would exist which is 100% sensitive and specific for consciousness). Furthermore, ideally any cut-off value should not be affected by patient physiology or the choice of anaesthetic agent.[7]

At present, the variables derived by commercially available monitors do not meet these ideals. Such monitors generally work on one of two principles:

1. spontaneous electroencephalography (EEG); and
2. auditory evoked potentials (AEP).

EEG

General principles, signal processing and artefact rejection

The EEG represents current flow in the cortical extracellular fluid, which is the result of post-synaptic potentials in cortical neurons. It is acquired through scalp electrodes. In a classical diagnostic EEG, more than 20 electrodes are required but in developing technology for use in anaesthesia, the tendency has been to limit the area of cortex over which the recording is made. Usually between one and four electrodes are used, depending on the device, together with a reference electrode. Impedance should be kept to a minimum (i.e. less than 5 kO). EEG voltage is measured as the potential difference between two electrodes.

The complex waveform of the EEG comprises many individual sine waves, whose frequencies lie from zero to approximately 50 Hz. (Fig. 19.5). Classically these are grouped into frequency bands (Table 19.1). For the purposes of analysis, the EEG is split into epochs of 1–4 ms.

In order to allow processing, the EEG is converted from a smooth continuous analogue signal into a digital one. The fidelity of this conversion depends on the degree of resolution for both voltage and time. The greater the number of bits used, the smaller the change in voltage that can be translated from analogue to digital. EEG monitors usually use 12–16 bits of resolution. The frequency at which the analogue signal is sampled is also important. Too slow a sampling frequency fails to take account of the fastest sine waves and results in 'aliasing', where the digital signal incorrectly identifies a low frequency

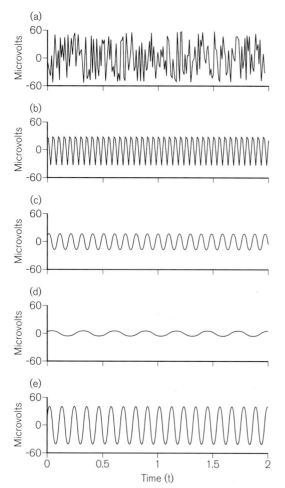

Table 19.1 Electroencephalographic frequency bands	
Band name	**Approximate frequency range (Hz)**
alpha	8–13
beta	13–30
theta	4–8
delta	<4

Figure 19.5 (a) A 2-second epoch from an unprocessed EEG. Also pictured are some of its constituent sine waves, whose respective amplitudes, phase angles and frequencies are **(b)** 30 µV, 60° and 20 Hz **(c)** 15 µV, 30° and 10 Hz **(d)** 4 µV, 15° and 4 Hz **(e)** 40 µV, 25 and 9 Hz.

cancels out that between negative and reference electrodes, assuming equal electrode impedance – see Chapter 16).

Time and frequency domain analysis and data presentation

Once artefact has been dealt with, the EEG is subjected to time-domain and frequency-domain analysis. The most widely used example of the former is the calculation of a burst suppression ratio (BSR). In deeply anaesthetized patients, the EEG may consist of isoelectric periods (suppression) interspersed with bursts of normal activity. The BSR is the fraction of time in an epoch in which the EEG is suppressed and is usually averaged over 60 seconds.

In frequency-domain analysis, each individual epoch is subjected to fast Fourier transformation. This mathematical process breaks down the EEG waveform into its constituent sine waves, from which a power ($µV^2$) vs frequency (Hz) histogram can be derived. On many monitors, the frequency histograms from sequential epochs can be presented as a compressed spectral array (CSA) or a density spectral array (DSA) (Fig. 19.7).

For the purposes of objective comparison, the frequency spectrum may be represented by a summary variable. Two commonly used variables are the median frequency (MF), which divides the power in the spectrum into two equal halves, and the 95% spectral edge frequency (SEF), below which 95% of the spectral power lies (Fig. 19.8). As anaesthesia deepens, lower EEG frequencies generally predominate and there is a concomitant fall in MF and SEF.

Despite this broad relationship, MF and SEF are unsatisfactory measures of consciousness during anaesthesia. They have not been related to clinical endpoints, nor are they independent of anaesthetic agents used.

Bispectral index

In calculating MF and SEF, much information in the spontaneous EEG is disregarded. For example, no data relating to burst suppression or to beta activation (a

waveform (Fig. 19.6). EEG monitors usually sample at frequencies above 250 Hz.

The commercially available EEG monitors described below process the signal to enable rejection of artefact. Artefacts due to the electrocardiogram, or to eye movement, have characteristic features enabling easy identification and exclusion. The scalp electromyogram typically contains higher frequencies than the EEG and can be screened out by band-pass filtering. Powerline pickup or 'mains interference' (at 50 Hz in the UK) is the largest source of artefact and is a common mode signal (i.e. the voltage difference between positive and reference electrodes

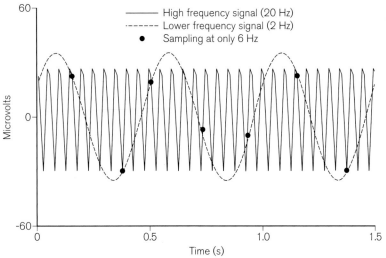

Figure 19.6 Aliasing. A high frequency signal at 20 Hz is incorrectly identified as a lower frequency signal at 2 Hz because the signal is sampled at only 6 Hz.

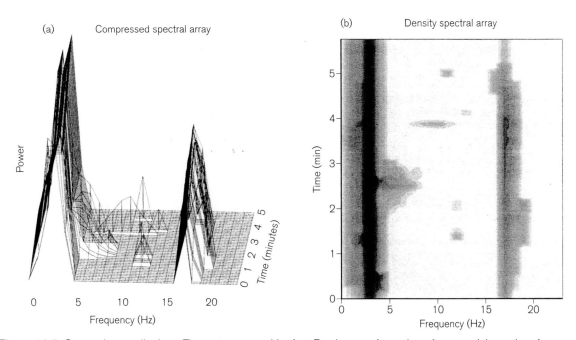

Figure 19.7 Spectral array displays. These are created by fast Fourier transformation of sequential epochs of raw EEG signal. Data from each epoch are transformed to produce a power *versus* frequency histogram. In the compressed spectral array (CSA) above, histograms derived from sequential epochs are plotted in pseudo-three-dimensional fashion. The density spectral array shown is derived from the same EEG data as the CSA. Each histogram is represented in grey-scale, with larger values depicted by darker shades. In each case, data from the most recent epoch are added to the bottom of the display. (Rampil IJ (1998) A primer for EEG signal processing. *Anesthesiology* **89:** 980–1002.)

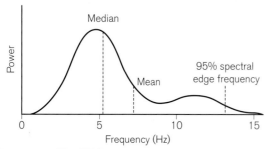

Figure 19.8 The EEG frequency spectrum and derived variables.

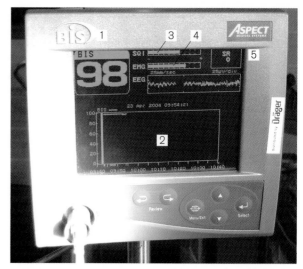

Figure 19.9 The display panel of the Aspect A-2000 bispectral index (BIS) monitor. (1) BIS; (2) BIS trend; (3) signal quality index indicator; (4) electromyogram interference indicator; (5) burst suppression ratio indicator.

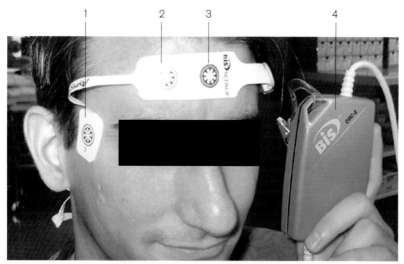

Figure 19.10 The sensor for use with the Aspect A-2000 bispectral index monitor. Applied to the skin are (1) recording, (2) ground, (3) reference electrodes. (4) digital signal converter.

paradoxical increase in relative beta power occurring at low brain concentrations of some anaesthetics) is utilized. Phase coupling of constituent EEG sine waves is also ignored.

Some of these issues are addressed by the *bispectral index* (BIS), an EEG-derived variable, which is calculated and displayed by the A-2000 EEG monitor (Aspect Medical Systems) (Fig. 19.9). The EEG is acquired from the BIS sensor: three electrodes embedded in an adhesive strip, which is applied to the forehead (Fig. 19.10). After the EEG signal is digitized and artefact-filtered, the BIS is calculated using a proprietary algorithm. This was originally developed using a prospectively collected database of EEGs, acquired during 1500 anaesthetics. EEG features correlating with clinical endpoints related to sedation were identified and incorporated into the algorithm, which was then tested prospectively. There have been several subsequent refinements.

The term 'bispectral' refers to bispectral analysis. This has some advantages over traditional frequency band analysis, including identification of non-linearities in the EEG signal and quantification of the degree of phase coupling between constituent sine waves. BIS incorporates:

(a) two time-domain features, the BSR and the QUAZI suppression index;

(b) two frequency-domain features, 'SynchFastSlow' (from bispectral analysis) and the 'BetaRatio' (the log ratio of power in the 30–47 Hz and 11–20 Hz frequency bands).[8]

The result is a dimensionless scale from 1 to 100, which indicates the likelihood of consciousness. During general anaesthesia, a BIS of less than 60 is said to indicate a negligible chance of recall. Recent developments include the incorporation of the BIS algorithm into a module for the Datex–Ohmeda anaesthetic monitors and the production of the BIS-XP sensor, which contains a fourth electrode applied over the eye. The additional information recorded at this point is fed into an updated algorithm and is said to reduce the influence of ocular artefact and improve calculation of the BSR.

Other EEG processing devices

Other monitors which record and process the EEG are available.

The Patient State Analyzer PSA-4000 (Physiometrix) has been developed in a broadly similar fashion to the BIS monitor, in that a database of EEGs from surgical patients with corresponding clinical correlates was examined for features apparently related to consciousness. Further information relating to age-dependent normative EEG variables and artefact characteristics was acquired from a large pre-existing EEG database. Finally, anaesthetic concentration-dependent EEG changes in volunteers were analyzed and used to assist in calibrating a patient state index (PSI), which ranges from 0–100. Most of the EEG descriptors used in the algorithm for PSI calculation relate to EEG power, though the suppression ratio is also taken into account. Four recording electrodes are used, one of which is on the posterior scalp. A PSI of between 25 and 50 is recommended for surgical anaesthesia.[9]

In the Narcotrend monitor (MonitorTechnik), the EEG is acquired from one reference and two recording electrodes on the forehead. Artefact is rejected, the data are analyzed and an algorithm applied in order to assign a Narcotrend stage. There are six such stages, A (awake) to F (general anaesthesia with increasing burst suppression).

The algorithm is distinct from the BIS and PSI algorithms in that it was developed purely as a means for objective analysis of the EEG waveform, using time and frequency domain information.[10] No clinical correlates were involved. Anaesthesia-induced changes in BIS values are accompanied by corresponding changes in Narcotrend levels in most patients.

Effective intraoperative titration of general anaesthetic has been demonstrated using all three of the monitors described above, with monitored patients recovering more quickly than controls.

Entropy

In 2003, Datex–Ohmeda released a depth of anaesthesia module for their anaesthesia monitor, based on the entropy of the EEG signal. If the awake EEG is characterized by a chaotic signal, then decreasing levels of consciousness are associated with a less disordered signal, as the number of signal generators diminish and slower wave activity becomes more dominant. By calculating the amount of disorder in the power spectrum of the EEG signal (cf. calculation of SEF and MF above) it is suggested that anaesthetic depth may be objectively estimated. A sensor similar in appearance and application to that for BIS is used and the numerical scale has deliberately been adjusted to correlate with BIS. The module displays a number for entropy over the frequency range 0.8 to 32 Hz and a second number for the range 0.8 to 47 Hz, to include components of frontalis muscle EMG. Clinical experience with this device is as yet limited,[11] although promising.[12]

Auditory evoked potentials

Loss of consciousness under general anaesthesia is accompanied by changes in the electrical response of the cerebral cortex to an auditory stimulus. The period of particular interest is the early cortical response, illustrated in Figure 19.11, which occurs approximately 10–100 ms after the stimulus (the mid-latency auditory evoked potential, or MLAEP). MLAEP waves are generated in the medial geniculate and primary auditory cortex. Anaesthesia increases the latency and decreases the amplitude of MLAEP waves. Threshold values for both Na and Pb latencies have been proposed as indicators of unconsciousness during anaesthesia. In recent research, indices have been mathematically derived, which incorporate several features of the MLAEP and reflect better its overall morphology.[13]

The A-Line monitor (Danmeter) is a commercially-available AEP monitor (Fig. 19.12). It administers

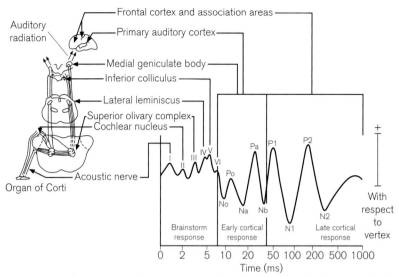

Figure 19.11 The auditory evoked response with its anatomical basis. (Thornton C, Sharpe RM (1998) Evoked responses in anaesthesia. *British Journal of Anaesthesia* **81**: 771–781. © The Board of Management and Trustees of the British Journal of Anaesthesia. Reproduced by permission of Oxford University Press/British Journal of Anaesthesia.)

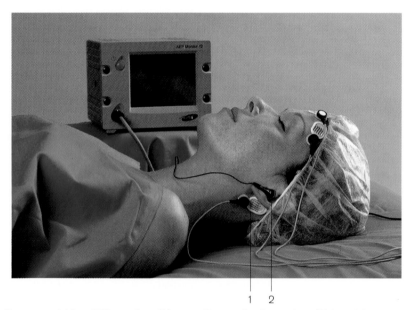

Figure 19.12 The Danmeter A-Line AEP monitor. (1) recording scalp electrodes; (2) headphones.

65–70 dB click stimuli at 9 Hz through headphones and records the response with scalp electrodes. The signal undergoes pre-processing, during which artefact is rejected and band-pass filtering applied.

The number of responses needed to permit AEP extraction from background cortical activity has recently been substantially reduced. The classical extraction method, moving time averaging, requires 256 responses with a resulting update delay of over 35 seconds. By using an autoregressive model with exogenous input (ARX), 15–25 responses are analyzed with an update delay of only six seconds. The A-line ARX index (AAI) is the sum of absolute differences in the 20–80 ms window of the AEP and is a unitless index ranging from 0 to 99. Under propofol anaesthesia, an AAI of 19 predicts unconsciousness (defined as the point at which physical stimulation is required to elicit a response from the subject) with a sensitivity of 100% and a specificity of 51%.[14]

At present, the most promising technologies for effective assessment of consciousness during general anaesthesia, appear to be BIS and AEP. In a direct experimental comparison during propofol sedation, an AEP-derived variable (the AEP index) was better than BIS at distinguishing the conscious from the unconscious state.[15] However, results from a recent large-scale trial indicate that BIS monitoring can reduce the incidence of intraoperative awareness in patients at risk of this complication.[16] At present, there is no corresponding evidence for the effectiveness of AA-guided general anaesthesia.

Alternative technology

Respiratory sinus arrhythmia

Depth of anaesthesia monitoring, based on the amount of respiratory sinus arrhythmia (RSA), was suggested nearly 20 years ago.[17] RSA is the high-frequency component of heart rate variability that is dependant on the phase of respiration. Different mathematical techniques for calculating the amount of RSA are possible and have been used in psychophysiological research into emotion and stress for some time, but a commercially available system for use in anaesthesia is yet to become a reality. The neurophysiology of RSA is explained on the basis of polyvagal theory which suggests that the nucleus tractus solitarii of the medulla receives afferent sensory information from stretch receptors in the lung, which then drive vagal inhibition of the heart via the nucleus ambiguus (as distinct from the dorsal motor nucleus vagal efferents of the baroreceptor reflex).[18] RSA can be estimated using ECG R–R interval and respiratory data, and alters with end-tidal isoflurane concentration[19] and propofol administration.[20] The relationship between RSA and clinical endpoints of consciousness is undefined. A key advantage of a monitor based on RSA would be the ease of data acquisition from existing standard monitoring (ECG) as opposed to the low signal to noise ratio of the EEG signal.

ASSESSMENT OF CEREBRAL BLOOD FLOW

During carotid endarterectomy (CEA), the adequacy of cerebral blood flow (CBF) may be assessed using a number of monitoring techniques. Their individual sensitivity and specificity in the detection of cerebral ischaemia, and their role in the prevention of adverse neurological sequelae, is disputed. Some of these techniques may have other surgical applications, for example, in cardiac or neurosurgery.

Methods include:

- Stump pressure measurement;
- Transcranial Doppler ultrasonography (TCD);
- EEG;
- SSEPs (Somatosensory Evoked Potentials); and
- Intraoperative jugular bulb oximetry (neurosurgery only).

Stump pressure

Immediately after clamping the carotid artery the surgeon may insert, distal to the clamp, a needle attached to a standard pressure transducer. In principle, the adequacy of collateral blood supply from the circle of Willis may be reflected in the pressure at this point. Typically, a shunt might be inserted for the duration of clamping if the stump pressure is less than 50 mmHg. There are a number of problems with stump pressure. It is a one-off measurement, it does not consistently reflect flow, and the relationship between stump pressure and ischaemic EEG changes is weak.

TCD

TCD is probably the most widely used continuous technique and requires an experienced operator. The principles of Doppler ultrasonography are covered in Chapter 18. Traditional 5–10 MHz ultrasound frequencies do not penetrate the skull and TCD usually involves pulses at 1–2 MHz, with the probe placed over the thin bone of the temporal region (Fig. 19.13). Even so, up to 30% of elderly patients cannot be insonated, even at the highest available energy output of relevant ultrasonographic devices.

During CEA, TCD is generally used to assess flow in the middle cerebral artery, which is found at a depth of about 50 mm from the temporal window. The probe emits ultrasound pulses and receives reflected frequencies, which are converted to electrical signals. These are subjected to fast Fourier transformation to produce a moving graph of flow velocity (cm s^{-1}) vs time. The waveform is characterized by its peak systolic velocity and its time averaged mean maximal velocity (Vmax). Vmax is typically 35–90 cm s^{-1}. Another useful variable is the

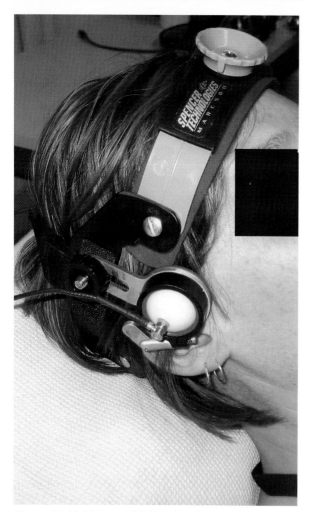

Figure 19.13 Transcranial Doppler ultrasound probe applied to patient's right temporal area.

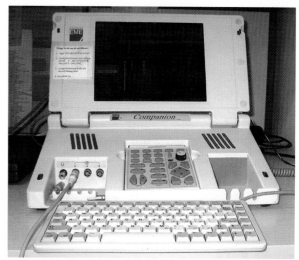

Figure 19.14 Transcranial Doppler ultrasound monitor.

As well as decreased CBF during surgery, TCD allows detection of increased flow postoperatively in hyperperfusion syndrome. This complication occurs in about 1% of patients undergoing CEA. Prompt recognition and administration of appropriate therapy may reduce the risk of cerebral haemorrhage.

Though TCD monitoring has been attempted in cerebral aneurysm surgery and resection of intracranial arteriovenous malformations, practical difficulties limit its usefulness. Given the high incidence of postoperative neuropsychiatric deficits after cardiopulmonary bypass, in which CBF changes and emboli have been implicated, there may be a role for TCD in cardiac surgery.

SSEPs

Cortical SSEPs are affected by large reductions in CBF. Median nerves may be stimulated bilaterally and evoked potentials recorded at scalp electrodes as described above. A baseline response is recorded before clamping and again about a minute after. Subsequent recording at regular intervals is recommended as delayed changes are occasionally seen. SSEPs have been used successfully as a basis for selective shunting in CEA.[22] On carotid clamping, a decrease in N20/P25 amplitude of greater than 50% from baseline has been proposed as an indicator of cortical dysfunction.[23]

EEG

Cerebral ischaemia occurring on carotid clamping may induce changes in ipsilateral EEG frequencies and ampli-

pulsatility index, which reflects the resistance to flow in the examined artery. A TCD monitor is illustrated in Figure 19.14 and typical intraoperative TCD data, taken from the monitor screen, in Figure 19.15.

Though changes in Vmax are widely regarded as being more significant than absolute values, it is unclear what constitutes a critical reduction. In one large study, ischaemia after clamping was considered severe if Vmax fell to 0–15% of baseline, mild if 16–40% and absent if greater than 40%.[21] A significant decrease on clamping may influence the surgical decision to shunt. Subsequent Vmax changes may allow detection of shunt occlusion and intraoperative emboli, the latter producing a characteristic sound.

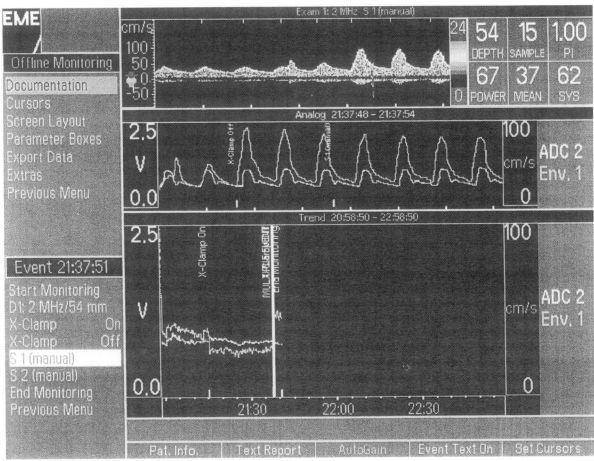

Figure 19.15 Intraoperative transcranial Doppler ultrasound recording. (1) Spectral Doppler trace (flow against time); (2) sample volume depth (mm); (3) sample volume size (mm); (4) pulsatility index; (5) percentage power; (6) mean flow velocity (cm s^{-1}); (7) systolic flow velocity (cm s^{-1}); (8) analogue recording of arterial pressure; and (9) arterial pressure and Doppler trends over time.

tudes. Raw EEG monitoring during carotid endarterectomy (CEA) has been advocated, although data interpretation requires considerable expertise. Processed EEG monitors may be more practical, e.g. CFAM4 (RDM Consultants Ltd), but the sensitivity of intraoperative EEG monitoring as a predictor of immediate postoperative neurological deficit has been shown to be only 50% in one study.[24]

Jugular bulb oximetry

This technique is more commonly associated with the intensive care unit than the operating theatre. However, it also allows intraoperative assessment of cerebral oxygen extraction and may be useful during cerebral aneurysm, tumour and haematoma surgery.[25] An oximetric catheter, e.g. Opticath (Abbott), is introduced into the internal jugular vein cranially until the jugular venous bulb is encountered. Jugular venous oxygen saturation (SjvO$_2$) reflects the oxygen supply:demand ratio and is usually 60–70%. Normal values give limited reassurance as they do not exclude focal cerebral ischaemia. An SjvO$_2$ of 90% or more is seen in hyperaemia – at less than 50%, SjvO$_2$ indicates increased oxygen extraction and impending ischaemia.

REFERENCES

1. Brull SJ, Silverman DG (1995) Pulse width, stimulus intensity, electrode placement, and polarity during assessment of neuromuscular block. *Anesthesiology* **83**: 702–709.

2. Kaiser H, Niesel HC, Klimpel L, *et al.* (1992) Prilocaine in lumbosacral plexus block – general efficacy and comparison of nerve stimulation amplitude. *Acta Anaesthesiologica Scandinavica* **36**: 692–697.

3. Hadzic A, Vloka J, Hadzic N, *et al.* (2003) Nerve stimulators used for peripheral nerve blocks vary in their electrical characteristics. *Anesthesiology* **98**: 969–974.

4. Nuwer MR, Dawson EG, Carlson LG, *et al.* (1995) Somatosensory evoked potential spinal cord monitoring reduces neurological deficits after scoliosis surgery: results of a large multicenter survey. *Electroencephalography and Clinical Neurophysiology* **96**: 6–11.

5. Hosking MP, Mongan PD, Peterson RE (1992) Removal of a large intrathoracic tumour in a child: neurogenic motor-evoked potential monitoring of spinal cord integrity and anesthetic management. *Anesthesia and Analgesia* **74**: 460–463.

6. Owen JH, Kostiuk JP, Gornet M, *et al.* (1994) The use of mechanically elicited electromyograms to protect nerve roots during surgery for spinal degeneration. *Spine* **19**: 1704–1710.

7. Drummond JC (2000) Monitoring depth of anesthesia. *Anesthesiology* **93**: 876–882.

8. Rampil IJ (1998) A primer for EEG signal processing. *Anesthesiology* **89**: 980–1002.

9. Drover DR, Lemmens HJ, Pierce ET, *et al.* (2002) Patient state index; titration of delivery and recovery from propofol, alfentanil and nitrous oxide anesthesia. *Anesthesiology* **97**: 82–89.

10. Kreuer S, Biedler A, Larsen R, *et al.* (2003) Narcotrend monitoring allows faster emergence and a reduction of drug consumption in propofol-remifentanil anesthesia. *Anesthesiology* **99**: 34–41.

11. Anderson RE, Barr G, Öwall A, *et al.* (2004) Entropy during propofol hypnosis, including an episode of wakefulness. *Anaesthesia* **59(1)**: 52–56.

12. Sleigh JW, Barnard JPM (2004) Editorial: Entropy is blind to nitrous oxide. Can we see why? *British Journal of Anaesthesia* **92(2)**: 159–161.

13. Mantzaridis H, Kenny GNC (1997) Auditory evoked potential index: a quantitative measure of changes in auditory evoked potentials during general anaesthesia. *Anaesthesia* **52**: 1030–1036.

14. Struys MMRF, Jensen EW, Smith W, *et al.* (2002) Performance of the ARX-derived auditory evoked potential index as an indicator of anesthetic depth. *Anesthesiology* **96**: 803–816.

15. Gajraj RJ, Doi M, Mantzaridis H, *et al.* (1998) Analysis of the EEG bispectrum, auditory evoked potentials and the EEG power spectrum during repeated transitions from consciousness to unconsciousness. *British Journal of Anaesthesia* **80**: 46–52.

16. Myles PS, Leslie K, McNeil J, *et al.* (2004) Bispectral index monitoring to prevent awareness during anaesthesia: the B-Aware randomised controlled trial. *Lancet* **363(9423)**: 1757–1763.

17. Donchin Y, Feld JF, Porges SW (1985) Respiratory sinus arryhthmia during recovery from isoflurane-nitrous oxide anaesthesia. *Anesthesia and Analgesia* **64**: 811–815.

18. Pomfrett CJD (1999) Editorial: Heart rate variability, BIS and 'depth of anaesthesia'. *British Journal of Anesthesia* **82**: 659–662.

19. Pomfrett CJD, Sneyd JR, Barrie JR, Healey TEJ (1994) Respiratory sinus arrhythmia: comparison with EEG indices during isoflurane anaesthesia at 0.65 and 1.2 MAC. *British Journal of Anesthesia* **72**: 397–402.

20. Pomfrett CJD, Barrie JR, Healey TEJ (1993) Respiratory sinus arrhythmia: an index of light anaesthesia. *British Journal of Anaesthesia* **71**: 212–217.

21. Halsey JH Jr (1992) Risks and benefits of shunting in carotid endarterectomy. The international transcranial Doppler collaborators. *Stroke* **23**: 1583–1587.

22. Schwartz ML, Panetta TF, Kaplan BJ, *et al.* (1996) Somatosensory evoked potential montoring during carotid artery surgery. *Cardiovascular Surgery* **4**: 77–80.

23. Horsch S, Ktenidis K (1996) Intraoperative use of somatosensory evoked potentials for brain monitoring during carotid surgery. *Neurosurgery Clinics of North America* **7**: 693–702.

24. McCarthy WJ, Park AE, Koushanpour E, *et al.* (1996) Carotid endarterectomy. Lessons from intraoperative monitoring – a decade of experience. *Annals of Surgery* **224**: 297–305.

25. Matta BF, Lam AM, Mayberg TS, *et al.* (1994) A critique of the intraoperative use of jugular venous bulb catheters during neurosurgical procedures. *Anesthesia and Analgesia* **79**: 745–750.

Atmospheric pollution

Chetan Patel

Exposure to a short duration of volatile anaesthetic agents in high concentrations: thousands of parts per million (ppm); has a therapeutic role in anaesthesia and has an excellent safety record. However, it is the chronic, cumulative exposure to relatively low concentrations (ppm in the hundreds) that has, for a number of years, raised concerns over the possible hazards to health. There have been many epidemiological studies, on the alleged adverse effects of chronic exposure to trace concentrations of anaesthetic gases and vapours in operating theatres and recovery rooms. The evidence is somewhat inconclusive and sometimes conflicting.

Some animal and human studies[1-5] have suggested that, as a result of chronic exposure to inhalational volatiles, there is an increased incidence amongst anaesthetic personnel of:

- spontaneous abortion;
- minor congenital abnormalities;
- subjective complaints (e.g. headaches, fatigue and nervousness);
- cancer (leukaemia and lymphoma);
- liver disease; and
- renal disease.

In several studies, chronic exposure to nitrous oxide has been shown to result in:

- reduced fertility in female dental assistants;
- litters that are reduced in number and size compared with control animals (rats);
- neurological symptoms suggestive of a vitamin B_{12} deficiency in dentists. This finding has been confirmed in rats chronically exposed to nitrous oxide.

The Health and Safety Commission's Advisory Committee on Toxic Substances reviewed the literature on the toxic effects of anaesthetic agents in the workplace in 1996.[6] They made the following conclusions based on the data available:

- There was no evidence in humans that exposure to nitrous oxide or volatile agents (halothane, isoflurane and enflurane) caused developmental defects in the foetus or other reproductive health effects.
- Animals (rats) continuously exposed to high concentrations of nitrous oxide (1000 ppm for over 8 hours), demonstrated developmental toxicity to the embryo/foetus, possibly by the inhibition of cell production by nitrous oxide. However, no adverse effects were seen when animals were exposed to nitrous oxide at lower concentrations (500 ppm).
- Pregnant animals exposed to high concentrations of halothane and isoflurane (1000 ppm) showed effects on the development of the foetus. However, there

was no convincing evidence when the concentrations of repeated exposure were lower – (100 ppm for halothane and 600 ppm for isoflurane).

- There was no evidence from animal studies that suggested enflurane had any adverse effect on the foetus. However, liver damage was demonstrated in mice when exposed to enflurane continuously (>700 ppm).
- Maximum exposure limits for volatiles have, therefore, been set at levels at which no adverse effects were seen in animal studies and thus represent levels at which there is no evidence to suggest the development of adverse effects in humans.

As a result of the inconclusive evidence on the adverse effects of volatile agents, the maximum exposure limits differ in each country (see below).

EFFECTS ON THE ENVIRONMENT

The contribution of halothane, enflurane, isoflurane and sevoflurane on the depletion of stratospheric ozone or on 'greenhouse warming', as with other chlorofluorocarbons (CFCs), is a function of the lifetimes of the volatile agents (Table 20.1). These lifetimes depend on the reaction of these agents with hydroxyl (OH) radicals in the troposphere.[8] The interactions of nitrous oxide in the atmosphere are more complicated and less predictable. Nitrous oxide does have an ozone depleting and greenhouse warming potential. Like the volatile anaesthetics however, the impact on the atmosphere is small when compared to other environmentally damaging gases, for example other

CFCs. This is due to the smaller quantities of the agents produced and their relatively shorter lifetime in the atmosphere. It takes about two years for the gases to reach the stratosphere, where they can begin to exert their effects on the ozone layer (Fig. 20.1).

Nonetheless, it would seem prudent to reduce levels of anaesthetic agents in the environment where they are used. This would include the operating theatre, recovery rooms, dental suites, maternity units, pharmacies and ambulances.

LEGISLATION

Various organizations in different parts of the world have introduced recommendations for maximum acceptable levels of pollution, to protect staff working in these areas.

In the USA, for example, several organizations, such as the Federal Occupational Safety and Health Administration (OSHA), the National Institute of Occupational Safety (NIOSH) and the American Conference of Industrial Hygienists (ACIGH) have this responsibility. In the UK, it is the responsibility of the Health and Safety Commission (HSC).

In the UK, it is a legal requirement that employers control industrial and medical pollution. The legislation takes the form of a government approved code of practice entitled, 'Control of Substances Hazardous to Health' (COSHH).[10] This was introduced in 1988, updated in 1994 and amended annually thereafter. The HSC's Advisory Committee on Toxic Substances has drawn up

Table 20.1 The effects of anaesthetic gases on the ozone layer and greenhouse warming

Compound	Lifetime in atmosphere (years)	Ozone depletion potential	Greenhouse warming potential	Global production (tonnes/yr)
CFC-11	76	1.00	0.390	350 000
CFC-12	140	1.00	1.000	400 000
Halothane	2	0.36	0.004	1000
Enflurane	6	0.02	0.040	220
Isoflurane	5	0.01	0.030	800
Sevoflurane	1.4	0.00	0.0005	–
*Nitrous oxide	120	0.15	0.040	–

The potential ozone depletion efficacy and greenhouse warming effect are normalized to the principle CFC-12.
(Halsey 1996, with permission of The Medicine Group (Education) Ltd[7] (based on original data from 1989)[8].)
*Represents data from the World Meteorological Organization[9]

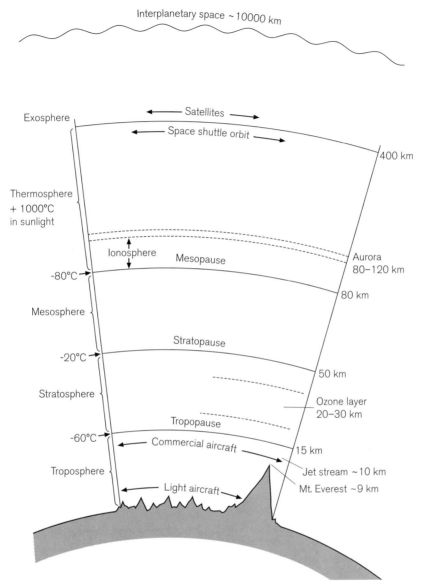

Figure 20.1 The Earth's blanket of air reaching approximately 10 000 km above its surface. Approximate temperatures are also shown.

this code of practice under Section 16 of the Health and Safety at Work Act (1974), for the purpose of providing practical guidance on the control of substances hazardous to health in the workplace. However, it is a separate organization, the Health and Safety Executive (HSE), that has the power to enforce the code of practice.

It was only in 1996 that COSHH defined the safe maximum exposure limits for a wide variety of substances, including anaesthetic gases and vapours (EH40/96 – updated annually).[11] COSHH recommends that:

'Exposure should be controlled to a level to which nearly all the population can be exposed day after day without adverse effect on health'. This reference to exposure is usually expressed as the upper acceptable limit for an agent averaged out in any 8-hour period of potential exposure (8-hour, time-weighted average, 8-hr TWA).

Recommended exposure limits for anaesthetic gases and vapours in some countries are set out in Table 20.2. No 8-hr TWA values are available for sevoflurane and desflurane, although both OSHA and NIOSH recom-

Table 20.2 Exposure limits to anaesthetic gases and vapours in parts per million (ppm) or as millilitres per cubic metre (ml m^{-3}) and expressed as 8-hour time-weighted averages (8-hr TWA)

Country		N$_2$O		Halothane		Ethrane		Isoflurane	
		ppm	ml m^{-3}	ppm	ml m^{-3}	ppm	ml m^{-3}	ppm	ml m^{-3}
UK	1996	100	180	10	80	50	380	50	380
USA	1994	50		50		75			
Switzerland	1994	100		5		10		10	
Sweden	1994	100		5		10		10	
Italy	1994	50		2		2		2	

mend ceiling limit (concentrations that must never be exceeded during any part of the day) of 2 ppm for both volatile agents. As a rough guide, substances with exposure limits below 100 ppm are considered highly toxic by inhalation, those substances with exposure limits of 10–500 ppm are considered moderately toxic by inhalation and those substances with exposure limits greater than 500 ppm are slightly toxic by inhalation.

When no steps are taken to avoid pollution, the exposure limits may be exceeded. One study from a 20-hospital survey, reported that the levels of halothane varied between 0.1 and 60 ppm (mean of 2.8 ppm) and for nitrous oxide between 10 and 3000 ppm (mean of 388.5 ppm) when scavenging systems were not used.[12] In the same study, the installation of an active scavenging system in one particular hospital reduced the anaesthetist's exposure to nitrous oxide (and halothane) from a mean value of 411 ppm (and 1.9 ppm) to a mean value of 24.5 ppm (and < 0.1 ppm).

COSHH also provides regulations that require an employer to protect employees by:

1. assessment of risk;
2. prevention or control of exposure;
3. installation and maintenance of control measures as well as regular examination and testing of the control measures;
4. monitoring of exposure at the workplace;
5. provision of health surveillance; and
6. provision of information and training.

CONTROL OF POLLUTION

The control of pollution should be tackled using the guidelines recommended in the COSHH in the UK and NIOSH in the USA,[13] namely:

- instilling awareness in personnel working in the potentially affected environment;
- installation of effective scavenging equipment (see below); and
- ensuring good working practices by:
  (a) always using the devices provided;
  (b) daily inspection of these devices to ensure that they are functioning;
  (c) considering the use of low-flow systems where appropriate;
  (d) checking for leaks in the breathing system;
  (e) flushing out the breathing system (including the reservoir bag) through the scavenging device provided, at the end of an anaesthetic;
  (f) considering capping off the breathing system at the end of an anaesthetic so as to prevent anaesthetic vapours that have impregnated the breathing hoses from polluting the environment;
  (g) the filling of anaesthetic vaporizers in a fume cupboard that includes a spill tray;
  (h) amending workplace practice by reviewing rotas so that the same personnel are not always working in those areas of highest pollution;
- efficient room air-conditioning so as to remove any pollutant that may have inadvertently escaped. (A minimum of 15 changes per hour with a balanced supply and extraction process); and
- regular monitoring of the theatre environment.

That which constitutes regular monitoring appears to be the most difficult issue to resolve. Monthly or fortnightly checks might miss a week in which the levels could, due to a fault, contravene COSHH/NIOSH guidelines. An employer (the hospital), if sued by an employee, could well find this case difficult to defend.

THE EXTENT OF POLLUTION

This depends on five factors:

1. the quantity of anaesthetic gases and vapours employed;
2. the employment of a scavenging system and its efficiency;
3. the amount of leakage from the anaesthetic equipment;
4. the efficiency of the air-conditioning and ventilation system in an operating theatre or anaesthetic room; and
5. the size and layout of the operating theatre and any other place where anaesthetic vapours are used.

Anaesthetic gases and vapours

The quantity of gases and vapours used may vary considerably, depending on the breathing system used. At one extreme is the Mapleson D System, where there may be a fresh gas flow of about $8 l min^{-1}$, of which 70% may be nitrous oxide, and to which other volatile anaesthetic agents may be added. At the other extreme is the low-flow circle system, where flows may be reduced to less than $1 l min^{-1}$. Also, there is substantial pollution from unscavenged Entonox demand valves used in maternity units.

The employment of a scavenging system and its efficiency

Surplus anaesthetic gases and vapours are vented from a breathing system or ventilator, via an expiratory valve and, if allowed to escape at this point, would pollute the immediate environment. The valve is normally adapted to discharge into a scavenging system, which collects the escaping gas and vents it to the atmosphere remote from a populated area. The efficiency of the scavenging system depends on its rate of extraction and the gas-tight fit of its components. The former must be greater than the discharge of pollutant gases, in order to be effective. These systems are discussed in greater detail later in the chapter.

Leakage

However efficient a scavenging system may be, its purpose will be defeated if gases and vapours are permitted to escape from the apparatus. Overt leaks from the high-pressure and regulated-pressure parts of the anaesthetic machine may be easily detected. Leaks from the breathing system may be less obvious, however, and may even be due to diffusion through the rubber or neoprene parts. The latter often absorb significant quantities of some of the volatile agents during the administration of one anaesthetic, only to release them during the next anaesthetic. For this reason, new and unused breathing attachments should be used for the administration of an anaesthetic to a patient who exhibits sensitivity to a particular anaesthetic agent, for instance in the case of malignant hyperpyrexia.

Leakage may also result from carelessness when vaporizers are refilled. It has been advocated that refilling of vaporizers should take place in a fume hood.

The efficiency of the air-conditioning system

The frequency of air changes is often quoted as a measure of the efficiency of an air-conditioning system. A figure of 20 changes per hour is usually considered satisfactory. However, the circulation of air throughout the theatre is often uneven. The recovery area, where the patient exhales anaesthetic agents, is often poorly ventilated and there may be no arrangements for scavenging. The nurse attending the patient is often in direct line with the exhaled gases.

There are two further considerations:

1. Some air-conditioning systems are wholly or partially recirculating, and may result in the vapours from one location polluting another.
2. Thought must be given to the siting of the external outlet of the extract system, which again may pollute other areas in which people work.

The size of the premises

'Dental chair' anaesthetics for dental extractions are frequently administered in small rooms. This, in itself, is probably of little importance, since the anaesthesia is of only short duration and most dentists employ general anaesthetics only occasionally, so exposure of the personnel is limited. However, the advent of inhalational methods for relative analgesia and sedation has resulted in much more prolonged exposure. In these techniques, high flow rates of nitrous oxide may be used.

MEASUREMENT OF POLLUTION

The extent of pollution in the theatre environment is now quantifiable. It may be measured by various methods, some of which are described below.

Operating theatres

With the introduction of low-cost non-dispersive, portable infrared analyzers, trace quantities of anaesthetic agents can be measured continuously. A direct reading

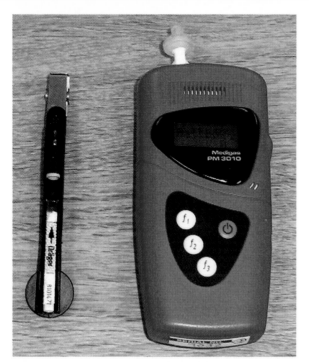

Figure 20.2 Nitrous oxide analyzers. On the right, a Medigas PM 3010 analyzer and on the left, a Dräger sampling tube and badge.

analyzer (Fig. 20.2) enables spot measurements to be taken at different sites, allowing the background level of nitrous oxide in a room to be assessed. Instant results of nitrous oxide levels (in the range of 0–1000 ppm with a resolution of 5 ppm) are displayed in real-time or as an 8-hr TWA. An alarm protects personnel against excessive levels of exposure.

Theatre personnel

Individuals can be issued with sampling tubes for nitrous oxide (Fig. 20.2) and sampling badges for volatile anaesthetics (Fig. 20.3) that are worn for approximately 8 hours. They are placed at shoulder height (to measure respirable exposure). The pollutants are adsorbed onto the material in the sampler in proportion to their concentration in the ambient atmosphere. For volatile agents, the material is based on activated charcoal, whereas for nitrous oxide, a molecular sieve is used. At the end of the passive sampling period, the samplers are sent to a specialist laboratory where the pollutants are measured using a gas chromatograph linked to an infrared detector.

Biological monitoring of post-volatile anaesthetic exposure, using urine samples analyzed by gas chromatography-mass spectrometry coupled with static headspace sampling, have been shown to be another useful tool to monitor the extent of exposure.[14]

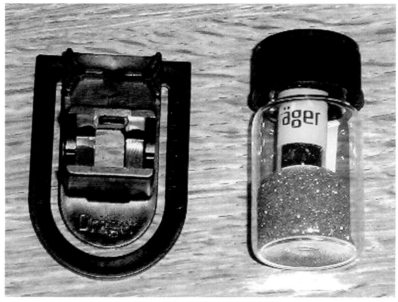

Figure 20.3 Dräger sampling badge for analyzing volatile agents.

SCAVENGING SYSTEMS

A scavenging system transports waste gases and vapours from a ventilator or breathing system and discharges them at a safer remote location. It includes several components, namely:

- *a collecting system*, which conveys waste gases from the breathing system to a transfer system;
- *a transfer system*, which consists of a section of flexible wide-bore hose linking the collecting system to the receiving system;
- *a receiving system*, which behaves as a reservoir to store surges in the flow of waste gas. From here, these gases have to pass via disposal tubing to a disposal system;
- *a disposal system*. This then transports the waste gases to a site on the outside of a building away from populated areas.

Two or more of these items may be embodied in a single item of equipment.

Waste gas normally passes through the collecting and receiving system to the disposal system, using only the power generated in exhalation by the elastic recoil of a patient's lungs. At this stage there is little difference between the various systems employed. It may then pass through the disposal system using this same power (*passive scavenging*). However, it maybe assisted by some form of gas or electrically powered apparatus, which generates a subatmospheric pressure (*active scavenging*). Only systems that employ active scavenging are able to deal with the wide range of expiratory flow rates (30–120 l min^{-1}) seen in anaesthetic practice, especially when certain ventilator systems are used. Active systems are, therefore, the only ones that can be recommended – provided that they also meet certain specification and performance criteria (BS 6834: 1987 UK).[1]

The collecting system

This has two components:

1. A 30 mm male conical connection (labelled M in Fig. 20.4) that is fitted either to the expiratory port of a ventilator, the demand valve (for Entonox) or to the APL valve of a breathing system. The version that fits the APL valve shrouds all the exit apertures on the body of the valve enclosing them in a gas-tight fit.
2. A 30 mm female conical connection (labelled F in Fig. 20.4) that fits over the male connector to form

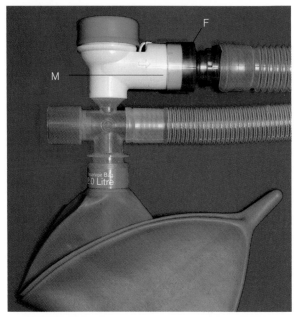

Figure 20.4 A collection system showing a shrouded APL valve encased in a gas scavenging collector system and terminating in a 30 mm conical male taper (M), and a 30 mm female conical taper (F) and 30 mm corrugated tubing for linking the former to a transfer system.

a gas-tight fit and is attached to the patient end of the transfer system.

Having two components in the collecting system allows the female part to be detached and reattached to different breathing systems as required. The selection of a unique 30 mm taper for this connection is intended to prevent other breathing system components from being attached to it in error.

The collecting system may also house an overpressure relief valve, which is normally set to blow off at 1 kPa (10 cmH$_2$0). This device (Fig. 20.5) prevents excessive pressure building up in the breathing system if the scavenging system becomes obstructed; for instance due to crushing or kinking of the transfer tubing.

The transfer system

This consists of a length of wide-bore, kink-resistant tubing that joins the collecting system to the receiving system.

The exhaled gases emerge intermittently from the breathing system, their volume and flow pattern varying according to the type of apparatus in use. For example, with spontaneous respiration there may be a fresh gas

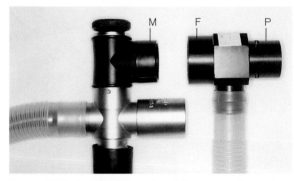

Figure 20.5 A collection system (M) and transfer system (F) incorporating an overpressure relief valve (P) (set at 1 kPa) in the female component.

flow of approximately $8 \, l \, min^{-1}$ which must be scavenged. However, the peak flow rate during the period when the APL valve is open, may be much higher (up to $45 \, l \, min^{-1}$). Furthermore, some ventilators that have gas-driven bellows discharge both driving gas and exhaled gas into the scavenging system. This might well produce intermittent flow rates in excess of $100 \, l \, min^{-1}$. It is important, therefore, to match the performance of the rest of the system to that of the anaesthetic equipment.

However, it would be dangerous to attach the collecting apparatus directly to a scavenging system that was actively extracting gas in excess of $120 \, l \, min^{-1}$, as this would suck gas out of both breathing system and patient.

The solution is to install a safety device (*receiving system*).

The receiving system

The receiving system (Fig. 20.6) consists of:

- a reservoir (normally a rigid material cylinder) for the expired and driving gases, from which they are passed to the disposal system. This may also temporarily store this gas if the extraction rate falls below the necessary level.
- an air break. The reservoir is open-ended at its base to allow entrainment of air when there is insufficient expired gas. This prevents the transmission of subatmospheric pressure from the scavenging system to the patient. It also provides an emergency escape route for the gas should the scavenging system fail.
- a flow indicator to show that the unit is working when connected to an active disposal system. There is normally a clear Perspex window sited near the top of the reservoir in which a coloured float appears when the extraction rate is normal (i.e. $120 \, l \, min^{-1}$). When

the flow drops below $80 \, l \, min^{-1}$ this disappears from view.

- a filter sited in the base of the unit to prevent debris entering and blocking the system, and
- an entry port on the side and an exit port on the top of the container.

The receiving system is connected to the disposal system via a wide-bore hose that is sufficiently strong to prevent collapse from the subatmospheric pressure within it. The hose terminates in a probe, which houses a screw-fit connection to the disposal system socket (terminal unit). The latter has a valve that is normally closed but opens when the male probe from the receiving unit is connected to it and screwed in (Fig. 20.7). The terminal unit may be sited on a wall or pendant.

The disposal system
Active disposal systems

The subatmospheric pressure required to power the disposal system is usually provided by an exhauster unit (Fig. 20.8). This works in a similar fashion to a fan and requires a low level of maintenance and no lubrication. The size of the unit depends on the number of scavenging sites to be supplied. Large exhauster units can provide waste gas flow rates of up to $2400 \, l \, min^{-1}$, servicing 20 sites. Large sites often have a 'duty' and a 'standby' unit, which are linked. The standby unit operates automatically if the duty unit fails, as well as during periods of high demand. Although the exhauster unit is sited outside the operating theatre suite (sometimes a considerable distance away), the operating control switch is sometimes located within the theatre suite.

Pressure fluctuations within the disposal system are controlled within precise limits by a vacuum/flow-regulating valve. It consists of an adjustable spring-loaded plate covering the valve aperture and behaves as an air-entrainment valve should the vacuum exceed a predetermined level. This level is set, by adjusting the spring tension, during commissioning of the system, to provide the correct flow rates. Several valves may be fitted to large scavenging systems, so as to protect and control specific areas.

The exhauster unit discharges the waste gas to a suitable outside location via rigid pipework. A water trap, with an isolating tap, is included in this pathway to drain any accumulated condensation.

The use of an existing hospital piped vacuum system has often been advocated in the past. However, these systems cannot be recommended for the following reasons.

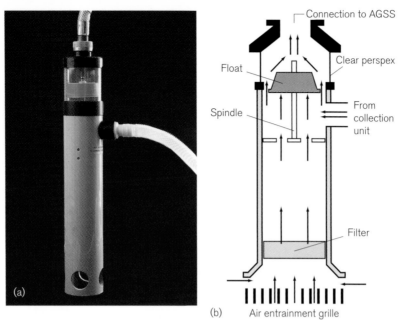

Figure 20.6 **(a)** An Ohmeda receiving system for use with active gas scavenging system (AGSS). **(b)** Internal arrangement of a receiving system.

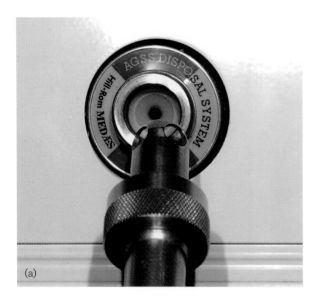

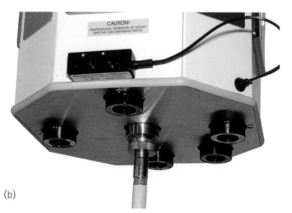

Figure 20.7 The probe from a receiver unit can be inserted into either. **(a)** A wall-mounted terminal or **(b)** a ceiling-mounted terminal.

- Scavenging requires a high-flow system with a small pressure gradient between the terminal unit and the exhaust unit, whereas the piped vacuum in a hospital uses a lower flow with a larger pressure gradient between the vacuum pump and the terminal unit.
- The extra demand upon the medical vacuum for this purpose may result in other users being deprived of an adequate medical vacuum in an emergency.

- The displacement (flow rate) of the vacuum line may be inadequate to cope with the high flow rate and the pulsating nature of the output of some ventilators.
- The outlet of the vacuum system may be so located that the expired gases would pollute areas where other personnel are working.
- More importantly, as vacuum lines do not contain safety valves (vacuum/flow-regulating valves, see above),

(a)

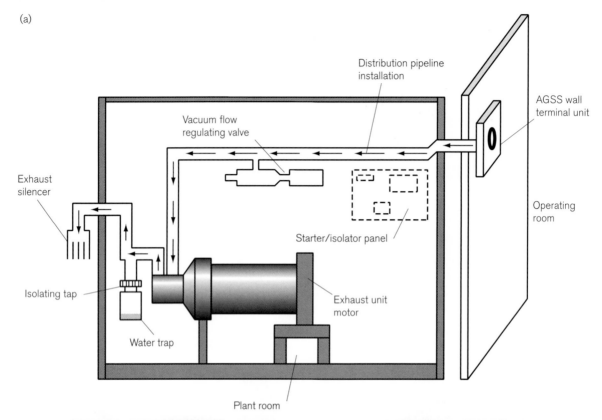

Distribution pipeline installation

AGSS wall terminal unit

Vacuum flow regulating valve

Operating room

Exhaust silencer

Starter/isolator panel

Isolating tap

Exhaust unit motor

Water trap

Plant room

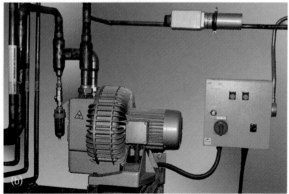

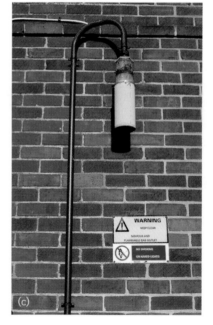

Figure 20.8 Active gas scavenging. **(a)** Schematic diagram of plant room, **(b)** The disposal unit in a plant room, **(c)** Exhaust silencer.

(a)

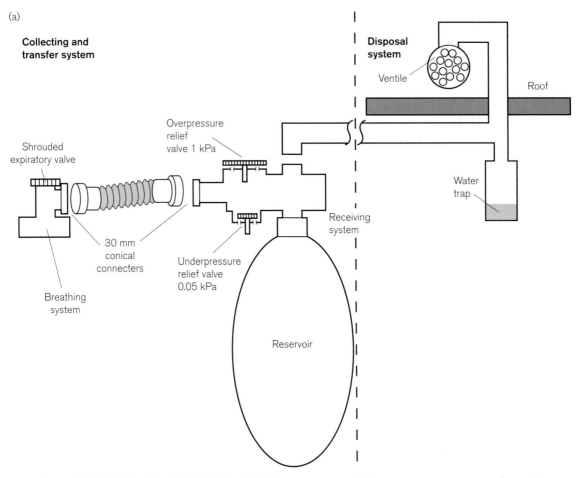

Collecting and transfer system

Disposal system

Ventile

Roof

Shrouded expiratory valve

Overpressure relief valve 1 kPa

Water trap

30 mm conical connecters

Receiving system

Underpressure relief valve 0.05 kPa

Breathing system

Reservoir

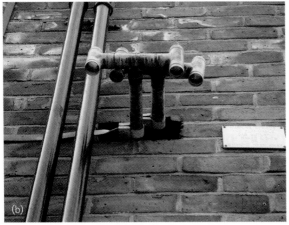

(b)

Figure 20.9 (a) A passive scavenging system. **(b)** A ventile for waste gas disposal emerging from the wall of an operating theatre suite.

there is a danger that an excessive 'vacuum' may be applied to a patient.

Collecting systems for scavenging in paediatric breathing systems are discussed in Chapter 14.

Passive disposal systems

Although these systems are not now recommended, a brief description is included to contrast the differences between passive and active systems.

In a passive system (Fig. 20.9), the receiver may house a 2-litre neoprene reservoir bag, an inlet and outlet and two relief valves. One of these valves opens at 1 kPa (10 cmH$_2$0) to prevent pressure build-up resulting from an obstruction in the scavenging system. The other valve can be opened if there is a subatmospheric pressure within the system greater than 50 Pa (0.5 cm H$_2$0) caused by excessive suction from the *ventile* (see below).

The outlet from the receiver is connected to a wide-bore tube, which passes through one of the walls or the roof of the building and terminates in a ventile. A ventile is a device that uses the wind to entrain the exhaust gases or air. Unfortunately, the passive system can be relied upon to operate satisfactorily only when the outlet is installed in a suitable position and when the wind is blowing from the desired quarter. It may be affected by the proximity of other buildings. Under adverse conditions, the flow may even be in the opposite direction. To prevent cross-contamination from one operating theatre to another, each point must have its own individual ventile. Cooling of the rising gas causes condensation and pooling, hence a water trap is essential. Alternatively, the wide-bore tubing from the receiver can be connected directly to a 'hole in the wall' (Fig. 20.10), although this is no longer advocated.

ABSORPTION SYSTEMS

Although these systems can remove the vapours of volatile anaesthetic agents from waste gases, they do not absorb nitrous oxide and, therefore, cannot be recommended as a scavenging system that meets current standards. They are included out of interest, as there may be occasions where they could be used with a low-flow breathing system where nitrous oxide is not employed and where scavenging is unavailable.

Most systems employ activated charcoal, in canisters of 1 kg, to absorb the volatile anaesthetic vapour efficiently. They have a low resistance and may be incorporated in the

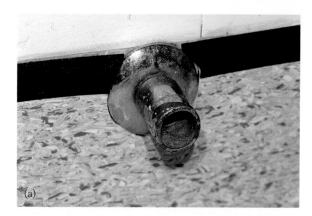

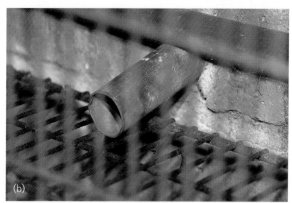

Figure 20.10 (a) Gas disposal via wall outlet on floor of theatre. **(b)** Exhaust pipe communicating to the outside.

expiratory limb of a breathing system (Fig. 20.11). The canister increases in weight as the vapour is absorbed, and this may be monitored by a spring balance on which it is mounted. When the weight reaches a stated level, it should be discarded. Care must be taken to ensure that it is disposed of in a safe location, where it will not permit the vapour to be released and pollute the atmosphere.

OTHER DEVICES

All the devices described are intended for use with adult breathing systems. Paediatric scavenging devices are described in Chapter 14. However, there are other situations where gaseous anaesthetic pollution can occur, notably in recovery rooms. Here, patients may continue to exhale anaesthetic agents postoperatively in close proximity to recovery room staff. The collecting systems described above cannot scavenge gas from many of the oxygen delivery devices often used on patients in these

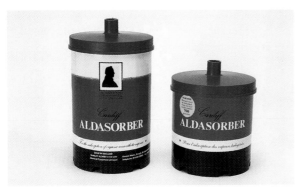

Figure 20.11 The Cardiff Aldasorber. (Photograph courtesy of Shirley Aldred & Co. Ltd. Sheffield, UK.)

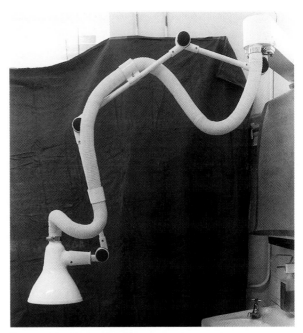

Figure 20.12 A collection system for use in recovery rooms.

sites. Devices such as that shown in Figure 22.12 are more suitable. A funnel attached to a wide-bore hose (which is then attached to a special active gas scavenging system) can be sited close to a patient's face to remove pollutants. The funnel is supported by a series of levers. For efficacy, the device requires a calm patient lying under the optimal extraction zone of the device. In practice, an efficient non-recirculating air-conditioning system in these areas would be more appropriate.

REFERENCES

1. Vaisman AI (1967) Working conditions in surgery and their effect on health of anesthesiologists. *Eksp Khir Anesteziol* **3**: 325–330.
2. Bruce DL, Bach MI (1976) Effects of trace anaesthetic gases on behavioural performance of volunteers. *British Journal of Anaesthesia* **48**: 871–876.
3. Guirguis SS, Pelmear PL, Riy ML, *et al.* (1990) Health effects associated with exposure to anaesthetic gases in Ontario hospital personnel. *British Journal of Industrial Medicine* **47**: 490–497.
4. Rowland AS, Baird DD, Weinberg CR, *et al.* (1992) Reduced fertility amongst women employed as dental assistants exposed to high levels of nitrous oxide. *New England Journal of Medicine* **327**: 993–997.
5. Deacon R, Perry J, Lumb M, *et al* (1978) Selective inactivation of vitamin B12 in rats by nitrous oxide. *Lancet* **2**(8098): 1023–1024.
6. Health and Safety Commission (1996) *Anaesthetic agents: Controlling exposure under COSHH*. Bristol: Health Services Advisory Committee.
7. Halsey MJ (1996) *Occupational exposure to anaesthetics. Anaesthesia Rounds*. Abingdon: The Medicine Group (Education) Ltd.
8. Brown AC, Canosa-Mas CE, Parr AD, *et al.* (1989) Tropospheric lifetimes of halogenated anaesthetics. *Nature* **341**(6234): 635–637.
9. Albritton DL, Auchamp PJ, Mergie G, *et al.* (1999) *Scientific assessment of ozone depletion: 1998*, World Meteorological Organization Global Ozone Research and Monitoring Project Report No.44, Geneva: WMO.
10. Health and Safety Commission (1988) *Control of Substances Hazardous to Health Regulations 1988. Approved Code of Practice*.
11. Health and Safety Executive (1996) *Occupational Exposure Limits*. Guidance Note EH40/96.12. Davenport HT, Halsey MJ, Wardley-Smith B, *et al.* (1980) Occupational exposure to anaesthetics in 20 hospitals. *Anaesthesia* **35**: 354–359.
12. National Institute for Occupational Safety and Health (1977) *Criteria for a Recommended Standard: Occupational Exposure to Waste Gases and Vapours*, DHEW Publication No. (NIOSH) 77–140 Cincinnati, Ohio, USA: NIOSH.
13. Accorsi A, Barbieri A, Raffi GB, *et al.* (2001) Biomonitoring of exposure to nitrous oxide, sevoflurane,

Isoflurane and halothane by automated GC/MS headspace urinalysis. *International Archives of Occupational and Environmental Health* **74(8):** 541–548.

14. British Standards (1994) *British Standard specification for active gas scavenging systems* (BS 6834). London: British Standards Institution.

Infusion equipment and intravenous anaesthesia

Ali Diba

The development of microprocessor-controlled volumetric infusion devices has brought about a significant change in UK hospital practice in the last ten years. No longer is it usual to see doctors and nurses with watch in hand, converting infusion rates from 'duration of infusion' to drops per minute and adjusting the roller clamp on an intravenous 'drip' set. It used to be commonplace to have infusates running through too fast or too slow, because the plastic tubing altered shape or the downstream resistance in the intravenous cannula altered for a number of reasons. Often it was simply the calculations that were wrong.

These techniques were superseded by electronic drip counters, which controlled the adjustable clamp on a gravity-fed giving set. This was before microprocessor-controlled volumetric and syringe pumps arrived, capable of sensing line pressure and of being programmed in a variety of units and languages to give stepped infusions based on patient weight.

1996 saw further progress with the commercial introduction of the Diprifusor™ system. This, a proprietary 'chip' added into a microprocessor-controlled syringe driver, allows drug delivery based on a pharmacokinetic algorithm aimed at controlling the infusion rate of the intravenous anaesthetic agent propofol, in order to achieve and maintain a given plasma concentration. To date this remains the only target-controlled infusion system widely available for clinical use. Although such systems would be logical for any drug (anaesthetic or otherwise) with a short half-life that needs to be given by continuous infusion, the development costs of achieving licensing for this route of administration for any given drug mean that it is only rarely commercially viable.

SIMPLE INFUSION SYSTEMS

In the operating theatre where there is closer observation of the patient's hydration and circulating volume as necessitated by their rapidly changing status, most intravenous fluids are still administered under gravity from flexible plastic containers using single-use fluid administration sets. These are of several types:
- simple fluid administration, no filter, droplet size approximately 15 drops/ml (0.07 ml);
- blood and fluid administration with clot filter at about 200 microns mesh size. These giving sets use a larger-bore tubing and a double drip chamber containing a float: on squeezing the bottom chamber the float acts as a one-way ball valve and allows fluid to be pumped.

Droplet size is usually approximately 15 drops/ml;
* burette, 100–150 ml in volume, droplet size either 15 drops/ml or, for paediatric usage, 60 drops/ml. A flap or ball valve at the bottom of the burette prevents air entering the drip chamber when the burette is empty;
* platelet giving sets, to reduce the risk of aggregation in the giving set as would occur with conventional blood giving sets.

Some giving sets are now designed so as to also be compatible with volumetric infusion pumps. This necessitates a narrower-bore tube made from softer plastic to function with the peristaltic pumps (see below). Flow rates are therefore lower and the tubing is less kink-resistant. These sets usually have a 15 micron filter at the base of the drip chamber and are not suitable for giving blood or for adult resuscitation.

The rate of infusion in a simple gravity fed system depends on:
* the height of the fluid container above the infusion site;
* the resistance to flow caused by the infusion set;
* occlusion of the tubing from a rate controlling device;
* the physical properties of the fluid to be administered;
* the bore of the intravenous cannula; and
* the hydrostatic pressure in the veins of the patient.

The manufacturers of giving sets quote the size of drops as number of drops per millilitre, usually between 10 to 60, but it must be remembered that the actual volume of the drops depends on the physical properties of the fluid being administered.

Rapid infusion

When rapid infusion of blood or other fluids is required, the rate of administration may be increased by the use of an inflatable pressure bag (Fig. 21.1), which may even be contained in a rigid box to increase the speed at which pressure may be applied.

When fluids are administered at a rapid rate, provision should be made for warming them to body temperature, otherwise significant cooling of the body may ensue.

Fluid warmers

Water baths with immersed coils of tubing were used initially for warming intravenous fluids. They are no longer acceptable as they were both inefficient and messy and were found to be ideal sites for bacterial growth.

Dry heat warmers may consist of two heated plates between which a plastic insert is sandwiched which carries the fluid pathway. Older types had a swing door

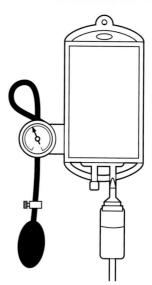

Figure 21.1 Pressure infusion device.

and could not be opened during use as the insert would swell with fluid and prevent the door closing again. Modern incarnations have a cassette, which inserts into the machine and in some models may be removed and reinserted (for example in a similar machine in the recovery ward). Figure 21.2 shows an insert heated by infrared radiation. Other dry heat warmers, consisting of a coil of plastic tubing, which is wrapped around a cylindrical hot 'plate', also exist but are laborious to use. A further development has been to introduce the pre-shaped heat exchange coil into the ducting of a forced air convective warmer (Fig. 21.3), creating a dry air 'water bath'. Here, although the heat capacity of air is quite low, the high airflow rates can bring about adequate heat transfer. In all these models, the increased length and hence resistance of the administration set from container to patient, necessitates the use of a pressurized bag to assist gravity. These types of warming system also suffer from a cooling of the infusate between heater and patient, which is more marked at low infusion rates. The device shown in Fig. 21.2 compensates by adjusting the output temperature, depending on the fluid flow rate and expected temperature drop. The flow rate is calculated from the temperature difference measured between two points on the cassette.

An alternative system is the Hotline® fluid warmer (Figs. 21.4 and 21.5) where heat exchange occurs across a water jacket enclosing the giving set (by use of a three lumen plastic tube) as far as the intravenous cannula. The central lumen carries the infusate to the patient, whilst

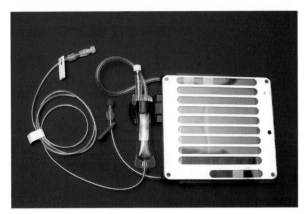

Figure 21.2 Fluido® S200 (The Surgical Company Group) insert for dry fluid warmer (see text for details).

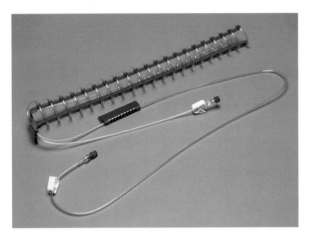

Figure 21.3 Dry air fluid warming coil.

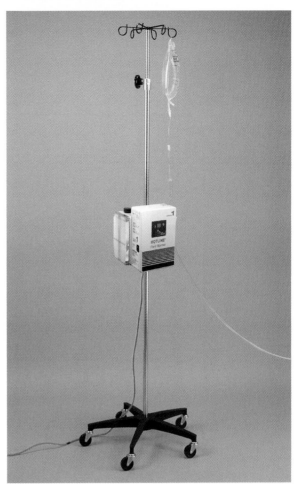

Figure 21.4 The Hotline® blood and fluid warming system. Photo courtesy Graseby Medical Ltd.

the other two lumens carry heated water. These systems are compact and efficient and do not suffer from heat loss from the giving set. The same manufacturer produces a high-flow fluid warming system incorporating two pressure infusers for uninterrupted flow and an aluminium heat exchanger for rapid warming at the higher flow rates (Fig. 21.6). The water jacket system is also retained and flow rates of up to 500 ml min^{-1} are claimed at temperatures above 38°C.

PRINCIPLES OF INFUSION PUMPS

Electronic drop counters do not control the infusion, but they do accurately inform the user of the infusion rate. A small beam of light, which may be infrared and thus invisible, is passed through the drip chamber of the giving

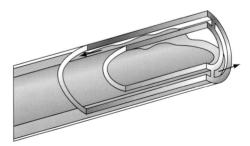

Figure 21.5 Heating jacket arrangement of Hotline® system. Arrows show flow of heated water in warming jacket.

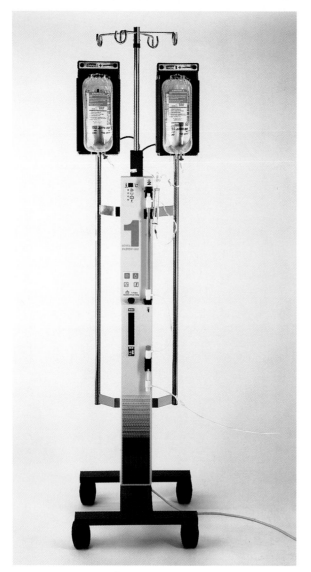

Figure 21.6 Level 1®, high flow fluid warming system. Photo courtesy Graseby Medical Ltd.

are not recommended now. Although manufacturers no longer sell these in the UK, they are still in use in some hospitals.

Infusion pumps are those devices capable of generating a flow, irrespective of the effects of gravity. Hence, they have to be driven by some form of motor.

The stepper motor

The driving force in the majority of infusion pumps and electronic syringe drivers is provided by an electronic stepper motor, which may be directly controlled from a digital microprocessor system. The speed of a conventional electric motor driven from either an AC supply or a DC supply may vary with mechanical load, the voltage or the frequency of the supply. It is therefore difficult, without electronic feedback, to control such a motor accurately. The stepper motor is designed so that a series of pulses applied to the stator windings of the motor cause the shaft to rotate by a fixed amount for each pulse, typically 1.8°, 2.5°, 3.75°or 7.5°, irrespective of the load, within certain limits. Infusion systems may be designed so that a pulse generator, whose frequency may be varied, can produce accurate control of an infusion and the frequency adjustment can be calibrated directly in millilitres per hour.

Infusion pumps

Pumped infusion systems overcome the variation in infusion rates caused by changes in back-pressure, tubing resistance and the vertical height of the fluid container above the patient.

The driving mechanism of infusion pumps may be a peristaltic arrangement, or may use a small syringe with associated valve in the manner of a conventional piston pump. Originally, the most accurate (and expensive) infusion pumps used syringes and were referred to as volumetric infusion pumps; the peristaltic pumps were less accurate as they depended on the quality of the infusion tubing and the constancy of the droplet size for the accuracy of their infusion rate. Most modern infusion pumps use the peristaltic principle, and as a result of using precision silicone tubing and not having to rely upon drop counters to judge the infusion rate are as accurate as the syringe type.

The principle of the peristaltic infusion pump is shown in Figure 21.8. The tubing of a giving set is compressed by a series of rotating rollers or by a wave of mechanical 'fingers ' or cam followers.

set and interruptions of this beam are detected by a photoelectric cell. By measuring the time between drops and given the size of drop, the rate of infusion is calculated by the device and displayed (Fig. 21.7).

Infusion controllers use an electronic drop counter in conjunction with some form of adjustable occlusion of the infusion tubing controlled by a microprocessor. The infusion is under gravity but the device is able to compensate, at least partially, for changes in resistance to flow. Devices of this type and electronic drop counters

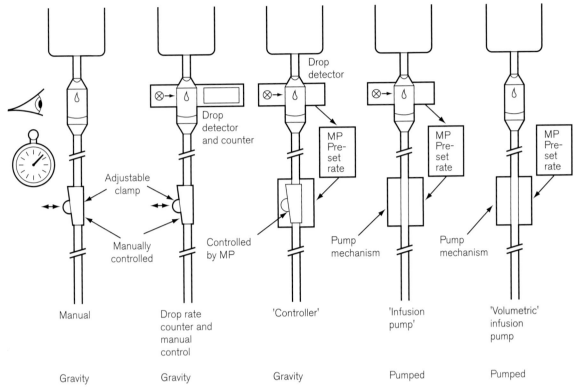

Figure 21.7 Types of infusion pumps. MP, microprocessor.

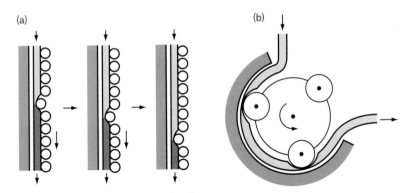

Figure 21.8 (a) linear and **(b)** rotary peristaltic mechanisms.

Figure 21.9 shows a typical syringe-type infusion pump mechanism. This, like the peristaltic pumps above, is driven by a stepper motor controlled directly by a microprocessor. The volume of the syringe is typically about 5 ml, with the dedicated disposable 'syringe cassette' for each manufacturers pump being supplied separately as a sterile product. Fluid is drawn rapidly from the reservoir bag into the syringe in less than 1 s. The valve is then actuated so that the syringe contents are expelled at the required rate into the patient, and then the process is repeated. Although effectively this produces an intermittent flow, it also gives overall extremely accurate infusion rates, with only infrequent 1 s interruptions.

Low budget infusion systems, that rely on drop counting to control the infusion rate (by comparing the desired rate with rate of drops passing the detector), are

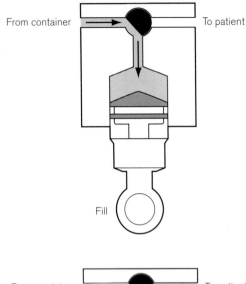

Fill

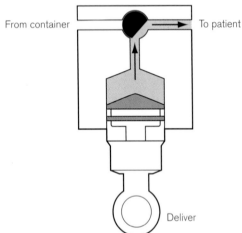

Deliver

Figure 21.9 Principle of a syringe-type volumetric infusion pump.

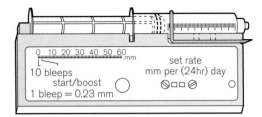

Figure 21.10 Graseby syringe driver.

Syringe drivers

The simplest mechanical syringe drivers are driven by clockwork mechanisms. These tend to work at a fixed rate only and are now rarely seen in UK hospital practice. There continues to be a range of small simple battery-operated syringe drivers (Fig. 21.10). The driving mechanism is a miniature DC motor that is switched on and off intermittently and drives a screw-threaded rod (lead screw), which is linked to the syringe plunger, causing its advancement. They may have a variable rate that is altered by adjusting a recessed control using a small screwdriver. These pumps are small and light enough to be worn in a holster by an ambulant patient and are now used chiefly for narcotic infusions for the relief of cancer pain. Great care must be taken in calculating drug dilutions and to ascertain that the correct units are used for setting the infusion rates, as the pumps are available in different models with rates set either as mm per 24 hr or mm per hr of plunger movement (Fig. 21.11).

Syringe drivers used in intensive care and anaesthesia normally use stepper motors, again connected to the syringe plunger by a lead screw. Thus, each pulse applied to the stepper motor causes the advancement of the syringe plunger by a known amount. The pulse generator may be calibrated from $0.1 \, \text{ml hr}^{-1}$ to $1200 \, \text{ml hr}^{-1}$, the higher rates being used only for delivering a bolus (often of predetermined volume) or for purging the infusion line.

Syringe pumps (the term is synonymous with syringe drivers) are now designed to automatically recognize a variety of syringes by virtue of the calibre of the barrel using some form of spring loaded arm; some manufacturers' models nonetheless require manual confirmation of the detector. Pressure sensors may be incorporated into the supports of the pusher operating on the syringe plunger to calculate line pressure and detect occlusion. This is a more popular option than the use of specialized infusion sets with in-built diaphragm and corresponding transducer housing on the syringe pump.

now rarely used in anaesthesia and acute areas of hospitals.

Because infusion pumps have the theoretical capacity to inject limitless quantities of air into a patient should its ingress occur upstream of the pump (for example due to an empty infusion bottle), these devices incorporate sophisticated ultrasonics or optics-based 'air in line' detection systems. These are usually placed downstream of the pump mechanism. Further protection is conferred by setting target delivery volumes smaller than the volume in the bag of infusate. Modern pumps are also able to detect line pressure and can be programmed to alarm for occlusion at different pre-set levels.

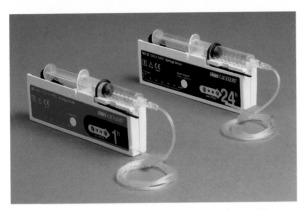

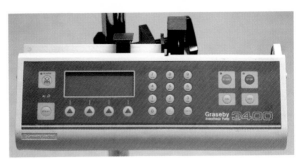

Figure 21.12 Graseby 3400 Anaesthesia Pump.

Figure 21.11 Graseby battery operated syringe drivers calibrated in mm per hr and mm per 24 hr. Photo courtesy M Stewart, Graseby Medical Ltd.

Because these pumps are software-driven, modern versions allow a multiplicity of units to be used for setting the infusion rate, including dosage on a mass of drug per weight per unit time basis. In such circumstances, great care again must be taken to ensure that unitary errors are not made when setting up the infusions. This risk is greater when the pump programmer is not the drug prescriber. For this reason pumps of this nature are often termed 'anaesthesia pumps' (Fig. 21.12) in order to restrict their usage. Other syringe drivers, and indeed infusion pumps, are also made with the ability to be pre-programmed with a library of drugs alongside their typical dilutions and infusion rates for use on the ITU. These devices can be configured to only allow the user to infuse drugs selected from the predetermined library (see below, Safety).

Rechargeable batteries

Although mains driven, electrical infusion devices must have battery back-up both to cover mains failure and for patient transfer and emergency situations. The perform-ance of the in-built rechargeable batteries is an important consideration when purchasing such equipment, but it must be remembered that this is also influenced by the battery maintenance procedures. Poor battery life can render otherwise excellent devices unreliable and un-usable. Pumps should be kept connected to the mains when not in use and batteries should be replaced appropriately. Microprocessor-driven infusion devices are susceptible to bizarre error conditions when rechargeable batteries begin to fail.

As with all rechargeable batteries, *Nickel-cadmium* (NiCd) rechargeable batteries should be periodically run down completely to prevent the development of 'memory', which renders them unable to discharge their full capacity. NiCd batteries are gradually being replaced by *nickel-metal hydride* (NiMH) batteries for environ-mental reasons (cadmium is a toxic heavy metal). In comparison to NiCd batteries, NiMH batteries have a higher-energy density, i.e. they can hold more charge per unit weight, but have a more limited service life. They are similarly prone to memory problems and need appropriate maintenance. *Lead acid* batteries, also called *'sealed lead acid'* to designate portability and to differentiate from the *flooded* type used in cars, have no 'memory', are cheap and reliable, but have long charging times. They are most often found on portable equipment such as ventilators and other heavy devices (e.g. wheelchairs and 'uninterruptible power supply' systems). Lead acid batteries, conversely, suffer by being allowed to fully discharge and must not be stored in this state as the process of *sulphation* can render them unusable. Lithium-ion (and to a certain extend lithium polymer) batteries have a high-energy density and no memory but are very expensive. The technology is currently confined largely to mobile telephones.

Battery maintenance is difficult in the hospital setting. Medical device batteries obviously cannot be safely run down whilst in use. Similarly, encouraging even partial discharge of a battery decreases the safety margins in the event of power failure or the need for transportation of a device.

Safety

Microprocessor-driven infusion devices have built-in alarms for occlusion, low battery, mains failure, dis-engagement of drive mechanism, failure to load infusion set and other common fault conditions. In spite of this, they remain high-risk devices capable ultimately of delivering drugs dangerously, they have a recognized associated morbidity and mortality. In at least 27% of the 1495 incidents involving infusion pumps reported to the Medical Devices Agency in the UK between 1990 and 2000, the cause was found to be user error (including failure to maintain the device appropriately). In a further 20% there were problems with performance, degradation and quality assurance with the device. The user must still be aware of the following possibilities:

- inadvertent administration with infusion pumps as a result of administration sets not being properly clamped off when the pump is not in operation or infusion set has not loaded into device properly;
- infusion of air;
- continued infusion after cannula has become extravascular;
- fault condition occurring in the pump device, caused by allowing intravenous liquids to spill on to the pump;
- rate of infusion upset by more than one infusion through the same cannula or catheter;
- siphoning – this is the term used to describe the uncontrolled flow of fluid from a syringe into the patient under gravity. Syringe drivers must have protection against the syringe plunger moving faster than the pusher attached to the lead screw. It is best, even with modern designs, to not have the syringe driver higher than the patient, as small amounts of siphoning can still occur. Anti-siphon valves, essentially a high-resistance one-way valve, may be incorporated into syringe pump giving sets (see below, Infusion lines);
- if syringe pumps are mounted with the syringe in the vertical position, the outlet of the syringe should be in the downward position so that bubbles formed by gas coming out of solution are not driven into the patient; and
- software revisions in microprocessor-driven devices can produce a wholly new machine within the familiar appearance of the old. Although features may be added or improved, there is also the possibility of introducing new problems and errors, particularly for those familiar to previous versions. Manufacturers should treat all but the most trivial revisions as new devices and issue new instruction and training/maintenance manuals.

Because of the huge flexibility of microprocessor-controlled infusion devices, it is increasingly important for users of these devices to have familiarized themselves specifically with the features and functions of each model before clinical application. Programming errors may potentially result in lethal overdosage. These devices are not always entirely intuitive to use, errors are commonplace with for example the 'hands free bolus' facility (a pre-programmable bolus dose that does not require the button to be kept depressed during delivery), which may give the option of a variety of unexpected units and infusion rates.

An approach to managing such risks is for the pumps to have pre-set limits for any given drug so that users must first choose a drug from a menu and can then only key in a limited range of infusion rates, bolus sizes and drug concentrations using predetermined units. Such a 'library' can be programmed into the device by a competent user with access codes to enter the 'set up' mode of the pump. This is often a laborious process given the limited keypads on devices and the fact that for each pump each drug may need upper and lower limits for patient weight, drug concentration, bolus size, bolus rate and infusion rates. It may be facilitated by downloading such libraries from a central computer.

The line pressure limit at which devices alarm for occlusion can usually be altered, for some models this is a user function whilst on others it must be performed by biomedical engineering departments. Limits must be set such that nuisance alarms do not occur due to the resistance of the giving set or 'stiction' at the syringe barrel/plunger interface. High-pressure limits, however, have two major disadvantages:

1. it will take longer to alarm for occlusion (alarm time is increased) particularly at low infusion rates and at the start of an infusion – most commonly due to leaving a stopcock closed; and
2. on release of the obstruction a proportionately larger bolus will be delivered to the patient; this may be clinically significant.

Microprocessors are susceptible to electromagnetic interference (EMI) from wireless telecommunication devices such as mobile telephones. EMI can cause serious malfunction in medical devices. The strength of the electromagnetic field is proportional to the power output of the telecommunication device and inversely proportional to the square of the distance from the source. The possibility of EMI is greatest with emergency radios (as used by ambulance, police and fire services) followed by security radios (as used by hospital maintenance and portering staff) and finally by cellphones (both analogue and digital type mobile phones). The Medical Devices Agency of the UK reports 41% of the medical devices they tested suffered interference from emergency radio handsets at a distance of 1 m with 49% of these being classed as serious. By comparison, the figures for security radio handsets were 35% and 49%, respectively, and those for mobile phones 4% and 0.1%.[1] It is important to note that these devices can cause interference even in standby mode and must therefore be fully switched off to be considered safe. Cordless telephones and wireless computer local area networks do not appear to cause significant interference.

Although most hospitals have policies demanding that mobile phones be switched off in clinical areas, clinicians must always bear in mind the potential for such malfunction, given the ubiquitous nature of mobile telephones and the increased risk of problems with the two-way radios used in hospitals.

TARGET CONTROLLED INFUSION

Intravenous anaesthesia, referring to anaesthesia maintained by continuous infusion of anaesthetic agents requires that consistent drug concentrations can be achieved which may be altered in response to the needs of the procedure. The term Total Intravenous Anaesthesia (TIVA) is used synonymously with intravenously-maintained anaesthesia but perhaps should be reserved for those scenarios where no inhalational agents (including nitrous oxide) are co-administered.

Although the drugs used for intravenously-maintained anaesthesia are of rapid onset and have short half-lives and durations of action, in order to rapidly achieve and maintain a given clinical effect it is still necessary with currently available agents to administer boluses and then to reduce progressively the infusion rate. Target Controlled Infusion (TCI) describes a system whereby a computer controls the rate of infusion of a drug to achieve (in as short a time as possible) and maintain any given target concentration. In use this means that the anaesthetist is relieved of having to continuously make complex calculations and adjustments of the infusion rate, thus lending the ability to endlessly vary the drug concentration to achieve the desired effect (Fig. 21.13).

Investigators in the fields of anaesthesia and pharmaco-kinetics have considerable experience in programming computers to achieve constant concentrations of drug by driving infusion pumps at variable rates. Many different terms have been used to describe this process since the description of the bolus elimination and transfer (BET) infusion scheme with a system called CATIA (Computer Assisted Total Intravenous Anaesthesia) in 1983.[2] The aim throughout has been to emulate the simplicity of administration of inhalational agents, in effect to design a 'calibrated vaporizer' for intravenous agents, i.e. a system akin to that for inhalational agents wherein a given setting on the 'vaporizer' will, within certain limits, result in a similar and constant drug concentration in the patient.

Although the original experimental systems were cumbersome, in 1990 workers from the University of Glasgow described a system for the delivery of propofol using a conventional syringe pump driven by a Psion II hand-held computer.[3] There was good correlation between measured and predicted plasma concentrations and users found the device easy to use. This was the basis for what remains still the only widely available commercial system for delivering a drug using a pharmacokinetic algorithm.

Key components

A TCI system must have the following key components:
- an infusion device;
- a computer and pharmacokinetic algorithm which translates predictions from the model into instructions to control the infusion device, the algorithm must have

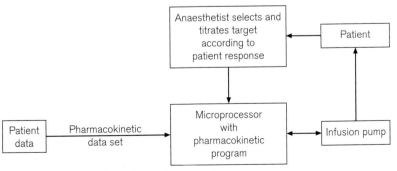

Figure 21.13 Relationships in a Target Controlled Infusion system.

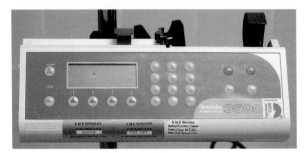

Figure 21.14 Graseby 3500 Anaesthsia Pump incorporating the Diprifusor™ chip.

the correct pharmacokinetic data set (constants) for the patient group in which it will be used;
- patient specific data, for example, weight, (currently the Diprifusor system does not alter the data set for patient age or circumstance);
- a user interface to allow and confirm data input and to inform the user of the algorithm's predictions; and
- a fail-safe system: a safety mechanism to shut down the system in the event of computer failure; this may be in the form of a second microprocessor calculating the drug concentration based upon the output of the pump and comparing this with the predicted value from the first microprocessor's control algorithm, with instructions to shut down the system if there is greater than a preset discrepancy (5% for Diprifusor).

It is important that the algorithm is not inadvertently reset as if for a new patient when renewing drug syringes during the course of an anaesthetic, as this will of course result in the delivery of a further loading dose.

Diprifusor™

In 1996 the manufacturer Graseby produced anaesthesia syringe drivers bearing the 'Diprifusor' TCI Subsystem (Fig. 21.14) licensed from Zeneca (now AstraZeneca), the makers of propofol. The Diprifusor chip has subsequently been incorporated into other makes of syringe driver. An advantage of this modular approach to the design of TCI systems, where the pharmaceutical company retains responsibility for the Diprifusor module, is the standardization of propofol delivery, such that all pumps bearing that module will deliver the same amount of drug for any given target setting because the same pharmacokinetic model is operating. To date, 15 000 such modules (Fig. 21.15) have been sold worldwide (personal communication, AstraZeneca). The Subsystem comprises components designed to:
- recognize electronically tagged pre-filled syringes of propofol produced by AstraZeneca in order to identify drug and concentration and enable TCI mode when appropriate; and
- control syringe pump in TCI mode to deliver propofol by Target Controlled Infusion (see above).

In order to ensure that the syringe driver operates in TCI mode only when loaded with the correct drug (proprietary propofol as Diprivan), the pre-filled syringes carry a small electronic tag in the finger grip of the barrel. When the syringe is correctly located the 'Programmable Magnetic Resonance' tag lies within a recess close to an aerial in the body of the pump. In response to signals from the aerial the magnets within the tag oscillate at particular frequencies generating a signal, which is picked up by the aerial. To discourage refilling of the syringe the tag is subsequently 'wiped' by the pump when the actuator pushing the syringe plunger reaches a pre-set travel.

The pharmacokinetic model used is based on the Marsh open three-compartment model[4] (Fig. 21.16) with parameters as shown in Table 21.1. Figure 21.17 shows a typical infusion scheme from a TCI device to

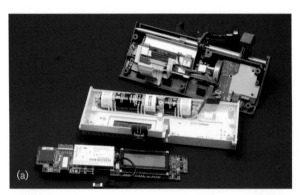

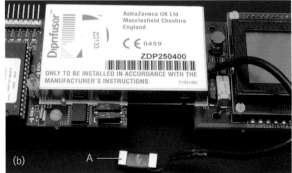

Figure 21.15 (a) The Diprifusor subsystem installed on the microprocessor control board of the Graseby 3500. **(b)** Note the 'aerial' (A) for recognition of the syringe tag.

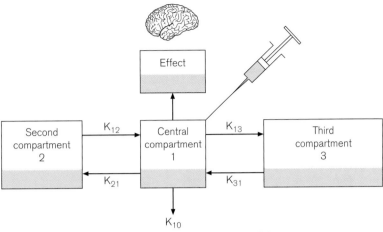

Figure 21.16 Schematic representation of open three-compartment model.

Table 21.1 Pharmacokinetic parameters for propofol incorporated in Diprifusor software

V_1 Volume of central compartment	228 ml kg^{-1}
Half life of delay central to effect site ($t_{1/2}$Keo)	2.6 min
Rate Constants:	
K_{10} (elimination rate constant)	0.119 min^{-1}
K_{12}	0.114 min^{-1}
K_{21}	0.055 min^{-1}
K_{13}	0.042 min^{-1}
K_{31}	0.003 min^{-1}

© University of Glasgow

demonstrate the bolus and decreasing infusion rate needed to maintain an increased concentration. Diprifusor software (which targets the plasma concentration as the control variable) also allows the predicted effect site concentration to be demonstrated at any time. This is a useful facility both in terms of demonstrating for impatient anaesthetists the magnitude of the time lag between the compartments and for correlating clinical effect with theoretical concentration when plasma compartment 'overpressure' is used to speed up the onset of effect.

Accuracy

Two independent factors contribute to the overall accuracy of a TCI system:

1. delivery performance of infusion system, how well the syringe pump outputs the desired volume of drug; and
2. predictive accuracy of pharmacokinetic model.

Syringe pumps incorporating Diprifusor are required by the manufacturer to have a performance such that the infusion error at specific time points is within $\pm 5\%$ of the ideal volume.[5]

In considering figures for the predictive accuracy of pharmacokinetic models, a number of issues must be borne in mind:

- inter-patient pharmacokinetic variability must always be expected and the need to titrate drug target concentration to achieve the desired effect is inescapable;
- performance is likely to vary with time and chosen target concentrations;
- errors in blood sampling technique or variability in the measurement of blood concentrations, this may at times be due to inadequate mixing at high infusion rates; and
- in clinical assessments of accuracy the co-administration of other drugs may affect the handling of the target drug.

There is an attempt to standardize measurement of the accuracy of computer-controlled infusion systems.[6] Performance error expressed as a percentage is calculated as shown below:

$$\text{Performance Error (\%)} = \frac{C_M - C_{Calc}}{C_{Calc}} \times 100$$

where C_M and C_{CALC} are the measured and calculated blood propofol concentrations. Other indices are derived

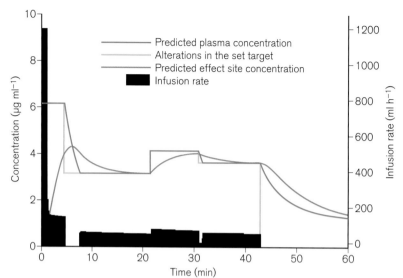

Figure 21.17 A typical infusion scheme from a TCI device, showing the predicted plasma concentration in response to alterations in the set target and the infusion rate.

from this. The median performance error (MDPE) is a measure of the tendency of the system to over or underestimate the measured blood concentration in a given patient or scenario. This is the degree of bias and has direction as well as value, thus if bias has a positive value the measured concentrations tend to be greater than predicted. The precision, or size of the error, is represented by the median absolute performance error (MDAPE). Divergence and wobble reflect on time-related changes in performance and intra-subject variability in performance respectively. Typical figures for MDPE of 16.2% and MDAPE of 24.1% were reported in one study,[7] with measured concentrations tending to be higher, particularly after induction or an increase in target concentration and at higher targets. In context these figures compare favourably with the performance of inhalational anaesthesia where after 15 min of isoflurane administration a ratio of 0.78 is reported between arterial and end-tidal partial pressures[8] with the concentration remaining 20% lower at 1 h. There is a greater difference between vaporizer setting and arterial concentration.[9]

Future developments

The introduction of the Diprifusor TCI system has been hugely successful and coincident with a substantial increase in the use of intravenous anaesthesia over the last five years, it remains to be seen if any new agents are

developed where a manufacturer feels the development costs of a commercial TCI system for the agent are worth the investment. Only very recently has the opioid drug remifentanil, in spite of its popularity and natural partnership with propofol, attracted this treatment, perhaps because the therapeutic window in anaesthetized and ventilated patients is large and wear off is not an issue due to its ultra–short and unchanging context sensitive half time.

A logical development from the TCI system, for maintaining constant concentrations of anaesthetic, has been to link this with some form of depth of anaesthesia monitor to automatically alter the chosen target to maintain a constant depth of anaesthesia. Such a set-up is termed Closed Loop Anaesthesia (CLAN) and has been successfully used to anaesthetize patients breathing spontaneously during surgery.[10,11]

TCI may also be used as the basis for an advanced form of Patient Controlled Analgesia (or Sedation). Here, the patient's button presses may, for example, result in an increase or prevent a decrease in the target concentration of drug rather than a drug bolus.[12] Such systems are so far experimental only.

An interesting consequence of the current popularity of Total Intravenous Anaesthesia has been the development in prototype of an integrated anaesthesia workstation comprising ventilator, two in-built syringe drivers and patient monitoring in one compact unit. The lack of volatile agents and N$_2$O negates the need to return patient gases to the machine for scavenging. The Aneo TIVAS has so far not progressed to the marketplace.

At least two manufacturers are producing syringe pumps that may be used individually or severally stacked together and controlled through one video control panel for use in anaesthesia and intensive care. Braun have their own TCI program which works with generic propofol but the usability of their system has still to be proved in the operating theatre. Fresenius have developed TCI programmes for both remifentanil and generic propofol. Ideally these systems will have the ability to output in real time, their target and predicted concentrations and infusion rates for the purposes of automated record keeping. Such a facility is currently lacking on Diprifusor. The Fresenius system offers a choice of different pharmacokinetic algorithms for propofol, and it is to be expected that those familiar with the clinical effects seen for a given target with one algorithm may see different effects when using an alternative algorithm due to differing amounts of drug being delivered.

PATIENT-CONTROLLED ANALGESIA

The quality of post-operative pain relief and patients' sense of autonomy have perhaps improved with the use of patient-controlled analgesia (PCA). Although intramuscular bolusing with opiates at 3–4 hourly intervals may provide good analgesia, the reluctance of patients to disturb hard-pressed nurses and the need for the increasingly rare presence of a second member of staff to administer 'controlled drugs' rarely resulted in optimal analgesia. The advantages of PCA are:

- patient autonomy;
- rapid relief of pain; and
- analgesia/dosage tailored to patient's requirements, with the patient able to balance analgesia and side effects.

For safety reasons most physicians are reluctant to use a background infusion alongside the patient-controlled bolus doses. This is the key disadvantage: bolus doses are necessarily small with a short duration of action resulting again in fluctuating analgesia levels, particularly at night-time where patients often complain of waking in pain and thus poor sleep.

Key points in any PCA system are:

- route of administration;
- type of administration (bolus, background infusion);
- ease of programming (dose, lock out);
- ease of priming;
- power source;
- safety;
- security;
- portability;
- display;
- printout.

PCA is most commonly delivered intravenously but may also be subcutaneous or into the epidural space, although this route of administration does have the theoretical problem of bypassing the safety feedback loop where the potentially overdosed patient becomes somnolent and unable to make further analgesic demands. The simplest method of administration is by bolus dosing; here a preset bolus, which may be programmed either by volume or in more complex systems by weight of drug in milligrams, is injected on demand. There is a pre-programmed lock-out time during which further demands are ignored, thus allowing for the time of onset of action of the previous bolus and protecting against overdosage.

A background continuous infusion may also be available with some devices. This militates against patients waking in pain due to protracted periods of no analgesic administration, although safety consideration make this a rarely-used facility (see above).

PCA devices (Fig. 21.18) are mostly variations of the infusion devices discussed earlier. They may be syringe drivers or peristaltic type volumetric pumps which are microprocessor-controlled, hence again the aspects of those devices mentioned elsewhere are still pertinent. Because of the trend towards increased patient mobility and Patient-Controlled Epidural Analgesia (PCEA), a number of manufacturers now produce miniaturized PCA pumps often using a small compressible pumping chamber designed as an integral part of the giving set (Fig. 21.19). Size and portability are limited by the size of the drug reservoir and the need to encase this in a lockable anti-tamper shell.

As with other microprocessor-controlled devices, there is a vast amount of information recorded by these newer devices, only some of which is presented to the clinician. This includes times of error messages, alarm conditions, 'power up' and 'power down' and rate or programme changes. There is usually a facility to view and/or download or print the 'patient history' so that pump settings may be tailored to the patient's needs. A further feature is the lockable control panel (this may be an actual key and lock in some machines) needing access codes and button presses of unlabelled 'soft-keys' to prevent unauthorized tampering with the pumps.

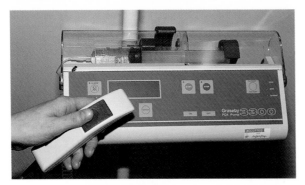

Figure 21.18 A Graseby PCA.

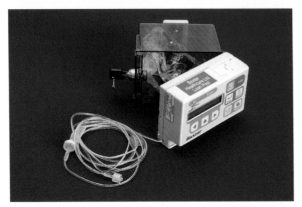

Figure 21.19 A Baxter PCA pump, which may be used for epidural and also epidural PCA.

A consequence of increasing functionality, together with miniaturization and the need for security, is that many of these devices are no longer intuitive to use and effectively need a dedicated 'pilot'. Disenfranchized staff become reluctant or unable to initiate and alter settings with the quality of analgesia suffering as a result. Uniformity of equipment in clinical areas helps but when deciding a purchasing policy, also to be considered are the considerable capital costs of these devices and the cost of initiation and maintenance of staff training and the sheer numbers of devices needed to provide the service.

There is much to be said for the use of simple disposable PCA devices, as shown in Figure 21.20. These elastomeric devices are in effect powered by the energy stored in the stretching of the balloon holding the reservoir of drug. A small compressible chamber of preset volume (usually 0.5 or 1 ml), on a wrist strap or attached to the reservoir, holds the bolus dose which is delivered to the patient through a one-way valve when the chamber is squeezed. The lock-out time is predetermined by a flow restrictor connecting the reservoir and chamber which

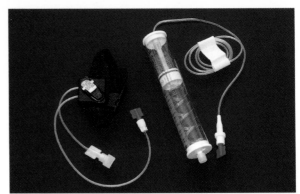

Figure 21.20 An elastomeric disposable PCA pump with the demand button worn as a 'wrist watch'.

governs the rate of refilling of the chamber, thus giving a maximal flow rate through the device, typically 5 ml hr^{-1}. Drug demands, before the effective lock-out time is reached, result in proportionately smaller doses. PCA regime alterations are therefore made by altering the drug concentration in the reservoir.

Of prime importance with PCA is safety and security. All devices must be safe against over-dosage, either caused by fault conditions or drug siphoning. There must also be security against tampering and adjustment of settings by unauthorized staff, patients or visitors.

FILTRATION

Intravenous fluids should be filtered to protect the patient from microscopic foreign material. Blood for transfusion that is more than 24 h old should be filtered (Fig. 21.21) to remove micro-aggregates that form from the breakdown products of the cellular components and platelets. Blood filters are of two basic forms: screen filters and depth filters. Screen filters function as 'sieves' and are usually constructed from a woven mesh. They have a regular pore size, often of 40 μm. The efficiency of a screen-type filter at removing foreign matter increases progressively with each unit of blood passed as the pore size tends to decrease progressively down to 20 μm. Screen-type filters are said to be less damaging to the red cells than are depth filters. Depth filters consist of a pack of synthetic fibre, often Dacron, not formed into a mesh. The mechanism of filtration is actually by adsorption of unwanted material, down to a size of about 10 μm onto the surface of the fibres. This adsorption is probably due to electrical charge differences between the particles and the fibres. With the depth filter, the efficiency at removal

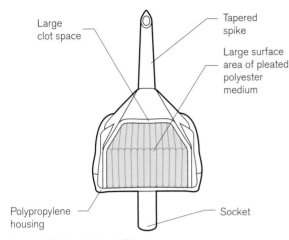

Large clot space

Tapered spike

Large surface area of pleated polyester medium

Polypropylene housing

Socket

Figure 21.21 A blood filter.

of unwanted material decreases with each unit of blood, probably as a result of channelling in the pack of fibres.

Intravenous crystalloids may be filtered with much finer sieve-type filters to remove foreign particulate matter, including bacteria. The Pall intravenous 'Site Saver' extends the life of the giving set, which should normally be replaced every 24 h, to up to 96 h. The construction of the 'Site Saver' is shown in Figure 21.22. All particulate matter larger than 0.2 μm is removed by the 0.2 μm filter membrane. Air can be vented through a hydrophobic membrane, which has 0.02 μm pores.

AUTOTRANSFUSION

When a large blood loss may be expected during surgery, it may be possible to re-use the patient's own blood,

provided that it is uncontaminated and free from clots. Uncontaminated blood is aspirated by the machine, red cells are washed, spun down and suspended in crystalloid solution with added anticoagulant and stored temporarily in a reservoir. It may then be transfused back into the patient via a filter. The operation of such machines needs a dedicated member of staff.

RELATED EQUIPMENT FOR TIVA

Infusion lines

When more than one fluid or drug is infused through a common intravascular device, alterations in the rate of infusion of one of these substances will temporarily affect the rate of administration of the remainder. The degree of perturbation is a function of the shared volume (dead-space) of intravenous device and the infusion rates (Fig. 21.23). For drugs with short half-lives this can have a dramatic effect. Ideally, each intravenous infusion of drug would be given through a dedicated infusion line so that alterations in the rate of infusion of one drug does not affect the others. For simplicity and patient comfort, it is preferable to insert only one intravenous catheter and use a many-tailed infusion set. Such infusion sets are available specifically for TIVA with one or two long narrow calibre 'pump lines' and one wider-bore line to connect to a giving set for fluid administration under gravity (Fig. 21.24). Each line should incorporate a one-way or anti-reflux valve to prevent backflow as well as anti-siphon valves on the pump lines. The shared volume, where the lines join before the intravenous catheter, should be as small as possible. Because such lines are made up of a number of

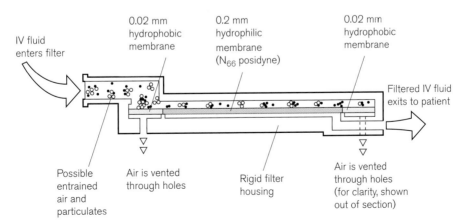

IV fluid enters filter

0.02 mm hydrophobic membrane

0.2 mm hydrophilic membrane (N_{66} posidyne)

0.02 mm hydrophobic membrane

Filtered IV fluid exits to patient

Possible entrained air and particulates

Air is vented through holes

Rigid filter housing

Air is vented through holes (for clarity, shown out of section)

Figure 21.22 Pall intravenous 'Site Saver'.

(a) Both infusions running

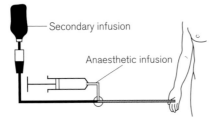

(b) Secondary infusion finished

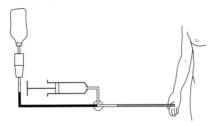

(c)

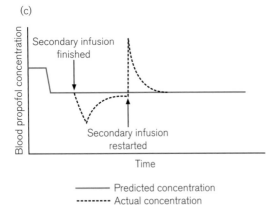

——— Predicted concentration
-------- Actual concentration

Figure 21.23 Changes in the flow rate of a secondary infusion influence the rate at which a drug is delivered to the body. For an infusion line with a volume of 5 ml between the connection of two infusions and the patient, if one infusion stops a considerable drop in drug concentration of the second may be expected. After restarting that infusion a bolus of the second drug is immediately administered, causing a peak in drug concentration. Redrawn with permission from Engbers F, Vuyk J (1996) *Anaesthesia Rounds, Target-controlled Infusion*. © The Medicine Group (Education) Ltd.

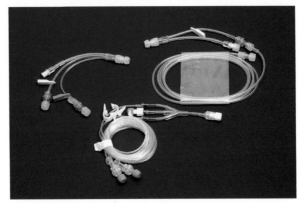

Figure 21.24 A selection of giving sets for intravenous anaesthesia (see text).

administration of epidural drugs. Demands in the lay and specialist press (in response to well-publicized cases of intra-thecal misadministration of cytotoxics) for the introduction of a new standard of non-interchangeable connections on equipment designed for centrineural access, have so far been met with silence. It is questionable whether such a massive sea change with its own unquantified risks is desirable.

TIVAtrainer©

For the purpose of understanding and predicting the disposition of intravenous drugs, no amount of theoretical knowledge of pharmacokinetics or practical experience of intravenous anaesthesia is as effective as seeing graphical representations of drug concentrations and the changes in response to interventions. TIVAtrainer (copyright F. Engbers, Leiden University Hospital) is a pharmacokinetic simulation programme for intravenous anaesthetics developed as shareware available from the web site for the European Society for Intravenous Anaesthesia – EuroSIVA. TIVAtrainer (Fig. 21.25) is not the first simulation software of this type,[13] but it is perhaps the most developed and 'user friendly'. It is an ideal teaching tool for use in the operating room or the lecture theatre, allowing simultaneous modelling of several different drugs used in anaesthesia.

The program can simulate manual and TCI infusion schemes demonstrating the infusion rates and associated plasma and effect site concentrations, as well as representing the amount of drug in each of the model's theoretical compartments, which are drawn to scale. A number of additional features permit the calculation of drug cost, the demonstration of Context Sensitive Half-

components assembled together it should be borne in mind that they may leak or be obstructed at the bonded junctions. This may not always be obvious.

There appears to be a general move towards using yellow-coloured or marked infusion lines for epidural infusions. This should help reduce the risk of intravenous

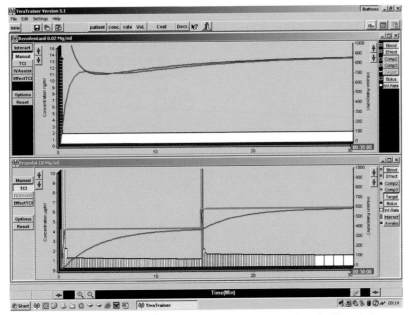

Figure 21.25 A screen shot from the TIVAtrainer©. Frank Engbers, Leiden University Hospital.

Time and the hypnotic interactions between opiates and anaesthetic agents. The 'Help' file is well referenced and the program provides a comprehensive teaching package. As with all mathematical modelling, extrapolations at the limits of the model must be interpreted with particular caution.

In use, a drug is chosen from the menu and a method of administration is chosen, which may be:

- manual bolus and infusion rates;
- TCI with targeting of either the plasma or effect site compartments; and
- a further mode called 'IV assist' is designed to present simplified stepped infusion rates for entry on a manual infusion pump in order to mimic TCI.

REFERENCES

1. Medical Devices Agency (1997) *Electromagnetic Compatibility of Medical Devices with Mobile Communications.* DB9702, Medical Devices Agency.
2. Schüttler J, Schwilden H, Stoeckel H (1983) Pharmacokinetics as applied to total intravenous anaesthesia. *Anaesthesia* **38(suppl)**: 53–56..
3. Kenny GNC, White M (1990) A portable computerized control system for propofol infusion. *Anaesthesia* **45**: 692–693.
4. Marsh B, White M, Morton N, Kenny GN (1991) Pharmacokinetic model driven infusion in children. *British Journal of Anaesthesia* **67**: 41–48.
5. Glen JB (1998) The development of 'Diprifusor': a TCI system for propofol. *Anaesthesia* **53(suppl 1)**: 13–21.
6. Varvel JR, Donoho DL, Shafer SL (1992) Measuring the performance of computer-controlled infusion pumps. *Journal of Pharmacokinetics and Biopharmaceutics* **20**: 63–94.
7. Swinhoe CF, Peacock JE, Glen JB, Reilly CS (1998) Evaluation of the predictive performance of a 'Diprifusor' TCI system. *Anaesthesia* **53(suppl 1)**: 61–67.
8. Frei FJ, Zbinden AM, Thomson DA, Reider HU (1991) Is the end-tidal partial pressure of isoflurane a good predictor of its arterial partial pressure? *British Journal of Anaesthesia* **66**: 331–339.
9. Dwyer RC, Fee JPH, Howard PJ, Clarke RSJ (1991) Arterial wash-in of halothane and isoflurane in young and elderly adult patients. *British Journal of Anaesthesia* **66**: 572–579.
10. Kenny GN, Mantzaridis H (1999) Closed-loop control of propofol anaesthesia. *British Journal of Anaesthesia* **83**: 223–228.
11. Morley A, Derrick J, Mainland P, *et al.* (2000) Closed loop control of anaesthesia: an assessment of the bispectral index as the target of control. *Anaesthesia* **55**: 953–959.

12. Irwin MG, Jones RD, Visram AR, Kornberg JP (1994) A patient's experience of a new postoperative patient-controlled analgesic technique. *European Journal of Anaesthesia* **11**: 413–415.

13. Stanford PK/PD server: http://anesthesia.stanford.edu/pkpd/_vti_bin/owssvr.dll?Using=Default%2ehtm

FURTHER READING

Medical Devices Agency (2003) *Infusion Systems*, Device Bulletin. MDA DB2003(02), Medical Devices Agency.

White PF (ed.) (1997) *Textbook of Intravenous Anaesthesia*. Baltimore: Williams & Wilkins.

Buchmann I (2001) *Batteries in a Portable World*: *A Handbook on Rechargeable Batteries for Non-Engineers*, 2nd edn. Cadex Electronics Inc. (also available on-line at http://www.buchmann.ca/default.asp accessed 05.10.2004).

Medical suction apparatus

John TB Moyle

Suction apparatus is vital to safe medical practice, especially anaesthesia, resuscitation and intensive care. It is used for the clearance of mucus, blood and debris from the pharynx, trachea and main bronchi. During surgery, suction is used to provide a clear operating field for the surgeon. Specially adapted suction apparatus can also be used for other procedures, such as gastrointestinal, wound and pleural drainage.

MAIN COMPONENTS

The main components of a medical suction system are:
* energy source;
* conversion of that energy to vacuum;
* filter; and
* collection vessel.

The schematic drawings in Figure 22.1 outline the methods used in suction apparatus, using internationally agreed symbols.

Energy source

Suction apparatus requires an energy source that generates a sub-atmospheric pressure. This is colloquially referred to as a *vacuum source*, despite the fact that a true (high) vacuum is rarely achieved. In fact, the pressure required is only a maximum of 60 kPa less than the normal environmental pressure (see Further Reading).

The energy sources most commonly used are mains electricity and pipeline suction. Pipeline suction, of course, is a source of vacuum generated by an electrically-powered vacuum pump at a distance from the user.

Portable suction apparatus may be battery driven, hand or foot operated, or make use of compressed gas as a source of energy.

Vacuum source

The sub-atmospheric pressure required may be generated by:
* An electric motor or other source of rotational energy that may be used to drive a mechanical pump, various forms of which are shown in Figures 22.2a–e.
* Pneumatically driven pumps that usually work on the venturi principle (Fig. 22.2f). The driving force may be air, oxygen, steam or water.
* A manually (or foot) operated spring-loaded bellows arrangement with unidirectional valves (Fig. 22.2g).

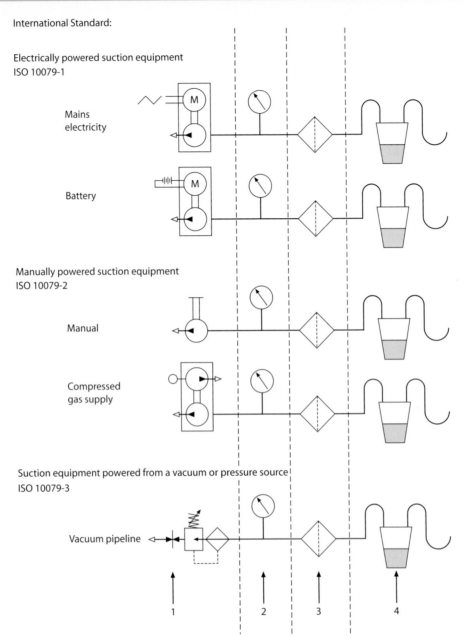

International Standard:

Electrically powered suction equipment
ISO 10079-1

Mains electricity

Battery

Manually powered suction equipment
ISO 10079-2

Manual

Compressed gas supply

Suction equipment powered from a vacuum or pressure source
ISO 10079-3

Vacuum pipeline

1   2   3   4

Figure 22.1 Suction equipment. Key: 1, Vacuum source/regulator; 2, vacuum indicator; 3, filter; 4, collection container. (See ISO documents in Further Reading.)

Pump types

Figure 22.2a shows a piston pump, which is capable of creating high vacuum but, in transportable models, has a relatively low displacement (i.e. can only sustain low flow rates). Figure 22.2b shows a diaphragm pump which is a variation of the piston pump. It is mechanically simpler but is also frequently much noisier. One reason for the increased noise is that often, rather than using a conventional rotating electric motor, a much simpler large electromagnet displaces the diaphragm. Figure 22.2c shows a form of rotary pump that can produce a high vacuum without conventional one-way valves. Figure 22.2d shows a rotary pump capable of producing very high flows, as would be required in a dental surgery. It

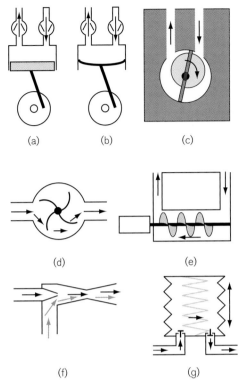

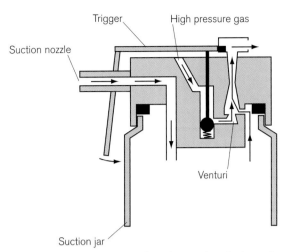

Figure 22.3 Working principles of a suction device using a Venturi injector.

Figure 22.2 Vacuum pumps. **(a)** Piston pump; **(b)** diaphragm pump; **(c)** high vacuum rotary pump; **(d)** low vacuum rotary vane pump; **(e)** rotary pump using an Archimedean wheel; **(f)** gas-powered pump using the Venturi principle; **(g)** a bellows pump.

works in the same way as a vacuum cleaner and has the disadvantage of being extremely noisy. Figure 22.2e shows a pump that works on the Archimedean principle. This type of pump can produce a high vacuum for a comparatively small size of machine. Figure 22.2f shows the principle of a Venturi pump which makes use of the Bernoulli effect. Compressed fluid (gas or liquid), passing through a narrow orifice, creates a region of negative pressure beyond that orifice, which can be used to entrain adjacent air/debris. The main disadvantage of this simple affair is that it uses and is thus wasteful of large volumes of driving fluid, which is usually oxygen from cylinders. However, it does have the virtue of being extremely portable (Fig. 22.3). Finally, Figure 22.2g shows a simple bellows mechanism with a pair of one-way valves, as would be used in manually operated suction apparatus.

The pump may be:

- *permanently sited* as in pipeline suction systems;
- *transportable*, usually powered by mains electricity and supported on castor wheels; or
- *truly portable*, powered by battery, a cylinder of gas or by human energy (hand or foot operated).

There are international standards for each type of suction apparatus and these are listed at the end of this chapter.

Internal connections

The vacuum source is connected to the filter and collection vessel by tubing, that is as rigid as possible to avoid collapse due to the vacuum. In pipeline systems the tubing can be made from metal or hard plastics but the internal tubing in transportable units has to be firm but flexible, as does the final connection to the collection vessel in all types.

Filter

This is fitted between the collection vessel and the vacuum source. It is to reduce the risk of contamination reaching the pipeline or pump or being expelled into the atmosphere. Filters should remain dry and must be replaced at intervals recommended by the manufacturer, otherwise there is risk of reducing suction efficiency and of the filter becoming an infection risk itself.

Collection vessel

The collection vessel stores the aspirate prior to its disposal. It needs to be of sufficient volume to hold enough aspirate so that it does not need emptying too often. However, the larger its volume, the greater the displacement that is necessary from the pump, in order to reduce the pressure in the vessel before aspiration can occur efficiently. It is important that the inlet to the collection vessel has an internal diameter sufficiently large to admit the largest particles expected in the particular application of the apparatus (see Further Reading).

To minimize risks of contamination to theatre staff, all suction apparatus, except portable emergency units, should make use of a disposable collection system (Fig. 22.4a.) This consists of a rigid outer transparent container with volume markings on its side and an inner (transparent) disposable plastic sleeve fitted with a lid. The aspirate is stored in the inner sleeve and when full is capped off and discarded. As it is disposed of with other clinical waste, a gelling agent should be added to the vessel so as to solidify the contents to prevent accidental spillage. Thus, staff should never come into contact with any aspirate.

Suction tubing to disposal

There must be a suitable length of *suction tubing*, the patient end of which is usually fitted with a detachable rigid suction hand-piece. This tubing is a compromise between rigidity to avoid collapse when the vacuum is applied and flexibility for ease of use. With portable hand-held apparatus, the hand piece may be connected directly to the collection vessel for ease of use.

Efficiency

The efficiency of suction apparatus depends upon:
- the degree of vacuum (*sub-atmospheric* pressure) that can be produced by the pump, with particular regard to the time taken to achieve it;
- the *displacement*, i.e. the volume of air at atmospheric pressure that the pump is able to move in unit time;
- the *internal resistance* of the suction apparatus as a whole. This is related not only to the length and diameter of tubing and other components, but also to the tubing and other accessories between the apparatus and the liquid being aspirated; and
- the *viscosity* of the matter being aspirated.

Different pump designs may have differing displacements and high-vacuum capabilities and, therefore, may be selected for specific tasks. For example, liposuction requires high vacuum to dislodge fat globules that have a

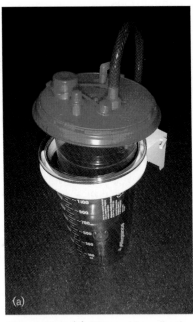

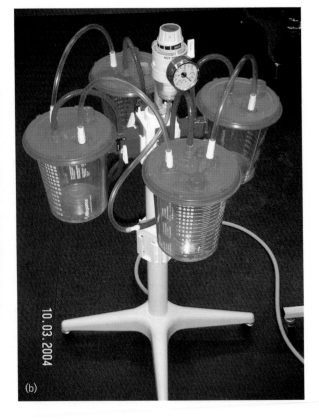

Figure 22.4 (a) Disposable collection vessel system. Note the outer container with volume markings and the inner sleeve fitted with a lid. **(b)** A disposable collection system with multiple collection vessels.

high viscosity but a small displacement because only a relatively small volume and no air are removed. In contrast, dental suction requires high displacement to remove large amounts of water spray, air and dental debris, but does not require a high vacuum. This type of apparatus must also have a low internal resistance and be connected to a relatively wide-bore hand-piece and tubing to maximize the rate of removal of debris.

OTHER COMPONENTS OF SUCTION APPARATUS

Vacuum gauge

The vacuum gauge is also placed between the vacuum source and the collection vessel. It is calibrated in mmHg or kPa or both scales. The purpose of the gauge is three-fold: to test the apparatus for efficiency and leaks, to allow for adjustment of the available vacuum during use and to warn of excessive suction being applied to tissues. Note that modern vacuum gauges indicate counter-clockwise.

Vacuum control valve or regulator

This may be fitted between the vacuum source and the collection vessel. A *vacuum control valve* is a bleed valve that when opened, admits air, thereby reducing the degree of vacuum. A *vacuum regulator* operates on a similar principle to a pressure regulator and so no energy is wasted from the system. Regulators are always used with pipeline systems, whereas control valves are common with transportable electrically driven units.

Cut-off over-flow valve

This is part of the collection vessel assembly and prevents any aspirate from leaving the vessel and entering the vacuum source or controller. It usually consists of a float, which is lifted by the rising level of aspirate when the vessel is full.

In order to test both the collection vessel and especially its inlet and also the cut-off over-flow valve, an international standard test vomit has been specified. It consists of food-grade xantham gum, water and 1 mm glass beads (see Further Reading).

Foam prevention

Foaming may be a problem in the collection vessel as it may cause premature closure of the over-flow cut-off valve. Foam may even pass beyond the valve and contaminate the filter or pump causing failure. Foaming also makes it difficult to estimate the amount of aspirate in the vessel. Foaming may be reduced by the addition of a small quantity of silicon-based emulsion or by silicon coating of the inside of the collection vessel.

Multiple collection vessels

Modern suction apparatus usually has two collection vessels with a manually operated valve, so that the vacuum source can be rapidly switched from a full vessel to a fresh one. Alternatively, where large volumes of aspirate are anticipated, a number of collection vessels are connected in series in a carousel and without valves. Here, aspirate overflows from the first vessel into the next and so on (Fig. 22.4b). When the accurate estimation of small volumes of aspirate is required, as in paediatric surgery, a small calibrated vessel may be used in addition to the main apparatus. This container is disposable and is usually close to the operative field.

The suction nozzle, catheter or hand-piece

The design of what is referred to in International Standards as the 'applied part' depends upon the application. The commonest examples of hand-held suction nozzles are shown in Figure 22.5. The key requirement of any suction 'applied part' is that the smallest internal diameter is at the very tip. If there are smaller diameters between the tip and the collection vessel, then blockages are likely to occur. The shape of the tip should be smooth so as to prevent damage to delicate tissues. The practice of allowing the tip to be occluded by any tissue, to reduce the noise of suction when not actually aspirating, must be deprecated as it causes tissue damage. Similarly, the noise of suction when using transportable, electrically powered suction machines should be reduced by switching off the motor rather than by occluding the suction tubing, as this may overload the motor. Hand-held suction nozzles of the Yankauer type (Fig. 22.5) often have a hole on the handle for fine control of suction with a finger.

Bronchial suction catheters should have smooth tips to avoid damaging delicate tissues and usually have several holes around the tip.

To protect staff, closed suction catheter systems are now commonly used (Fig. 22.6). The catheter is enclosed in a flexible sheath, which is permanently attached to a special 15 mm-taper adapter which is left in circuit

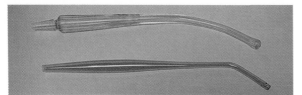

Figure 22.5 Two examples of hand-held Yankauer suction nozzles.

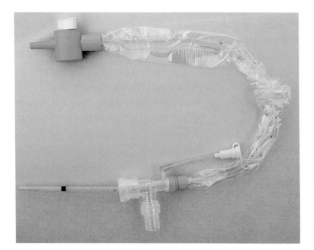

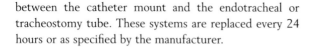

Figure 22.6 Closed bronchial suction system.

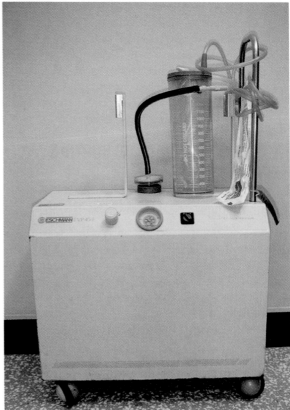

Figure 22.7 Free-standing medical suction unit.

between the catheter mount and the endotracheal or tracheostomy tube. These systems are replaced every 24 hours or as specified by the manufacturer.

LOCAL VACUUM UNITS

Piped vacuum systems are now installed in most hospitals. The 'behind the wall' equipment and terminal outlets are described in Chapter 3. Medical suction apparatus may be connected into this system wherever there is a terminal outlet.

There are two main types of 'local' apparatus:

1. *Free-standing floor units*, mains electricity powered and often with two collection vessels used for surgical purposes in the operating theatre (Fig. 22.7). Small, 'low-suction', low displacement units are also available for bedside use for intracavitary and continuous wound drainage. Generating typically 5 to 50 mmHg subatmospheric pressure, these devices are usually mains and rechargeable battery powered piston pumps.

2. *Wall mounted units* are local suction controllers for connection to central piped vacuum source (see Chapter 3). These have a single collection vessel as shown in Figure 22.8. There are two types of controller: conventional 'high-suction' and also 'low-suction'. Low suction controllers are deliberately limited to provide safe suction for intra-pleural drainage or nasogastric suction. Confusion between the two types of suction controller can have disastrous consequences, hence the resurgence of free-standing 'low-suction' units.

CHOICE OF SUCTION APPARATUS

When selecting a suction apparatus for a particular purpose, the following points need to be considered:
- must it be portable? If so, should it be hand/foot operated (Fig. 22.9)? If not, should it be powered by electricity (mains or battery) or is pipe-line vacuum

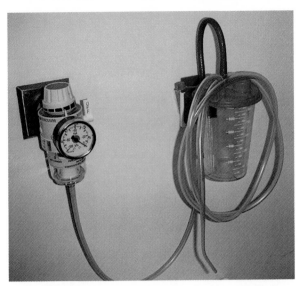

Figure 22.8 A pipeline vacuum unit. On the right is the controller, which is plugged directly into a flush-fitting outlet (obscured in this picture). On the left is the reservoir jar.

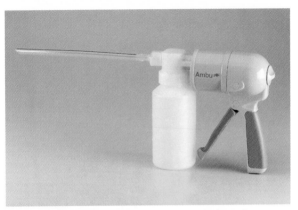

Figure 22.9 Ambu ResCue hand-operated suction apparatus. Courtesy of Ambu International Ltd.

available? Could it be powered from a gas cylinder using a Venturi injector?
* is a high displacement needed?
* is a high vacuum needed? and
* what size should the collection vessel be?

It is important to ascertain, for an electrically driven suction machine, whether it is rated for continuous or intermittent use.

High-volume aspirators, as used in dental surgery, use a pump similar to that used in a vacuum cleaner (Fig. 22.10a). They usually have several suction tubes of different diameters for different applications (Fig. 22.10b). These tubes and their nozzles should never

be obstructed, as a high flow of air is required to cool the motor, which would otherwise overheat. This type of high-flow suction is needed in dental surgery to aspirate the spray of water used to cool the tooth during high-speed drilling.

STANDARDS AND TESTING

As with all other medical equipment, there are published standards for design and manufacture. These standards, now, not only relate to safety but also to function and use. Typical ranges of volume for the collection container for specific uses are listed, as are standards for levels of suction and flow.

Previous editions of this book suggested methods of testing equipment including suction apparatus; however, as all equipment has become more complex, only tests recommended by the manufacturers should be carried out.

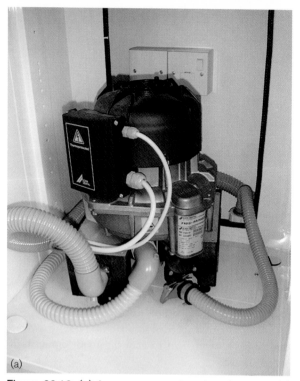
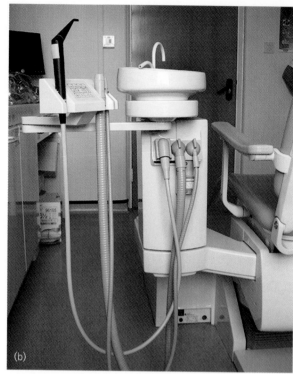

Figure 22.10 **(a)** A vacuum pump in a dental surgery. **(b)** A high-volume aspiration unit in a dental surgery. Note the different-sized suction tubes.

FURTHER READING

Medical suction equipment – Part 1 Electrically powered suction equipment – Safety requirements. British Standard BS EN ISO 10079-1:2000, BS 5724-2.28:2000, London: British Standards Institute.

Medical suction equipment – Part 2 Manually powered suction equipment. British Standard BS EN ISO 10079-2:2000, London: British Standards Institute.

Medical suction equipment – Part 3 Suction equipment powered from a vacuum or pressure source. International Standard EN ISO 10079-3:2000, London: British Standards Institute.

HTM 2022 (1994) (Suppl.) Permit to Work Systems. London: HMSO.

Cleaning, disinfection and sterilization

Trevor A King and Richard P D Cooke

Numerous case reports have demonstrated the risk of hospital-acquired infection from anaesthetic equipment, for example, cross-infection with *Pseudomonas aeruginosa* from laryngoscope blades.[1] This can occur outside the theatre complex and more commonly involves vulnerable patient groups, as in, *Streptococcus pneumoniae* transmission from resuscitaires[2] within neonatal units.

Consequently, all staff involved with anaesthetic equipment have a duty of care to ensure that this risk is kept to an absolute minimum. For this to be achieved, all reusable anaesthetic equipment must be appropriately decontaminated prior to patient use and single-use items must be discarded immediately following use. Unfortunately, wide variation in decontamination practices between anaesthetic departments is well recognized. This can be avoided by ensuring that every hospital has a comprehensive infection control policy in place for all anaesthetic equipment, with a nominated Anaesthetist and Infection Control Doctor (ICD) taking lead responsibilities.[3] Such a policy should be evidenced-based and subject to periodic audit and review. Guidance is available from various authorities in different countries (e.g. the Association of Anaesthetists of Great Britain and Ireland (AAGBI) publication[4] on the prevention of blood borne virus (BBV) and prion disease transmission during anaesthesia). Key areas requiring risk assessment are listed in Table 23.1.

The aim of this chapter is not to be prescriptive but to provide the necessary background information for a hospital to formulate its own anaesthetic equipment infection control policy, incorporating local risk assessments.

RISK ASSESSMENT AND THE DECONTAMINATION PROCESS

Contaminated medical devices are typically classified into three infection risk categories:[5]

1. *High Risk (critical) devices* – items in contact with a break in the skin, mucous membranes or intro-

Table 23.1 Clinical areas where anaesthetic equipment is used

Theatres	Special Care Baby Units
Day Surgery Units	Accident and Emergency
Endoscopy Suites	Departments
Maternity Units (including neonatal resuscitaires)	Radiology Suites
Coronary Care Units	Electroconvulsive Therapy Suites
Intensive Care and High Dependency Units	Ward Resuscitation Stations
	Ambulances

duced into a sterile body area. Such items must be sterile at the time of use. Examples include surgical instruments, dressings, catheters and prosthetic devices.

2. *Intermediate Risk (semi-critical) devices* – items in contact with intact mucous membranes or contaminated with readily transmissible organisms (which do not penetrate skin or enter sterile parts of the body). Disinfection is required though sterilization is preferred if the devices are heat-stable. Examples include endoscopes and respiratory equipment.

3. *Low Risk (non-critical) devices* – items in contact with healthy intact skin. Cleaning, typically using hot water and a neutral detergent or a disposable detergent wipe, and drying are adequate for such items. Examples include ECG electrodes, sphygmomanometer cuffs and stethoscopes.

If disposable anaesthetic equipment is chosen (Fig. 23.1), then a risk assessment may not be required. However, it is important to remember that disposable equipment will be for 'single use' or 'single patient use' only. 'Single use' indicates that the manufacturer intends the item to be used once only on an individual patient and then discarded. The packaging will be labelled either 'Single use', 'Do not re-use' or with the symbol ②.

'Single patient use' indicates that the manufacturer advises that the item may be used more than once on the same patient.[6] Examples of 'single patient use' items in anaesthesia include ventilator tubing and bacterial/viral filters used in critical care units.

By its nature, re-usable anaesthetic equipment poses an intermediate or high (if used on broken mucous membranes or skin) risk of infection. Consequently, decontamination by sterilization or disinfection is required. However, the responsibility for choosing the correct decontamination method lies with the Sterile Services Department (SSD) manager, supported by the ICD, lead Anaesthetist and the relevant manufacturer's guidance. This is because the choice of decontamination method will depend on a number of factors, including the nature of the contamination, the time required for processing, the heat, pressure, moisture and chemical tolerance of the item, the availability of the processing equipment and the risks associated with the decontamination method. Furthermore, decontamination performed in SSDs will ensure that procedures are undertaken in a controlled and standardized manner, as well as being subject to audit review. Consequently, detailed knowledge of decontamination processes is not required by anaesthetists and their assistants. However, a sound understanding of the principles and level of decontamination required is essential, to ensure that a local infection control policy is both practical and supported by all staff involved in anaesthetic practice. This also applies to the purchase or loan of any new anaesthetic equipment, since a preliminary decontamination assessment must be made prior to its use on patients.

Terminology[4,5]

Decontamination

Removal or destruction of contaminants (infectious or otherwise). The levels of decontamination are either cleaning followed by high-level disinfection or cleaning followed by sterilization.

Bioburden

The population of viable infectious agents contaminating a medical device. This should be routinely assessed by SSDs.

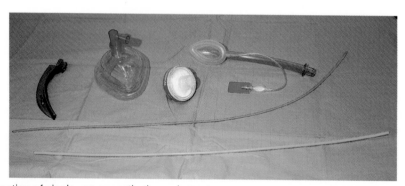

Figure 23.1 A selection of single use anaesthetic equipment.

Cleaning

Physical removal of infectious agents or organic matter. It involves washing with a solvent (usually water and detergent), which may be heated (e.g. thermal washer disinfection). This process does not necessarily destroy infectious agents. It is an essential process prior to disinfection or sterilization to remove bioburden.

Disinfection

This process reduces the number of viable infectious agents but does not inactivate all microbial agents or bacterial spores. Low-level disinfection kills most vegetative bacteria (except mycobacteria and endospores), some fungi and some viruses. High-level disinfection kills vegetative bacteria (but not endospores), mycobacteria, fungi and viruses.

Sterilization

A validated process used to render a device free from infectious agents, including viruses and bacterial spores. Prions, which are recognized to cause Transmissible Spongiform Encephalopathies (TSEs), are resistant to deactivation by disinfection methods and by most sterilization procedures.

Sterilant

A liquid chemical agent, which can kill bacteria, fungi, viruses and bacterial spores (e.g. gluteraldehyde, chlorine dioxide, peracetic acid). However, this term is not precise and is not generally used. The term high-level disinfectant is preferred.

A flow chart of appropriate decontamination methods is shown in Figure 23.2.

Dry saturated steam

Saturated steam that contains no water particles in suspension.

INFECTION CONTROL STRATEGIES

Factors to be considered

Single use versus re-usable anesthetic equipment

Infection control measures have been greatly simplified with the introduction of single-use anaesthetic equipment. Decontamination issues, already outlined with re-usable equipment, will not be relevant. However, when preparing an option appraisal, the revenue, procurement and waste disposal costs of single-use equipment needs to

be balanced against capital procurement costs for new equipment and SSD charges for reprocessing items. In addition, careful thought needs to be given to where disposable equipment will be stored. To avoid compromising environmental cleaning standards, good communication is required between theatre and supply managers. An example of a local infection control policy for anaesthetic equipment is shown in Table 23.2.

Disinfection or sterilization

Decontamination by heat rather than by chemicals is always preferred. Disinfection by washer-disinfectors or low temperature steam is commonly employed, since autoclaving (with dry saturated steam) may damage anaesthetic equipment that is repeatedly processed.[3] Equipment used for invasive procedures or those that come into contact with broken skin or mucous membranes always require sterilization.

Centralization of decontamination services

When preparing an infection control action plan, it should be agreed at the outset with all relevant parties, that reprocessing of contaminated anaesthetic equipment should, whenever possible, be undertaken outside the clinical environment in central decontamination units or SSDs (Fig. 23.5).[4,5] Stand-alone autoclaves in theatres are not acceptable. Their use necessitates instrument cleaning (the most important component of the decontamination process) within the theatre complex. Furthermore, the scrupulous quality control measures required for the safe use of autoclaves cannot be guaranteed outside non-specialist areas.

Heat-labile instruments

Equipment needing high level disinfection but unable to tolerate high temperatures, such as endoscopes, pose particular infection control problems. Their decontamination should be undertaken in designated endoscopy units with appropriately trained personnel[7] (Fig. 23.6). The use of chemical disinfectants, because of their toxicity, needs to be strictly controlled and subject to risk assessments in accordance with the Control of Substances Hazardous to Health Regulations, COSHH.[8]

Standard precautions

Universal infection control precautions should be used for the prevention of hospital-acquired infection between patients and staff. Classification of patients into high- and low-risk groups is inappropriate, since carriers of BBVs may be asymptomatic and unknown to staff. The same principles apply to the decontamination of medical

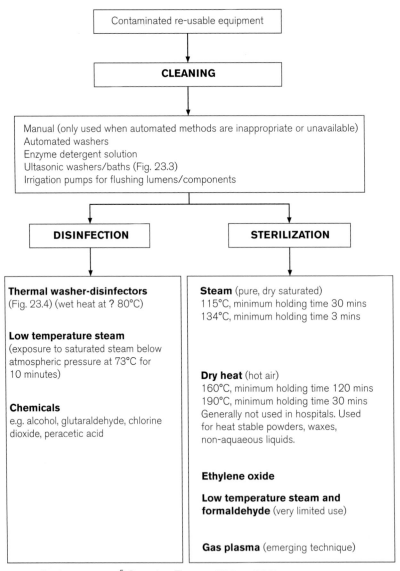

Figure 23.2 The decontamination process.[5] See also Figures 23.3 to 23.5.

equipment, the one exception being the prevention of prion related diseases (see below).

Tracking of re-usable anaesthetic equipment

SSDs must have tracking systems in place to enable re-usable instruments to be traced to an individual patient in the event of a 'clinical incident', for example, failure of the decontamination process or instruments being used on a patient with unsuspected Creutzfeldt–Jakob Disease (CJD).[9] Furthermore, some anaesthetic equipment (e.g. laryngeal masks, gum elastic bougies) can only be reprocessed a finite number of times according to the

manufacturers' instructions. A suitable tracking system therefore needs to be agreed between SSD and theatre staff, so that specific items of equipment are discarded after the maximum permitted number of uses. Single-use equipment overcomes the need for tracking systems to be in place.

Damage caused by the decontamination process

Some anaesthetic equipment, made from rubber or plastics, may be destroyed by autoclaving at 115°C to 134°C. Use of washer-disinfectors operating at lower temperatures may then be the preferred option.

Table 23.2 An example of a local Infection Control Policy for anaesthetic equipment

Equipment	Action	Comment

Airways
   Oral/nasopharyngeal
   Plastic endotracheal
   Tracheostomy tubes
	Single use
	Single use
	Single use	

Angle pieces	Single use	
Catheter mounts	Single use	
Red rubber endotracheal	Return to SSD	
Laryngeal masks	Return to SSD	40 uses maximum*
Anaesthetic breathing systems (theatres)	Disposable	Change weekly provided new bacterial/viral filter used with every patient. Change sooner if visibly contaminated. If filter not used, discard after single use.
Circle absorbers	As for ventilators (see below)	Single use bacterial/viral filter for each patient
Anaesthetic masks	Return to SSD or single use	

Bougies
   Gum elastic
   Others
	Return to SSD
	Single use
		5 uses maximum*

Entonox delivery system (including mouthpiece/mask, tubing, one-way expiratory demand valve)	Single use	
Laryngoscope blades	Return to SSD or single use	
Manual resuscitators (self-inflating bags used at resuscitation)	Single use	
Oxygen mask and tubing	Single use	
Paediatric resuscitaire, facemask and tubing	Single use	
Temperature probes	Single use	
Ventilators	Routine disinfection not required. Follow cleaning and maintenance policies for specific ventilators	In ICU, bacterial /viral filter placed on ventilator expiratory port and changed daily* or sooner since single patient use only.
Ventilator tubing (ICU)	Disposable	Change weekly[13] or sooner since single patient use only.

* = Manufacturers' recommendation
SSD = Sterile Services Department
ICU = Intensive Care Unit
(After King and Cooke 2001[3] with permission from The Hospital Infection Society.)

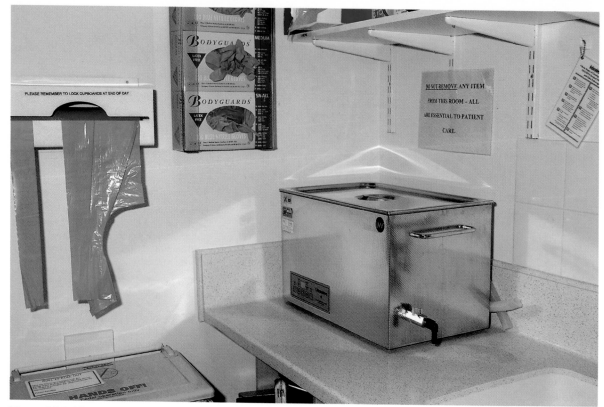

Figure 23.3 Ultrasonic washer used for endoscope accessories.

Manufacturers will provide written instructions on the decontamination of re-usable equipment and it is important that these are followed to avoid instrument damage. Some light sources for metal laryngoscope blades lose luminance with repeated high temperature autoclaving.[10] This may influence the decision to procure single-use items.

Bacterial/viral filters and anaesthetic breathing systems

Bacterial/viral filters can be used to protect anaesthetic breathing systems from contamination. Although their role in the prevention of nosocomial pneumonia is controversial,[11] the AAGBI do recommend that a new bacterial/viral filter be used for every patient.[4] Similarly, implementation of a local policy on the re-use of breathing systems in line with manufacturers' instructions is recommended. Some breathing systems are marketed with instructions which permit re-use for a period of up to one week, if a new bacterial/viral filter is used with every patient.

Prion disease

Abnormally shaped prion proteins are implicated as the causative agents in transmissible spongiform encephalopathies, of which variant (v) and sporadic CJD are examples. Both result in progressive neurological symptoms and death. By 2003, vCJD had caused the death of 137 people in the UK, whilst sporadic CJD effects one person per million each year in the UK. There are a number of uncertainties concerning diagnosis, transmission and incubation periods for prion-related diseases. In both types of CJD, the highest concentration of prion protein occurs in the brain, spinal cord and posterior eye. With vCJD, abnormal prion protein has been detected in the appendix, tonsils, spleen and gastrointestinal lymph nodes.

The prion protein is remarkably resistant to conventional methods of disinfection and sterilization.[12] Standard washing techniques do reduce the concentration of prions in an exponential fashion but 10 to 20 cycles are required to produce negligible levels. Standard decontamination methods will not protect against

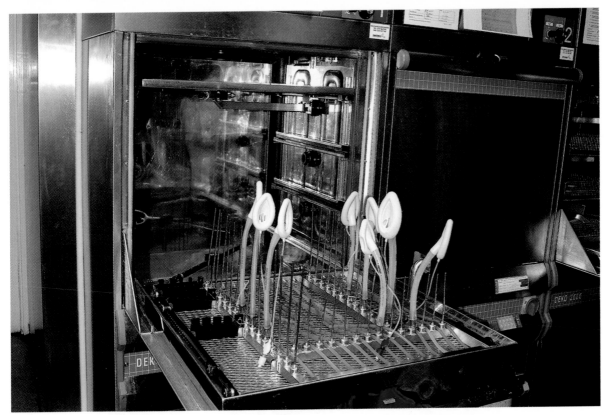

Figure 23.4 Laryngeal masks going into washer-disinfector.

transmission of prion proteins, although the risk of transmission by surgical equipment from patients with undiagnosed CJD is thought to be minimal. Specific decontamination processes, which are the specialist realm of SSDs, have been recommended by the Advisory Committee on Dangerous Pathogens.

From the anaesthetic viewpoint, disposable equipment is preferred for tonsillar surgery. To avoid contamination by tonsillar tissue, laryngeal masks, bougies and other intubation aids should not be re-used.[4]

Equipment used on definite, probable, possible or 'at risk' CJD patients should be dealt with as follows:[12]

1. If used on patients with *definite or probable* CJD, the instruments should not be reused and must be destroyed by incineration.

2. If used on patients with *possible* CJD, re-usable equipment should be quarantined until the diagnosis is either confirmed (when equipment must be destroyed) or excluded (following which equipment may re-enter general use). Suspect patients are defined as having clinical symptoms suggestive of CJD but have not yet had the diagnosis confirmed.

3. For '*at risk*' patients, single-use equipment should be used wherever possible. Asymptomatic patients, who are potentially at risk of developing CJD or a related disorder, include recipients of hormones derived from human pituitary glands, recipients of human dura mater grafts and those with family history of CJD. For procedures involving high or medium risk tissues (i.e. brain, spinal cord, anterior and posterior parts of the eye, lymphoid tissue, olfactory epithelium), instruments should be disposed of by incineration. However, for procedures on low risk tissues, normal reprocessing guidance should be followed.

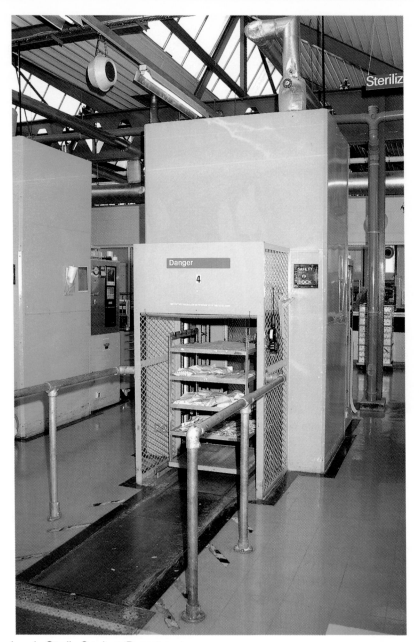

Figure 23.5 Autoclave in Sterile Services Department.

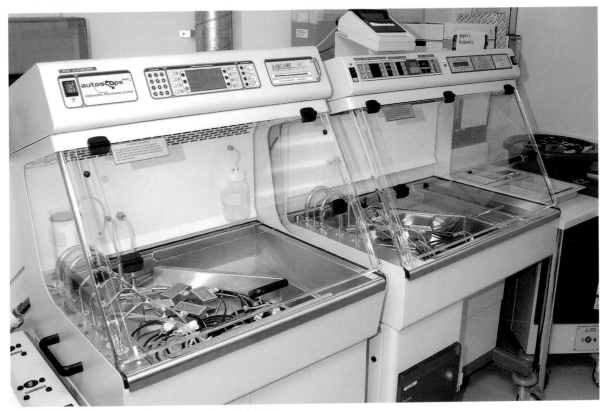

Figure 23.6 Automated endoscope washer-disinfector.

REFERENCES

1. Neal TJ, Hughes CR, Rothburn MM, Shaw NJ (1995) The neonatal laryngoscope as a potential source of cross-infection. *Journal of Hopsital Infection* **30**: 315–317.

2. Mehtar S, Drubu YJ, Vijeratnam S, Meyet F (1986) Cross-infection with *Streptococcus pneumoniae* through a resuscitaire. *British Medical Journal* **295**: 25–26.

3. King TA, Cooke RPD (2001) Developing an infection control policy for anaesthetic equipment. *Journal of Hospital Infection* **47**: 257–261.

4. The Association of Anaesthetists of Great Britain and Ireland (2002) *Infection control in anaesthesia* www.aagbi.org

5. Medical Devices Agency (2002) *Sterilization, disinfection and cleaning of medical equipment: guidance on decontamination from the Medical Advisory Committee to Department of Health*. Parts 1, 2 and 3. Department of Health.

6. Medical Devices Agency (2000) *Single-use medical devices: implications and consequences of reuse*. Medical Devices Agency DB2000(04).

7. Medical Devices Agency (2002) *Decontamination of endoscopes*. MDA DB 2002 (05).

8. Health and Safety Executive (1999) *Control of Substances Hazardous to Health Regulation: General COSHH ACOP and carcinogens ACOP and biological agents ACOP (Approved Code of Practice)*. HSE Books.

9. NHS Estates (2003) A guide to the decontamination of reusable surgical instruments. Leeds: NHS Estates.

10. Bucx MJL, Veldman DJ, Beenhakker MM, Koster R (1999) The effect of steam sterilisation at 134°C on light intensity provided by fibrelight Macintosh laryngoscopes. *Anaesthesia* **54**: 875–878.

11. Lorente L, Lecuona M, Málaga J, Revert C, Mora ML, Sierra A (2003) Bacterial filters in respiratory circuits: an unnecessary cost? *Critrical Care in Medicine* **31**: 2126–2130.

12. Advisory Committee on Dangerous Pathogens and the Spongiform Encephalopathy Advisory Committee (2003) *Transmissible spongiform encephalopathy agents: safe working and the prevention of infection.* Department of Health.

13. Hess D, Burns E, Romagnol D, Kacmarek RM (1995) Weekly ventilator circuit changes: a strategy to reduce costs without effecting pneumonia rates. *Anaesthesiology* **82:** 903–911.

Information technology and the anaesthetic workstation

Chris J Barham

Anaesthetists perform the majority of their clinical work in the operating theatre, and the anaesthetic machine, therefore, acts as their desk and office, as well as a device for delivering anaesthesia. It is essential that it is equipped with all the tools to provide care, record activity, provide information and enable communication.

This chapter will consider, not only how information technology can assist in maintaining a record of the anaesthetic, but also its wider use in the theatre environment.

RECORD KEEPING

The earliest anaesthetic records date from 1894, although over 80 years later 3.4% of records in the UK were still merely an entry in the operating theatre register. It is now a requirement of a number of accrediting bodies (e.g. in the United Kingdom: Royal College of Anaesthetists, Clinical Negligence Scheme for Trusts, Commission for Health Audit and Inspection, etc.) that an anaesthetic record is kept.

The majority of anaesthetists in the UK still create a hand-written record, which may be augmented by a print-out from the trend screen of the monitoring systems, both only being stored in paper format. The advantages and disadvantages of manual records, compared with computerized records, are listed in Table 24.1. The report of the National Confidential Enquiry for Perioperative Deaths for 2000[1] showed that 5% of case notes were lost, and in 3% of those present, the anaesthetic record was missing. Nevertheless, it concluded that 'Improvements in Information Technology can make retrieval of patient information more, rather than less, difficult.' This must be viewed in the context of a time when records were almost all paper-based, and the majority of information systems did not communicate with each other.

Functions of the anaesthetic record

CLINICAL   The following records must be available for subsequent review by other clinicians involved in the care of the patient:
- pre-assessment;
- pre-operative evaluation and investigations;
- intra-operative record; and
- post-operative instructions and progress.

ADMINISTRATIVE   Data from the anaesthetic record can provide valuable information on anaesthetic and surgical workload. This can assist in the management of the surgical process, and provide statistics for both

Table 24.1 Comparison of manual and computerized records

	Manual Records	**Computerized Records**
Advantages	Familiar structure Easy navigation Portable Versatile and flexible Good 'user interface'	Available anywhere Available anytime Can be viewed by several users at the same time Accuracy of captured data On line decision support Integration with medical record No need to enter data already present (e.g. medications) Ease of aggregate reporting
Disadvantages	Legibility Availability Accuracy Comprehensiveness Fragmentation No decision support Difficult to aggregate	Inflexibility Training required Update – new drugs, operations Data entry may be difficult Duplication of entries Distraction Different systems Artefacts

local and national use. Appraisal requires some record of clinical workload, which will ultimately be obtained from the clinical record.

EDUCATIONAL Records can be used both as an educational tool, and to assess the adequacy of training. Trainees maintain logbooks to demonstrate their experience, and this information will be derived from the record.

MEDICOLEGAL The record should be accurate, complete and legible, and its quality may be seen as a reflection of the quality of care given.

RESEARCH Extraction of information from clinical records is often essential in research. The system introduced by Michael Nosworthy was an early and effective means of extracting data from a large number of records. Holes around the edge of a record card could be opened up with a ticket punch, and then records could be sorted by inserting a knitting needle through a particular hole.

COMPUTERIZED ANAESTHETIC RECORDS

Computerized anaesthetic record systems have been available for many years, but despite their benefits and the sophistication of modern systems, they have yet to gain widespread acceptance. One of the major impediments to

their introduction has been the lack of a 'business case' for their introduction, despite the fact that anaesthetists are involved in 60% of inpatient hospital activity, and that many studies have shown their benefits.[2,3]

The National Health Service in England is currently making a major investment in information technology for medical records – the NHS Care Record (NCRS). This will include integrated records for all patients and all specialties – including anaesthesia.[4] One of the core features of the NCRS is the 'spine' record, which will carry summary information from the patient's medical record, and this will be accessible at any site. The anaesthetist will ultimately have online access to key features of the patient's medical history, including previous surgery, medications and allergies. This should be available at any point of care, including the anaesthetic workstation.

Features

The key features of a computerized anaesthetic system are listed in Table 24.2. Figures 24.1 and 24.2 show a well-established system in place, together with the 'splash' screen and some screen shots.

Firstly, there should be comprehensive links to other clinical information systems, to ensure that up-to-date information is available, and to avoid duplicate entry of pre-existing information (e.g. demographic details, proposed surgery, etc.)

Table 24.2 Criteria for Anaesthetic Record Systems

Should link to	Pre-assessment information Electronic clinical record Electronic prescribing system Pathology Radiology and PACS (public access computer system) Theatre system for operating list information, personnel
Peri-operative record should have	Appropriate user interface Anaesthetic pre-operative assessment record Validation of staff Capture of all patient monitor data Capture of all machine monitor data Configurable display of all trend data Comprehensive data dictionary Rapid entry of narrative from menus Automatic coding Free text entry Drugs/Fluids/Infusions (including calculations) Critical incidents Post-operative instructions Recovery progress Key outcomes (death, pain, PONV, etc.) Audit trail
Reporting should include	Staff logbooks Activity analysis Performance indicators Data for audit Financial analysis

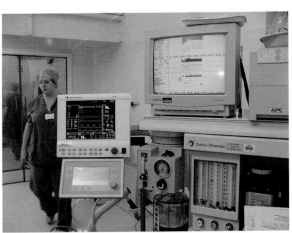

Figure 24.1 An established networked anaesthetic record keeping system in place on the workstation

Secondly, all displayed data from patient and machine monitoring systems (including infusion pumps, ventilators, etc.) should be captured by the system. In the past, this was another major obstacle to implementing automated record keepers, due to the difficulties of interfacing. Now, most record keeping software incorporates interfaces to common monitoring and other equipment, and equipment manufacturers publish the structure of the output messages of their machines.

Thirdly, there should be an appropriate method of entering information to the system. This will normally be a keyboard or touch screen, together with some pointing device. These must all be suitable for use in the theatre, and should be easy to clean to avoid cross-infection. For this reason, a sealed plastic covered keyboard (Fig 24.3) may often be the most appropriate solution.

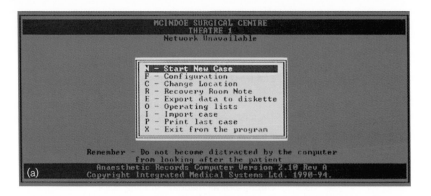

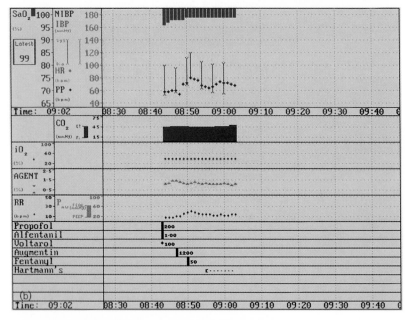

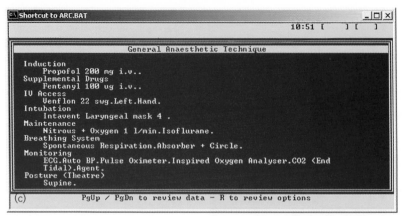

Figure 24.2 Screen shots from the type of workstation seen in Figure 24.1. **(a)** the splash screen; **(b)** the trend page in use; **(c)** a summary screen.

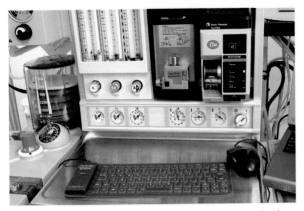

Fig 24.3 A keyboard suitable for use on an anaesthetic machine should have a wipe clean surface and be affordable enough to be disposed of when no longer able to be decontaminated.

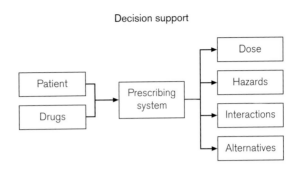

Decision support

Figure 24.4 The process of decision support from a prescribing system based on embedded knowledge.

Data entered should conform to the standards recommended by the Royal College of Anaesthetists (Table 24.3),[5] and the system should be capable of attributing each procedure to individual members of staff.

Finally, the data should be stored in an appropriate format for retrieval, and production of reports such as logbooks and audit studies.

OTHER INFORMATION AND COMMUNICATION SYSTEMS

Decision support

Electronic record systems can be made to incorporate *decision support*. This can be defined as any method that takes input information about a clinical situation and then produces inferences that can assist practitioners in their decision-making. For example, a prescribing system (and hence also an anaesthetic system) should be able to give the clinician information about dosage, interactions and alternatives, on the basis of embedded knowledge about the patient and drug (Fig 24.4).

Decision support can take a number of forms, and is classified into three levels (Table 24.4):

Level 1 clinical decision support is provided by access to online information systems, that the clinician can interrogate as required. This includes the local intranet for policies and procedures, and the Internet for sources such as the National Electronic Library for Health (NELH), or guidelines from the National Institute for Clinical Excellence (NICE).

Level 2 provides information in the context of the clinical situation. This may either be passive, where it is accessed as required (for example, information about a drug about to be administered) or active, where the system will warn of a potential hazard (for example a drug interaction).

Finally, with *level 3* decision support, the system can intelligently take account of all data available about the clinical situation, and suggest the best course of action.

Communication

Commonly, the only method of communication for the anaesthetist in the UK is a message via a third party, or possibly through an intercom system with, for example, the recovery ward. Other more complex communications will normally be handled by the anaesthetist leaving the theatre (and hence the patient) to speak on a telephone elsewhere in the theatre suite. The other alternative is the use of mobile phones, but their use is frequently prohibited in clinical areas.

The best solution would be for all anaesthetic machines to be fitted with some form of communication system that allows the anaesthetist to receive and send messages without leaving the patient. This could either be by the use of a fixed telephone (as is used in many countries by nurse anaesthetists to communicate with the physician anaesthetist) or by the use of e-mail. The latter has the advantage of being less intrusive, and capable of being dealt with at the most appropriate moment.

Table 24.3 Suggested Anaesthetic Record set. (Royal College of Anaesthetists Newsletter 36 (1997) – reproduced with permission.

PRE-OPERATIVE INFORMATION

PATIENT IDENTITY
Name / ID No. / Gender
Date of Birth

ASSESSMENT AND RISK FACTORS
Date of Assessment
Assessor, where assessed
Weight(kg), [height(m),optional]
Basic Vital Signs (BP,HR)
Medication incl. Contraceptive drugs
Allergies
Addiction (alcohol, tobacco, drugs)
Previous GAs, family history
Potential Airway Problems
Prostheses, teeth, crowns
Investigations
Cardiorespiratory fitness
Other problems
ASA +/– comment

URGENCY
Scheduled – listed on a routine list
Urgent – resuscitated, not on a routine list
Emergency – not fully resuscitated

CHECKS
Nil by mouth
Consent
Premedication, type and effect

PLACE AND TIME
Place
Date, start and end times

PERSONNEL
All anaesthetists named
Qualified assistant present
Duty consultant informed
Operating surgeon

OPERATION PLANNED / PERFORMED

APPARATUS
Check performed, anaesthetic room, theatre

VITAL SIGNS RECORDING / CHARTING
Monitors used and vital signs (specify)

DRUGS & FLUIDS
Dose, concentrations, volume
Cannulation
Injection site(s), time & route
Warmer used
Blood loss, urine output

AIRWAY AND BREATHING SYSTEM
Route, system used
Ventilation: type and mode
Airway type, size, cuff, shape
Special procedures, humidifier, filter
Throat pack
Difficulty

REGIONAL ANAESTHESIA
Consent
Block performed
Entry site
Needle used, aid to location
Catheter y/n

PATIENT POSITION AND ATTACHMENTS
Thrombosis prophylaxis
Temperature control
Limb positions

POST-OPERATIVE INSTRUCTIONS
Drugs, fluids and doses
Analgesic techniques
Special airway instructions, incl oxygen
Monitoring

UNTOWARD EVENTS
Abnormalities
Critical Incidents
Pre-op, per-op, post-op
Context, cause, effect

HAZARD FLAGS
Warnings for future care

Table 24.4 Levels of clinical decision support

Level	
1	• **Elective Decision Support – Knowledge Management:** delivery on request of evidence-based information to support clinical decisions
2	• **Passive Decision Support – Embedded Guidance:** e.g. order sets, formularies, protocols and pathways describing best practice but for guidance only
	• **Active Decision Support – Alerts:** alerts to any event or combination of events that is pre-determined to lead to a serious clinical outcome
3	• Collates clinical history, physical findings, physiological parameters and the results of investigations, links the collated data directly to clinical decision making and **informs/suggests integrated care pathways and care programmes**

REFERENCES

1. Then and Now (2000) *The 2000 Report of the National Confidential Enquiry into Perioperative Deaths.* London: NCEPOD. p. 29
2. Devitt JH, Rapanos T, Kurrek M, *et al.* (1999) The Anaesthetic Record: accuracy and completeness. *Canadian Journal of Anaesthesia* **46(2):** 122–128.
3. Byrne AJ, Sellen AJ, Jones JG (1998) Errors in Anaesthetic Record Charts as a Measure of Anaesthetic Performance During Simulated Critical Incidents. *British Journal of Anaesthesia* **80(1):** 58–62.
4. Integrated Care Records Service Output Based Specification, Second Iteration. http://www.dh.gov.uk/assetRoot/04/07/16/32/04071632.pdf accessed 7th June 2004.
5. Smith A (1997) New College Guidelines for Anaesthetic Records. Newsletter 36. *London: Royal College of Anaesthetists* September 1997: p. 3.

Electrical hazards and their prevention

Patrick T Magee

THE MAINS ELECTRICITY SUPPLY

Most electromedical devices, including anaesthetic apparatus and monitors, are powered by mains electricity. It is therefore important for the anaesthetist to have an understanding of the principles of its provision and its hazards. For reasons of efficiency of power transmission, the mains provides *alternating current* (AC) rather than *direct current* (DC), as is provided by batteries. In DC, current flows steadily in one direction, while in AC, it flows rapidly back and forth at a frequency of 50 Hz in the UK, Europe and elsewhere in the world, and at 60 Hz in the USA. These frequencies may be a good choice for power transmission, but they are more hazardous to the user than other frequencies, including DC (see later).

In cables carrying DC, one cable is designated positive and the other negative, which is not the case with AC cables. Figure 25.1a shows how a three phase, 16 kV primary winding of a power station transformer steps the voltage down to a three phase 240 V root-mean-square supply (325 V peak). It also shows how these secondary 240 V windings are linked together and connected to earth at the 'star point' (Fig. 25.1b). For each 240 V supply, therefore, one end is deemed 'live' and

the end connected to earth at the star point is deemed 'neutral'.

Because of this earthing of the neutral conductor at the power station, any person or object who is also connected to earth, would complete an electric circuit by touching the live conductor, even if no contact were made with the neutral one. Figure 25.2 shows how, under certain conditions, the circuit connecting a patient to a live lead may be completed by, for example, an earthed diathermy plate, resulting in fatal electrocution. However, in most modern diathermy machines, this plate is isolated from earth as far as mains current is concerned (see Chapter 26). Furthermore, here in this example of a faulty monitor, an additional interruption of the neutral cable would result in the apparatus not working. However, because the live cable is still functioning, any contact with the ('live') casing would lead to electrocution of an inadvertently earthed user.

Stringent precautions should be taken to ensure that the polarities are correctly defined and connected for all mains electrical apparatus. Electrical accidents can be minimized by careful, regular maintenance by qualified personnel. It cannot be overemphasized that, if a fault exists, the apparatus should be removed

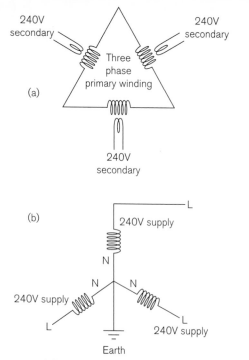

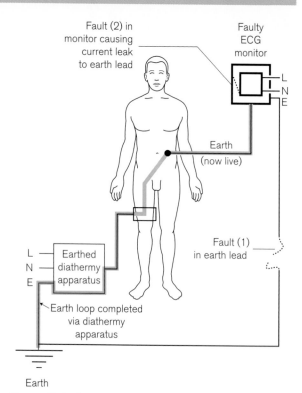

Figure 25.1 (a) Power station transformer reduction of three phase 16 kV supply to 240V supply. **(b)** 240V supply circuit at power station with neutral end of supplies connected to earth. L, live; N, neutral.

Figure 25.2 A fault in a monitor can cause electrocution by completion of a circuit through another electromedical device.

from use and the services of a competent technician sought.

The inclusion of a lead, which connects the metal chassis, frame and enclosure of the apparatus to earth, ensures that under faulty conditions, the enclosure is prevented from becoming live, and is thus called the 'earth' lead. The faults in Figure 25.2 show a break in the earth lead to the metal enclosure of the monitor (1); this allows a second fault within the monitor (2) to render the apparatus dangerous to the patient. This is discussed further in the section below, on Class I equipment.

Apparatus can be rendered safer by the inclusion of a fuse in the electrical circuit. They may be installed either in the mains supply circuit, in the plug of the electrical lead to the apparatus, or in the apparatus itself. They usually consist of a fine gauge wire, which melts if the current passing through exceeds that against which they are intended to offer protection. So, in Figure 25.2, if the earth lead of the monitor were intact, the fault consisting of a current leak between the apparatus and its enclosure, assuming adequate leak current and low enough fuse rating, would result in a fuse in the live wire melting,

breaking the continuity of the electrical circuit and the apparatus being rendered harmless. However, there is a risk that the fuse may not protect against electric shock. This can happen if someone is in contact with the equipment as the fault develops and before the fuse has time to melt (see below). Fuses are used mainly to interrupt the electric supply in the event that the current passing through the equipment exceeds a predetermined level that might cause overheating or damage.

PATHOPHYSIOLOGICAL EFFECTS OF ELECTRICITY

The pathophysiological effects of electric current passing through the human body include:
- resistive heating of the tissue and burns;
- electrical stimulation of excitable tissues;
- electrochemical effects; and
- ignition of flammable material in contact with the body.

The factors that determine the severity of electrical injury are tissue resistance (R), current (I), potential

Table 25.1 Electrical resistance of skin

Skin type	Electrical resistance $k\Omega\ cm^{-2}$
Mucous membranes	0.1
Vascular areas (volar aspect of arm, inner thigh)	0.3–10
Wet skin: in the bath	1.2–1.5
Sweat	2.5
Dry skin	10.0–40
Sole of the foot	100–200
Heavily calloused palm	1000–2 000

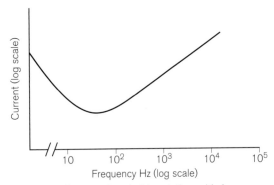

Figure 25.3 Current threshold variation with frequency for pathophysiological effects.

Table 25.2 The pathophysiological effects of 50 Hz AC current

current mA	Pathophysiological effect
1	Tingling
5	Pain
15	Severe pain and muscle contraction
30	'Let go' threshold
50	Respiratory muscle contraction, asphyxia
70	Multifocal beats, cardiac failure
100	Local burns, ventricular fibrillation
1000	Extensive burns, charring

difference (V), current frequency, current pathway and duration and current density. The thermal energy delivered to the tissues depends on the power dissipated (P), which can be calculated from:

$$V \times I = I^2\,R$$

The body may be considered electrically to be an electrolyte (a good conductor) in a leathery bag (a poor conductor, an insulator). However, the resistance of the integument is very variable (Table 25.1).

Other tissues have diverse electrical resistances, which can be grouped as follows:
- *low*: nerve, blood, mucous membrane, muscle;
- *intermediate*: dry skin; or
- *high*: tendon, fat, bone.

There is, however, an idiosyncratic relationship between whole body electrical impedance (AC resistance) and the applied voltage. At low voltages, 25–100 volts, it depends on the state of the skin and area of contact. At 250 volts and higher, the total body impedance falls to 2000–5000 ohm, irrespective of the contact area and the current pathway.[1]

The effects of electric current upon excitable tissues such as muscle and nerve depend not only on current and time, but also on the frequency.[2,3] It is one of the ironies of life that that the commonly used mains frequencies of 50 Hz (UK, Europe) or 60 Hz (US) are the frequencies at which the excitable tissues are at greatest risk of excitation and damage (Fig. 25.3).

In greatest danger is the heart, as it is susceptible to induced arrhythmias as well as permanent damage. The direction of the current pathway through the heart is also important. Clinical studies suggest that sudden death from ventricular fibrillation is more likely with current passing 'horizontally' from hand to hand, whereas heart muscle damage is more often associated with a 'vertical' current pathway.[4]

The effects of hand-to-hand 50 Hz AC on the body are shown in Table 25.2 and Figure 25.4. Figure 25.5 shows a plot of current magnitude against duration in relation to pathophysiological effects.

Direct current (DC) electric shock tends to produce:
- single muscle spasm;
- the victim thrown from the source;
- blunt mechanical trauma; and
- disturbance of heart rhythm.

Even very low imperceptible DC may produce electrochemical burns if the current is allowed to pass for

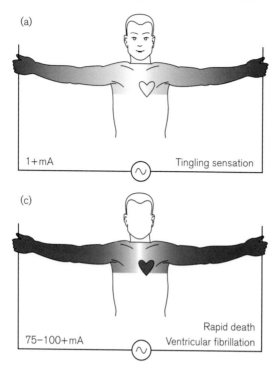

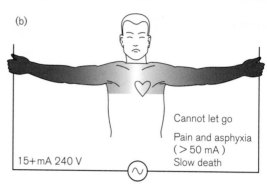

Figure 25.4 **(a)** A current in excess of 1 mA passing through the body may produce a tingling sensation. **(b)** If the current exceeds about 15 mA, muscles are held in tonic spasm, the victim cannot let go and will eventually die of asphyxia. **(c)** When the current exceeds 100 mA, ventricular fibrillation and rapid death will occur.

long enough, for example from swallowed button-sized 1.5V hearing aid type batteries.[5]

Alternating current (AC) electric shock:

- is about three times more dangerous than DC, at similar current flows;
- produces continuous muscle contractions (tetany) with AC at 40–110 Hz;
- induces grip and pull as flexor muscles are much stronger than extensor muscles. If a person were to be holding onto a faulty conductor, they would be unable to let go. This prolongs the duration of the effect of the current; and
- induces local sweating, which reduces skin resistance.

ACCIDENTS ASSOCIATED WITH THE MAINS ELECTRICITY SUPPLY

There are four ways in which the mains electric current, or equipment powered by it, endanger the patient:

1. electrocution;
2. burns;
3. electrochemical effects; and
4. ignition of flammable materials leading to fire or explosion.

Electrocution

As shown in Figure 25.4, electrocution can cause death relatively slowly by tonic contraction of the respiratory muscles, leading to asphyxia, or more rapidly by ventricular fibrillation. The onset of ventricular fibrillation may be delayed, being preceded by ventricular tachycardia, which causes circulatory failure, but which may revert to normal rhythm, if stopped in time.

As discussed earlier, the neutral pole of the mains electricity supply is connected to earth at the star point, a point at the power station and thus remote from the patient. Since all conductors have some resistance, however low, there is therefore a small voltage drop between the patient end of the neutral conductor and the star point, i.e. they represent non-identical earth points. The patient end of the neutral conductor may therefore not be exactly at earth potential. This difference in potential along the neutral lead may facilitate stray capacitative or inductive currents in a circuit, which includes the patient connected to earth. Similarly, earthed electrodes may be attached to more than one part of the patient and from more than one piece of equipment supplied by different mains sockets, which may also facilitate stray capacitative or inductive currents in a circuit, which includes the patient. This is shown in Figure 25.6 and it is recommended that that the earth connections on all the socket outlets in a single clinical area be interconnected by a low resistance conductor to minimize voltage differences between them. Similarly, all exposed metal objects, such as metal pipes and radiators, should be interconnected to a good earth.

Microshock

So far only *macroshock* has been discussed. Figure 25.4 shows the effect of a current passing between the extremities. When it passes across the patient's trunk, only a small part of it passes through the heart. However, many modern medical, surgical and critical care procedures involve the placement of electrodes on, within or close to the heart, e.g. a pulmonary artery catheter or even a transduced arterial line by virtue of its column of electrolyte. Under these circumstances, a very much smaller current, possibly as low as 100 µA, can result in ventricular fibrillation (Fig. 25.7) because all the current passes through the heart. A very small potential, such as the stray voltage in the mains neutral lead, could be

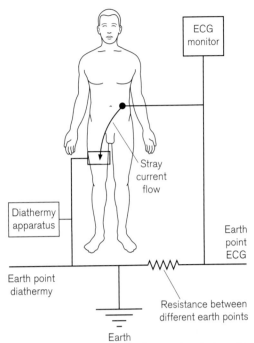

Figure 25.6 Stray current flow in a patient induced by earthing devices at different points.

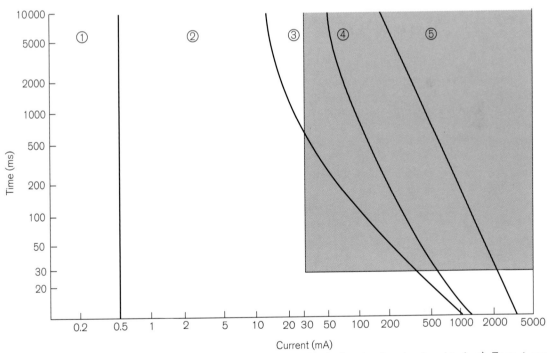

Figure 25.5 The effects of a current passing through the human body (hand to hand or hand to foot). Zone 1, usually no effect; zone 2, usually no dangerous effect; zone 3, usually no danger of ventricular fibrillation; zone 4, ventricular fibrillation possible; zone 5, ventricular fibrillation probable. The shaded area denotes the protection given by a current-operated earth-leakage circuit breaker (COELCB).

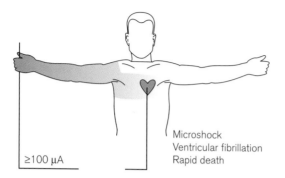

Figure 25.7 If one electrode is applied to the right ventricle of the heart itself, a very small current can result in ventricular fibrillation.

≥100 µA

Microshock
Ventricular fibrillation
Rapid death

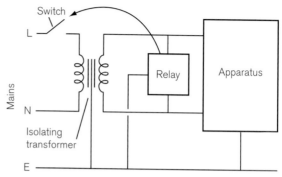

Figure 25.8 Safe patient power. The output of the isolating transformer is free from earth. Should earth leakage occur above a pre-arranged level, the relay will either disconnect the supply to the input of the transformer or sound a warning device. L, live; N, neutral; E, earth connectors.

sufficient to produce electrocution in this way. This phenomenon is known as *microshock*.

Shock protection

There are two ways of preventing accidents caused by unwanted currents returning to earth:

1. install an isolating transformer, the output of which is carefully isolated from earth;
2. detect unwanted currents passing earth by a device that will sound a warning or automatically switch the supply.

Both have advantages and disadvantages. An isolating transformer may supply all the outlets for a whole operating room or theatre suite. It works on the principle that the output from the transformer is free from earth. Should the apparatus develop a fault, the earth leakage current is sensed almost instantaneously by a relay which then trips a switch in the transformer input (Fig. 25.8). Apart from the expense, problems arise if there are several appliances in use and each of these has a small earth leakage current that is harmless in itself. The sum of all these currents may be sufficient to trip the relay and cut off the power to a monitor or other mains powered anaesthetic equipment. Likewise, a fault in one piece of apparatus may cause the power to another be cut off. If the relay operates an alarm rather than a circuit breaker, it may be ignored by staff. A better alternative is to include a small isolating transformer in the circuitry of each individual item of mains operated electromedical equipment, which can be connected to the patient. The patient circuit is, therefore, earth-free and said to be *fully floating*. The enclosure of the equipment may be earthed (or completely insulated see below).

The second method of improving safety is to install a *current-operated earth-leakage circuit breaker* (COELCB, also known as an '*earth trip*' or *residual current circuit breaker* or *RCCB*) (Fig. 25.9). This may be installed in the electric supply to the whole operating room or theatre suite, or may be installed in each item of equipment. The live and neutral conductors each take a couple of turns or so (both exactly the same) around the core of a toroidal transformer. A third winding is connected directly to the coil of the relay that operates the circuit breaker. If the current in the live and neutral conductors is the same, the magnetic fields cancel themselves out. If they differ, there is a resultant magnetic field, which induces a current in the third winding and this causes the relay to operate and break the circuit. A difference of as little as 30 mA can trip the COELCB in as little as 30 msec or be used to operate an alarm. It may be manually reset and may also have a test button to check its operation. COELCBs may have similar problems to isolating transformers but are less expensive. They operate so quickly and at such low earth leakage currents, that they greatly reduce the possibility of serious electric shock. The shaded area of Figure 25.5 shows the protection afforded by a COELCB.

In the UK electrical safety in clinical areas is achieved by a high standard of earthing of the fixed wiring, by good earthing of enclosures and fully floating patient circuits where appropriate. Safety may be further improved by using battery-operated equipment. In some cases the battery may be recharged from the mains between uses.

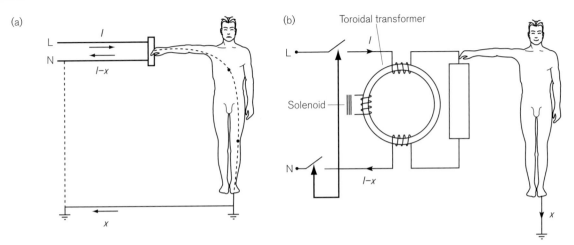

Figure 25.9 (a) If a load is taking a current of *I* amps from the live conductor L and *x* amps is returning via the patient and earth, then the current in the neutral conductor N will be (*I* − *x*) amps. **(b)** A current-operated earth-leakage circuit breaker (COELCB). The imbalance between the currents in the live L and neutral N conductors is sufficient to set up a field in the toroidal transformer sufficient to induce in the third, winding a current that will trip the solenoid and therefore disconnect both the live and neutral supply.

Classification of electromedical equipment to ensure electrical safety[7,8]

Class I equipment

This includes household electrical items. The electrical apparatus itself is connected to live and neutral conductors and insulated from the metal casing. The casing, which can be touched by the user, is connected to the earth lead. In the event of a fault in the apparatus in which there is current leakage from the apparatus to its casing, the earth connection grounds this 'earth leakage current'. A fuse in the live wire plug connection (UK) melts and the apparatus becomes disconnected from the mains. The user is thus protected from electric shock. However, if the earth connection is also faulty, such protection is lost (Fig. 25.2).

Class II equipment (Fig. 25.10a)

Both the apparatus and its casing are insulated – 'double insulated equipment'. There is no need to earth such equipment.

Class III equipment

This equipment is designed to operate from a power source not exceeding 24 V AC. The apparatus may either have its own internal power source or be connected to the mains by an adaptor containing a transformer. Although macroshock is unlikely with such equipment, microshock is still possible.

Class I, II, and III equipment may be subdivided into the following:

Type B equipment (Fig. 25.10b)

This defines a device in which the earth leakage current is restricted to 0.05 mA in Class I equipment or 0.1 mA in Class II equipment. It may refer to Class I, II or III, which is mains powered or internally powered. Although the equipment can be connected to the patient externally or internally, such equipment shall not be connected to the heart.

Type BF equipment (Fig. 25.10c)

This is as type B equipment, except that the part applied to the patient is isolated from the rest of the apparatus. This confers a degree of safety such that the maximum earth leakage current under a single fault condition is not exceeded, even if 1.1 times the maximum rated voltage is applied between earth and the patient attachment. It is still not safe enough for direct attachment to the heart.

Type CF equipment (Fig. 25.10d)

This provides the highest measure of protection against electric shock and can be connected to the heart. Thus earth leakage currents of up to 0.05 mA per electrode for Class I equipment and up to 0.01 mA per electrode for Class II equipment will not result in electrocution.

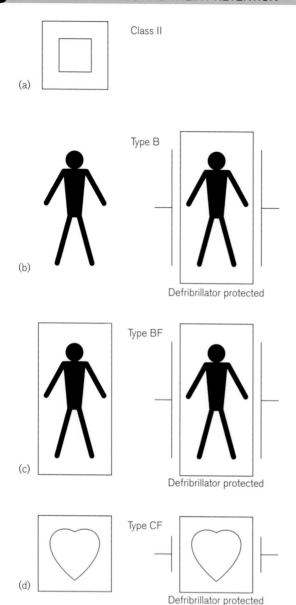

(a) Class II

(b) Type B

Defribrillator protected

(c) Type BF

Defribrillator protected

(d) Type CF

Defribrillator protected

Figure 25.10 Symbols indicating degrees of protection in electromedical equipment. See text.

Burns

Where electric current is passed through the skin, the heat generated is proportional to the square of the current flow and the electrical resistance of the surface area of skin involved, as indicated above. Depending on the amount of heat produced, the area over which it is applied and the rate of cooling by the circulation, burns may

result. This is discussed further in Chapter 26, in connection with diathermy.

Sparks and static electricity

Sparks occurring at switches or from the interruption of the supply by the removal of a plug could ignite flammable vapours. They may be prevented by the installation of spark proof switches and electrical sockets which 'capture' the plug, preventing its withdrawal while the switch is turned on. All electrical apparatus in the operating room, which does not comply with these precautions, is kept outside the 'zone of risk', described below. Sparks may also occur when metal strikes metal or stone, such as when a metal component from a breathing system is dropped on to a terrazzo floor. Chromium plating of metallic components reduces the likelihood of sparking and was extensively used on anaesthetic equipment for this purpose.

Static electrical discharges have probably been responsible for most of the explosions that have occurred in the past. Just as static electricity is discharged from nylon and other man-made materials, similar static charges are developed on dressing trolleys, operating tables and anaesthetic machines.

Although the quantity of static electricity generated in the operating room is relatively small, there is sufficient energy in the spark, when it is rapidly discharged, to ignite flammable anaesthetic vapours. It is therefore important, not only that the generation of static electricity is prevented, but also that the slow discharge to earth is allowed for any that does occur.

There is, therefore, an upper and a lower limit to the permissible electrical resistance between any part of the antistatic floor of the operating room and earth. The resistance between two electrodes set 60 cm apart should nowhere be less than 20 kilo ohm (kΩ) or more than 5 mega ohm (MΩ). All mobile operating equipment in the operating room and anaesthetic room should make electrical contact with the floor. Anaesthetic machines and trolleys have wheels whose tyres are constructed of antistatic (conducting) rubber. In the absence of such precautions a metal chain, one end of which is attached to the frame of the trolley, is allowed to dangle on the floor so that at least three links are in contact with the floor. The chains can be damaged or kept off the floor and are therefore a poor substitute for conducting rubber wheels. Similarly, all footwear worn by staff should contain conducting material. Periodic tests should be carried out to ensure that the resistance of the above items remains within prescribed limits.

If flammable anaesthetic agents are used, the most important precaution, however, is the use of antistatic (conducting) rubber or neoprene in the components of the breathing systems and other tubing components in the anaesthetic machines. As recently as 1982, an explosion occurred when a co-axial breathing system, part of which was made of a non-conducting material, was used with cyclopropane.

Fire and explosion[9-11]

For these to occur, there are three prerequisites: combustible material (fuel), oxidant to support combustion and a source of ignition. These risks arise from the following sources:
- the use of high partial pressure of oxygen (pressurized oxygen and high oxygen concentrations); and
- the use of flammable anaesthetic agents and of solvents for cleaning and skin preparation, such as alcohol.

Burning consists of the chemical combination of a 'combustible' material with oxygen. Energy is liberated in the form of heat and if it takes place in a confined space the pressure may increase greatly. Rapid liberation of heat and the rise of pressure result in an explosion.

High oxygen partial pressure

When there is a rise in the pressure of a gas, heat is generated. If a flammable material, such as oil or grease, in a confined area, is suddenly subjected to a high partial pressure of oxygen, such as 140 000 kPa in a full oxygen cylinder, the heat generated is sufficient to ignite it and cause an explosion. (This is the principle of the compression-ignition (diesel) engine). Therefore, oil, grease or other flammable materials should be kept away from apparatus in which high oxygen partial pressures exist.

Under some conditions, nitrous oxide may dissociate into nitrogen and oxygen and the latter gives rise to risk of explosion. Hence nitrous oxide sources should be treated with similar care.

Volatile anaesthetic agents and flammable solvents

Cyclopropane, most ethers and ethyl chloride are explosive in anaesthetic concentrations. They are no longer in common use in the developed world.

Carbon dioxide, halothane, enflurane, isoflurane, sevoflurane and desflurane are not flammable, nor is nitrous oxide at atmospheric pressure. However, nitrous oxide does support combustion even more fiercely than oxygen. Trichloroethylene is also non-flammable under conditions in which it is used by an anaesthetist. Halothane is flammable in oxygen, but at much higher concentrations than are used clinically.

Fire or explosion may be caused by the ignition of gases or vapours within the anaesthetic equipment, or escaping from it, or of the vapour of a flammable substance that is used for skin cleaning, such as alcohol.

Although naked flames are seldom employed in the operating rooms nowadays, they may be encountered elsewhere. However ignition of flammable mixtures may be caused by sparks from static electricity, from electric motors, faulty electrical apparatus or from diathermy apparatus, electrical cautery (as used in ENT surgery), or from the electric plug top being pulled out of the socket when the switch is turned on and the current is flowing.

Other causes of fire

There are two other modern causes of burns and fire in the operating room: these are fibreoptic light sources and surgical lasers. Powerful visible light sources are now commonplace in the operating room to provide illumination for endoscopic procedures. These sources, even at the patient end of a fibreoptic light cable, produce a concentrated amount of heat as well as light. The carelessly placed end of the cable may cause a burn directly or set fire to the drapes or other flammable material. This situation is even more dangerous if the drapes have a high concentration of oxygen or flammable material beneath them.

Zone of risk

This is a term used to denote the area in which explosive mixtures are deemed liable to exist during anaesthesia. Within the zone of risk, the following precautions are advised:
- there should be no naked flames;
- all electric switches should be spark proof and electric plugs should be 'captive' while the switch is turned on; and
- all parts, especially rubber tubing, etc. of anaesthetic apparatus, should be constructed of conductive (antistatic) rubber or other material, and the operating room floor should be antistatic. Antistatic rubber, containing carbon, has sufficient conductivity to leach away static electricity, and yet sufficient resistance to prevent so fast a discharge that a spark occurs.

All trolleys, stools and other mobile equipment should have tyres or feet of a conducting material. These are painted yellow or have a yellow flash or label to indicate that they are antistatic.

In 1956 in UK, the original working party looking into the risks of explosion in clinical settings, defined the zone of risk as the whole anaesthetic room and operating room where the anaesthetic machine was mobile. Since 1956, with the replacement of cyclopropane and ether with non-flammable anaesthetic agents, there was a dramatic fall in the number of explosions. Subsequently, in 1970, the Association of Anaesthetists of Great Britain and Ireland changed the definition of the zone of risk to 25 cm around the gas pathways of the anaesthetic machine and breathing system. Non-spark proof switches and sockets are permissible outside the zone of risk, providing they are permanently attached to the wall of the operating room, and that electrical outlets are 40 cm above the floor to prevent damage to cables. Breathing systems should still be constructed of anti-static material.

Classification of anaesthetic equipment and zone of risk (Fig. 25.11)

Anaesthetic Proof equipment

AP equipment standards are based on the energy required to ignite the most flammable mixture of ether and air. AP equipment can be used within 5 to 25 cm range of flammable gas escaping from a breathing system, and its temperature should not exceed 200°C.

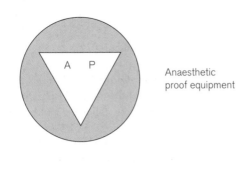

Anaesthetic proof equipment

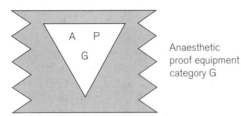

Anaesthetic proof equipment category G

Figure 25.11 Symbols indicating 'zone of risk' classification for anaesthetic equipment.

APG equipment

These standards are based on the ignition energy, which should not exceed 1 µJ, required to ignite the most flammable mixture of air and oxygen. APG equipment can be used within 5 cm of gas escaping from a breathing system, and its temperature should not exceed 90°C.

REFERENCES

1. Beiglemeyer G (1987) 'Effects of Current passing through the Human Body and the Electrical Impedance of the Human Body'. In: *A guide to IEC Report 479*. Berlin: vde Verlag gmbh.
2. IEC (1984) 'Effects of Current passing through the human Body'. In: *IEC 479-1 General Aspects*. Geneva: Bureau Central de la Commission Electrotechnique Internationale.
3. IEC (1987) 'Effects of Current passing through the human Body'. In: *IEC 479-2 Special Aspects*. Geneva: Bureau Central de la Commission Electrotechnique Internationale.
4. Fontanarosa PB (1993) Electric Shock and Lightening Strike. *Annals of Emergency Medicine* **22**: 378–387.
5. Yoshikawa T, Asai S, Takekawa Y et al (1972) Experimental investigation of battery induced esophageal burn injury in rabbits. *Critical Care Medicine* **25**: 2039–2044.
6. Hull CJ (1994) 'The electrical hazards of patient monitoring'. In: *Monitoring in Anaesthesia and Intensive Care*. London: Hutton & Prys Roberts Saunders.
7. Al-Shaikh B, Stacey S (2002) *Essentials of Anaesthetic Equipment*. 2nd edn. London: Churchill Livingstone; 175–180.
8. British Standard (1989) *Medical Electrical Equipment Part l. General Requirements for Safety*, BS5724: Part 1 (IEC 60101: 1988) Milton Keynes, UK: BSI.
9. MacDonald A (1994) A short history of fires and explosions caused by anaesthetic agents. *British Journal of Anaesthesia* **72**: 710–722.
10. MacDonald A (1994) A brief historical review of non-anaesthetic causes of fires and explosions in the operating room. *British Journal of Anaesthesia* **73**: 843–846.
11. Vickers MD (1973) Hazards in the operating theatre. Fires and explosions. *Annals of the Royal College of Surgeons of England* **52**: 354–357.

Surgical diathermy

Patrick T Magee

The anaesthetist and assistants may sometimes find themselves responsible for the correct connection of the diathermy machine. Therefore, they should know something of the principles and problems of diathermy.

PHYSICAL PRINCIPLES

Radio frequency (RF) surgical diathermy or electrosurgery uses the heat generated by an electric current,[1] often delivered at more than 200 V, passing through a small amount of tissue to cut, destroy or vaporize that tissue and to create haemostasis by causing coagulation and sealing of small blood vessels. Passing an electric current through the body causes all the tissue through which it passes to heat up. For this effect to be clinically useful, the current must pass through a small area of tissue at the active electrode. In contrast, at the indifferent electrode of the diathermy plate, which completes the electrical circuit, the current must pass from the skin surface to a large area to prevent burns where they are undesirable. This is the concept of *current density*.

Current density

Current density refers to the current per unit cross-sectional area. With a large conductive area, such as at the patient plate, there is a low current density and although the amount of heat generated is the same at the active electrode, the heat is rapidly conducted away. At the contact point of the active electrode, the current density is high, the heat being generated over a small area, thus creating the desired surgical effect (Fig. 26.1).

It is necessary to pass considerable currents through the human body to produce enough heat to have this effect. Under normal circumstances, the accidental passage of electric current at mains frequency (50 Hz) through the body has several highly undesirable effects, including burns, muscle spasm leading to asphyxiation and ventricular fibrillation. However, it was found experimentally years ago, that although living tissues, especially conducting and contractile tissues, are maximally sensitive to electric current at mains frequency, this sensitivity decreases at lower frequencies (including direct current (DC)), and decreases markedly at very high frequencies (Fig. 25.3 in the preceding Chapter).

Diathermy frequencies used in surgery are in the region of 0.4–1.5 MHz. RF diathermy machines are, in fact, powerful radio transmitters and would cause severe interference to radio receivers, even at some distance. Without good screening, RF diathermy signals can capacitatively couple with ECG or other amplifiers and grossly interfere

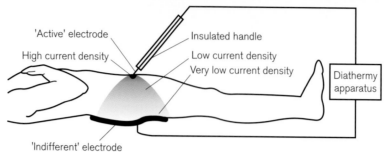

Figure 26.1 The concept of 'current density' or the current per unit cross-sectional area. In areas of low current density the heat generated is quickly dissipated, whereas in the area of high current density the heating effect is very high.

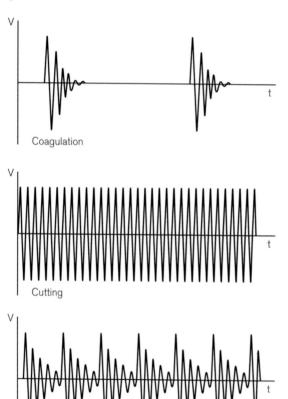

Figure 26.2 The waveforms commonly used for surgical diathermy.

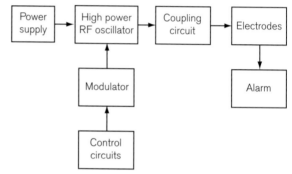

Figure 26.3 Block diagram of a surgical diathermy unit.

usually referred to as 'blend', which is commonly used during cystoscopic resections of tumour or prostate.

A block diagram of a RF diathermy machine is shown in Figure 26.3. A high-power, high-frequency oscillator or generator is controlled by a modulator to produce the necessary waveforms. The output of the generator is led through coupling circuits to optimize impedance matching between the generator and the 'indifferent' and the 'active' electrodes. The circuitry normally contains a 0.01 μF capacitor from the indifferent electrode to earth. It will be recalled that the electrical impedance (the term used to describe electrical resistance at different frequencies of current) is inversely proportional to both the frequency of the current and the magnitude of the capacitance; therefore this capacitor in the diathermy circuit provides a low impedance (20 Ω) route to earth for the high-frequency diathermy current, but a high impedance (300 kΩ) to any incidental low-frequency mains current. This effectively isolates the circuit from earth against mains leakage current. The risk of electrocution from a diathermy apparatus is therefore much reduced, but the risk of burns should not be underestimated (see below). Where the indifferent lead (i.e.

with the biological signal being monitored. For this reason, by international agreement, only certain narrow frequency bands are used. A sine waveform has been found to be better for cutting and a damped waveform for coagulation (Fig. 26.2). A combined waveform is also available, the plate) socket is at earth potential, as it is in many older diathermy sets, it is vitally important that the lead is connected to the correct terminal of the diathermy apparatus. If the plate were accidentally connected to the active terminal, when the foot switch is depressed the patient may be burned at all points connected to earth (i.e. where the body is in contact with those parts of the operating table at earth potential).

The above description is of a unipolar arrangement. However, some diathermy sets are capable of being used with a bipolar system in which the current passes from one blade of a pair of forceps to the other. The circuit is earth-free and the current does not pass through any part of the patient's body, other than that grasped by the forceps (Fig. 26.4). The power required is small and electrically safer, but it is suitable only for the coagulation of small pieces of tissue or blood vessels. It is particularly suitable for ophthalmic or neurosurgical procedures, and is also more acceptable in the presence of a cardiac pacemaker. From a safety point of view, it should be used whenever possible.

ACCIDENTS DUE TO DIATHERMY

Electrical burns

These may be divided into two groups; first, where the patient receives electrical burns; second, where the diathermy causes fires or explosions in the presence of flammable vapours (see Chapter 25). Hot wire cautery is also a cause of fire.

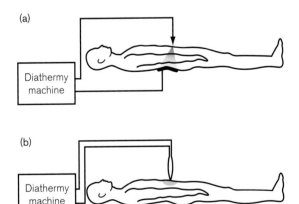

Figure 26.4 (a) Unipolar and **(b)** bipolar diathermy. Note that the current passes through a much smaller volume of tissue with bipolar diathermy.

Electrical burns occur with diathermy use in the following ways:

- Accidental depression of the foot switch when the forceps or cutting electrode is inadvertently in contact with some part of the patient can result in significant burns. This may be prevented by keeping the forceps in an insulated quiver when not in use; it is also minimized by the installation of an audible alarm which sounds when the foot switch is depressed. This must never be turned down to inaudible levels. The indicator light on the machine is useful as a confirmation that the machine is working, but cannot warn of unintentional activation.
- Burns can arise where there is intermittent or partial contact of the plate surface and the skin resulting in areas of high current density due to the small area of contact at these points. Some diathermy machines give an audible warning if the plate lead is not plugged in, or if the electrical continuity of the lead is broken. However, an absence of the audible warning is not proof that the plate has been correctly applied to the patient. Some diathermy sets incorporate an isolating transformer which allows them to have a fully floating output; the patient is then unharmed if the indifferent electrode is neglected, providing it is not inadvertently connected to earth.
- Burns can also be caused, even if the patient plate is not applied, by the electrical circuit being completed via the operating table and the floor, or other points through which a patient may be inadvertently earthed. Although ECG leads represent the most likely pathway to earth to allow diathermy burns, other monitors can also provide an earth route resulting in burns from radio frequency currents; these can include temperature probes[2] and Doppler probes.[3] It is also possible, for example, for the tracheal mucosa to be severely damaged if the patient is inadvertently earthed through the damp endotracheal tube and the anaesthetic machine.
- Another danger, which is seldom appreciated, is the risk of infarction when unipolar diathermy is used on an organ, which has been temporarily raised on its vascular pedicle. The classical injury is that caused to the testis, when raised from the scrotum on its vas deferens. Figure 26.5 shows that the current density is greatly increased in the vas, thus causing its destruction. For this reason, bipolar diathermy is by far the preferred option. The same applies to diathermy for use in appendages such as digits. If unipolar diathermy

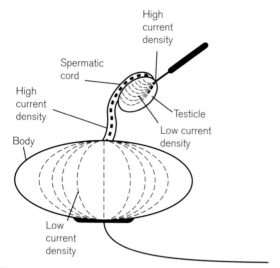

Figure 26.5 The testis elevated from the body on the spermatic cord generates unintentional areas of high current density (thick dashed lines) during unipolar diathermy.

must be used, then the exposed testis must remain in contact with the rest of the body; its electrical conduction must be improved by the interspersion of a saline soaked swab.

- Burns can be caused by capacitative coupling through intact insulation. The concept of capacitative coupling is shown in Figure 26.6. Any two electrical conductors separated by an insulator form a capacitor. Such a capacitor can be formed in the space between, for example, the lighting over an operating table and the patient on the table. One property of a capacitor is an infinitely high resistance to direct current and progressively lower resistance (impedance) as the frequency of the current is increased. Burns caused by capacitative coupling can occur to the surgeon's gloved fingers in contact with another conductive surface such as an active electrode[4] to the vaginal wall during cervical cautery; and during laparoscopic surgery (see below).

DIATHERMY AND LAPAROSCOPIC SURGERY

In the same way as external diathermy has hazards, laparoscopic surgery also has electrical hazards associated with its use.[5] There is a danger of current leakage to the

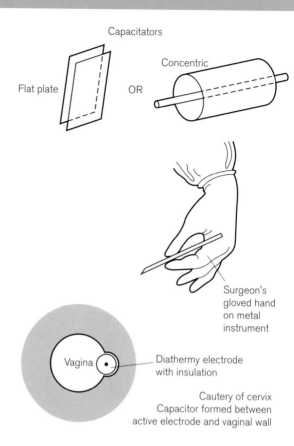

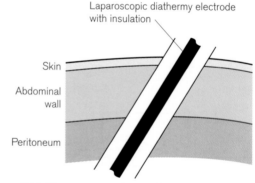

Figure 26.6 The concept of capacitative coupling. A capacitor is formed between any conductive surfaces separated by an insulator (dielectric). At DC, a capacitor is a pure insulator; as the frequency increases, its resistance (reactance, impedance) decreases. Inadvertent capacitors may be formed between an instrument and the surgeon's fingers, the active electrode and other tissue (e.g. the vaginal wall) or between the (insulated) active electrode and the abdominal wall during laparoscopic surgery.

patient from laparoscopic instruments, causing either apparent malfunction of laparoscopically applied unipolar diathermy, or tissue damage at the cannula site or other sites outside the operator's field of vision.

The stray current pathways may be due to:
- insulation breaks in the diathermy applicator;
- capacitative coupling through intact insulation; or
- direct coupling between the active electrode and other organs or metal instruments outside the field of vision.

Major insulation breaks may be obvious. However, small cracks in insulation of the diathermy electrode may be invisible, but their effect may be magnified by conducting fluids such as saline, peritoneal fluid or blood.

Capacitative coupling between a laparoscopic cannula and electrically isolated but adjacent tissues is shown in Fig. 26.6. The problem is aggravated by the use of plastic coated cannulae of small diameter, which are used to produce smaller scars;[6] the smaller the cannula, the greater the capacitance and the larger the stray current passed at a given frequency

To guard against inadvertent direct coupling to tissues outside the field of vision, instruments may be used, which are insulated along the entire length except at the tip.

All of the problems described here can be avoided by the use of bipolar diathermy and such laparoscopic instruments are available.

DIATHERMY AND PACEMAKERS

The use of RF diathermy should be avoided in patients with internal or external pacemakers as there is a risk of inhibition of or damage to the pacemaker, either of which can cause its failure to function.[7] There is also the risk of causing burns to cardiac tissue at the conductive sites of the pacemaker wire. Bipolar diathermy is much preferred if diathermy must be used and then only at sites well away from the pacemaker and its connections. This is further discussed in Chapter 27.

FIRES AND EXPLOSIONS

The causes of fires and explosions, of which diathermy may be one, are discussed in Chapter 25. The external cases of diathermy machines are made to be gastight. Pressure gradients can develop across the gas-proof seal: if, due to an internal electrical fault, the inside of the device is heated and fumes are generated, rupture of the device can occur.

REFERENCES

1. Haag R Cuschieri A (1993) Recent Advances in high frequency electrosurgery: development of automated systems. *Journal of the Royal College of Surgeons Edinburgh* **38**: 354–364.
2. Parker EO (1984) Electrosurgical burn at the site of esophageal temperature probe. *Anaesthesiology* **60**: 93–95.
3. Block EC, Burton LW (1979) Electrosurgical burn using a battery operated Doppler monitor. *Anaesthesia and Analgesia (Cleve)* **58**: 339–342.
4. Tucker RD, Ferguson S (1991) Do surgical gloves protect staff during electrosurgical procedures? *Surgery* **110**: 892–895.
5. Department of Health (1994) *Safety Action Bulletin – Diathermy injury during laparoscopic surgery* SAB (94)38 September 1994. London: Department of Health.
6. Voyles CR, Tucker TD (1992) Education and engineering solutions for potential problems with laparoscopic monopolar electrosurgery. *American Journal of Surgery* **164**: 57–62.
7. Kellow NH (1993) Pacemaker failure during TURP. *Anaesthesia* **48**: 136–138

FURTHER READING

Watticz A, Khandwala S, Maurice-Antoine B (1995) *Electrosurgery in operative endoscopy.* Oxford: Blackwell Scientific.

Pacemakers and defibrillators

Nicholas P Gall and Mark T Kearney

BASIC CARDIAC ELECTROPHYSIOLOGY

While pacemakers and defibrillators are not strictly anaesthetic equipment, they are frequently encountered, both in the elective and emergency situation. An understanding of their hardware and software is important, not least because of their interaction with strong electromagnetic fields that may be encountered in anaesthetic practice.

To understand pacemaker and defibrillator functioning, an understanding of normal cardiac electrophysiology is necessary. The myocardium consists of an interconnected network of myocytes. At rest, the myocyte interior is maintained at a negative potential (–80 mV) in relation to the extracellular fluid. This is due to the relative impermeability of the plasma membrane, differential intra- and extracellular ion concentrations and active ion transporters. Either because of the spontaneous inward leak of positively charged ions, in the sinus node for example, or because of an external electrical stimulus, the potential difference across the membrane decreases. At a threshold potential (approximately –70 mV in ventricular myocytes) various ion channels become activated, producing further ion influx. This leads to myocyte depolarization and the *action potential* (Fig. 27.1). Calcium influx leads to the release of additional intracellular calcium stores activating the contractile apparatus, a process described as *excitation-contraction coupling*.

Further ion movements, particularly potassium efflux, restore the myocyte's potential to its resting value. During the early part of the action potential, the myocyte cannot be induced to depolarize again – *the absolute refractory period*. Later, a stimulus of sufficient strength can induce further depolarization – *the relative refractory period*.

Myocytes in different areas of the heart have different ion channels and therefore different action potentials. Some cells spontaneously discharge due to a resting inward leak of positively charged ions, with some cells discharging at a faster rate than others, for example, the sinus node; this is known as *automaticity*. Due to the inter-linked nature of myocytes, the cells with the fastest rate of depolarization set the heart rate.

Pacemakers

The association between a slow pulse and syncope was recognized up to 300 years ago. With the development of the electrocardiogram at the turn of the twentieth century, the various forms of bradycardia were defined. At the same time, experimental electrical stimulation of cardiac cells was first studied, followed soon after by the first descriptions of the use of cardiac electrical stimulation as a therapeutic modality. Dramatic improvements in battery, capacitor and electronic technology, driven particularly by the Second World War, followed. On 8 October 1958, the first entirely implantable epicardial cardiac pacemaker was inserted. A transvenous device

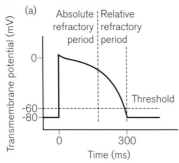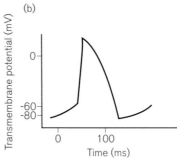

Figure 27.1 An action potential of: **(a)** a ventricular myocyte, **(b)** that of a sino-atrial myocyte.

followed in 1962. Multiple technological advances have followed, leading to the complex and reliable pacemakers we have today.

Pacing essentially involves passing a small electric current into the myocardium, usually with a wire placed endocardially. The stimulus, if of sufficient strength and outside the absolute refractory period, can induce myocyte and subsequently chamber depolarization.

The NASPE/BPEG code

With the increasing complexity of pacemakers, a three-letter code was designed in 1974, by the Inter-Society Commission for Heart Disease Resources, to define a pacemaker's characteristics. This was refined in 1981 and subsequently led to the 1987 North American Society of Pacing and Electrophysiology (NASPE)/British Pacing and Electrophysiology Group (BPEG) five-letter generic code.

The first letter of this code denotes the chamber(s) paced, the second letter the chamber(s) sensed, the third letter the response to sensing and the fourth letter programmability and rate response. The fifth letter, rarely used, denotes anti-tachycardia functions. NASPE/BPEG defibrillator (1993) and lead (1996) codes, have also been designed.

In general terms, five forms of pacing are likely to be encountered clinically, the first four being available for both temporary and permanent pacing:

1. VVI – A single lead is placed in the ventricle, for pacing (**V**VI) and sensing (V**V**I). If the ventricular rate is above the minimum set (*the base rate*), pacing is *inhibited* (VV**I**). Otherwise pacing occurs.
2. AAI – A single lead is placed in the atrium. It functions in a similar way to the VVI and is used for sick sinus syndrome, where AV nodal conduction is normal.
3. DDD – Leads are present in the atrium and ventricle. Both chambers (hence *dual*) can be paced

(**DDD**) and sensed (D**DD**). If activity in either chamber is sensed, a pacing stimulus will be inhibited. If no ventricular QRS wave follows atrial activity, ventricular pacing will be *triggered* (DD**D** representing the dual responses of inhibition or triggering).

4. VOO/AOO/DOO – These are the simplest pacing modes. No sensing occurs (_O_) and, therefore, there can be no response to sensing (_ _O); the chamber(s) is paced at a fixed rate. This mode is used temporarily where the sensing of external noise could lead to the inappropriate inhibition of pacing, e.g. diathermy. It is also known as *asynchronous pacing*.
5. VDD – Only one lead is used which paces the ventricle (**V**DD). An electrode further up the lead is positioned in the atrium allowing dual chamber sensing (V**DD**). This allows physiological pacing, i.e. ventricular activity follows atrial at a physiological PR interval as long as atrial pacing is unnecessary. This mode is uncommon and is used as an alternative to DDD pacing in order to reduce system complexity.
6. The presence of an (R) as the fourth letter denotes a pacemaker able to increase the paced heart rate in response to the patient's activity (see below, Software).

Pacing terminology

A number of pacing terms require explanation:

1. *Threshold* (Fig. 27.2) – the minimum stimulus needed to capture the heart. It is given as current (amperes) or voltage (volts) over a time period (pulse width, milliseconds).
2. *Unipolar/bipolar* – refers to the pacing or sensing circuit (Fig. 27.3). The pacing circuit involves a negatively charged cathode and a positively charged

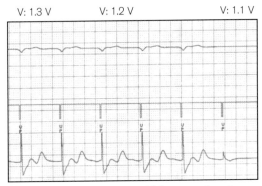

V: 1.3 V   V: 1.2 V   V: 1.1 V

Figure 27.2 A print-out from a VVI pacemaker. A standard ECG lead is seen at the top. The pacemaker marker channel is seen beneath, VP indicating ventricular pacing. The bottom line shows the electrogram seen by the bipolar lead. Loss of capture is seen at 1.1 Volts.

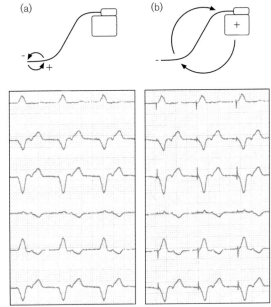

Figure 27.3 Bipolar **(a)** and unipolar **(b)** pace/sense circuits are shown. Representative ECGs are shown beneath; note the larger pacing artefact on the unipolar ECG, due to the larger pacing circuit.

anode. In the bipolar circuit, the cathode and the anode are separated by a short distance at the pacing lead tip. The circuit is localized to the immediate myocardium. In the unipolar circuit, the cathode is at the pacing lead tip with the anode at a distance; in the permanent pacing system it is found in the pacing box. The unipolar pacing circuit is larger and therefore produces a larger pacing artefact on the ECG. While there is little difference between the pacing characteristics of these two conformations, bipolar sensing is less susceptible to external noise.

3. *Impedance* – this represents the total resistance to current flow in the pacing circuit. This resistance occurs in the leads, at the lead-myocardial interface for endocardial leads and in the tissue between the cathode and the anode. Fractures in the leads increase impedance, while insulation breaks reduce it.

Temporary pacing

Temporary pacing is used in emergency situations of life-threatening bradycardia or where a bradyarrhythmia could occur temporarily.

Transvenous pacing

This is the usual method for temporary pacing. A thin, semi-flexible, shaped, bipolar pacing lead is normally used. The central circulation is accessed via the internal jugular, subclavian or femoral veins, the first of these being preferable, as there is a lower risk of complications (pneumothorax with the subclavian route, infection and deep vein thrombosis with the femoral). Furthermore, with the internal jugular approach, the veins used for

possible subsequent permanent pacing are not directly punctured. The lead is manipulated into position at the right ventricular apex under X-ray guidance. Some leads may have a central shapeable stylet to allow more accurate positioning. Others have a tip-mounted flotation balloon to allow non-radiographic positioning. Active fixation (screw tipped) leads are also available to prevent lead displacement. In most cases one ventricular lead is used. Atrial pacing and dual chamber pacing is also possible. Due to the risks associated with temporary transvenous pacing, its use should be avoided where possible. Various guidelines are listed in the bibliography section at the end of this chapter.

The pacing lead is connected to an external box, which allows various programming options:

1. *Mode*: usually VVI ('demand') or VOO ('asynchronous' or 'fixed rate').

2. *Output*: either the output voltage or current is programmable, the pulse width being fixed. Maximum outputs are higher than with permanent systems as battery size is unimportant and the pacing threshold is more often unstable.

3. *Sensitivity*: the threshold above which electrical activity will be detected as cardiac. This is usually

measured in millivolts, a higher value indicating less sensitivity.

4. *Rate*: usually 30 to 150 or even higher for the overdrive pacing of tachyarrhythmias.

Transgastro-oesophageal pacing

An electrode (on a device similar to an oesophageal stethoscope or nasogastric tube),placed oesophageally, can capture the left atrium, while in the stomach ventricular pacing may be possible. Transoesophageal atrial pacing (TAP) is a simple and safe method for temporary treatment of bradyarrhythmias and is particularly applicable to use during anaesthesia. Because voltages of up to 20 V or more may be required to achieve capture (Fig. 27.2), a signal amplifier is needed if using an ordinary external (transvenous) pacing box (signal generator). TAP, like transgastric pacing, is rarely used because of unfamiliarity with the technique and scarcity of the equipment.

Transcutaneous pacing

In the peri-arrest situation it may be difficult to position a transvenous temporary wire. It is possible to capture the ventricle by passing a large enough current through the chest using specially-designed electrodes (Fig. 27.4). These electrodes may also be used for monitoring and defibrillation.

There is significantly greater impedance in the transcutaneous pacing circuit than with endocardial stimulation, due to the additional significant impedances of the electrode-skin interface, the lung and the pericardium. High currents are required, usually 50–90mA, at pulse widths of 10–20 ms. Pacing thresholds may be further increased by poor electrode-skin contact, metabolic disturbance (hypoxia, acidosis) and pericardial effusion. Unpleasant cutaneous nerve and skeletal muscle stimulation occur at currents as low as 10 mA, making this method of pacing, without sedation, short-lived by necessity. Pulse widths of the order of 10 ms produce optimal pacing thresholds and reduce patient discomfort. Significant pacing artefacts occur on the ECG, making myocardial capture difficult to assess without pulse or blood pressure monitoring.

Another form of transcutaneous pacing is also used by cardiothoracic surgeons. Wires are implanted directly into the myocardium, atrial and ventricular, at the time of operation and brought out through the skin. Two wires can be used per chamber to allow bipolar pacing. These can be connected to a temporary pacing box. Similar to temporary wires, they are prone to infection and thresholds can rise without warning. They are normally used to await recovery of the normal conducting system. Atrial pacing may also reduce the incidence of post-operative atrial fibrillation.

Permanent pacing

The principles of permanent pacing remain the same as temporary pacing; the indications continue to expand and have been recently updated. Following significant improvements in battery and lead technology, devices are now small enough to be placed subcutaneously in the pre-pectoral region, the leads passed via the subclavian or cephalic veins. Other routes including the femoral veins and epicardial systems may also be used where subclavian access is impossible or due to previous pacemaker infection.

Hardware

An implantable pacemaker box consists of:

1. *The battery*. This forms a major part of the volume

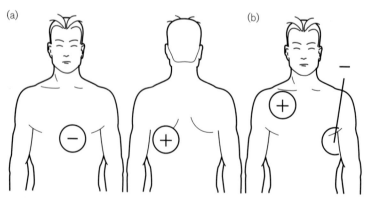

Figure 27.4 The suggested positioning for transcutaneous pacing electrodes is shown, antero-posterior **(a)** and antero-lateral **(b)**. There is no significant difference in pacing thresholds between the two conformations.

of the pacemaker. It has a number of important requirements including:

a) small size;

b) the ability to produce small amounts of current reliably and consistently over long periods;

c) a low self-discharge rate so that it does not wear out without use;

d) a predictable discharge rate so that replacement can be planned in advance;

e) lack of gas production to allow hermetic sealing; and

f) significant longevity to allow infrequent box changes. It is not unusual for batteries to require replacement only once a decade.

A number of different power sources have been used, including nuclear devices. However the lithium-iodine battery is currently the industry standard.

2. *Voltage/Output circuits*. Various circuits are required to allow the battery voltage (usually 2.8 V at implant) to be altered to produce a range of programmable outputs, according to the threshold, to prolong battery life.

3. *Telemetry circuits*. These allow an external computer to communicate and program the pacemaker using radio frequency signals.

4. *Pacing circuits*. These control all aspects of pacemaker function including the timing circuits, diagnostics and the rate response circuitry.

5. *Sensing circuits*. These allow sensing of intrinsic cardiac activity with filtering allowing exclusion of external electromagnetic noise.

6. *Memory*. Modern pacemakers are able to store significant quantities of data, for example on arrhythmias and heart rate variability.

7. *Reed switch*. This is activated by the magnet, completing a circuit allowing a particular predefined program to start.

In contrast to temporary leads, permanent pacing leads are expensive, highly engineered multi-component devices, required to be *in situ* for several decades, without failing or producing significant local damage. Their components include:

1. *Electrode*. Most newly-implanted leads are bipolar with a cathode tip and a larger anode further back. The cathode is surprisingly complex – it is small, producing a high charge-density, thus improving myocardial capture, and a high pacing impedance which reduces battery drain. Platinum, titanium or activated carbon are used for their good conducting properties and durability. A small reservoir of steroid is also found in the lead tip to reduce the inflammatory reaction at the lead-myocardial interface, maintaining lower stimulation thresholds.

2. *Fixation mechanism*. It is necessary to secure the lead in the myocardium, thus maintaining capture. Passive fixation is achieved with small flexible protrusions from the lead tip, *tines*, which hook into the trabeculated muscle. For less stable positions, active fixation mechanisms are available, often a small retractable screw (B, Fig. 27.5).

3. *Lead conductor*. This is the wire, often made of a complex alloy, which transmits the electrical current. Bipolar leads require two, one each for the cathode and the anode. Coiling the wires produces great lead flexibility, the anodal conductor being wound inside the cathode (*coaxial wire*), separated by an insulator. A recent advance involves coating each individual conductor with insulation (*coated wire technology*) which allows the anodal and cathodal conductors to run together producing leads with even smaller diameters.

4. *Lead insulation*. Silicon was used initially; polyurethane is used today; it allows flexibility, resistance to damage, biocompatibility and good handling characteristics.

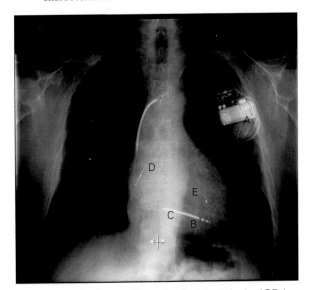

Figure 27.5 A chest radiograph of a biventricular ICD is shown. A number of the components are visible: the box **(A)**, the screw tip of the active-fixation ventricular lead **(B)**, the distal shocking coil **(C)**, the atrial lead **(D)** and the coronary sinus left ventricular pacing lead **(E)**.

5. *Lead connector.* The metal connectors, which link the conductor to the pacemaker. There is now an industry standard, *IS-1*.
6. *Central lumen.* A central lumen runs the length of the lead allowing the passage of a stylet that can be shaped to allow accurate positioning. A number of leads are also shaped to allow positioning in certain positions, e.g. the coronary sinus or the right atrial appendage.

Software

Pacemakers are becoming increasingly complex, with multiple programmable parameters and functions, including:

1. Mode (see The NASPE/BPEG code, above);
2. Base rate – the minimum paced rate;
3. Hysteresis rate – it is possible to allow the intrinsic heart rate to drop to a lower value, say 40, before pacing is initiated at a higher rate, say 60;
4. Maximum paced rate – the maximum rate above which pacing will not occur, either driven by the patient's atrial rate or by the rate sensor;
5. AV delay – the paced equivalent of the PR interval;
6. Rate response functions. An increase in heart rate is a prime mechanism through which cardiac output is increased during both physical and mental activity. To allow a more physiological heart rate response in paced patients with abnormal sinus node function, many pacemakers sense this requirement; motion sensors, changes in transthoracic impedance as a marker of respiratory rate and QT interval are used. The pacing response can then be tailored to each patient.
7. Sensitivity. The signal amplitude above which electrical activity will be 'seen'; and
8. Mode switch. Pacemakers should not track atrial tachycardias. Modern pacemakers can detect these arrhythmias and change mode accordingly.

The evolving complexity of the programmable parameters (the most important of which are summarized above) has made it increasingly difficult to diagnose pacemaker malfunction from the surface ECG without knowledge of the pacemaker set-up. In general terms 'pacemaker malfunction' due to software or hardware failure is a rare event.

Future directions

Pacemaker therapy for traditional bradycardic indications is currently underused in the UK; implant rates are likely to increase. Furthermore, pacemaker indications are expanding beyond bradyarrhythmias, for example:

1. pacing to prevent atrial tachyarrhythmia;
2. pacing to prevent ventricular tachyarrhythmia in long QT syndrome;
3. pacing to treat vasovagal syncope; and
4. pacing to improve symptoms and prognosis in heart failure. Many patients with heart failure have conducting system abnormalities; e.g. left bundle branch block which produces disco-ordinate contraction of the right and left ventricles. Biventricular pacing (E, Fig. 27.5) in which both the right and left ventricle, via the coronary sinus, are paced, can restore co-ordinated ventricular activation and has been shown to improve symptoms and potentially reduce mortality.

In addition, we will have the ability to monitor pacemaker function remotely. Device-treated patients in the future are likely, therefore, to be an expanding, increasingly heterogeneous group requiring highly individualized care.

Defibrillators

To understand defibrillator design and function, and why defibrillation may fail, requires some understanding of the pathophysiology of fibrillation and defibrillation.

Ventricular fibrillation (VF) is a complex arrhythmia consisting of random, discoordinate, three-dimensional waves of depolarization, thus producing the loss of cardiac output and allowing arrhythmia persistence.

The mechanisms through which a shock of sufficient strength allows the return of spontaneous, co-ordinated electrical activity remains incompletely understood. A shock can have three effects, depending on its timing in the action potential. Early on, during the absolute refractory period, no effect occurs. Later on, action potential prolongation is seen. Later still, a new action potential is induced. It is hypothesized that a shock of sufficient strength and appropriate timing will extend the refractory period in enough of the myocardium to allow the waves of depolarization to die out. Subsequently, cardiac automaticity allows the return of normal electrical activity, depending upon the underlying cardiac condition.

The amount of current required to produce defibrillation is known as the defibrillation threshold (DFT). For historical reasons, this is given in terms of energy (joules). Its determinants explain the success or failure of a shock.

As with the pacing threshold, there is a minimum current below which defibrillation will not occur. Above a certain level, detrimental effects may occur, reducing the likelihood of success. Between these values, success is most likely. However, as the waves of depolarization in VF are entirely random, an element of chance exists that the shock is delivered at the optimal time to defibrillate a critical mass of myocardium. This concept is known as the *probabilistic nature* of DFTs.

Factors affecting DFTs include:

1. *Charge characteristics*. A monophasic shock is one where the polarity of the shock remains constant throughout its delivery (Fig. 27.6a). In biphasic shocks (Fig 27.6b), the polarity is reversed during delivery. In general terms, DFTs are lower and there is less post-shock myocardial depression with biphasic shocks. The shape and time-course of the shock can also be varied to produce optimal effects.

2. *Electrode position*. In implantable systems shocks can occur in a number of configurations, which may affect the DFT (*see* Hardware, below). Altering the position of the endocardial coils can also have some effect. External paddle positions may also have an effect.

3. *Shock polarity*. Which electrode is used as the anode and which the cathode, can affect DFTs, particularly with monophasic shocks.

4. *Underlying cardiac condition*. The more severe cardiac conditions as assessed using heart size, ejection fraction, QRS width or heart failure symptoms, predict higher DFTs. Furthermore, the time spent in VF prior to defibrillation adversely affects DFTs.

5. *Metabolic disturbance*. DFTs are higher in hypoxic and acidotic patients.

6. *Medication*. DFTs can be affected by numerous medications. Of note, intravenous amiodarone reduces DFTs, whereas its chronic administration increases them. Fentanyl reduces DFTs. Common

inhalational anaesthetic agents do not appear to have significant effects.

7. *Shock impedance*. Shock impedance affects current delivery to the myocardium. The transthoracic impedance for external defibrillation is dependent on lung volume, skin contact and tissue thickness.

External defibrillation

In the cardiac arrest situation and with external cardioversion for non-arrest arrhythmias, the energy is applied from the outside, positioned as for transcutaneous pacing. To improve current flow, gel or gel pads are used between the paddles and the skin. This allows better contact, reducing impedance and the incidence of skin burns. Downward pressure on the paddles serves a similar purpose. Some defibrillator pads can also be used for monitoring and pacing. Smaller paddles for use during cardiac surgery are also available.

Current resuscitation recommendations are for the use of 200–360 J monophasic shocks for the defibrillation of VF and pulseless ventricular tachycardia. Biphasic shocks may allow the use of lower energies with less post-shock cardiac dysfunction. For the cardioversion of more co-ordinated, non-arrest arrhythmias, e.g. atrial flutter, it may be possible to use lower energies, whether mono- or biphasic.

The implantable cardioverter defibrillator

Implantable cardioverter defibrillators (ICDs) have been commercially available since 1985, for the treatment of those at risk of recurrent life-threatening ventricular tachyarrhythmias. Over recent years, technological improvements have allowed improved defibrillation success, easier implantation, greater longevity and increased programmability. Initially, the devices were large and required abdominal placement and epicardial patches. In 2003, devices as small as 33 ccs became available and can be implanted in the same manner as pacemakers.

Hardware

The ICD system (Fig. 27.5) consists of a box containing:

1. **Battery.** The defibrillator battery has a number of requirements in common with pacemaker batteries:
   a) small size;
   b) low self-discharge rate;
   c) predictable discharge rate; and
   d) good longevity.
   However, it is also required to produce a large current over a short period to produce the shock,

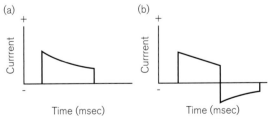

Figure 27.6 Diagrams showing the change of current with time for a monophasic **(a)** and a biphasic shock **(b)**.

something the lithium-iodine battery is incapable of. The lithium silver vanadium oxide battery is used instead. Of note, because of its differing electrochemistry, ICD batteries are much less efficient for pacing, a feature reducing their longevity.

2. *Capacitor*. The ICD battery is unable, by itself, to produce sufficient charge quickly enough to allow defibrillation. It is necessary to store the charge produced over a few seconds so that it can be discharged effectively. It is stored in a capacitor, which consists of two conductors, an anode and a cathode, separated by an insulator (see Chapter 2). A battery connected to the capacitor increases the potential difference between these conductors, thus storing charge. This is discharged by completing the circuit between the conductors via the myocardium. Modern ICD capacitors consist of thin films of aluminium, separated by a non-conducting layer of aluminium oxide.

3. *Voltage/Output circuits*. These allow different voltages to be produced for pacing and for capacitor charging. In addition the capacitor output can be controlled to produce the biphasic shock.

4. *Telemetry circuits*;

5. *Pacing circuits*;

6. *Sensing circuits*;

7. *Memory*; and

8. *Reed switch*.

Defibrillator leads are constructed in a very similar way to pacing leads, with some added complexity:

1. *A pace/sense electrode*. This is essentially identical to a normal lead for a pacemaker. The cathode is found at the tip, with the anode either separate from or integrated with the distal shocking coil.

2. *One/two shocking coils*. The distal lead coil is positioned in the right ventricle and the proximal coil in the superior vena cava. They are constructed of similar material to pacing electrodes, but with a large surface area to improve current delivery. It is through these coils that the charge is distributed. A number of shock pathways are possible, which may produce varying DFTs. The most common is between the coils and the ICD box; it is also possible to shock between the box and one coil or between one coil and the other.

3. *A fixation mechanism*;

4. *Lead conductor*. The conductors are of similar construction to those of pacing leads. With a dual coil, bipolar defibrillator lead four are necessary –

one per coil and one each for the pacing anode and cathode.

5. *Lead insulation*;

6. *Lead connector*. An IS-1 connector is used for the pace/sense functions. An industry standard connector for the defibrillator coils, *DF-1*, has been defined.

7. *Central lumen*.

Software

The first generation of ICDs were only able to give therapy above a non-programmable ventricular rate, defined prior to device manufacture. As time has progressed, the complexity and programmability has increased to give the current third generation devices:

1. Up to three zones for the detection and treatment of different ventricular tachyarrhythmias,

2. Multiple electrogram characteristics can be used to improve the sensitivity and specificity of differentiating ventricular arrhythmia from other rhythms (rate, onset characteristics, rate stability, ECG morphology, relationship of atrial to ventricular activity, etc.).

3. Varying treatment options are programmable including anti-tachycardia pacing, low energy cardioversion and defibrillation.

4. Aspects of shock characteristics are programmable including varying energies, shock pathways, polarity, timing, etc.

5. Single, dual or biventricular pacing functions are available.

6. Some devices can also detect and treat atrial tachyarrhythmias.

7. Electrophysiological studies can be performed non-invasively.

Future directions

As time goes on and as our understanding of VF and defibrillation improves, it is likely that both external and internal defibrillation will change. Important changes in the short term will include the remote monitoring of ICD function and a dramatic expansion in ICD indications. The population with these devices will greatly increase.

Electromagnetic interference

Pacemakers are required to detect low-amplitude electrical signals and communicate with pacemaker programmers with radio-frequency transmissions. They are, therefore, susceptible to interference from external sources of electromagnetic radiation. As pacemaker and

ICD design has progressed and with the increased use of bipolar leads, electromagnetic interference is now less of an issue.

Frequencies between 0 and 10^{11} Hz, representing radio frequency and microwave energies, can affect pacing systems. Pacemakers respond to electromagnetic interference in different ways. If the device recognizes the signal as noise it can react by turning off its sensing circuits during the noise (VOO/DOO), resetting permanently to a default mode (often VVI) or by triggering a paced beat to prevent noise inhibiting its output. Clearly, if the signals are not recognized as noise, pacemaker inhibition, reprogramming or ICD shock therapy may be triggered.

There are many sources of electromagnetic interference that can affect pacemakers and ICDs. However, those that are likely to influence anaesthetic practice include:

1. *Diathermy* – diathermy can affect pacemakers in a number of ways, as discussed above. In addition, the diathermy current can activate the rate-response circuitry, damage the pacing circuits or pass via the lead, damaging the lead-myocardial interface, thus affecting pacing thresholds. Bipolar pacemakers are much less susceptible to this. Suggested management includes:

   a) pre-operative consultation with the pacing technicians to enable programming alterations (asynchronous mode, rate response and magnet functions off, ICD tachyarrhythmia therapy off);

   b) the use of bipolar diathermy or unipolar diathermy as far as possible from the device, in short bursts only. Urgent pacemaker interrogation may be required. A magnet can be used in an emergency but may, in some circumstances, start automatic threshold testing or open the device to reprogramming; and

   c) post-surgery, a further pacemaker test is recommended.

2. *External Cardioversion/Defibrillation* – like diathermy, the considerable current can overwhelm the protective circuitry and reprogram or damage the device or the lead-myocardial interface. Management includes device interrogation pre and post-procedure. Paddles should be placed at least 10 cm from the box and at 90 degrees to the axis of box to lead tip (preferably AP).

3. *MRI* – the MRI scanner can interact in a number of ways with pacing systems, not least because of the ferromagnetic components of old devices. Strong electrical signals are also produced, which can either inhibit or induce rapid pacing. In general terms, an MRI is contraindicated in pacemaker/ICD patients, although case reports exist of patients undergoing this investigation without ill-effect.

4. *Lithotripsy* – the shock can trigger arrhythmia, cause mode switch or pacemaker inhibition or damage the box and, in particular, the piezoelectric crystals used for activity sensing. The manufacturer should be consulted particularly for abdominally-placed systems. Devices should be programmed to an asynchronous mode and ICDs should be disabled.

5. *Radiotherapy* – radiotherapy, if directed at the pacing box may destroy the circuitry. Pacing systems require repositioning.

6. *Electro-convulsive therapy* – adverse effects are unlikely but pacemaker checks and asynchronous pacing are suggested.

In general terms, consultation in advance with the pacing technicians for up-to-date advice is strongly recommended. Magnet placement may not be sufficient and may even be detrimental.

FURTHER READING

Crockett PJ, Droppert BM, Higgins SE, *et al.* Defibrillation. What you should know; www.medtronic.com/physician/cardiology

Cummins RO, Hazinski MF, Kerber RE, *et al.* (1998) Low-energy biphasic waveform defibrillation: evidence-based review applied to emergency cardiovascular care guidelines. *Circulation* **97**: 1654–1667.

De Latorre F, Nolan J, Robertson C, *et al.* (2001) European Resuscitation Council Guidelines 2000 for Adult Advanced Life Support. *Resuscitation* **48**: 211–221.

Del Monte L, Gamrath B. Non-invasive pacing. What you should know. www.medtronic.com/physician/cardiology

Ellenbogen KA, Kay GN, Wilkoff BL (2000) Clinical cardiac pacing and defibrillation. 2nd edn. Philadelphia: WB Saunders.

Gammage MD (2000) Temporary Cardiac Pacing. *HEART* **83**: 715–720.

Gregoratos G, Abrams J, Epstein AE, *et al.* (2002) ACC/AHA/NASPE 2002 guideline update for implantation of cardiac pacemakers and antiarrhythmia devices: summary article. *Circulation* **106**: 2145–61.

Gold MR (2001) Permanent Pacing: new indications. *HEART* **86**: 355–360.

Murphy JJ (2001) Problems with temporary cardiac pacing. *British Medical Journal* **323**: 527.

28

Lasers

Patrick T Magee

PRINCIPLES

The increasing surgical use of lasers, with their inherent potential hazards to patients and operating room staff, mandates an understanding of their physical principles by anaesthetists.[1]

The word *laser* is an acronym for 'Light Amplification by Stimulated Emission of Radiation'. The laser produces an intense beam of pure monochromatic light (one wavelength, one colour). The output beam is likely to be of a very small cross-sectional area and is virtually a non-divergent parallel beam. These properties mean that energy may be delivered to very small areas of tissue with great accuracy, and the intense parallel beam of light constitutes a very large amount of power per unit area of tissue. The wavelength of a laser is determined by the lasing medium used. Although described as mono-chromatic, most laser media produce light within a narrow waveband consisting of a number of discrete frequencies.

Although there are many more complex laser systems,[2] the basic components of a laser are shown in Figure 28.1. The lasing medium may be a solid, liquid or gas. The atoms of a lasing medium are excited to high energy levels by a 'pumping' source, which may be a high voltage discharge in the case of a gas, an intense flash of light from a flashtube or the energy from a radio frequency power source. Figure 28.2 shows the excitation and emission process possible in a gaseous lasing medium. A photon of energy from the pumping source may be absorbed by a stable atom in its so called 'ground state', which then becomes an atom in an excited state, with an electron or electrons in an orbital shell at a higher energy level.[3] Spontaneous emission of a photon of energy occurs as the electrons fall back to shells of a lower energy state and the excited atom reverts to the ground state.

If a further photon of pumping energy, at the correct wavelength, is applied to an atom in its excited state, then as it falls to the ground state, two photons of energy will

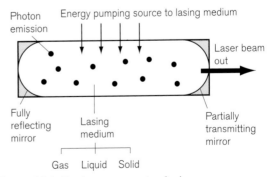

Figure 28.1 Basic components of a laser.

(a) Absorption

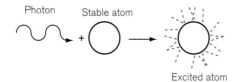

(b) Spontaneous emission

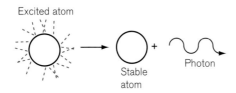

(c) Stimulated emissions

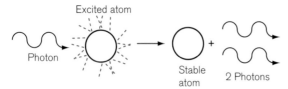

Figure 28.2 Absorption, excitation and emission processes.

be emitted instead of one. This is known as stimulated emission, originally described by Einstein in 1917 as the basis for laser technology[4] and the inversion of the energy states is referred to as *population inversion*. The emitted photons thus produced are in phase with, have the same polarization as, and travel in the same direction as the stimulating radiation. This mechanism is amplified by many of the escaping photons being reflected back into the lasing medium by the mirrors. Thus a chain reaction occurs, and this can be thought of as a positive feedback system. The process produces an intense source of light energy, some of which is allowed to escape through the partially reflecting mirror at the output end of the lasing medium. The output beam of the laser is usually directed to the tissues through a fibreoptic light guide. However, the wavelength of the carbon dioxide laser is so long, at 10.6 μm, that there is no fibre currently available to transmit energy, so that it has to be directed by a series of mirrors instead.

CLINICAL APPLICATIONS

The clinical use of lasers depends on a compromise between:

- laser-tissue interaction;[5]
- absorption and penetration depth;
- availability of a laser of the correct wavelength and power; and
- availability of a suitable method of transmission.

The extent of the effect of a laser on human tissues depends primarily on the intensity and the frequency of the light being used.[6] At low light intensity, stimulation occurs within the cell and this is exploited in physiotherapy applications. At slightly higher intensity, attenuation of cellular activity occurs. At still higher intensity levels, about 40 J cm^{-2}, sensitizing agents in tissue become activated (this is the basis of protecting the skin from the sun's ultraviolet rays using suntan lotions). By the time the light intensity has risen to 400 J cm^{-2}, the tissue temperature has risen to 60°C and protein denaturation and photocoagulation predominate. Further large increases in light intensity result in a tissue temperature rise to 100°C, vaporization of tissue fluids and destruction of cell structures. In order to control the destructive power of a laser, most systems can be pulsed, the light is emitted in short bursts, to allow heat dissipation between bursts and reduction of thermal damage to neighbouring tissues. 'Q *switching*' of a laser refers to a device which allows aliquots of laser light to be stored and released in bursts of even higher energy and shorter duration. Such a technique is used in ophthalmology to cause photoablation and to minimize thermal damage to the eye. With Q switching, while collateral thermal damage may be reduced, the frequency of switching is such that vibration and therefore mechanical damage may predominate.

The penetration of light energy into body tissues depends on the wavelength of the light. Far infrared and ultraviolet light has little penetration because it is rapidly absorbed near the surface of the tissue, by tissue water. Maximum penetration of light occurs at the red end of the spectrum.

The graph in Figure 28.3 shows the spectrum of absorption of light at different wavelengths by haemoglobin, melanin and water. Monochromatic light energy is absorbed by tissue of complementary colour and reflected by substances of the same colour.

Carbon dioxide laser energy at 10.6 μm is absorbed by water within 1 mm depth, causing rapid vaporization of intracellular water. The main use of the carbon dioxide laser is, therefore, as a bloodless cutter and vaporizer. The blue-green argon laser beam penetrates to about 2 mm depth and is maximally absorbed in the 500 nm waveband by substances of a complementary colour (red), such as

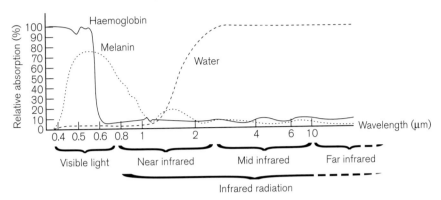

Figure 28.3 Absorption characteristics of tissue constituents.

Table 28.1 Some currently available medical lasers

Lasing medium	Wavelength, nm	Colour	Transmission
Krypton	476, 521, 568, 647	Blue to red	Optical fibre
Argon	488–515	Blue-green	Optical fibre
Nd-YAG-KTP	532	Green	Optical fibre
Helium-Neon	633	Red	Optical fibre
Nd-YAG	1064	Near IR	Optical fibre
CO_2	10 600	Far IR	Mirrors

haemoglobin. Thus, the argon laser is used to coagulate blood in small vessels with very little effect on other more transparent tissues, for example, the retina. The Nd:YAG (neodymium: yttrium-aluminium garnet) laser has a solid lasing medium and produces energy in the near infra-red region of the spectrum, which has maximum penetration, being absorbed at 3–5 mm depth, by haemoglobin, melanin and water. When invisible infrared lasers are used (e.g. CO_2 laser), it is common practice to make use of a low powered, visible-light laser, such as a helium:neon laser at the same time, in order to aid in aiming the therapeutic laser accurately. Table 28.1 shows the currently available lasers in medical use.

SAFETY ASPECTS

Apart from the danger to the patient from the beam of laser energy if it is misused, there is a risk to the operator and other persons in the operating environment.[7] This is because of the long range of laser light due to the virtual non-divergence of the beam; thus, in contrast to a collimated X-ray beam for example, increased distance from the source has very little safety benefit. Even reflected laser light may be very dangerous to the eyes. Visible laser light transmitted to the retina of the eye may burn it irreparably, leaving a blind spot in the field of vision. A similar lesion over the optic nerve may result in total blindness of that eye. The cornea, lens and aqueous and vitreous humours partially or totally absorb far-infra-red laser radiation; these tissues, therefore, are more susceptible to damage than the retina.

Laser radiation on the skin may be felt as a burning sensation, which is therefore self-protective, provided that the victim is conscious and has not received analgesia.

In terms of the danger that lasers pose to humans, there is a complex relationship between power, frequency and time of exposure. There is an international classification for lasers, shown in Table 28.2, where Class I lasers are inherently safe and Class IV lasers are, broadly speaking, hazardous if misused. Most lasers, in medical use, are in Class IV. No one should use a laser who is not trained to

Table 28.2 International classification of continuously working lasers

Class I	Powers not to exceed maximum permissible exposure for the eye
Class II	Visible laser beams only; powers up to 1 mW; eye protected blink-reflex time of 0.25 s
Class IIIa	Relaxation of class II to 5 mW for radiation, provided beam is expanded so that the eye is still protected by the blink-reflex
Class III b	Powers up to 500 mW; direct viewing hazardous
Class IV	Powers over 500 mW; extremely hazardous

do so, and everyone who is working in the vicinity of a laser should be trained in the safety aspects of its use. This includes the anaesthetist, who is often standing in the line of fire of the laser.

Anaesthetic related risks

As with electrical apparatus and diathermy, laser use carries the risk of fire, particularly when the immediate environment in which it is being used is oxygen enriched. This problem occurs not only during airway surgery, but also when the laser is inadvertently directed towards drapes under which high concentrations of oxygen and nitrous oxide may be present. The following precautions should be taken:

* No flammable anaesthetic agents or nitrous oxide should be used; nitrous oxide supports combustion better than oxygen under some circumstances.[8]
* Non-reflective (matt-black) instruments should be used, since the reflected laser beam is almost as powerful as the main beam.
* The oxygen concentration in the immediate vicinity of the laser beam should not exceed 25% where possible.
* Non-flammable endotracheal tubes constructed from special materials (see Chapter 8) should be used. Plastic endotracheal tubes should be avoided. The cuff of a LMA is more vulnerable to laser damage than the shaft and should be filled with saline as a protective measure.[9] Other tissues should be protected with wet swabs.
* Protective goggles fitted with specific lenses that absorb the wavelength of the laser in use, should be worn by everybody in the operating theatre, including the patient. Goggles give better protection than spectacles. They should also be kept with the laser for which they are relevant.
* Doors to the operating area should be locked and all windows should be covered to protect those outside

the operating area. Warning signs should be posted outside doors.

Safety codes

In the UK, the Medical Devices Agency[10] has published guidance (1995) on laser safety, both in medical and increasingly in dental practice. This guidance should form the basis of a set of local rules and a Safety Code. It specifically recommends the appointment of a Laser Protection Supervisor, who should not be the laser operator, who should ensure all staff are wearing correct eye protection, and who should be available in every area where a laser is in use. Additionally, the guidelines recommend that a Laser Protection Advizer be identified, who advises on the risk management aspects of a laser to be installed, and on the drawing up of local safety policy and rules.

REFERENCES

1. van der Speck AFL, Spargo PM, Norton ML (1988) The physics of lasers and implications for their use during airway surgery. *British Journal of Anaesthesia* **60:** 709–729.
2. Houssin M, Courteille P, Champenois C, *et al* (2003) Linewidth reduction by 6 orders of magnitude of a broad area 729 nm diode laser. *Applied Optics* **42:** 4871–4876.
3. MT Tooley (2003), personal communication.
4. Graudenz K, Raulin C (2003) From Einstein's quantum theory to modern laser therapy: a history of lasers in dermatology and aesthetic medicine. *Hautarzt* **54:** 575–582.
5. Jacques SL (1992) Laser-tissue interactions. *Surgical Clinics of North America* **72:** 531–558.
6. Parsons R (2002) 'Basic Principles of Lasers'. In: *Anaesthesia and Intensive Care Medicine* Abingdon: The Medicine Publishing Co. pp. 419 –421.

7. Sliney DH (1995) Laser Safety. *Lasers in Surgery and Medicine* **16:** 215–225.

8. MacDonald AG (1994) A short history of fires and explosions caused by anaesthetic agents. *British Journal of Anaesthesia.* **72:** 710–722.

9. Pandit JJ, Chambers P, O'Malley S (1997) KTP laser resistant properties of the reinforced LMA. *British Journal of Anaesthesia.* **78:** 594–600.

10. The Medical Devices Agency (1995) *Guidance on the Safe Use of Lasers in Medical and Dental Practice.* London: Department of Health

Provision of anaesthesia in difficult situations and the developing world

John A Carter

The provision of anaesthesia in modern well-equipped operating theatres is dependant on sophisticated electronic equipment that requires an uninterrupted supply of both electricity and compressed gases. Such equipment is not readily transportable, although it may be moved within a hospital facility. There are many locations throughout the world where anaesthesia is administered to facilitate surgery, investigations or other forms of treatment outside this generally accepted 'safe' environment.

The following are examples of locations and situations away from hospital operating theatres where anaesthesia may be required, and where simpler or alternative means of providing anaesthesia may need to be employed:

- within hospitals away from operating theatres:
  - Accident and Emergency Departments;
  - Radiology Departments;
  - Magnetic Resonance Imaging Suites;
  - Radiotherapy Departments;
  - Intensive Care Units;
  - Coronary Care Units – e.g. for Cardioversion; and
  - Psychiatric Units – for Electroconvulsive Therapy:
- site of an accident or major disaster;
- the battlefield; and
- developing countries:
  - hospitals, medical centres; and
  - self-contained visiting surgical teams.

Domiciliary anaesthesia, as in kitchen table appendicectomy and obstetric flying squad interventions, has long been abandoned on safety grounds and, more recently, anaesthesia in dental surgeries is no longer practised in the UK.

All of these situations are remote from the relatively safe, comfortable and familiar operating theatre anaesthetic environment, and the following problems may be encountered to a greater or lesser degree:

- lack of continuous electricity supply;
- lack of continuous supply of oxygen and nitrous oxide;
- difficulty with storage of drugs and equipment;
- difficulty in transport and supply of drugs and equipment;
- lack of maintenance of equipment;
- lack of skilled assistance;
- lack of control of environment; and
- financial restrictions.

Where possible, on grounds of safety, patients should be transferred to medical facilities capable of providing the appropriate level of care. For example, electroconvulsive therapy for the psychiatric patient with severe aortic stenosis and depression would be better managed (from their cardiac status) in the operating suite of the main hospital rather than in a room off the psychiatric ward. Non-essential surgery should not be undertaken at the site of a major disaster or on the battlefield, and the use of local, regional or sedative techniques should be considered where appropriate.

The overriding principle in providing anaesthesia under any of these conditions should be to use a simple, safe technique, familiar to the practitioner. To reduce complexity and avoid the potential administration of a hypoxic gas mixture as well as reducing the need for scavenging, (and for many other well-rehearsed reasons), there is a case for avoiding the use of nitrous oxide entirely. Training and practice in such techniques is invaluable for the time when they may be required. Even within a modern operating theatre environment, a 'difficult situation' may arise due to failure of a sophisticated electronic anaesthetic workstation, a major power cut with failure of back-up generators or a disruption to piped gas supply. The use of total intravenous anaesthesia (TIVA) and a self-inflating bag with a separate oxygen cylinder, combined with practical clinical monitoring, will allow adequate and safe anaesthesia in such a situation, and a torch may be the most essential item of additional equipment.

DIFFICULT SITUATIONS WITHIN HOSPITALS

Sites away from the operating theatres often have anaesthetic equipment that is used only occasionally. Piped oxygen and suction facilities may be absent. The equipment in such areas must be maintained and checked adequately, with basic monitoring meeting the standard recommended by the Association of Anaesthetists.[1] Since January 2003, all anaesthetic machines in use in the UK should be incapable of delivering a hypoxic mixture. There must be immediate access to resuscitation equipment and drugs, and a means of summoning additional assistance (i.e. telephone or intercom). The anaesthetist and his or her assistant should have sufficient experience and be familiar with both the environment and the equipment.

Some specific problems posed to patients, medical attendants and equipment within particular areas are detailed below.

Radiology departments

- ionizing radiation risk;
- long procedures – e.g. coiling of intracerebral aneurysms;
- low levels of lighting;

- restricted access to patient or patient's head; and
- there may be a requirement to stop ventilation briefly to avoid image blurring.

Radiotherapy units

- intense ionizing radiation requiring patient isolation from the medical attendants;
- closed circuit television or glass-liquid-glass window to view patient causing colour and image distortion;
- multiple frequent treatments over a few weeks; and
- radiotherapy applicators may obstruct access to the patient's head.

Magnetic resonance imaging (MRI)

- intense magnetic field with the ability to cause equipment made of ferromagnetic material to be attracted at projectile velocity into the scanner. There is, however, a rapid decrease in field strength with distance.
- electrical inductance – potential thermal injury from electrical conducting leads;
- electromagnetic interference leading to equipment malfunction – e.g. syringe drivers;
- noise from vibration of switched gradient coils – ear protection for patients; and
- theoretical risk of hypoxia if quenching of the superconducting magnets with cryogenic gases (usually helium) occurs. Quenching may occur as a fault condition or be initiated for emergency shutdown of the magnet.

These factors pose risks to patients and potential occupational hazards to staff. Patients and staff must be screened before access is granted to an MRI scanner, to exclude ferromagnetic implants such as aneurysm clips or pacemakers. Anaesthetic equipment taken into the vicinity of the MRI scanner must be MR-compatible.[2]

Remote anaesthesia

Anaesthesia for MRI, radiotherapy and some radiological procedures may necessitate the anaesthetist and the bulk of the anaesthetic equipment being remote from the patient. This may be either to ensure all ferromagnetic equipment is outside the magnetic field, or to remove anaesthetic personnel from ionizing radiation.

- TIVA may be employed using long infusion lines on pumps which must be able to cope with the increased resistance to flow caused by the increased length. This usually means setting to maximum the pressure limit for sensing an occlusion.

- Whilst sedation may be sufficient for some patients, the airway may need to be secured with a laryngeal mask airway (LMA) or tracheal tube.
- Intermittent positive pressure ventilation through a long co-axial breathing system such as a 9.6 to 10 metre Bain circuit and Nuffield Penlon series 200 ventilator, has been shown to provide safe anaesthesia[3]. With this system, there is an increase in the static compliance in proportion to the length of the tubing (see Compression Volume, Chapter 11). This is caused by expansion of the breathing hose and compression of the volume of gas during positive pressure ventilation and will result in a lower tidal volume being delivered than is set on the ventilator. This is insignificant in adults. In children, if a Newton valve is used, the ventilator becomes a pressure generator, and the increased resistance and compliance of the long system results in the pressure delivered being significantly less than that selected. (23% less with a 10 kg child). This compares to a 6 to 11% reduction when using a long rubber Ayre's T-piece.[4]
- The capnography signal is delayed due to the length of the sampling line but provides a guide for adjustment of the tidal volume.

MAJOR ACCIDENTS AND DISASTERS

These may occur in any part of the world at any time, and are by definition unexpected. All medical services should have a plan to deal with major disasters. A typical approach is to have a mobile medical team that can be rapidly deployed to the disaster site and a receiving hospital capable of dealing with the retrieved casualties. In the event of the number of casualties overwhelming the initial response, there should be a means of either escalating the number of teams or hospitals deployed. In developing countries, there may be a need to seek international assistance. Many countries have teams available for worldwide deployment at short notice. Particular problems encountered include:

- unfamiliar territory;
- unfriendly environment:
  - extremes of hot and cold and altitude, even in normally temperate climates;
  - dark, wet, cramped conditions.
- unfamiliar injuries:
  - blast and crush injuries;
  - delayed extrication.

- risk to rescuers:
  - nuclear, biological or chemical incidents;
  - terrorism;
  - fire, explosion risk;
  - continuing disaster (e.g. earthquake);
  - unstable buildings.

The predominant anaesthetic contribution to a major disaster is resuscitation and stabilization prior to transfer to the receiving medical facility. Exceptionally, to aid extrication of casualties, amputation of trapped limbs may be required. This is best achieved using ketamine, either intravenously or intramuscularly. Equipment for intubation, self-inflating bag, fluid and cannulae for intravenous fluid resuscitation should be available. Oxygen and Entonox should be used cautiously in such conditions as they support and accelerate combustion of flammable materials, and whilst the latter has excellent analgesic properties, it may not be suitable in very cold conditions (see Poynting Effect, Chapter 1) or in the presence of a head injury or pneumothorax.

THE BATTLEFIELD

Mobile Field Hospitals are deployed as close to the battlefront as safety will allow, and receive casualties who will normally have had only life-saving first-aid treatment at a Regimental Aid Post or equivalent. In addition to military casualties from both sides of the conflict, there are frequently civilian casualties, which may include children. This poses a problem if paediatric equipment is not available. Large numbers of casualties may arrive simultaneously, and require triage on arrival. In some, immediate surgery is required as part of the resuscitation process. Some of the features of military anaesthesia are as follows:

- equipment must be air portable;
- oxygen cylinders or concentrators are usually readily available;
- cost constraints for drugs and equipment is minimal;
- resupply not usually a problem – unless supply lines are cut.

Electricity is required for lighting, monitoring, suction, heating, refrigeration (for blood storage and some drugs) and will usually be supplied from generators that must be of sufficient power to cope with maximum demand. Vital equipment should have an independent battery back-up. Many modern pieces of equipment have a back-up supply of only 10 minutes. Sensitive equipment should have surge protection to limit voltage spikes from erratic power supplies.

Draw-over anaesthesia is the most suitable inhalational technique for use in the field.[5] It can be employed for both spontaneous and controlled ventilation, is not dependent on compressed gases and requires only light portable equipment. The basic equipment required comprises:

- non-rebreathing valve;
- self-inflating bag;
- low-resistance vaporizer; and
- means of giving supplemental oxygen (T-piece, length of tubing to use as oxygen reservoir and source of oxygen – i.e. cylinder or concentrator).

Several draw-over vaporizers are available, including the Epstein-Macintosh-Oxford (EMO) (Fig. 29.1), Oxford Miniature vaporizer (OMV) (Fig. 29.2), the Dräger Afya vaporizer (Fig. 29.3) and the Ohmeda PAC (Fig. 29.4).

The equipment in use at the moment, by the British military medical services, is the Triservice Anaesthetic Apparatus (Fig. 29.5). This consists of two modified OMVs connected to a self-inflating bag, which leads to a non-rebreathing valve connected to a facemask or airway device. Supplemental oxygen may be delivered upstream of the vaporizers by a T-piece with a length of corrugated tubing acting as a reservoir. This complete apparatus, including an oxygen regulator and cylinder yoke, comes securely packed in foam within an air portable container, all weighing less than 25 kg, and can be safely dropped by parachute.

The OMVs used in this apparatus have been modified by incorporating three folding feet to enable them to stand on a flat surface. Additionally, the capacity of the chambers has been increased to 50 ml. The wicks within the vaporizing chamber are of metal gauze, so that a different agent may be used by simply draining the

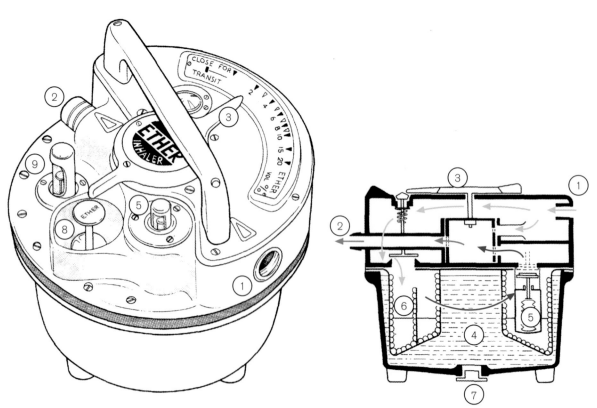

Figure 29.1 EMO ether vaporizer. (1) Inlet port, (2) outlet port, (3) concentration control, (4) water jacket, (5) thermocompensator valve, (6) vaporizing chamber, (7) filling port for water, (8) filling port for anaesthetic, (9) anaesthetic-level indicator. (Reproduced with permission of WHO from Dobson MB (1988) *Anaesthesia at the District Hospital*. Geneva: World Health Organisation.)

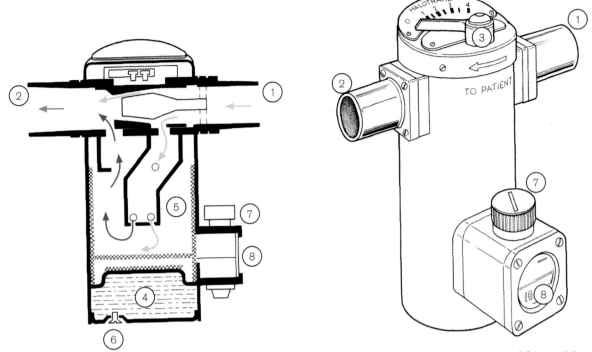

Figure 29.2 Oxford Miniature Vaporizer (OMV). (1) Inlet port, (2) outlet port, (3) concentration control, (4) heat sink (5) vaporizing chamber, (6) filling port for water, (7) filling port for anaesthetic, (8) anaesthetic-level indicator. (Reproduced with permission of WHO from Dobson MB (1988). *Anaesthesia at the District Hospital*. Geneva: World Health Organisation.)

vaporizer and rinsing the chamber (with a little of the new agent, which is then discarded), before properly charging the vaporizer for use.

Detachable calibration scales are supplied for different agents. When the control is turned to '0' (off), the contents will not spill if the vaporizer is accidentally inverted, although it is recommended that the vaporizer should be drained for transport. If it is tipped or inverted during use, the vaporizer must be kept upright for a few minutes before use to allow agent that may have entered the bypass or the control mechanism to drain back into the chamber, otherwise very high concentrations of vapour may be initially delivered. The OMV is not temperature-compensated, and although its body acts as a small heatsink, the vapour output concentration will decrease with time. By having two OMVs in the circuit, it is possible to switch between them as the output from one starts to fall off, to switch between different agents, or to use both in series to deliver a higher concentration for induction of anaesthesia.

The Triservice apparatus may be used in spontaneously breathing patients, or IPPV may be instituted either using the self-inflating bag, or by replacing the bag with a suitable ventilator. Originally the CapeTC50, which consists of a bellows expanded and contracted by an electric motor, was used, but this has been replaced by the Pneupac CompPAC ventilator (Fig. 29.6). The Triservice apparatus may also be used in 'push-over' or continuous flow mode using the Pneupac CompPAC ventilator, which may be either gas-driven or operated by a 24 volt or 240 volt electrical supply. When used in pushover mode, the pumping effect causes a slight to moderate increase in delivered vapour concentration. Capnography, end expired agent concentration monitoring and pulse oximetry should all be available at the Mobile Field Hospital, and will enable safe anaesthesia to be provided with such equipment.

The Tri-Service Apparatus, and the OMV vaporizer itself, are not CE marked as the problems of poor calibration, lack of temperature compensation and inherent risk of spillage of agent into the breathing circuit are insurmountable. This causes difficulty in attempts to gain experience with the equipment in the modern hospital environment, as patients are entitled to receive the

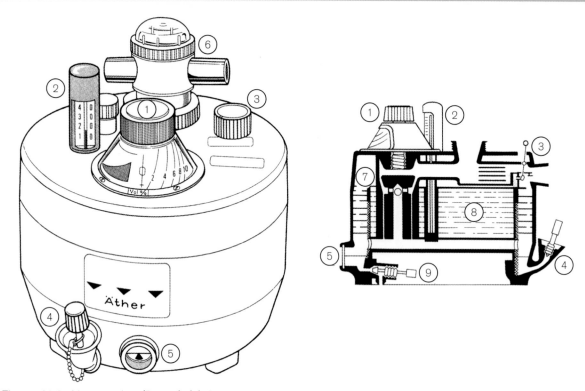

Figure. 29.3 Afya vaporizer (Dräger). (1) Concentration control, (2) thermometer, (3) on/off control, (4) filling port for ether, (5) ether-level gauge, (6) outlet and one-way valve, (7) vaporizing chamber, (8) water-filled heat reservoir, (9) drainage port for ether. (Reproduced with permission of WHO from Dobson MB (1988). *Anaesthesia at the District Hospital.* Geneva: World Health Organisation.)

highest standard of available care. There are, however, courses available to demonstrate the use of such draw-over apparatus, using highly sophisticated anaesthetic simulators.

Nuclear biological chemical (NBC) capability

Under conditions of NBC warfare, Mobile Military Operating Theatres are designed, by the use of air filters, to provide a protected environment. For additional patient protection, an NBC filter may be placed on the end of the inlet tubing of the Triservice apparatus, and if an oxygen concentrator is used as the source of supplemental oxygen, this can also be provided with an NBC filter.

Equipment for other battlefield anaesthetic techniques

Total intravenous anaesthesia is also advocated for military anaesthesia as it can simplify equipment requirements. Ketamine/midazolam and propofol/alfentanil (either

combination with vecuronium added for controlled ventilation) have been used very successfully, and requires little more than a self-inflating bag and oxygen source, together with an infusion bag (or syringe) with the mixed combination of drugs, and an infusion pump if available.[6]

ABNORMAL AMBIENT PRESSURES

Altitude

It may be necessary to use anaesthetic equipment at low ambient pressures, as in the transfer of patients by aircraft and in high-altitude locations. The highest human habitation is at about 5000 m or 16 000 ft, giving an atmospheric pressure of about 400 mmHg. Commercial aircraft, however, usually have cabin pressure maintained at 640 mmHg minimum, which is equivalent to 5000 ft, despite flying at heights of over 30 000 ft. In order to provide safe anaesthesia, a knowledge of the altered performance of anaesthetic equipment at different ambient pressures is essential.

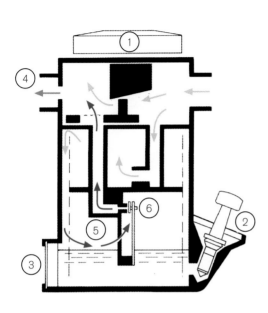
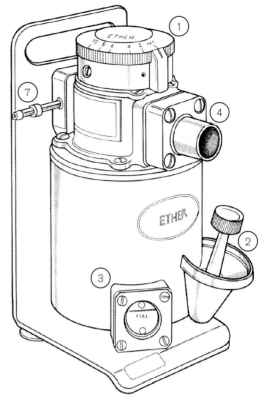

Figure. 29.4 PAC (Portable Anaesthesia Complete) vaporizer (Ohmeda). (1) Concentration control, (2) filling port for ether, (3) ether-level gauge, (4) outlet and one-way valve, (5) vaporizing chamber, (6) thermocompensator valve, (7) port for oxygen enrichment. (Reproduced with permission of WHO from Dobson MB (1988) *Anaesthesia at the District Hospital*. Geneva: World Health Organisation.)

- *Vaporizers.* Saturated vapour pressure is a function of temperature, not ambient pressure. Hence, the concentration delivered by a vaporizer is inversely proportional to the ambient pressure as the vapour pressure takes up a higher proportion of the ambient pressure at altitude, and a lesser proportion under hyperbaric conditions. However, the partial pressure of the agent, which determines the clinical effect, remains constant. Therefore, when vaporizers are used at a given setting, the anaesthetic will be delivered at a constant potency or effect, regardless of concentration changes with altitude (or depth). A vaporizer set at 1% at sea level will deliver 1.7% at 15 000 feet, but the clinical effect will be unaltered.

- *Flowmeters.* The reduction in gas density at altitude results in under-reading of variable orifice, constant differential pressure flowmeters. The error is about 20% at 10 000 ft. Under hyperbaric conditions, these flowmeters will over-read.[7]

- *Venturi-type oxygen masks.* These will entrain less air at altitude and so deliver higher concentrations of oxygen. A 35% mask will deliver approximately 41% oxygen at 10 000 ft.

- *Ventilators.* Volume or time-cycled ventilators may be preferable to pressure-cycled ventilators, but capnography and other monitoring will assist in adjusting ventilator settings under these conditions.

- *Pressure gauges.* These are calibrated at sea-level and so over-read at altitude. The error is negligible, as the pressures measured are so much greater.

- *Gas analyzers and capnography.* Gas analyzers measure the partial pressure of the gas under test but are calibrated in percentage at sea-level. They will, therefore, under-read at high altitude. Reduction of atmospheric pressure may also affect capnography in the following ways:[8]
  - pumping of gas through sample chamber – more powerful pump may be required to maintain flow rates;

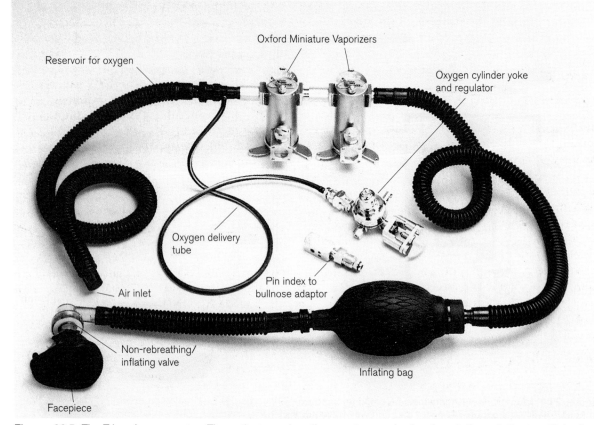

Figure. 29.5 The Triservice apparatus. The patient may breathe spontaneously, drawing air through the two Oxford Miniature vaporizers and the inflating bag. There is a valve mounted on the facepiece that prevents rebreathing. The air drawn in through the inlet may be enriched with oxygen from a cylinder, which is attached to the cylinder yoke, with the pin index to bullnose adaptor if required. During expiration, the oxygen is stored in the reservoir tubing. The two Oxford Miniature Vaporizers may be used for a variety of anaesthetic agents, there being interchangeable calibration labels for each. In the case of induction with ether, with spontaneous ventilation, both vaporizers will be required so as to produce an adequate vapour concentration. However, with spontaneous ventilation, if halothane is employed in the first vaporizer, it may be found convenient to use trichloroethylene in the second in order to make good the deficiency of analgesia caused by the exclusion of nitrous oxide. These vaporizers may be easily cleaned to remove traces of previous anaesthetic agents. For controlled or assisted ventilation, the inflating bag may be squeezed manually or it may be replaced by a mechanical ventilator of the bag-squeezing type. The choice is dictated to some extent by the type of power source available. As an alternative to the inflating bag shown, the Laerdal folding silicone rubber bag may be used.

– calibration inaccuracies may occur – this may be corrected by recalibration at altitude; and
– fall in barometric pressure may be electronically sensed as a gas leak within the monitor.

Hyperbaric chamber and anaesthetic equipment

A brief synopsis of some issues specific to high ambient pressure environment is given below:

- Gas diffusion into gases or liquids causes bubbles on decompression. Rapid decompression with gas expansion may result in breakages of sealed, and particularly glass containers.
- Oxygen-rich environment under hyperbaric conditions increases the risk of fire; normally non-flammable materials may become flammable.
- During decompression, humidity increases, causing water condensation.
- The combination of increased water vapour and

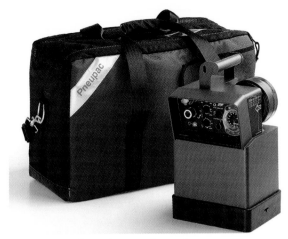

Figure. 29.6 CompPac ventilator, Pneupac. Photo courtesy of Smiths Medical International.

metallic walls and equipment increases the risk of electrocution and short circuits.

Most anaesthetic equipment is at best untested under these conditions, and at worst dangerous. The following issues should be considered:

- Batteries – risk of bursting or leaking.
- Endotracheal tube cuffs should be liquid filled.
- Intravenous lines must be primed without air.
- Chest drains must be vented to chamber air through flutter valves (not bottles, as water seals may be problematic, particularly during rapid transition to different pressures).
- LCD monitor screens may crack or break due to gas bubbling out of solution during rapid decompression.
- Pressure transducers may malfunction.
- Simple minute volume divider ventilators may function better than other types of ventilators.
- Defibrillators are extremely hazardous due to the risks of electrocution and fire (see above). The metal floors and walls of the chamber mean that patient and operator are permanently earthed. Sparking may be disastrous under hyperbaric conditions in an atmosphere which may be contaminated with additional oxygen from the patient.

DEVELOPING COUNTRIES

There are two extremes of conditions that may be met in providing anaesthesia in developing countries. The anaesthetist may be totally dependant on the equipment, drugs and personnel provided within the healthcare system of that country, or they may be part of a visiting team that is totally self-contained. Visiting teams may be very 'operation specific' (e.g. Project Orbis, Operation Smile and other eye or cleft palate teams), or they may have a much wider remit. These teams usually have rigid pre-assessment protocols, ensuring that standard operations are carried out on fit patients, enabling the greatest good to be done to the largest number of people. Some visiting teams may bring everything they need to perform a certain number of standard operations and anaesthetics (in which case the equipment may be very similar to that for battlefield anaesthesia, i.e. OMV based draw-over or TIVA), whilst others opt to mainly use local equipment, adding only their own disposable equipment.

'District hospital'-based anaesthesia

Many small hospitals in developing countries rely on non-medically qualified assistants to deliver anaesthesia under the supervision of the doctor who will also be performing the surgery. Under these conditions, anaesthetized patients are more likely to be intubated to ensure a secure airway. Most anaesthetists in developing countries work in larger hospitals, but even here they may be responsible for the training and supervision of medical assistants giving anaesthesia. Many such hospitals, large and small, will have storerooms which have become graveyards of anaesthetic machines and other equipment donated by well-meaning organizations or countries, without consideration for spare parts or expertise needed for their maintenance. There will often be continuous flow (Boyle's) machines, discarded as the necessary compressed medical gas supply is absent or erratic. In addition, such machines may not have anti-hypoxia devices and vaporizers may be outdated, unserviceable or grossly inaccurate.

For all these reasons, local anaesthetic techniques (nerve blocks, spinals and epidurals) should be used where appropriate.

Draw-over apparatus

The unreliability of supply of pressurized gases favours the use of air with supplemental oxygen when available and draw-over type vaporizers. A combination of the EMO vaporizer or the OMV (calibrated and used for both halothane and trichloroethylene), together with a means of inflation such as a manual resuscitator or Oxford bellows; a Ruben, Ambu E or similar non-rebreathing valve, and a facemask or endotracheal connector and tube, may be the most practical equipment for safe anaesthesia under these circumstances. The facility for giving supple-

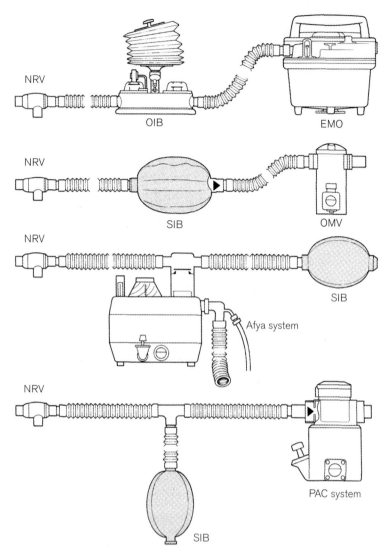

Figure 29.7 Several arrangements of draw-over apparatus: OIB, Oxford inflating bellows (Penlon); EMO, Epstein Macintosh Oxford ether vaporizer (Penlon); NRV, non-rebreathing valve (e.g. Ruben); SIB, self-inflating bag (Laerdal, Ambu, etc.); PAC, Portable Anaesthesia Complete (Ohmeda). (Reproduced with permission of WHO from Dobson MB (1988). *Anaesthesia at the District Hospital*. Geneva: World Health Organisation.)

mentary oxygen, using a T-piece and reservoir tubing as with the Triservice apparatus (see above), is desirable.

Various arrangements of draw-over apparatus are shown in Figure 29.7, and the working principles of the commonly available draw-over vaporizers are shown in Figures 29.1–4

Supplemental oxygen

Medical oxygen may be available in cylinders, but these may not follow international standards of cylinder identification, and apparently full cylinders may be found to be empty. Industrial oxygen may be available, but be aware that there may be an increased level of impurities in such supplies. Up to 95% high-quality oxygen may be obtained from an oxygen concentrator (see Chapter 3). Oxygen concentrators are relatively maintenance-free but require a source of electrical power to run a compressor and a switching device. A concentrator the size of a small domestic fridge will produce an inexhaustible supply of oxygen at the rate of about 4 litres a minute.

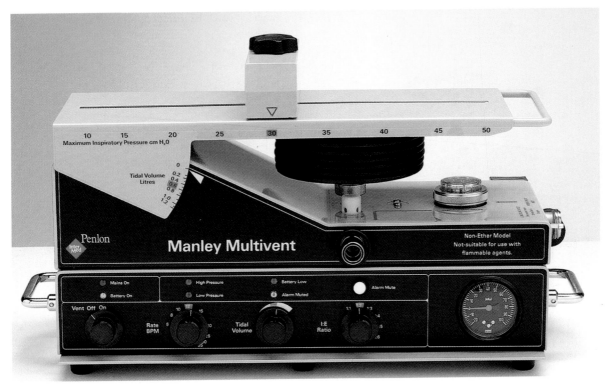

Figure 29.8 Manley Multivent. Photo courtesy of Penlon Ltd UK.

Ventilators suitable for developing countries

Manley Multivent Ventilator

This ventilator was developed by the late Roger Manley, specifically for use in developing countries (Fig. 29.8).[9] It differs from most other gas driven ventilators, in that the volume of gas required to drive the ventilator is only one tenth of the patient's minute volume. Furthermore, if the driving gas is oxygen it may be automatically collected and used to supplement the inspired oxygen concentration. Used in this way, set at a minute volume of 4 litres per minute, an E size oxygen cylinder containing 680 litres would drive the ventilator and supply 35% oxygen in air for a period of 28 hours. The ventilator consists of a weighted beam, attached at one end to a fulcrum and at the other end to the top of the bellows. The beam is pushed upwards by the driving gas under a pressure of at least 140 Kpa acting on a piston. When the set tidal volume is reached, the flow of driving gas is interrupted and the weight of the beam compresses the bellows, delivering the mixture of anaesthetic gases to the patient. The economy of driving gas is achieved by the relative distances of the piston and the bellows to the fulcrum.

Should the supply of pressurized gas fail completely, the bellows can be operated manually.

Combination anaesthetic equipment

A number of ingenious machines incorporating an oxygen concentrator, oxygen cylinders, a ventilator, and vaporizers, which can be used in either draw-over or continuous flow mode, assembled on a mobile trolley, have been produced. The advantage of such equipment is that it is permanently assembled and available and recognized as the complete versatile anaesthetic machine. If monitoring equipment is available, this can be incorporated as well. Two examples of these are the 'Glostavent' (Fig. 29.9), which was developed by Roger Eltringham in Gloucester, UK,[10] and is based on the Manley Multivent Ventilator, and the 'Fentolator' developed by Paul Fenton in Malawi.[11]

Finally, the other essential piece of equipment is suction apparatus. In areas where electricity supply may be unreliable, it is advisable to have manual or foot-operated suction apparatus.

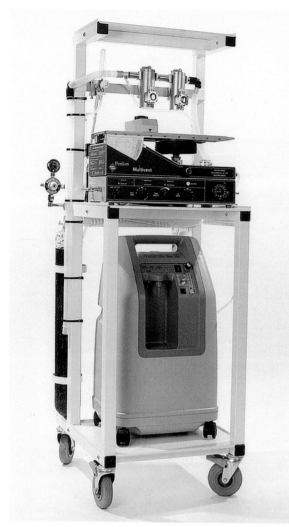

Figure 29.9 Glostavent Anaesthetic Machine (supplied by Dr Roger Eltringham).

Essential equipment to pack

When going to work as an anaesthetist in a developing country, there is a limit to the amount of equipment that can be taken. Excess baggage is currently charged at £22/kg on British Airways flights, although many airlines will waive charges if contacted in advance and charitable status established. Communication by the now ubiquitous e-mail will determine what equipment is available. Examples of equipment to take include:

- Bodok seals;
- assorted connectors and adaptors;
- basic airway equipment – self-inflating bag, mask,

guedel airways, laryngoscope (including spare batteries and bulbs);
- stethoscope;
- peripheral nerve stimulator needles, nerve stimulator and batteries;
- selection of emergency drugs, relaxants and local anaesthetics, preferably in plastic ampoules (a Home Office visa is required to take controlled drugs); and
- rolls of adhesive tape.

Monitoring

The minimum standards of monitoring for safe anaesthesia have been recommended by the Association of Anaesthetists. These include:

- Pulse oximetry;
- Electrocardiogram;
- Arterial blood pressure;
- Capnography and gas analysis

In developing countries, various local factors may make this ideal difficult to attain, in particular:

- capital cost of equipment;
- reliable power source;
- availability of disposables – electrodes, tranducers, etc.;
- maintenance of equipment;
- transportability of equipment;
- user ability to interpret results.

In the absence of electronic equipment, relatively safe anaesthesia may still be achieved using minimal equipment and observations, for example:

- pre-cordial stethoscope;
- sphygmomanometer;
- finger on pulse;
- patient's colour (mucous membranes);
- capillary refill time;
- other clinical observations.

However, in remote situations, there is no doubt that both the safety and quality of anaesthesia depends upon the ability of anaesthetists to adapt techniques and equipment appropriate to the local resources, and to their skill and attention to respond rapidly to clinical signs where monitoring may be minimal by comparison with standards of practice in the developed world.

REFERENCES

1. The Association of Anaesthetists of Great Britain and Ireland (2000) Recommendations for Standards of Monitoring during Anaesthesia and Recovery. 21 Portland

Place, London W1B 1PY: www.aagbi.org

2. The Association of Anaesthetists of Great Britain and Ireland (2002) Provision of Anaesthetic Services in Magnetic Resonance Units. 21 Portland Place, London W1B 1PY: www.aagbi.org

3. Sweeting CJ, Thomas PW, Sanders DJ (2002) The long Bain breathing system: an investigation into the implications of remote ventilation. *Anaesthesia* **57**: 1183–1186.

4. Jackson E, Tan S, Yarwood G, Sury MRJ (1994) Increasing the length of the expiratory limb of the Ayre's T-piece: implications for remote mechanical ventilation in infants and children. *British Journal of Anaesthesia* **73**: 154–156.

5. Adley R, Evans DHC, Mahoney PF, *et al.* (1992) The Gulf war: anaesthetic experience at 32 Field Hospital Department of Anaesthesia and Resuscitation. *Anaesthesia* **47**: 996–999.

6. Restall J, Tully AM, Ward PJ, Kidd AG (1988) Total intravenous anaesthesia for military surgery. A technique using Ketamine, Midazolam and Vecuronium. *Anaesthesia* **43**: 46–49.

7. McDowall DG (1964) Anaesthesia in a pressure chamber. *Anaesthesia* **19**: 321-336.

8. Pattinson K, Myers S, Gardner-Thorpe C (2004) Problems with capnography at altitude. *Anaesthesia* **59**: 69–72.

9. Manley R (1991) A new ventilator for developing countries and difficult situations. *World Anaesthesia Newsletter* **5**: 10–11.

10. Eltringham RJ, Fan Qui Wei (2001) The Glostavent – an anaesthetic machine for difficult situations. *ITACCS* **Spring/Summer:** 38–40.

11. Fenton PM (2003) Inhalation anaesthesia in developing countries: the problems and a proposed solution – 3. *Anaesthesia News* **191**:8–9. Association of Anaesthetists of Great Britain and Ireland, UK. (ISSN 0959-2962). www.aagbi.org/anaesthesia_news_2003.html

FURTHER READING

Dobson MB (1988) *Anaesthesia at the District Hospital.* Geneva: World Health Organisation.

Ezi-Ashi TI, Papworth DP, Nunn JF (1983). Inhalational anaesthesia in developing countries. The problems and a proposed solution. *Anaesthesia* **38**: 729–47.

Magee PT, Tooley M (2004) *The Physics, Clinical Measurement and Equipment of Anaesthetic Practice.* Oxford: Oxford University Press.

The anaesthetist and the Medicines and Healthcare products Regulatory Agency

Stephen Fenlon

The Medicines and Healthcare products Regulatory Agency (MHRA) is the government body responsible for regulating the use of all healthcare devices and medicines within the UK. For practitioners outside the UK, an understanding of the role and function of the MHRA, as a case study in medical devices regulation, will hopefully serve to inform and educate the individual as to the purpose and likely process of any local authorities.

The MHRA was formed in April 2003 by the amalgamation of the Medical Devices Agency and The Medicines Control Agency. It is an executive agency of the Department of Health and has a large body of personnel, including many health professionals, dealing with a wide remit within the healthcare sector. This chapter will concentrate on the responsibilities of the MHRA as a regulator of medical devices. Regulation of clinical trials, licensing of medicines and pharmaceutical surveillance are just some examples of the many other areas in which anaesthetists may have intimate involvement with the MHRA.

All products, except medicines, used in healthcare for the diagnosis, prevention, monitoring, treatment or alleviation of illness or handicap are medical devices. There are thus, about half a million items falling under the jurisdiction of the MHRA. While some, such as syringes, ventilators and tracheal tubes, are in routine use by anaesthetists, many other medical devices (e.g. artificial eyes, condoms and surgical supports) have little impact on our professional life. Unregulated manufacture and use of medical devices, much like unregulated medical practitioners, have the capacity to inflict great harm, both on patients and on those operating the device (Fig. 30.1).

As a regulatory body, the MHRA in effect oversees manufacture of all medical devices. It also provides a wealth of information and advice to health professionals in the UK and beyond, which aims to disseminate the manufacture and principles of safe use of medical devices. As part of this process the MHRA remain dependent on consumers and manufacturers to provide further details of how products perform in use; this information may subsequently modify device form, function and application.

A glossary of terms used in regulation of medical devices is given in Appendix 1.

STANDARDS

To ensure suitability for a given task, any device must be manufactured according to verified standards.

Healthcare professionals are by no means the first group to recognize and demand the need for consistent and universal standards in the equipment and materials they

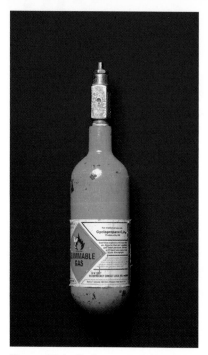

Figure 30.1 Cyclopropane. Used correctly, causes a rapid and smooth beginning to many anaesthetics; used incorrectly, can bring about a rapid and violent end. Misuse can have catastrophic consequences, and this agent is no longer available.

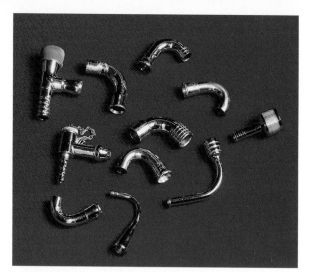

Figure 30.2 A selection of connectors from older breathing systems showing the lack of uniform dimensions. (Compare with Fig. 30.3.)

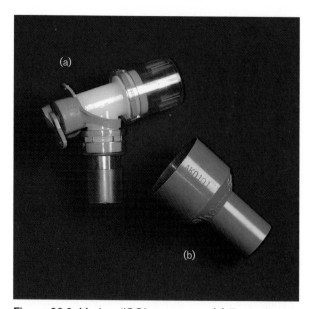

Figure 30.3 Modern 'ISO' connectors. **(a)** Tracheal tube connector with 15 mm/22 mm diameter fittings. (b) Gas scavenging connector with 30 mm diameter fitting.

work with; in other industries this process dates back many years. An essential requirement for mass distribution of goods is independent manufacturing specifications, not just for safety but also to allow widespread usage and hence economically viable production. During the early industrial revolution, widely-used items were custom-built by many manufacturers. The chaos this caused, when trying to put different components together, led to the birth of the standard setting body. The first of these, the British Standards Institute (BSI), began work in 1901 specifying dimensions of rails and steel plate, and now encompasses a wide range of standards from heavy engineering to good employment practice. Attempts at international standardization commenced soon after in the electrotechnical field and culminated ultimately in the establishment of a new body: the International Organization for Standardization based in Geneva, which started work in 1947 (in the spirit of standardization, the abbreviation ISO is retained across all languages). The ISO will be familiar to many anaesthetists as the body that resolved the seemingly random sizes of breathing system connectors (Fig. 30.2) into the universal system we have today (Fig. 30.3).

These organizations produce the standards but do not enforce them; in the majority of cases the application of standards is voluntary. Organizations can, however, provide independent inspection of products covered by a

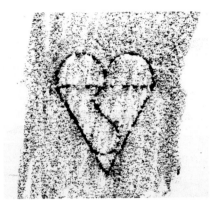

Figure 30.4 British conformity assessment: a reproduction of the BSI Kitemark™ taken from a drain cover.

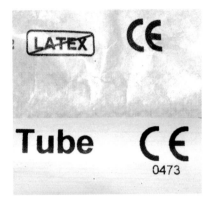

Figure 30.5 CE marks on two items of anaesthetic equipment, the lower mark also has a number with it to identify the Notifying Body employed for part of the conformity process.

standard: a process termed conformity assessment. In the UK, BSI also has a conformity assessment function as well as being a standards body. Where BSI carries out such an assessment and a product meets the appropriate standards, the manufacturer may be entitled to affix the familiar BSI Kitemark™ to its product as a sign of manufacturing conformity (Fig. 30.4).

The ISO has also published generic standards for quality management systems. This is the ISO 9000 family of standards (ISO 9001, ISO 9002, ISO 9003). Manufacturers and many other organizations and businesses may choose, as a marker of quality, to be certified by an independent organization as meeting the requirements of the appropriate ISO 9000 standard. This should not be confused with conformity assessment of the finished product.

Interrelationship of standards

The European Committee for Standardization (CEN, for Comité Européen de Normalisation) can be mandated by the European Union (EU) to produce standards for the member states. This may be carried out in conjunction with ISO and national standards bodies or by wholesale endorsement of ISO standards. These are then termed European Standards and identified with the designation EN (for Norme Européenne). CEN member bodies, who are not necessarily EU members, are obliged to give such standards national status. As such, standards may often bear any or all of the prefixes BS, EN or ISO (e.g. BS EN ISO 10993-1:2003 for Biological evaluation of medical devices – Part 1).

CE MARKING

As the EU expands and integrates, there is a need for harmonized conformity assessment of many of the goods passing across the borders of member states. The items deemed to require this are described in a number of directives; all medical devices are encompassed within three directives. Within each directive, essential requirements specify the standards for each item. A manufacturer confirms compliance with the essential requirements of a directive by placing the CE (Conformite Européene) mark on their product, once they have followed and complied with an appropriate conformity assessment route (Fig. 30.5). There are certain exceptions from CE marking for 'custom made' and investigational devices. Apart from these exceptions, any item specified within a directive cannot be sold within the EU without a CE mark. Regardless of which member state authorizes the manufacturer to place the mark, the item can be marketed in all member states, thus marking achieves both product regulation and compliance with the EC single market. It is inherent in the regulations that products imported from outside the EU are subject to the same set of rules.

Competent authorities and notified bodies

CE marking is of great importance to the healthcare sector. Following the incorporation of the medical devices directives, it is now a legal requirement for all medical devices purchased for use in the UK to have a CE mark. A major role for the MHRA is to oversee this process; it is therefore termed the *Competent Authority* for the UK, with other European countries having similar organizations. Exchange of information between Competent Authorities ensures a common approach throughout Europe. Hence, in essence, the MHRA acts as if it were the UK arm of a large pan-European organization responsible for regulating medical devices available throughout the EU. The directives and the standards within are produced by mutual agreement of EU member states, possibly incorporating standards from organizations such as the BSI or ISO (see above). The manufacturer is ultimately responsible for placing the mark and verifying that their product meets essential requirements. For simple low risk items, the manufacturer can directly place the CE mark. More complex devices, such as pacemakers, require detailed independent verification and certification by an independent organization, termed a *Notified Body*, who then issue certification to allow the placing of the CE mark. A flow chart illustrates how the system works and where the MHRA may be involved (Fig. 30.6).

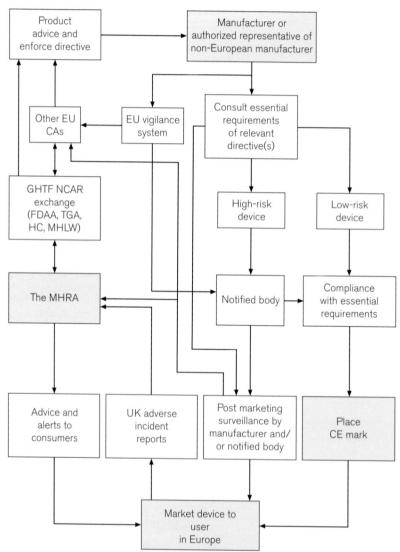

Figure 30.6 The process of placing a CE mark on a medical device, and the interrelationships of various agencies (EU, European Union; CAs, Competent Authorities; GHTF, Global Harmonization Task Force; NCAR, National Competent Authority Report, a term coined by GHTF for international reports; FDA, Food and Drug Administration of the USA; TGA, Therapeutic Goods Administration, Australia; HC, Health Canada; MHLW, Ministry for Health Labour and Welfare, Japan).

The implications of this whole process, for the anaesthetist in particular, and for those involved in producing and modifying medical devices, are discussed in greater detail elsewhere.[1] Although recently passed into UK law, it may only be a short time before a CE mark is detectable on every piece of medical equipment in UK hospitals. In fact, spring has clearly arrived in the garden of European product regulation; the eagle-eyed can detect an abundance of CE marks on everything from refrigerators to dynamite and children's toys.

Limitations of CE marking

To the end user, the CE mark implies that the product is made to a Europe-wide standard; is compliant with the regulations; its manufacturer can be traced and is liable for the product within the terms of its prescribed use, and in correct use the benefits should far outweigh any risks. Medical devices placed on the market in the UK are regulated by the MHRA. They investigate whether essential requirements are met, that UK Notified Bodies are suitably qualified, and rarely they may take action against manufacturers who fail to comply with the directive. Despite offering this reassurance, the Medical Devices Directive is not perfect and modification is needed in some areas. Devices may need to be classified into a different risk group needing more intensive pre-marketing testing, or the essential requirements may even need to be redrafted to reflect problems discovered in use.

Essential requirements may focus on such manufacturing specifications as tissue compatibility and decontamination, rather than clinical efficacy of the device when in use; the implications of this for the paediatric anaesthetist have been discussed in Chapter 14. This situation is also well illustrated by anaesthetic breathing system filters. Produced to the same essential requirements, and appropriately CE marked, filters from different manufacturers may still show wide variation in performance when subject to more intensive testing. This is acceptable under the regulatory system. However, MHRA reported an independent investigation of the performance of breathing system filters, allowing practitioners a more informed choice of which product they wish to use.[2] Another example of varying clinical performance by similarly marked products is the group of supraglottic airway devices (see Chapter 8, Supraglottic Airway Devices). Again, they bear the appropriate CE mark, but may lack adequate clinical testing prior to market release, with some performing inadequately.[3]

Products may meet or even exceed the standards specified by the medical directive but still be found wanting in clinical use. Some manufacturers choose to go beyond the requirements of the relevant standard prior to CE marking with further clinical testing and perfection. This is done both to increase product safety and to avoid the costly launch of a device that subsequently fails commercially.[4]

The MHRA fosters a close relationship with manufacturers aiming to promote the sharing of product information and reported difficulties. As a regulatory body, they may occasionally need to enforce the law for breaches of the Medical Devices Directive. Ideally, most problems are resolved by mutual consent prior to this stage. The MHRA is in a position to encourage necessary changes to the European Medical Devices Directives using information from manufacturers, from its own work or clinical trials or from other bodies, to ultimately improve the level of assurance provided by CE marking.

In summary, although a useful, legally binding regulatory mechanism generally contributing greatly to device safety, the CE mark cannot be taken as a guarantee of the clinical effectiveness of all devices.

GLOBAL HARMONIZATION

As well as its role in Europe, the MHRA is also active on the wider international scene participating in the Global Harmonization Task Force (GHTF) along with Australia, Canada, the US, other European countries and Japan. The work of the GHTF is to harmonize some of the more important regulatory aspects of medical devices, such as nomenclature and surveillance and vigilance protocols. The value of such work is evident, but it also provides a starting point for developing countries, allowing them to adopt standards that are time-consuming and difficult to set initially and are already in place around the world.

The lack of universal consent can be startling: as a professional group, we cannot agree the simplest things such as the best colour to paint oxygen cylinders (*ISO R 32/BSS 1319, first published in 1955, specified colours for medical gas cylinders – the fact that the standards have not been internationally adopted illustrates the voluntary nature of standards*) or even how to diagnose death.[5] Perhaps we should not feel too bad about this wasteful disunity; we are not alone. Despite a huge global market, the alcoholic beverage industry has no single standard for gauging the alcohol content of their tempting wares, the

UK staunchly relying on an ancient system based on igniting gin-doused samples of gunpowder. *This test was used originally to determine a concentration of alcohol and was subsequently called 'proof spirit' and equates to 57.1% ethanol v/v. Proof spirit in the USA contains 50% ethanol v/v.*

UK CONSUMER ADVISORY ROLE

The wider role of the MHRA on the European and international scene has a direct impact on the working life of the anaesthetist. Practising clinicians in the UK will be familiar with its work at a national level, covering the entire process of medical equipment use from purchase through to disposal. The MHRA has issued wide-ranging guidance for hospitals to improve the management of equipment within the NHS[6,7]; some is more specific, such as that covering anaesthesia workstations.[8] Despite this, a recent examination by the National Audit Office identified deficiencies and inconsistency of practice by trusts in the areas considered.[9] Partly as a result of this, national audit has been initiated under the auspices of the Controls Assurance Support Unit (CASU) to whom trusts are obliged to provide regular audit returns, based on details within the MHRA recommendations above.

ADVERSE INCIDENT REPORTAGE

Problems with medical devices for one reason or another are common. Adverse incident reporting generates a large amount of information from various sources. Collating, analyzing and disseminating this data is a major role of the MHRA. Concerns about medical devices arrive through a wide network:

- other Competent Authorities in the EU;
- through the obligatory vigilance system followed by manufacturers;
- voluntary reporting by manufacturers;
- and in the UK, from the users' voluntary reporting system.

Medical device-related adverse incidents are also reported to other bodies, such as the newly formed National Patient Safety Agency (NPSA). Data provided to the NPSA is sourced from anonymous critical incident reporting and analyzed to detect trends and identify areas to improve practice. Unfortunately, such overlap between authorities can be counter-productive, for example NPSA data cannot be traced to source, and thus faulty equipment reports cannot be explored further with the

reporter. Ideally, all medical device-related adverse incidents should be reported to the MHRA primarily and other authorities as thought necessary; it may be insufficient to depend on channels of communication between organizations after the report is received. Electronic reporting by all parties is encouraged; the Manufacturers' On-line Reporting Environment (MORE) enables rapid communication of alerts from companies. Adverse incident reports are investigated according to the level of risk and its frequency. The investigation may lead to design changes and/or improved advice to users.

SAFETY ADVICE

Information is disseminated in a number of formats to every UK hospital via its liaison officer. From 2003, the previous Hazard Notice, Device Alert, Safety Notice and Pacemaker Technical Note were replaced by a single format of notice: the Medical Device Alert. Details of the device concerned, the problem, who to distribute to, who must take action and what action to take are all included. Each alert is assigned one or more of the following categories:

- immediate action;
- action;
- update;
- information request.

Since 2004, a new system the Safety Alert Broadcast System (SABS) sends out alerts by e-mail and requires a liaison officer to send confirmation of receipt and subsequent action. SABS may also contain alerts from the NPSA, NHS Estates and patient safety specific guidance from the Department of Health (Fig. 30.7). The advice contained within safety alerts is not enforceable but should be viewed as reflecting best practice. As such, a decision not to heed all or part of a warning may require a robust defence.

Trusts must have in place a system ensuring appropriate and timely dissemination of the alert; failure to do this and to ensure that subsequent practice does not regress may result in repetition of harmful incidents and unnecessary injury.[10]

OTHER MHRA PUBLICATIONS

One liners

An outlet for less urgent information from the MHRA is the 'one liner'. These are single sheet publications

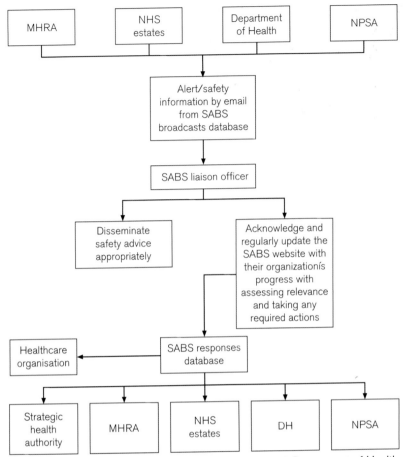

Figure 30.7 The function of SABS, the Safety Alert Broadcast System. DH, Department of Health.

containing a number of problems in a short note format providing adverse incident updates to all practising healthcare workers.

Evaluation reports

Evaluation reports compare manufacturers' specific models of a device to assist with decision making when considering purchasing equipment. They are a source of technical information, giving product specification as well as 'in use' appraisal of the device.

Device bulletins

Device bulletins are produced periodically and include an annual adverse incident report as well as bulletins dedicated to specific issues (e.g. MDA DB2003 (02) on Infusion Systems). They give general information and advice on classes of devices and aim to educate and inform professionals.

Annual adverse incident report

The annual report on adverse incidents contains figures for the number of incidents reported, their outcome, and their subsequent risk management. The causes of adverse incidents are categorized as follows:

- before delivery – design, manufacture, quality control and packaging;
- after delivery – performance and/or maintenance failures and device degradation;
- user error – where the device itself was not at fault;
- no established link to device – where the device was subsequently found to work as intended (possibly due to an intermittent fault, tampering or user error) or the device was not available for inspection.

For example, in 2003, there were 8,795 incidents reported and of these 7% involved serious injury or fatality. The categories of 'user error' and 'no established link to device' (which is likely to be unascribed user

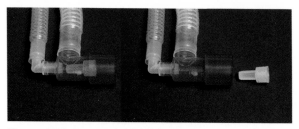

Figure 30.8 A recently highlighted cause of equipment failure. Though topical, the occlusion of anaesthetic breathing systems with extraneous items has been reported before.

error) usually account for up to 50% of causes. It bears repetition to state here that user error, especially when commonplace, is likely to be a consequence of poor design (see Chapter 31, Error and Man/Machine Interaction) or poor instructions for use and on its own does not absolve the MHRA or manufacturers of the need for further examination of the device. If reported, these will be investigated in the same way as a defect in the device itself.

THE ANAESTHETIST'S ROLE

The main aim of incident reporting is to identify the potential for harm before actual harm occurs. The importance of prompt reporting and prompt action on device alerts is self-evident. Healthcare workers in the UK are encouraged to report any device failure to the MHRA who aim to recognize patterns of problems or particularly serious isolated issues worthy of action. There is a natural tendency to under-report adverse incidents, particularly when the practitioner perceives some element of personal responsibility. This undermines the value of a system that is not seeking to apportion blame, but to learn from such problems and to direct manufacturers or practitioners in such a way that safe use of all devices is maximized. Reports can be communicated to the MHRA by e-mail, telephone, fax or post (see Appendix 2).

The reader may wonder whether anaesthetists feature with greater frequency in reports of equipment misuse and failure than other specialists. Certainly anaesthetists work in a device rich environment, but are generally well-trained and examined in the correct function and application of a wide range of equipment and are aware of the consequences of device failure or abuse. Just occasionally items neither directly connected to administration of anaesthesia nor operated by an anaesthetist can present us with a major problem.[11] However, continued

vigilance is required from us and our colleagues, to provide the information necessary to alert others to any potential hazard from an increasingly complex array of medical equipment. The application of numerous safety and conformity marks to an item does not mean it is incapable of being dangerous given incorrect use or unanticipated malfunction (Fig. 30.8). The MHRA provides an invaluable resource, aiming to promote the safe and effective use of medical devices within the UK and beyond.

ACKNOWLEDGEMENTS

The author would like to thank the following people for their support: Miss Katie Taylor BA MIMI, Medical Photographer, QVH; Clive Bray BSc (Pharm) MSc MRPharmS and Tony Saint BSc MSc, both of the Medicines and Healthcare Products Regulatory Agency.

REFERENCES

1. Grant LJ (1998) Regulations and safety in medical equipment design [editorial]. *Anaesthesia* 53(1): 1–3.
2. MHRA 04005 (2004) *Breathing system filters: an assessment of 104 breathing system filters.* London: Medicines and Healthcare products Regulatory Agency.
3. Cook TM (2003) Novel Airway Devices: Spoilt for Choice? [editorial]. *Anaesthesia* 58: 107–110.
4. Benumof JL (2003) New airway devices [letter]. *Anaesthesia* 58: 810.
5. Park GR (2004) Death and its diagnosis. *British Journal of Anaesethia 92(5):* 625–628.
6. Medical Devices Agency (2000) *Equipped to Care. The safe use of medical devices in the 21st Century.* London: Medical Devices Agency.
7. Medical Devices Agency (1998) DB9801 – *Medical device and equipment management for hospital and community based organizations.* London: Medical Devices Agency.
8. Medical Devices Agency Evaluation (2000) 00374 – *Anaesthesia workstations.* London: Medical Devices Agency.
9. The National Audit Office (1999) *The management of Medical Equipment in NHS Acute Trusts in England* HMSO.
10. Carter JA (2004) Checking anaesthetic equipment and the Expert Group on Blocked Anaesthetic Tubing (EGBAT). *Anaesthesia* 59: 105–107.
11. Chawla AV, Newton NI (2002) Machine and monitoring failure from electrical overloading. *Anaesthesia* 57: 1134–1135.

FURTHER READING

Bridgeland IA, Menon DK (2001) Monitoring Medical Devices: the need for new evaluation methodology [editorial II]. *British Journal of Anaesthesia* **87(5):** 678–681.

MHRA website: *www.mhra.gov.uk*

APPENDIX 1

Glossary

Adverse Incident: An event that causes, or has the potential to cause, unexpected or unwanted effects involving the safety of patients, users or other persons.

Authorized Representative: A body within the EU appointed by a manufacturer from outside the EU to enable them to meet the requirements of conformity assessment.

BSI: The British Standards Institute, the oldest such organization in the world responsible for a wide range of standards, they are also a recognized Notified Body.

CASU: The Controls Assurance Support Unit, soon to become the Healthcare Standards Unit, this body implements controls assurance and maintains and evaluates new healthcare standards.

CE mark: (Conformite Européene) confirms compliance with product directive standards for the EU; the size and form in which the mark appears are closely specified in Council Decision 93/465/EC.

CEN: (Comité Européen de Normalization) European Committee for Standardization. One of three standards organizations for the EU with CENELEC (electrotechnical) and ETSI (telecommunications) they develop European standards and consider applications for standards.

CNST: The Clinical Negligence Scheme for Trusts provides guidance and incentive for trusts, to improve their risk management and insures them against claims for damages arising from clinical negligence.

Committee on Safety of Devices: Set up to complement the work of the MHRA by advising ministers and overseeing strategic direction in improving medical device safety and the work of the MHRA.

Competent Authority: A national organization overseeing the Medical Devices Directive; the MHRA is the Competent Authority for the UK.

Conformity Assessment: Testing of a product or process and certification that it meets a particular set of standards, usually confirmed by placing a mark somewhere on that product.

EGBAT: The Expert Group on Blocked Anaesthetic Tubing, a UK body set up to investigate the reasons for these untoward incidents and to suggest how they may be prevented.

Essential Requirements: Those agreed standards specified within a directive that a product must meet to gain a CE mark.

GHTF: The Global Harmonization Task Force, a multinational body currently chaired by the EU, which aims to harmonize features of medical devices on a worldwide scale.

ISO: International Organization for Standardization, founded in 1947, determines a wide range of international standards.

Liaison Officer: Person within a healthcare organization responsible for receiving alerts from and communicating with the MHRA, it is anticipated that most liaison officers will take on the role of SABS liaison officer.

NAO: The National Audit Office is the non-governmental auditor of public spending.

Notified Body: An institution recognized by the Competent Authority of that state for the purposes of carrying out CE conformity assessment procedures.

NPSA: The National Patient Safety Agency is a special health authority created by the Department of Health as part of its drive to produce 'an organization with memory', to report and learn from problems affecting patient safety.

Patient Safety Research Programme: Undertake to research the safety of practice in certain areas, for example, a current programme is examining the risks of reuse of single-use products.

SABS: The Safety Alert Broadcast System, an initiative by the MHRA employing electronic communication to improve the flow of information for safety alerts.

Standards: Documented voluntary agreements which establish important criteria for products, services and processes. For a standard to be European, it must be adopted by one of the European standards organizations and made public.

APPENDIX 2

Adverse Incident Reporting

Advice on reporting adverse incidents with medical devices is updated and re-issued annually. The latest version can be found on the MHRA website: *www.mhra.gov.uk*

In England:
On Line: *www.mhra.gov.uk*
Telephone (urgent reports only): 0207 972 8080
Fax: 0207 972 8109
Post to:
Adverse Incident Centre Medicines & Healthcare products Regulatory Agency
Hannibal House
Elephant and Castle
London SE1 6TQ
Forms for reporting specific or general problems are available on the website above.

In Wales:
E-mail *haz-aic@wales.gsi.gov.uk*
Tel: 029 2080 1438
Fax: 029 2082 5479
Post to:
HIMT Division,
National Assembly for Wales,
Cathays Park,
Cardiff CF10 3NQ

In Scotland:
E-mail *iric@shs.csa.scot.nhs.uk*
Tel: 0131 551 8333
Fax: 0131 559 3922
Post to:
Incident Reporting and Investigation Centre
Scottish Healthcare Supplies
Trinity Park House
Edinburgh EH5 3SH

In Northern Ireland:
e-mail *niaic@dhsspsni.gov.uk*
Tel: 028 9052 3868
Fax: 028 9052 3900
Post to:
Northern Ireland Adverse Incident Centre (NIAIC)
Health Estates, Estate Policy
Stoney Road
Dundonald
Belfast BT16 1US

31

Error and man/machine interaction

Nicole Svatek

Over 3000 years ago, when Icarus flew too close to the sun, the wax on his wings melted and he crashed. The accident was the first recorded case of pilot error. The next person to try flying kept the wings but declined the wax. This canny individual had learnt from someone else's mistake. 'To err is human' – we accept that error is, and always has been, ubiquitous; error is all around us: it is described in our literature and embedded in our lives. It is only recently, however, that we have started to examine why human beings make mistakes, in what context mistakes occur, and to ask if by understanding the context we can reduce the error rate, or better still, prevent errors from occurring at all.

Just over 50 years ago, aircraft gear levers were located behind the pilot's seat, along with various other handles that were indistinguishable on a dark and stormy night. Mis-selection caused so many accidents that a mirror was installed on the forward panel, in an attempt to help the pilot see. It was not until Boeing realized that the levers should be at the front and visible that these particular accidents ceased. The design was further modified by varying the shape of the individual levels, thus providing the pilot with additional tactile confirmation. An extra margin of safety had thereby been introduced into the critical function of gear selection.

For the anaesthetist, some understanding of the approach to error management in an analogous system where safety is critical, such as in the aviation industry, should both instruct and enhance awareness.

HUMAN FACTORS IN AVIATION

Today, almost 80% of aircraft accidents are due to human performance failures; and the introduction of human factors into *safety critical* systems has stemmed from the recognition of human error as the primary cause in a significant number of catastrophic events worldwide. In the late 1970s, a series of aircraft accidents occurred where, for the first time, the investigation established that there was nothing wrong with the aircraft and that the causal factor was poor decision making and lack of situational awareness. The nuclear industry (Three Mile Island, Chernobyl) and the chemical industry (Piper Alpha, Bhopal) suffered similar accidents, where it became evident that the same issues, i.e. problem solving, prioritizing, decision making, fatigue and reduced vigilance, were directly responsible for the disaster.

It was clear, however, that the two-word verdict, 'Human Error', did little to provide insight into the reasons why people erred, or what the environmental and systems influences were that made the error inevitable. There followed a new approach to accident investigation that aimed to understand the previously under-estimated influence of the cognitive and physiological state of the individuals involved, as well as the cultural and organizational environment in which the event occurred. The objective of 'Human Factors' in aviation, as elsewhere, is to increase performance and reduce error, by understanding the personal, cognitive and organizational context in which we perform our tasks.

Human factors bring into focus the fact that people are active participants in whatever they are doing, that they 'do' whatever makes sense at the time – based on the circumstances surrounding them. Individuals bring their own perspective, their own level of interest and their own state of well-being on the day. In many instances, they also have an emotional investment in the outcome in terms of professional pride. In other words, whereas it was once assumed that effective decision making was the product of mechanistically making the correct choice in a rational, predictable manner every time; current understanding is that even the most superior decision makers are vulnerable to the weaknesses of the systems in which they operate. Error is a product of the context in which it occurs.

A commonly-used diagram, which is useful in forming a basic understanding of the man/machine interface and Human Factors, is the SHEL model, first described by Edwards in 1972 and later refined by Hawkins in 1975 (Fig. 31.1). Each block represents one of the five components in the relationship, with liveware (human) always being in the central position. The blocks are, however, irregular in shape and must be carefully matched together

in order to form a perfect fit. A mismatch highlights the potential for error.

For example:

- *Liveware–Environment* errors could be the product of extremely rushed procedures and items being missed. Long flights and excessive fatigue, or multiple, short busy flights could also incur error as a direct product of the environment.
- *Liveware–Software* errors would naturally occur where information is delivered in a misleading or inaccurate manner, i.e. cluttered computer screens, or wrongly-calculated weights and loads in published charts.
- *Liveware–Hardware* errors caused by poor design or equipment location, critical knobs, levers, wiring or plugs that are too similar or indistinct in shape, size and colour.
- *Liveware–Liveware* errors as a direct by-product of the quality of the team relationship, interaction, leadership and information flow

Decision making

Decision makers are critically dependent on the quality of information they receive, be it verbal, computerized, or in the form of checklists or procedures. If the information is wrong, or delivered late, the decision and subsequent action will be incorrect. Decision making is also dependant upon training, experience and situational awareness (see below).

Psychological research has shown that the human brain is able to make only a single decision at any one instant. The individual can, therefore, attend to only one process at a time and although he can change from one process to another extremely rapidly, the danger of preoccupation is obvious. Computers (rationality) ignore the impact of time and emotion in the decision-making process. The attraction of computers to assist in collating information and decision making is therefore evident.

Advanced technology has, in many instances, brought increasing complexity in the machinery, whilst at the same time seductively simplifying what is seen on screen. For instance, in older aircraft, the flight crew are surrounded by a vast number of dials, bars and indicators that provide a continuous source of raw data, which they interpret and formulate into a mental model of the aircraft's position and status. However, notwithstanding the banks of visible instrumentation, there is relatively little going on 'behind' and the logic of the systems is fairly transparent: it is quite manageable for the human brain to visualize, to interpret and to understand. Any discrepancies, either between

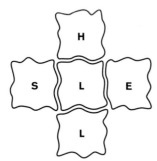

Figure 31.1 SHEL model as modified by Hawkins. **S**, software (procedures, Standard Operating Procedures Checklists, etc); **H**, hardware (machine); **E**, environment (external, internal); **L**, liveware (human).

instruments or between the instruments and the pilots' own mental model, immediately trigger investigation.

Conversely, one of the most striking features of the highly automated flight deck is the tidiness and absence of dials. The logic of the systems is now hidden deep in the computers and easy access to the 'visualization' or the 'conceptualization' of the big picture is lost. This complexity is potentially very fragile: a small problem can collapse a whole system and lure the pilot down deceptive and unnecessary computerized pathways. Equally, complexity can also provide safeguards that we simply never see. Either way, *system action* has become invisible. Software programmes are opaque and decision making has changed because of it. It could be said that the relationship between man and machine is defined by physical and environmental qualities on the part of the human and autocratic and opaque qualities on the part of the machine – differences that do not make for an ideal rapport, particularly when tired or under stress. Perhaps the irony of our relationship with technology is that the more advanced the systems, the more we need the human being to solve all the problems we unwittingly designed into them in the first place.

Situational awareness

Effective decision making is based on judgement, which in turn is based on good-quality information and accurate situational awareness. In aviation decision making, calls for a three-dimensional appreciation of the environment (considered a hostile environment), travelling at speeds of up to 500 miles per hour. There is the added pressure that the consequence of error can be catastrophic. In order to minimize the potential for error, human factors training has provided flight crews with a basic understanding of the significance of mental models, perception and where and how error is most likely to occur.

The term '*situational awareness*' describes a dynamic state of (cognitive) awareness that integrates information and uses it to anticipate changes to the current environment. Every individual has his or her own 'picture' or, perception, of the environment. This mental model is informed by culture, training and previous experience. But no matter how familiar the territory, an individual's perception of a situation may not be the right one and, if left unchallenged, could lead to faulty decisions and serious consequences. Crews are, therefore, taught to confer and cross check their mental models before making assumptions or decisions that give rise to mistakes. They are thus enhancing their situational awareness and using this knowledge to make predictive judgements on the progress of the flight (Fig. 31.2).

In a dynamic, fluid environment, where there is little time to go back and correct errors, it has long been appreciated that it is better to spend time making accurate decisions than to be caught in a reactive mode of trying to correct error. Errors inevitably give rise to more errors, a process that can suck its victim down a root and branch corridor of mistakes literally miles away from the original task at hand.

Vigilance and arousal

Decision-making ability relies on vigilance to detect pertinent information and, along with vigilance itself, is dependant on the individual's level of arousal.

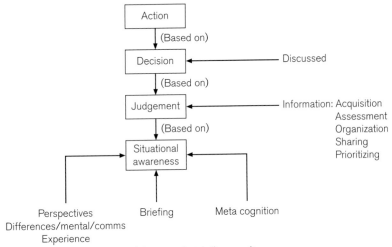

Figure 31.2 The decision-making process and factors that influence it.

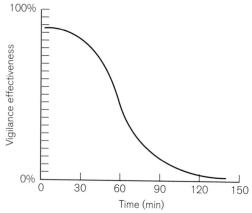

Figure 31.3 The kind of vigilance effect that can be expected in the performance of passive tasks with a low signal rate. This shows a notable decline in performance after about 30 min. (Reproduced from Hawkins FH (1987) *Human Factors in Flight*, London: Gower Technical Press.) This would occur over a similar period of uneventful anaesthesia.

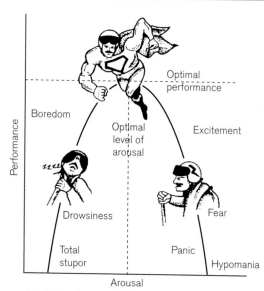

Figure 31.4 The inverted 'U' curve of arousal. Optimum performance for a particular task does *not* occur at maximum arousal. The optimum level varies depending upon the task.

Vigilance, from the Latin *vigilantia* for watchfulness, is defined in the dictionary as 'being keenly alert to danger'. In 1943, research by the Royal Air Force showed that vigilance, requiring continuous monitoring and detection of brief low-intensity and infrequently occurring events over long periods, is poor. This is illustrated in Fig. 31.3, which shows rapid fall-off in vigilance after a period as short as half an hour. In acknowledgement of this, modern anaesthesia machines and monitors allow alarm parameters to be set for all measured variables; this level of *vigilance monitoring* was unheard of 25 years ago (see Chapter 6: The Anaesthesia Workstation).

Arousal is the level of 'wakefulness'. For any task there is a level of arousal at which one performs most efficiently, as shown in Figure 31.4. Surprisingly, this optimal level decreases as the difficulty of the task increases. As such, overarousal often occurs in emergency situations when difficult tasks may need to be carried out rapidly. Underarousal for a particular task slows decision making and makes it less accurate and also reduces vigilance. Underarousal occurs with boredom and sleep deprivation.

Table 31.1 shows some common stressors, which adversely affect performance.

Understanding error

Aircraft accidents are seldom due to one single catastrophic failure. Investigations invariably uncover a chain of events – a trail of errors, where each event was inexorably linked to the next and each event was a vital contributor to the outcome. The advantage in this truth is that early error detection and containment can prevent links from ever forming a chain. Errors can be defined as lapses, slips and misses, or errors of omission and errors of commission (see Appendix 1 for definition of these terms in the context of the study of error). Some errors occur as a direct result of fatigue, where maintaining vigilance becomes increasingly difficult. Conversely, others are a product of condensed time frames, where items are simply missed. Whatever its source, it must be recognized that error is forever present in both operational and non-operational life. High error rates tell a story, they are indicative of a system that either gives rise to, or fails to prevent them. In other words, when errors are identified, it should be appreciated that they are the symptoms and not the disease.

The 'Swiss Cheese analogy' is often used to explain how a system that is full of holes (ubiquitous errors, systems failures, etc) can appear solid for most of the time. Thankfully, it is only rarely that the holes line up or cluster (e.g. adverse environmental circumstance + error + poor equipment design + fatigue) such that catastrophic failure occurs (Fig. 31.5). Error management aims to reduce the total number of holes, such that likelihood of clustering by chance is reduced (see below).

Table 31.1 Stressors contributing to reduction in performance

Environmental stresses	Domestic stresses	Professional stresses
Heat	Marriage	Colleagues
Noise	Divorce	Management
Vibration	Birth	Legal problems
Low humidity	Bereavement	Lack of sleep
	Financial problems	Hunger and thirst
	Health	Lack of rest

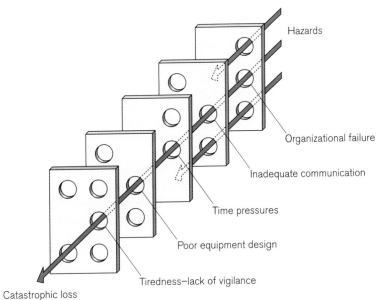

Figure 31.5 The Swiss Cheese Model, originally by James Reason,[2] demonstrates the multifactorial nature of a sample 'accident' and can be used to explain how latent conditions for an incident may lie dormant for a long time before combining with other failures (or viewed differently: breaches in successive layers of defences) to lead to catastrophe. In this example the organizational failure may be the expectation of an inadequately trained member of staff to perform a given task.

ERROR MANAGEMENT

Helmreich defines error management as 'the process of correcting an error before it becomes consequential to safety'.[1]

One of the principal methods of error avoidance/containment enshrined in flight safety is the use of 'briefing' and an understanding of its role in threat and error management. Every critical aspect of flight, and the conditions along the way, represent a potential threat that could cause the pilots to err. Such threats are referred to as 'red flags'. Early identification and planning against threats reduces the likelihood of error. It also increases vigilance at those times when threats are anticipated.

Every flight begins with planning and briefing. This is a process of evaluating the weather on departure and en route, calculating the various weights and load of the aircraft, the fuel, the runway conditions at take-off and take-off speeds. This information then forms the basis of the briefing. The details of the flight plan and the reasons behind each decision are fully discussed and understood by everyone. The core purpose of the briefing is to establish a *mutual mental model* between crew members prior to departure and, equally importantly, to provide the opportunity for any additional information, relevant experience, or even subjective opinion, to be aired and added to the crews' collective situational awareness. It is recognized here that a steep authority gradient stifles information flow and a 'superior' attitude can induce stress and provoke errors in the subordinate. This level of preparedness affords the crew more mental capacity when variances occur, as they inevitably will and do

Briefings continue throughout all major phases of flight. Human factors training has taught flight crews that enhanced communication and information exchange increases the quality of decision making and helps to reduce error rate. At particularly crucial phases of flight, i.e. approach and landing, the briefing rate increases and the 'challenge/response' use of checklists becomes more critical in error capture and mitigation. In this instance, the external environment, for example all the conflicting priorities of landing at a busy foreign airport in poor weather conditions, is considered replete with potential 'threats' which, if they do not recognize and manage, will cause the crew to make errors. Hence, the greater the understanding of the threat posed by the circumstances, the less the likelihood of error arising. It is perhaps this discipline; of briefing, conferring and cross checking, that most markedly distinguishes the aviation industry from anaesthesia and medicine.

Additional protocols also aid in the reduction (and/or capture) of error. Aviation is highly procedurally driven and the use of checklists and standard operating procedures governs most aspects of flight. Aircrews visit the simulator every six months to maintain a state familiarity with aircraft systems, procedures and handling skills. Perhaps one of the most successful training initiatives has been the introduction, in the late 1980s, of 'real time' flying scenarios, known as Line Orientated Flight Training (LOFT), which has enhanced the *meta cognitive* (awareness of one's own thinking process) aspect of aircrew training. These simulator scenarios are less technical and instead present the crews with situations that have many options and/or priorities of varying complexity. The 'consequences' are the product of the quality of the decisions and subsequent actions. It is virtually certain that successively poor decisions will result in a technical failure. Crews experience the outcome of their own decision pathways in a non-jeopardy, learning environment. The crews debrief the simulator session using human factors guidelines as performance criteria, with an instructor who is specifically accredited in this process.

Teaching meta-cognitive (human factors) strategies helps crews understand how current information fits into the larger picture and how best to utilize that information to reach the desired end – reduced error, a safe and effective relationship between man and machine and many happy landings.

APPENDIX 1

Glossary of Error Terms

Error of commission: generic term for error arising from an intended act against recommended procedure.

Error of omission: generic term for error arising from an item or action being unintentionally missed.

Slips: unintended actions/inactions occurring during the execution of familiar or pre-planned procedures, (slip of memory).

Lapses: unintended 'oversight' of information after the planning stage and before action.

Misses: errors arising from items overlooked at planning stage.

Mistakes: error incurred when a properly selected and applied action will not result in the desired outcome.

Mishaps: generic term for an unfortunate event.

Violation: a deliberate action against the recommended procedure, which may, however, be the safest choice at the time. These occur when there is a conflict between the task and the recommended procedure versus the safest outcome.

REFERENCES

1. Helmreich RL, Merritt AL (1998) *Culture at Work in Aviation and Medicine*. Aldershot: Ashgate.
2. Reason JT (1997) *Managing the Risks of Organizational Accidents*. Aldershot: Ashgate.

FURTHER READING

Billings CE (1997) *Aviation Automation*. Lawrence Earlbaum Association.

Hawkins FH (1993) *Human Factors in Flight*. London: Gower Technical Press.

Kantowitz H, Sorkin RD (1983) *Human Factors: Understanding People– System Relationships*. New York: Wiley & Sons.

Klein GA, Orasanu J, Calderwood R, Zsambok CE (1993)

Decision Making in Action. Norwood: Ablex Publishing Corporation.

Lawton R, Parker D, Reason J (1998) *Bending the Rules II, The Violation Manual.* Manchester: Manchester University.

Orlady W, Orlady LM (1999) *Human Factors in Multi-Crew Flight Operation.* Aldershot: Ashgate.

Reason JT, Hobbs A (2003) *Managing Maintenance Error.* Aldershot: Ashgate.

Strauch B (2002) *Investigating Human Error.* Aldershot: Ashgate

Toft B, Reynolds S (1994) *Learning from Disasters.* Oxford: Butterworth-Heinemann.

Wiener EL, Kanki BG, Helmreich RL (1993) *Cockpit Resource Management.* San Diego: Academic Press Inc.

Wiener EL, Nagel DC (1988) *Human Factors in Aviation.* San Diego: Academic Press Inc.

Appendix: SI unit and conversion tables

Chetan Patel

SI UNITS

In 1960, the Conference Generale des Poids et Mesures (11th CGPM), which is the international authority on the metric system, replaced all previous systems with the modern metric system officially named the Système International d'Unités, abbreviated to SI. Over the years, this metric system has been adopted throughout the world and is continually being revised to parallel developments in science and technology.

The SI is founded on seven base units (Table App.1). Other derived units are defined in terms of the seven base units and, for ease of understanding and convenience, may have special or compound names and their own symbols (Tables App.2 and App.3). There are also 20 SI prefixes used to form decimal multiples and submultiples (Table App.4).

Table App.1 The seven base units of the SI		
Physical Quantity	**Base Unit**	**Symbol**
Amount of substance	mole	mol
Electric current	ampere	A
Length	metre	m
Luminous intensity	candela	cd
Mass	kilogram	kg
Thermodynamic temperature	kelvin	K
Time	second	s

Table App.2 Examples of SI derived units with special names

Physical Quantity	Unit Name	Symbol	Expressed in base units
Plane angle	radian	rad	$m\ m^{-1} = 1$
Solid angle	steradian	sr	$m^2\ m^{-2} = 1$
Frequency	hertz	Hz	s^{-1}
Force	Newton	N	$m\ kg\ s^{-2}$
Work/Energy	joule	J	$m^2\ kg\ s^{-2}\ (N\ m)$
Pressure/Stress	pascal	Pa	$m^{-1}\ kg\ s^{-2}\ (N\ m^{-2})$
Power	watt	W	$m^2\ kg\ s^{-3}\ (J\ s^{-1})$
Electric charge	coulomb	C	$s\ A$
Electric potential difference	volt	V	$m^2\ kg\ s^{-3}\ A^{-1}\ (W\ A^{-1})$
Electric capacitance	farad	F	$m^{-2}\ kg^{-1}\ s^4\ A^2\ (C\ V^{-1})$
Electric resistance	ohm	Ω	$m^2\ kg\ s^{-3}\ A^{-2}\ [V/A\ ]$
Electric conductance	siemans	S	$m^{-2}\ kg^{-1}\ s^3\ A^2\ [A/V]$
Magnetic flux	weber	Wb	$m^2\ kg\ s^{-2}\ A^{-1}$
Magnetic induction	tesla	T	$kg\ s^{-2}\ A^{-1}\ (Wb\ m^{-2})$
Inductance	henry	H	$m^2\ kg\ s^{-2}\ A^{-2}\ (Wb\ A^{-1})$
Luminous flux	lumen	lm	$cd\ sr$
Illuminance	lux	lx	$cd\ sr\ m^{-2}$

Table App.3 SI units with compound names

Physical quantity	Name of unit	Symbol
Area	square metre	m^2
Volume	cubic metre	m^3
Speed / velocity	metre per second	$m\ s^{-1}$
Acceleration	metre per second squared	$m\ s^{-2}$
Density	kilogram per cubic metre	$kg\ m^{-3}$
Electric field strength	volt per metre	$V\ m^{-1}$
Magnetic field strength	ampere per metre	$A\ m^{-1}$
Current density	ampere per metre squared	$A\ m^{-2}$
Specific heat capacity	joule per kilogram per kelvin	$J\ kg^{-1}\ K^{-1}$

Table App.4 The 20 SI prefixes

Prefix	Symbol	Ordinary Notation	10^x
yotta-	Y	1,000,000,000,000,000,000,000,000	10^{24}
zetta-	Z	1,000,000,000,000,000,000,000	10^{21}
exa-	E	1,000,000,000,000,000,000	10^{18}
peta-	P	1,000,000,000,000,000	10^{15}
tera-	T	1,000,000,000,000	10^{12}
giga-	G	1,000,000,000	10^{9}
mega-	M	1,000,000	10^{6}
kilo-	k	1,000	10^{3}
hecto-	h	100	10^{2}
deca-	da	10	10^{1}
		1	10^{0}
deci-	d	0.1	10^{-1}
centi-	c	0.01	10^{-2}
milli-	m	0.001	10^{-3}
micro-	μ	0.000 001	10^{-6}
nano-	n	0.000 000 001	10^{-9}
pico-	p	0.000 000 000 001	10^{-12}
femto-	f	0.000 000 000 000 001	10^{-15}
atto-	a	0.000 000 000 000 000 001	10^{-18}
zepto-	z	0.000 000 000 000 000 000 001	10^{-21}
yocto-	y	0.000 000 000 000 000 000 000 001	10^{-24}

CONVERSION TABLES

French/Gauge

By convention single lumen catheters, like needles, are identified by Gauge (G) as a contraction for Imperial Standard Wire Gauge (SWG). Multi-lumen catheters and other larger diameter devices (particularly where there is a non-circular cross section, e.g. double lumen tracheal tubes) are labelled by French Gauge (Fr). French Gauge is also referred to as Charriere Gauge (CH) after the 19th century Parisian surgical instrument maker and corresponds to the external circumference in millimetres which approximately equates to three times the maximal external 'diameter'.

Each lumen of a multi-lumen catheter is by convention referred to by a nominal Gauge (G) derived from the observed flow rate. It should be noted that American Wire Gauge (AWG) is not the same as SWG.

REFERENCES

1. http://physics.nist.gov/cuu/Units/prefixes.html (07/08/2004)
2. www.arrowintl.com/products/critical_care/faqs2/faq17.asp (02/09/2004)

Table App.5 French and Gauge cross reference (1 inch = 25.4mm)

French	Inches	mm	Gauge (SWG)
	0.016	0.406	27
	0.018	0.450	26
	0.020	0.508	25
	0.022	0.559	24
	0.024	0.610	23
	0.028	0.711	22
	0.032	0.813	21
	0.035	0.889	20
3	0.039	0.975	
	0.042	1.067	19
	0.049	1.245	18
4	0.053	1.346	
	0.058	1.473	17
	0.065	1.651	16
5	0.066	1.676	
	0.072	1.829	15
6	0.079	2.001	
	0.083	2.108	14
7	0.092	2.337	
	0.095	2.413	13
8	0.105	2.667	
	0.109	2.769	12
9	0.118	2.997	
	0.120	3.048	11
10	0.131	3.327	
	0.134	3.404	10
11	0.144	3.658	
12	0.158	4.013	
13	0.170	4.318	
14	0.184	4.674	
15	0.197	5.004	
16	0.210	5.334	

Table App.6 Useful conversions

1 metre	= 1.0936 yards = 3.2808 feet = 39.3696 inches
1 kilogram	= 2.2046 pounds = 35.2736 ounces
1 litre	= 0.22 (imperial) gallons = 0.27 (US) gallons = 1.76 pints
1 kilopascal (100 N m^{-2})*	= 0.146 psi = 7.50 mm Hg = 10.20 cm H$_2$O
1 mmHg**	= 1.36 cmH$_2$O = 133.3 N.m^{-2} ($\equiv$ 0.1333 kPa) = 0.0194 psi
1 psi	= 6.89 kPa = 51.71 mm Hg = 70.33 cm H$_2$O
1 joule	= 107 ergs = 0.239 calories
0 K	= −273 °Celsius ('absolute zero')
273.15 K	= 0 °C = 32 °F
373.16 K	= 100 °C = 212 °F
K → °C	= −273.15
°C → K	= +273.15
°C	= (°F − 32) × 5/9
°F	= (°C × 5/9) +32

* See Table App.2: 1 pascal = 1 N m^{-2}

** This unit may also be referred to as torr.

Index